Medical Neurosciences

An Approach to Anatomy, Pathology, and Physiology
by Systems and Levels

Fourth Edition

D1002405

Medical Neurosciences

An Approach to Anatomy, Pathology, and Physiology by Systems and Levels

Fourth Edition

Eduardo E. Benarroch, M.D.
Consultant in Neurology, Mayo Clinic and Mayo Foundation;
Associate Professor of Neurology, Mayo Medical School, Rochester, Minnesota

Barbara F. Westmoreland, M.D.
Consultant in Neurology, Mayo Clinic and Mayo Foundation;
Professor of Neurology, Mayo Medical School, Rochester, Minnesota

Jasper R. Daube, M.D.
Consultant in Neurology, Mayo Clinic and Mayo Foundation;
Professor of Neurology, Mayo Medical School, Rochester, Minnesota

Thomas J. Reagan, M.D.
Former Consultant in Neurology, Mayo Clinic and Mayo Foundation;
Former Associate Professor of Neurology and Assistant Professor of Anatomy,
Mayo Medical School, Rochester, Minnesota; Presently, Neurologist,
Newport News, Virginia

Burton A. Sandok, M.D.
Consultant in Neurology, Mayo Clinic and Mayo Foundation;
Professor of Neurology, Mayo Medical School, Rochester, Minnesota

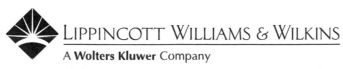

LIPPINCOTT WILLIAMS & WILKINS
A **Wolters Kluwer** Company
Philadelphia · Baltimore · New York · London
Buenos Aires · Hong Kong · Sydney · Tokyo

Acquisitions Editor: Richard Winters
Developmental Editor: Delois Patterson
Manufacturing Manager: Kevin Watt
Production Manager: Robert Pancotti
Production Editor: Jeff Somers
Indexer: Mary Kidd
Compositor: Lippincott Williams & Wilkins Desktop Division
Printer: Courier Kendallville

Copyright © 1999 by Mayo Foundation, Rochester, Minnesota.

Fourth edition

Previous editions copyright © 1978 by Little, Brown and Company (Inc.); 1986 and 1994 by Mayo Foundation.

All rights reserved. No part of this book may be reproduced in any form or by any electronic or mechanical means, including information storage and retrieval systems, without permission in writing from Mayo Foundation, except by a reviewer who may quote brief passages in a review.

Printed in the United States of America

9 8 7 6 5 4 3 2 1

Library of Congress Cataloging-in-Publication Data
Medical neurosciences : an approach to anatomy, pathology, and physiology by systems and levels.—4th ed. / Eduardo E. Benarroch . . . [et al.]
    [p.   cm.
  Includes bibliographical references and index.
  ISBN 0-7817-1426-5 (alk. paper)
  1. Nervous system—Diseases—Diagnosis.   2. Neurosciences
I. Benarroch, Eduardo E.
  [DNLM: 1. Nervous System Diseases. 2. Nervous System—anatomy & histology. 3. Nervous System Physiology. 4. Neurologic Examination. WL 140 M489 1999]
RC348.M43   1999
616.8—dc21
For Library of Congress   98-24218
                                                     CIP

Care has been taken to confirm the accuracy of the information presented and to describe generally accepted practices. However, the authors and publisher are not responsible for errors or omissions or for any consequences from application of the information in this book and make no warranty, expressed or implied, with respect to the contents of the publication.

The authors and publisher have exerted every effort to ensure that drug selection and dosage set forth in this text are in accordance with current recommendations and practice at the time of publication. However, in view of ongoing research, changes in government regulations, and the constant flow of information relating to drug therapy and drug reactions, the reader is urged to check the package insert for each drug for any change in indications and dosage and for added warnings and precautions. This is particularly important when the recommended agent is a new or infrequently employed drug.

Some drugs and medical devices presented in this publication have Food and Drug Administration (FDA) clearance for limited use in restricted research settings. It is the responsibility of the health care provider to ascertain the FDA status of each drug or device planned for use in their clinical practice.

Contents

Preface

The first edition of *Medical Neurosciences*, published in 1978, presented a way to organize knowledge of the nervous system based on the physician's approach to clinical problems. For medical students and residents alike, this organizational framework served as an effective foundation on which to build knowledge, and it required only an updating in the second edition.

In the last 20 years, our understanding of the normal function and pathophysiology of the nervous system has rapidly increased, adding immeasurably to the range and depth of information vital to comprehending neural function. This change required a reorganization of the text as well as the addition of a new chapter in the third edition. Nonetheless, the basic framework remains valid, and systems and levels continue to be the book's guiding principles. The expanding knowledge of the molecular and biochemical basis of neural organization and disease has led us to incorporate, in this fourth edition, brief discussions on neuronal development, apoptosis, and molecular mechanisms of some neurologic disorders and their pharmacologic treatment. We have also updated and increased the number of illustrations.

We sincerely hope that these additions and changes will allow *Medical Neurosciences* to better serve as an introduction to the neurosciences for new students, as a review and update of the knowledge of basic neuroscience for more experienced students, and as a framework for an organized approach to the principles of neurologic diagnosis for all who attempt to evaluate clinical problems.

This edition, like its predecessors, is the product of the authors. However, many others have contributed significantly to its development and evolution, and we are grateful to the students and faculty, both at the Mayo Clinic and elsewhere, who have taken the time to share their suggestions with us. In particular, we acknowledge the faculty consultants at Mayo who contributed to this edition: Charles F. Abboud, M.D., Division of Endocrinology, Metabolism, and Internal Medicine; Arnold D. Aronson, Ph.D., Section of Speech Pathology; Robert C. Benassi, Section of Visual Information; Shelley A. Cross, M.D., Department of Neurology; Clifford R. Jack, M.D., Department of Diagnostic Radiology; Terrence D. Lagerlund, M.D., Department of Neurology; Jay W. McLaren, Ph.D., Section of Ophthalmology Research; O. Eugene Millhouse, Ph.D., Section of Publications; Ronald C. Petersen, M.D., Department of Neurology; Michael H. Silber, M.B.Ch.B., F.C.P. (SA), Department of Neurology; and Jerry W. Swanson, M.D., Department of Neurology. We also thank Roberta J. Schwartz, Sharon L. Wadleigh, and Dorothy L. Tienter of the Section of Publications for their help in preparing the manuscript.

This is an exciting time in the world of neuroscience; we hope our readers will be stimulated to explore it further.

Integrated Neuroscience for the Clinician

Objectives

1. Define: problem solving, pattern recognition, inductive reasoning, and hypothesis.
2. Given any clinical problem, develop a series of hypotheses that will allow you to understand its cause. Identify and describe the type of reasoning used to generate and test these hypotheses.

Introduction

Neurologic disorders are common, and clinicians must be capable of dealing confidently with them. Many steps are required in accomplishing this task. Patients seldom present to their physician with a well-defined diagnosis for which appropriate therapy can be readily dispensed. Instead they arrive with a vast array of symptoms and signs that constitute a clinical problem the physician must attempt to resolve.

In solving problems, one generally approaches them by using one of two well-known methods. First, if the problem is similar to or identical to one encountered previously and the person is able to recall the answer or solution, he or she may move quickly and rapidly to an answer. This method is called *problem solving by pattern recognition.* A second approach is that of *logical analysis,* or *inductive reasoning.* In using this method, one traces the problem to its source

by a series of steps based on knowledge of the underlying structure and function. Both methods have a critical step in common that will be used throughout your medical career—hypothesis testing. When a problem looks like one seen before, one can hypothesize that the solution is likely to be the same and develop a scheme to test the hypothesis. When a problem is not clearly understood or familiar, but some of the underlying components are understood, one can propose a hypothesis about the mechanism of the problem based on an analysis of that knowledge.

The solution of a clinical problem in neurology, as in any area of medicine, requires a knowledge of anatomy, physiology, and pathophysiology. This book is an attempt to organize the body of information contained in the basic neurologic sciences into the format used by clinicians in dealing with diseases of the nervous system.

The process used by a clinician who examines a patient with a neurologic disorder (that is, one involving the brain, spinal cord, nerves, or muscles) may involve either pattern recognition or inductive reasoning. The latter is a familiar process in which a number of distinct pieces of information are put together to reach a general conclusion. For example, if a woman has a 1-year history of slowly progressive numbness and weakness of the left side of her face, left arm, and left leg, the physician concludes that the patient may have a neoplastic lesion at the supratentorial level on the right side. The physician uses the data obtained by interviewing and examining the patient to produce a history that is a chronologic account of the patient's symptoms and their evolution with time (the temporal profile). The specific symptoms in the history can be categorized into broad groups and related to particular anatomical structures and certain disease categories. In a patient with neurologic disease, these symptoms often are identified with changes in sensation, activity, movement, thinking, or consciousness. Often the physical examination of a patient with neurologic disease allows an even more precise definition of abnormal function, which, based on the clinician's knowledge of anatomical structure and function, can be related to specific areas of the nervous system.

Throughout the interview and the examination, the clinician is constantly organizing and reorganizing the collected data to arrive at hypotheses about the nature of the disorder. In the previous example, the hypothesis of a right cerebral tumor was reached because the temporal profile of slow progression is common with neoplastic disorders, and weakness and numbness on the left side of the body often are due to disease of structures that are controlled at the supratentorial level on the right.

The physician must answer three questions: Is there disease involving the nervous system? If so, where is the disease located? And what kind of disease is it (that is, what is the pathologic nature of the disease)? The first question is often one of the most difficult to answer, because an answer depends not only on the knowledge to be presented in this book but also on experience with disease involving all other body systems. This book focuses primarily on answering the two simpler questions: Where is the lesion located? and What is its pathologic nature?

Objectives

Neurologic diseases include all the major pathologic categories seen in other organ systems and can involve one or several areas in the complex human nervous system. However, adequate management of neurologic problems can be based on answering two questions: Where is the problem? and What is the problem? The elaboration and analysis of these specific questions form the major objectives in the study of neuroscience. The answers to these questions are based on a knowledge of the gross anatomical structures of the nervous system (Fig. 1), their function, the usual patterns of disease, and the forms of treatment available. This simplified approach to neurologic disease is the one customarily used by many neurologists, and it includes four questions:

1. Is the responsible lesion located at
   a. the supratentorial level?
   b. the posterior fossa level?
   c. the spinal level?
   d. the peripheral level?
   e. more than one level?
2. Is the responsible lesion
   a. focal, and located on the right side of the nervous system?
   b. focal, and located on the left side of the nervous system?
   c. focal, but involving midline and contiguous structures on both sides of the nervous system?
   d. diffuse, and involving homologous, symmetric, noncontiguous areas on both sides of the nervous system?
3. Is the responsible lesion
   a. some form of mass lesion?
   b. some form of nonmass lesion?
4. Is the lesion most likely
   a. vascular?
   b. degenerative?
   c. inflammatory-immunologic?
   d. neoplastic?
   e. toxic-metabolic?
   f. traumatic?
   g. congenital-developmental?

Therefore, the major objective of this text is to provide the information necessary to answer these questions for any clinical problem involving the nervous system and to provide a description of the mechanism by which the patient's symptoms and findings are produced by the underlying disorder.

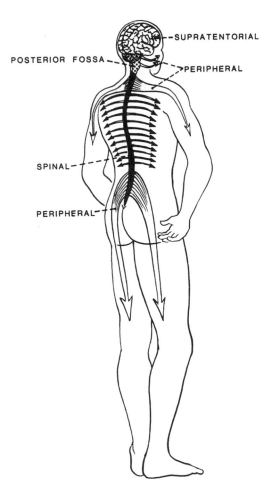

FIG. 1. Levels of the neuraxis. The supratentorial level includes the cerebral hemispheres and portions of cranial nerves I and II within the skull. The posterior fossa level includes the brainstem, cerebellum, and portions of cranial nerves III through XII within the skull. The spinal level includes the spinal cord and portions of nerve roots contained within the vertebral column. The peripheral level includes portions of both cranial and peripheral nerves that lie outside the skull and spinal column, and structures innervated by these nerves.

Organization ▪

The solution of a neurologic problem requires three levels of knowledge; therefore, this text is organized into three sections. Section I provides general information necessary to understand how neurologic disorders are diagnosed. The remainder of the text is organized

to enable a precise topographic and etiologic diagnosis. Topographic localization initially requires relating the patient's functional impairment to one of the major longitudinal systems (Section II) and then localizing the lesion at a well-defined level of the nervous system (Section III).

Each chapter begins with a list of objectives, an introduction, and an overview and ends with clinical problems for self-assessment. A list of additional readings is provided.

Survey of the Neurosciences

The clinician must first have an understanding of the methods utilized in diagnosing a neurologic disorder. How is a lesion localized, and to what do the general anatomical terms used to describe localization refer? How is a pathologic or etiologic diagnosis determined, and what do the terms used to describe them mean? These questions require a general knowledge of the diagnostic principles of neurologic disorders as these principles relate to the anatomy, physiology, and pathology of the nervous system. Chapters 2 through 5 provide the basic vocabulary and the background knowledge necessary to begin solving clinical problems. These chapters cover the following subjects:

Chapter 2: Developmental Organization of the Nervous System: Neuroembryology
Chapter 3: Diagnosis of Neurologic Disorders: Anatomical Localization
Chapter 4: Diagnosis of Neurologic Disorders: Neurocytology and the Pathologic Reactions of the Nervous System
Chapter 5: Diagnosis of Neurologic Disorders: Transient Disorders and Neurophysiology

Longitudinal Systems

Increasingly detailed knowledge of the anatomy and physiology of the nervous system is required for a precise diagnosis of a neurologic disorder. The clinician usually first identifies the patient's symptoms and signs as indicative of disease involving one or more of the major longitudinal subdivisions of the nervous system. These longitudinally organized groups of structures are called *systems* within the nervous system, each subserving a specific function. In Section II the anatomy, physiology, and clinical expression of disease as it affects the following major longitudinal systems are described:

Chapter 6: The Cerebrospinal Fluid System
Chapter 7: The Sensory System
Chapter 8: The Motor System
Chapter 9: The Internal Regulation System
Chapter 10: The Consciousness System
Chapter 11: The Vascular System
Chapter 12: The Neurochemical Systems

The name of each system characterizes its function. Correlation of the symptoms and signs with the appropriate system permits localization of the disease process in one dimension.

Chapter 12 examines the functional organization of the systems in terms of the chemical agents used for the transmission and modulation of neural activity and provides an additional method of classifying neurologic function.

Levels of the Neuraxis

The final step in localizing a lesion requires identification of an additional dimension—determining its location along the length of the systems involved. Although a precise localization can be made in many cases, most clinicians classify the disorder according to one of four major regions defined by the bony structures surrounding much of the nervous system. Section III explores the ways in which functions in each major system are integrated and modified at each of the following levels:

Chapter 13: The Peripheral Level
Chapter 14: The Spinal Level
Chapter 15: The Posterior Fossa Level
Chapter 16: The Supratentorial Level

In all three sections, there is repetition of material, with each subsequent section building on the basic information presented earlier

to provide amplification and emphasis. This approach to clinical neurologic problems can be used with any of the problems that may be encountered and is particularly useful in problems that are new, unfamiliar, or unusual to the clinician. Although the identification of diseases by recognition of a particular syndrome sometimes can be very efficient, the method of hypothesis testing and inductive reasoning presented herein is consistently more accurate and more reliable.

Clinical Problems   ■

1. You walk into a room and find your friend lying limp and motionless on the floor. As you approach and attempt to assess the situation further and offer aid, several thoughts go through your mind about what might have happened. Describe the thoughts and the reasoning that contributed to each of them.

2. You sit quietly in a chair with your legs crossed and begin to notice a numb-tingling feeling in your right lower leg. On attempting to rise from the chair, you are unable to move the right leg normally. What hypotheses have you developed about the possible cause of this dysfunction?

Additional Reading   ■

Albanese, M. A., and Mitchell, S. Problem-based learning: A review of literature on its outcomes and implementation issues. *Acad. Med.* 68:52, 1993.

Barrows, H. S., and Tamblyn, R. M. *Problem-Based Learning: An Approach to Medical Education.* New York: Springer, 1980.

Eddy, D. M., and Clanton, C. H. The art of diagnosis: Solving the clinicopathological exercise. *N. Engl. J. Med.* 306: 1263, 1982.

Engel, G. L. Clinical observation: The neglected basic method of medicine. *JAMA* 192:849, 1965.

Kassirer, J. P., and Gorry, G. A. Clinical problem solving: A behavioral analysis. *Ann. Intern. Med.* 89:245, 1978.

Larkin, J., McDermott, J., Simon, D. P., and Simon, H. A. Expert and novice performance in solving physics problems. *Science* 208:1335, 1980.

ONE

SURVEY OF THE NEUROSCIENCES

two

Developmental Organization
of the Nervous System: Neuroembryology

Objectives

1. Describe the formation of the primitive streak, notochord, neural plate, neural folds, neural tube, and neural crest.
2. On a transverse section of the neural tube, identify the ventricular, subventricular, intermediate, and mantle zones and the alar and basal plates.
3. Name the major functional systems of the brain and spinal cord, and describe their origin in terms of their relationship to the components of the wall of the neural tube mentioned above.
4. List the five major subdivisions of the cephalic portion of the neural tube, their associated central cavities, and major adult structures derived from them.
5. Name the major immature cytologic elements in the ventricular and subventricular zones and their derivatives in the mature central nervous system.
6. Describe the major processes involved in forming the mature pattern of synaptic connections between distant neuronal groups.
7. Describe the formation of the peripheral nervous system and how its connections with the central nervous system are formed.
8. List two major types of developmental abnormalities of the nervous system, and give examples of each.

Introduction

The study of neuroscience begins with a survey of neuroembryology because it provides a framework and background for understanding the anatomy of the nervous system in the adult. The eventual location of the structures in the brain is not a random occurrence but a reflection of the orderly development of the primitive nervous system. Neuroembryology also serves as an aid in understanding the pathogenesis of developmental neurologic abnormalities that are encountered not only in the newborn and pediatric periods but also in later life.

Overview

The formation of the neural tube begins on the 18th day of gestation. By this day of embryonic development, the early stage of gastrulation is completed. The two-layered embryo consisting of ectoderm and endoderm is transformed into a three-layered structure by the outgrowth of mesoderm from the midline primitive streak into the area between the original layers. The notochord, a specialized column of mesodermal cells, grows forward from the anterior end of the primitive streak (Hensen's node). The ectoderm overlying the notochord is induced to form the neural plate, which thickens and folds into the neural tube. The entire central nervous system develops from this tube. Cell columns, called the neural crest, derived from the junction of skin ectoderm and neuroectoderm separate from the neural tube and form a major portion of the peripheral nervous system.

Throughout the length of the neural tube, primitive neuroectodermal cells proliferate, differentiate into neurons and supporting cells (ependyma, astrocytes, and oligodendrocytes), migrate to their genetically coded location, and develop specific intercellular connections and relationships. The cells of the neural crest differentiate into dorsal root ganglia, autonomic ganglia, and Schwann cells.

The neural tube undergoes transverse differentiation (Fig. 1), with formation of a dorsal region, the alar plate, which subserves sensory functions, and a ventral region, the basal plate, which subserves motor functions. Also, at all levels, structures that develop in close proximity to the cavity of the neural tube—that is, in the inner tube or core—give rise to primitive functional systems (the consciousness system and the internal regulation system). Structures that develop in the outer regions of the tube (outer tube), at a greater distance from the neural canal, generally belong to higher level functional systems (the motor system and the sensory system). Even within systems, such as the motor system, this concentric relationship pertains, with older and less discrete components of the system located in the inner tube and newer and more highly developed components in the outer regions of the tube. The neurochemical system develops in parallel with the development of functional systems as outlined above, with different sets of excitatory and inhibitory neurotransmitters acting at synapses in different systems.

The cavity of the tube forms the central canal at the spinal cord level and more complex fluid-filled spaces, the ventricular system, at cephalic levels. Mesodermal tissues surround the neural tube and form the meninges, which in conjunction with the ventricular system form the cerebrospinal fluid system. Mesoderm that surrounds and grows into the neural tube forms the vascular system.

The neural tube undergoes differentiation into six regions: telencephalon (cerebral hemispheres), diencephalon (thalamus and hypothalamus), mesencephalon (midbrain), metencephalon (pons and cerebellum), myelencephalon (medulla), and spinal cord. These subdivisions of the neural tube are the precursors of three of the four major anatomical levels in the adult: supratentorial (telencephalon and diencephalon), posterior fossa (mesencephalon, metencephalon, and myelencephalon), and spinal (spinal cord). The fourth, or peripheral, level is composed of a combination of efferent fibers growing outward from the posterior fossa and spinal levels and neural crest derivatives, including somatic and visceral afferent neurons and postganglionic autonomic neurons.

Disorders of development of the nervous system may occur at any embryonic step. They generally are classified according to the dominant process occurring at the time they

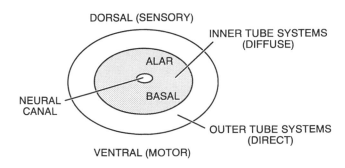

FIG. 1. Functional organization of the neural tube.

are thought to arise. The most common are failures of fusion (dorsal induction) of the neural tube (for example, spina bifida and meningomyelocele) and failures of proliferation and migration (for example, pachygyria and microgyria).

Formation of the Neural Tube

The nervous system is commonly divided into central and peripheral components. The central nervous system is that part located within the spinal column and skull. It is formed from the neural tube between the 18th and the 25th day of gestation. Before these structures are formed, at the end of the second week of gestation, gastrulation has been completed. The longitudinal axis of the two-layered embryonic disk is established by the formulation of an area of rapidly proliferating cells, the *primitive streak*. The midline of the embryo is defined by the growth of the *notochord,* a group

of mesodermal cells that grow forward from one end of the primitive streak (Hensen's node) in a plane between the ectoderm and the endoderm. The mesoderm of the rest of the embryonic disk is formed by the outgrowth of mesodermal cells from the lateral margins of the primitive streak. As the notochord and mesodermal tissues grow forward, the primitive streak becomes incorporated into the tailbud, and a three-layered embryo with a clearly delineated longitudinal axis is formed. These early changes set the stage for the subsequent events that establish the *neural tube,* the morphologic substrate of the adult nervous system.

The neural tube is formed in approximately 1 week, beginning on the 18th day. The initial step in its formation is a thickening of the ectoderm in the dorsal midline overlying the notochord to form the *neural plate* (Fig. 2A,B). The lateral edges of the neural plate thicken more rapidly than the center and begin to roll toward the midline, creating the *neural groove,* which has lateral margins, the *neural*

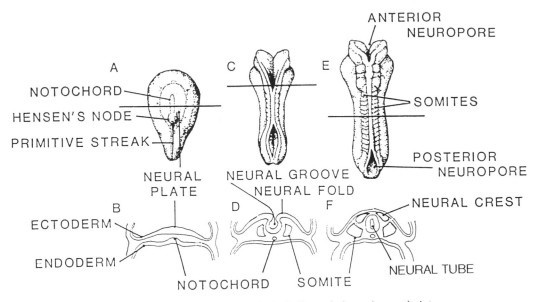

FIG. 2. Formation of neural tube (18th to 25th day). **A:** Dorsal view of neural plate forming over notochord, which has grown forward from Hensen's node between ectoderm and endoderm. **B:** Cross section through neural plate shown in **A. C:** Dorsal view of early closure of neural tube. **D:** Cross section through neural tube shown in **C. E:** Dorsal view of almost complete closure of neural tube and formation of well-defined somites. **F:** Cross section through **E.**

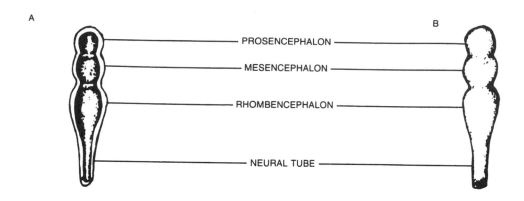

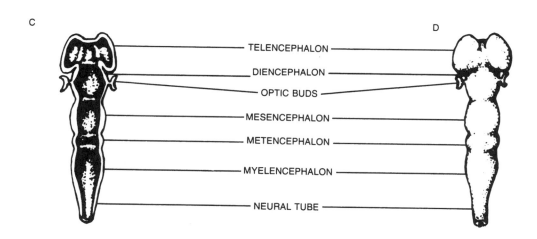

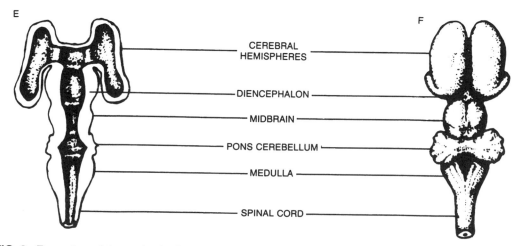

FIG. 3. Formation of the major brain vesicles of the neural tube (25th to 30th day) in horizontal section *(left)* and dorsal view *(right).* **A,B:** Stage of three primary vesicles. **C,D:** Stage of five major vesicles. **E,F:** Differentiation of specific structures by cell migration and overgrowth.

TABLE 1. *Major elements in adult nervous system derived from the neural tube*

Level	Primary divisions	Subdivisions	Major derivatives	Cavities
Supratentorial	Prosencephalon	Telencephalon	Rhinencephalon Basal ganglia Cerebral cortex	Lateral ventricles
		Diencephalon	Thalamus Hypothalamus Optic nerves and retina Neurohypophysis Pineal body	Third ventricle
Posterior fossa	Mesencephalon Rhombencephalon	Mesencephalon Metencephalon	Midbrain Cerebellum Pons	Aqueduct of Sylvius Fourth ventricle
Spinal Peripheral	Primitive neural tube	Myelencephalon Neural tube Neural crest	Medulla Spinal cord Peripheral nerve Ganglia	Fourth ventricle Central canal None

folds. With continued growth, the neural folds meet in the midline to form a hollow tube, the neural tube, which closes first in the middle of the embryo (Fig. 2C,D) (the future cervical region) and then proceeds toward the head (cephalad) and toward the tail (caudad), until the entire tube is closed. The unfused areas at the two ends of the tube before complete closure are *neuropores* (Fig. 2E). As the neural tube is being formed by the fusion of the margins of the neural folds, the skin ectoderm also fuses and covers its dorsal surface. Ultimately, the two ectodermal derivatives, neural tube and skin, become further separated by the growth of intervening mesodermal derivatives, bone and muscle. Cell columns derived from the original junction of skin and neuroectoderm form the neural crests, which later differentiate into important components of the peripheral nervous system.

Even before the neural tube is entirely closed, longitudinal differentiation begins. Parallel to the neural tube, the mesodermal cells on each side segment into aggregates, the *somites,* from which bone and muscle arise (Fig. 2E,F). At the same time, the cephalic, or head, end of the neural tube becomes larger than the caudal end, resulting in an irregularly shaped tubal structure. Continued differential growth along the length of the neural tube results in the formation of three cavities at the cephalic end of the tube. These

are the primary brain vesicles: the *prosencephalon, mesencephalon,* and *rhombencephalon* (Fig. 3A,B). These three vesicles further differentiate into five subdivisions, which persist in the brain of the mature nervous system (Fig. 3C,D). The remaining caudal end of the neural tube undergoes much less modification as it forms the spinal cord. A central remnant of the internal cavity of the tube remains in each of these derivatives.

The subdivisions of the primitive neural tube evolve, through the processes of cellular proliferation, migration, and differentiation (described in the next section), into the major elements in the adult nervous system listed in Table 1.

Differentiation of the Central Nervous System

Cytologic Differentiation

Through four processes that occur in concert, the cells that make up the mature nervous system accumulate in sufficient numbers, develop into the appropriate type of cells, move to their assigned places, and make the proper connections with other cells. These four processes are called proliferation, migration, differentiation, and maturation (Fig. 4).

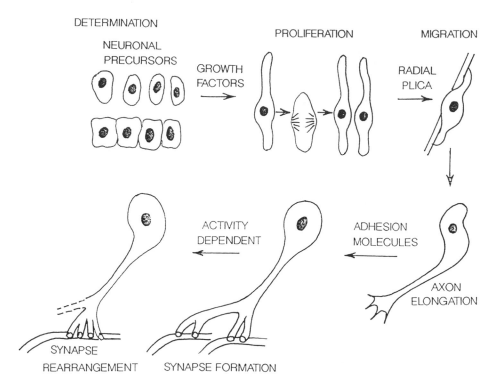

FIG. 4. Steps in the development of the mature nervous system. The first step is cellular determination, that is, determining which cells in the ectoderm will become neuronal precursors, a process called neural induction. During and after determination, the cells begin to divide, a stage referred to as proliferation. After their final division, most cells migrate a considerable distance to their final destination. During migration, cells are exposed to adhesion molecules and diffusible factors that allow interactions among neurons, glial cells, and extracellular matrix proteins. During development of the different layers of the cerebellum and cerebral cortex, migration is directed by radial glial cells with processes that span the entire width of the neural tube. After an immature neuron has reached its final location, it establishes contacts with its appropriate partners, by extending axonal and dendritic branches. In most cases, this is guided by a specialized region of the growing process, the growth cone. After the processes of cellular determination, migration, and neurite elongation, developing neurons form specific synaptic connections. This occurs in two phases. The first phase is target selection; it is closely related to the process of axonal pathfinding. The second phase entails extensive remodeling of the original pattern of connections. This is determined by the pattern of electrical activity that occurs in the synaptic pathway. Only those inputs whose activity is correlated in time with that of the postsynaptic target are stabilized.

Proliferation

The wall of the primitive neural tube consists of multipotential neuroepithelial cells derived from ectoderm. Initially, the neural tube is a single layer of pseudostratified epithelium. As the tube thickens and other layers

form, the initial and innermost layer is called the ventricular layer (Fig. 5). (Earlier textbooks refer to it as the ependymal layer, but this term is now reserved for the single layer of fully differentiated ciliated cells that line the ventricular cavity of the developed central nervous system.) The cytoplasmic processes

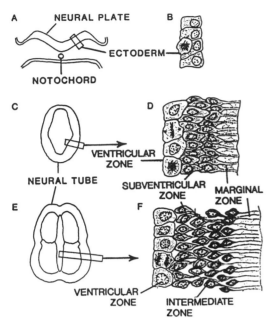

FIG. 5. Differentiation of cell layers in the primitive neural tube, with a high-power view on the *right* and a cross section of the tube shown on the *left*. **A,B:** The early neural plate is a single layer of cells. **C,D:** Formation of layers of cells by outward migration of cells proliferating in the ventricular zone. **E,F:** Formation of the outer acellular marginal zone by the growth of processes (axons) peripherally from cells.

processes that compose it increase. Cells migrating from the subventricular to the marginal zone make up the fourth, or intermediate, zone of the tube. The prominence of the zones varies at different levels and during different stages of development. For example, the subventricular zone of the telencephalic level, called the germinal matrix, is conspicuous until late in gestation.

Many neuronal precursors created during the proliferative phase are removed through programmed cell death, or apoptosis (see Chapter 4). Briefly, neuronal survival and maturation depend on exposure to trophic factors released by target and glial cells, including nerve growth factors and other neurotrophins. These factors act on neurons in a manner that promotes expression of survival genes as well as growth, differentiation, and sprouting of processes. The absence of these trophic factors, or perhaps exposure to death-inducing molecules such as tumor necrosis factor, can trigger the molecular cascade that leads to apoptosis. Neuronal survival is also dependent on the establishment of functional synaptic contacts, as described below.

of these ventricular cells extend radially from the ventricular surface to the outer surface of the tube. During the intermitotic phase of the cell cycle, the nuclei migrate from the ventricular surface toward the outer surface. As the nucleus enters the mitotic phase, it migrates back to the ventricular zone and the cytoplasmic processes retract. After cell division, these processes again extend radially. This process may be repeated for several cell cycles.

The nuclei of the proliferating cells eventually accumulate in the subventricular zone and most of them lose the capacity for further division. The cytoplasmic processes still extend radially to the outer limits of the tube, forming the marginal zone. This zone increases in width and definition as the number and complexity of neuronal and glial

Migration

The migration of neurons to their ultimate location in the central nervous system, that is, where they mature and develop their functional connections, is not random but programmed by the genetic code. A physical superstructure for directing neuronal migration is established by the differentiation of glial cells and their radially arranged processes. These glial cells constitute the radial glia. The process of migration and the interactions among neurons, glial cells, and the extracellular matrix are controlled at the molecular level by the expression of adhesion molecules and by soluble factors that act through receptors on the cell membrane to direct the cell to its final destination.

An anatomically conspicuous and functionally critical result of migration is seen at the prosencephalic level. A vast number of postmitotic cells migrate from the subventricular zone (germinal matrix) to the outer limits of the intermediate zone, where they accumulate in what constitutes, at this level, a fifth zone called the cortical plate.

Differentiation

The earliest processes involved in the differentiation of the neuroectoderm are *neural induction* and *neural determination.* Shortly after the formation of the neural plate, the capacity of neuroectodermal cells to become anything other than neurons or glial cells is restricted. The source of this restriction is derived from the underlying mesoderm in the form of diffusible molecules that switch on, or induce, differentiation into specific neuroectodermal components. These molecules act via transcription factors in the target cells, which decode incoming messages and effect changes in gene expression. The gene expression thus induced determines the ultimate lineage (neuronal or glial) of the cell. Precisely what factors determine whether a given primitive neuroectodermal cell differentiates into a neuronal or glial precursor and subsequently into a specific type of neuron or glial cell (astrocyte, oligodendrocyte, or ependymal cell) is a subject of active research.

Maturation

After a neuron has reached its final location in the central nervous system, it establishes appropriate contacts with other neurons, both locally and at a distance. It does this by extending processes called neurites, most of which become dendrites, to receive information coming from other nerve cells. One neurite, the axon, ultimately reaches a specific target. The growth of the axon and target selection are closely controlled and directed by adhesion molecules, nerve growth factors, and other extracellular molecules that either attract or repel it, ultimately directing the axon to its target cell, where it makes synaptic contact on a dendrite or cell body.

The initial synaptic contact, established by target selection, is followed by a protracted process of refinement and remodeling that involves the expansion of some contacts and the elimination of others. This depends on the pattern of synaptic activity. This process, called *synaptic plasticity,* is retained to some extent even in the adult nervous system. Immature neurons that do not establish appropriate functional contact are eliminated through programmed cell death.

Transverse Differentiation

The anatomical and cytologic events described in the preceding section apply to the entire transverse area of the neural tube in the earliest stages of development. However, as the neural tube enlarges, it undergoes anatomical and functional differentiation in the transverse plane.

In transverse section, the region of the neural tube nearest the thoracic and abdominal cavities is described as *ventral (anterior)* and the region farthest from them, as *dorsal (posterior).* As the neuroblasts proliferate, most of them accumulate laterally in the wall of the neural tube so that the middorsal and midventral areas are relatively thin. These thin areas are the *roof plate* and the *floor plate* (Fig. 6). Differential proliferation of cells in the dorsal and ventral regions of the ventricular zone on each side results in the formation of a longitudinal groove, the sulcus limitans, on each lateral wall of the neural canal. The *sulcus limitans* divides the neural tube into dorsal and ventral regions.

The portion of the intermediate zone that is dorsal to the sulcus limitans is the *alar plate* (Fig. 6). Neurons in this area form pathways related primarily to sensory function. They serve either as receiving stations for sensory information transmitted from the periphery or as relay stations passing the information to higher levels of the central nervous system. The term *afferent* is used to describe nerve fibers conducting information from the periphery toward the central nervous system. They receive information from somite derivatives (skin, muscle, joints, and bone) or endodermal derivatives (internal organs). These

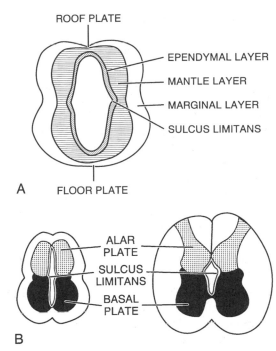

FIG. 6. A: Transverse section of the neural tube at 30 days, with early regional differentiation. **B:** Transverse section of the spinal cord at 4 *(left)* and 15 *(right)* weeks.

neurons and pathways constitute the sensory system.

The part of the intermediate zone that is ventral to the sulcus limitans is the *basal plate.* Under the influence of factors that are secreted by the notochord and floor plate, and that act through transcription factors, neurons in this area differentiate into motor neurons and interneurons that control such activities of the body as limb movement. These neurons are efferent, that is, they conduct impulses away from the central nervous system. Neurons and pathways concerned with the control of striated skeletal muscle constitute the somatic motor system.

Afferent and efferent neurons concerned with the control of internal organs and homeostasis are derived from portions of the alar and basal plates close to the sulcus limitans and constitute the *visceral,* or *internal regulation, system.* They are functionally distinct from the afferent and efferent neuronal aggre-

gates that develop in the intermediate zone further from the central canal. The latter aggregates are concerned with the innervation and control of somite derivatives and make up the somatic sensory and somatic motor systems.

The functional organization of the nervous system at each level may be viewed in terms of the relationship of neuronal groups to the central canal and the ventricular system (Fig. 1). Neuronal aggregates that reside close to the wall of the canal or ventricular system constitute the *core region* (or *inner tube*) of the neural tube and, in general, are interrelated by diffuse multisynaptic (indirect) pathways, and display a particular profile of neurochemical transmitters, which include acetylcholine, monoamines, and neuropeptides. Neuronal aggregates in regions further removed from the central canal, that is, in the *outer region* (or *outer tube*) of the wall of the neural tube, tend to form more direct pathways or relay systems and to use excitatory amino acids, especially L-glutamate, as neurotransmitters.

When the central nervous system is viewed in this manner, there are two systems that are derived primarily from the inner tube, or core, of the neural tube, namely the *internal regulation system* and the *consciousness system.* Structures related to the consciousness system are largely elaborated from neurons in the alar plate. The two systems related primarily to the outer portions of the tube, or the outer tube, are the motor and somatosensory systems. Furthermore, as will be apparent when each of these systems is studied, older and newer functional components in each system follow the same general pattern.

In addition to these four longitudinal systems (motor, sensory, internal regulation, and consciousness), two essential support systems are formed during embryogenesis of the central nervous system. These are the *cerebrospinal fluid system* and the *vascular system.* The primitive neural tube is surrounded by mesoderm from which are derived layers of connective tissue that encase the tube. The innermost layer, the pia mater, is intimately adherent to the outer wall of the tube. Angiogenic mesodermal elements penetrate the substance of the neural tube through this layer and form an extensive vascular network. Surrounding the pia mater is a layer of loose connective tissue called the *arachnoid*. This, in turn, is surrounded by a thick tough layer, the *dura mater*. In certain areas of the thin roof plate of the rhombencephalon, diencephalon, and telencephalon, the pia mater and its accompanying blood vessels grow into the ventricular cavity and carry a layer of ependyma with them to form the *choroid plexuses*. Choroidal epithelial cells are specialized ependymal cells. Filtration of plasma through the choroid plexus leads to the formation of the *cerebrospinal fluid,* which fills the central canal and ventricular system. This fluid, in turn, leaves the ventricular system through the caudal fourth ventricle and enters the space between the pia mater and the arachnoid, the *subarachnoid space*. These structures and spaces together constitute the cerebrospinal fluid system.

With further development, the basic plan of organization of the central nervous system is modified at each level of the neuraxis (Fig. 7). The modifications that occur at each level are considered in the following section.

Longitudinal Differentiation

Between the third and the fifth weeks of gestation, development differs significantly along the length of the neural tube. The most complex changes occur at the cephalic end, where the brain is forming. These changes are the result of three processes: flexure formation, development of special structures in the head, and differential growth rates.

As the major anatomical features of each level are described, it will be helpful to keep in mind the general principles that govern the location of functional systems, that is, the relationship of motor and sensory functions to the basal and alar plates, somatic and visceral motor neurons to the sulcus limitans, and old (indirect) and new (direct) systems to the inner tube and outer tube of the central nervous system.

Three bends, or flexures, occur in the neural tube (Fig. 8). The *cervical flexure* occurs between the spinal cord and the myelencephalon in a ventral direction, the *pontine flexure* occurs in the metencephalon in a dorsal direction, and the *midbrain flexure* occurs in the mesencephalon in a ventral direction. These flexures produce a widening in the transverse configuration of the neural tube in the rhombencephalon, with lateral displacement of the alar plates (Fig. 7C,D). The sum of the three flexures leaves only slight bends in the mature brain at the diencephalon-mesencephalon junction and at the medulla-spinal cord junction.

Two types of specialization occur in the cephalic region of the embryo. The first of these is the development of *branchial arches,* phylogenetic remnants of the gill system in lower animals. These arches contribute to the formation of structures in the head and neck, such as the facial muscles. The motor and sensory neurons that provide innervation to structures derived from the branchial arches are located in the rhombencephalon but are aggregated in groups distinct from the somatic and visceral sensory and motor neurons. The second specialization is the appearance of complex sensory structures such as the eyes, ears, balance receptors (vestibular), and smell and taste receptors. Separate groups of sensory neurons develop for each of these structures. Neurons concerned with vision and smell are located in the prosencephalon, and those concerned with balance, hearing, and taste are located in the rhombencephalon.

Finally, certain areas of the cephalic portions of the neural tube undergo marked proliferation of cells, with exuberant growth of related structures. This overgrowth and accompanying migration of cells produce complex rearrangements of the basic plan of the neural tube. For example, growth of the alar plate of the prosencephalon results in large cerebral hemispheres, which almost completely surround the derivatives of the diencephalon. The cerebellum also arises by proliferation of cells of the alar plate in the metencephalon and eventually covers the dorsal surface of the entire rhombencephalon.

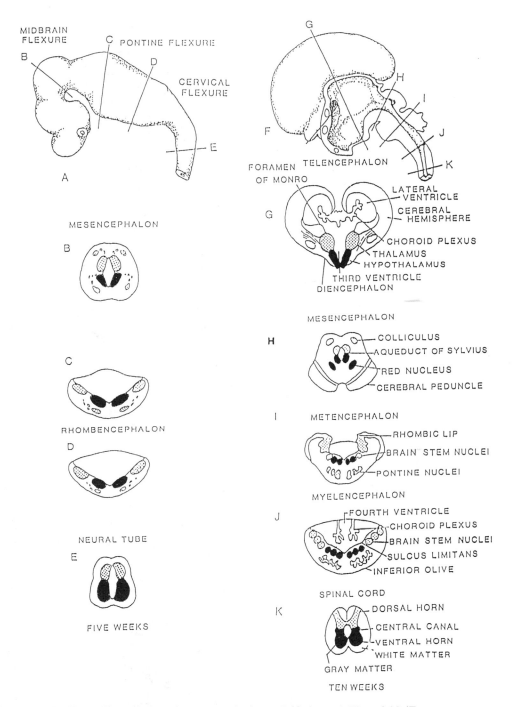

FIG. 7. Longitudinal differentiation along neural tube at 5 (**A** through **E**) and 10 (**F** through **K**) weeks seen in whole embryo and transverse section. (**F–J** modified from Moore, K. L. *The Developing Human: Clinically Oriented Embryology* [2nd ed.]. Philadelphia: W. B. Saunders, 1977. With permission.)

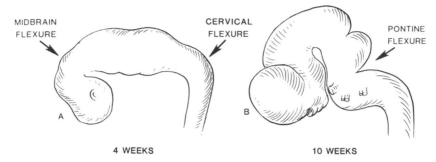

MIDBRAIN FLEXURE   CERVICAL FLEXURE   PONTINE FLEXURE

A   B

4 WEEKS   10 WEEKS

FIG. 8. A,B: Flexures *(arrows)* of the neural tube as primary brain vesicles are forming.

The unique changes that occur at each major level during the fourth to sixth weeks of development are considered below for each level.

Spinal Level

As the caudal end of the neural tube develops into the spinal cord, it remains basically the same as that seen in the primitive nervous system (Fig. 7E,K). The central canal becomes obliterated, and the shape of the cellular areas of the intermediate zone, now called *gray matter,* is modified. The marginal layer becomes the *white matter,* a dense layer of nerve fibers or tracts carrying axons longitudinally. The meninges surround the spinal cord and form a subarachnoid space. Bone surrounding the cord forms the spinal column. Therefore, at the spinal level, the sensory, motor, internal regulation, cerebrospinal fluid, and vascular systems are all present.

As the spinal cord develops, it is surrounded by the vertebral column, but there is a notable difference between the growth rate of the spinal cord and that of the vertebral column, with the latter growing faster. As a result, in the third fetal month, the spinal cord completely fills the vertebral canal; at birth, it terminates at the lower border of the third lumbar vertebra; and in adults, it terminates near the upper border of the second lumbar vertebra (Fig. 9). Therefore, a lumbar puncture in newborn infants must be done at a

very low level to avoid puncturing the spinal cord.

The differential rate of growth of the cord and the spinal column also places the spinal cord segments, particularly in the lower half of the body, above the vertebral segments of the corresponding number. Because the spinal nerves emerge between the embryologically established vertebral bodies, there is progressive elongation of the lower nerve roots that is known in the adult as the *cauda equina* (Fig. 9).

Posterior Fossa Level

The mesoderm that surrounds the cephalic end of the embryonic nervous system forms the skull and meninges that enclose and protect the brain within the cranial cavity. In concert with the formation of the primary brain vesicles and flexures, folds of meninges that ultimately become tough dural septa are formed. A major horizontal fold of dura mater forms at the level of the mesencephalon. This fold eventually covers the dorsal surface of the cerebellum and is called the tentorium cerebelli. The region of the cranial cavity below the plane of the tentorium is the posterior cranial fossa and contains the mesencephalon, the rhombencephalon, and their derivatives.

As the flexures occur in the rhombencephalon, the alar plates of the myelencephalon and the metencephalon rotate laterally, the roof plate becomes greatly thinned, and the central cavity opens out into a rhom-

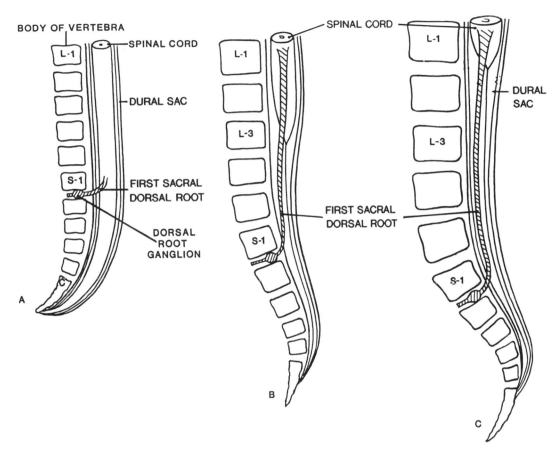

FIG. 9. The location of the caudal end of the spinal cord in the vertebral column at 12 weeks **(A)**, birth **(B)**, and adulthood **(C)**. The first sacral dorsal root in **B** and **C** is representative of the spinal roots that form the cauda equina. (Modified from Moore, K. L. *The Developing Human: Clinically Oriented Embryology* [2nd ed.]. Philadelphia: W. B. Saunders, 1977. With permission.)

bic-shaped space, the *fourth ventricle.* This rotation results in a change in the relationship of the alar and basal plates, so that the alar plate lies lateral to the basal plate, with the sulcus limitans marking their junction in the floor of the fourth ventricle in the adult derivatives, the medulla and pons (Fig. 7C,D,I,J). The junction between the thinned roof plate and the alar plate is the *rhombic lip.* Proliferation and migration of cells from the rhombic lip result in the formation of the *inferior olives,* the nuclei of the base of the pons, and portions of cerebellum that come to overlie the entire fourth ventricle and rhomben-

cephalon. The neurons innervating branchial arch derivatives and the special sensory structures for hearing, balance, and taste also are located at this level.

In the mesencephalon, which becomes the midbrain, the basic relationships seen in the spinal cord persist (Fig. 7B,H). The central cavity here is a small canal, the *aqueduct of Sylvius.* As the alar and basal plates differentiate into specialized sensory and motor structures, they become known as the *tectum* and *tegmentum,* respectively. Dense bundles of longitudinal axons beneath the tegmentum become the cerebral peduncles, part of the motor system. In addition to the motor system, other longitudinal systems in the posterior fossa are the sensory, cerebrospinal fluid, internal regulation, consciousness, and vascular systems.

Supratentorial Level

The portion of the cranial cavity located above the tentorium cerebelli contains the two derivatives of the prosencephalon, the *diencephalon* and the *telencephalon.* The general rule, that the sensory structures are dorsal and arise from the alar plate and the motor structures are ventral and arise from the basal plate, does not hold true in the diencephalon and telencephalon because most of the structures that arise from these regions are derived from the alar plate. Only some of the ventral diencephalon (hypothalamus and subthalamus) is derived from the basal plate. Nevertheless, other general features of the developmental relationships of functional systems mentioned above hold true. The more primitive, indirect, multisynaptic systems occupy the inner core of the cerebral hemispheres, and the more recently evolved direct relay systems subserving higher level functions occupy the outer region, especially the cerebral cortex.

The neural canal in the diencephalon becomes a slitlike cavity, the *third ventricle.* Only a small portion of the telencephalon remains as a midline structure, its neural canal becoming the anterior third ventricle. Most of the telencephalon develops from paired lateral evaginations that undergo tremendous growth to become the largest portion of the

mature brain, the cerebral hemispheres (Fig. 7F,G). The orifice of each lateral evagination is the *foramen of Monro,* which leads into the *lateral ventricles,* the cavities in the cerebral hemispheres (Fig. 7G).

The cerebral hemispheres are seen initially as two lateral evaginations of the prosencephalon. However, the rapid rate of proliferation of the cells in the dorsal parts of these outpouchings results in a sweeping of tissue posteriorly, laterally, and ventrally. This broad sweep and cellular migration give the hemispheres and ventricles a C-shaped configuration. As these cellular areas form the major lobes of the cerebral hemispheres, they pull along with them deep midline groups of cells and fiber pathways connected to the hypothalamus in the diencephalon. These cells and pathways become the limbic system, which is also C-shaped. Continued proliferation of cells in the enclosed space of the skull leads to the complex folds in the surface of the hemispheres known as *gyri* (ridges) and *sulci* (grooves).

Two specialized cranial structures are derived from the diencephalon, and each depends on an interaction of neural tissue with other tissue. The eye develops from tissue that is derived from paired lateral outgrowths of the diencephalon and from the overlying ectoderm in contact with these outgrowths. The pituitary gland, an endocrine gland, is derived from a midline ventral outgrowth of the diencephalon, the *infundibulum,* a ventral neuron ridge, and oral ectoderm, *Rathke's pouch* (Fig. 10). The mature pituitary gland has two

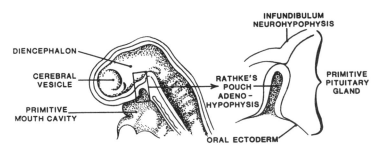

FIG. 10. Embryogenesis of the pituitary gland at the junction of invaginated oral ectoderm and evagination of the diencephalon.

divisions, the *adenohypophysis* (anterior pituitary gland) and the *neurohypophysis* (posterior pituitary gland).

The group of specialized sensory structures concerned with olfaction is derived from the telencephalon. As at the posterior fossa level, all the major longitudinal systems are represented at the supratentorial level.

Postnatal Development of the Central Nervous System

Birth is an artificial landmark in the process of growth and development of the central nervous system. The process is a continuum that begins with formation of the neural plate and proceeds late into the second decade when the brain reaches its maximum weight.

Cellular proliferation makes a minor contribution to brain growth after the second trimester of gestation. The number of neurons in the adult nervous system is determined by about 36 weeks of gestation, when the source of the neuroblasts (the germinal matrix or the primitive subventricular layer) is depleted of undifferentiated cells. The increase in brain weight, from about 380 g at 40 weeks of gestation to about 1,400 g at 18 years of age, is accounted for by two major factors.

One factor is the progressive increase in the volume of individual cells, especially neurons. An increase in the diameter of a 5-μm neuroblast to a 50-μm mature neuron results in as much as a 1,000-fold increase in cell body volume. The overall effect of the increase in length, diameter, and complexity of cell processes on the volume of the central nervous system is enormous. Similar considerations apply to glial and other supporting cells.

The other important influence on both the anatomical growth and physiologic maturation of the central nervous system is progressive myelination. The formation of myelin sheaths around central nervous system axons begins early in the second trimester and continues into early adult life. The period of most rapid myelination occurs between the third trimester and about 2 years of age. This corresponds to the period of most rapid brain growth and most rapid physiologic maturation. The myelination of the various tracts and regions of the central nervous system follows a well-defined, orderly sequence. The progression of this sequence correlates well with the progression of physiologic maturation and the development of specific functions and skills. For example, in the corticospinal tract (the major direct projection from the cerebral cortex to the motor neurons of the spinal cord), the proximal portions of the axons begin to myelinate at about 36 weeks of gestation. However, the cerebral cortex has almost no control over motor function at birth. Myelination of this tract progresses in an orderly fashion from the cerebral hemispheres through the sacral spinal cord during the first 2 years of life and correlates well with the progressive acquisition of motor skills, first of the upper extremities (grasping, manipulating objects) and then of the lower extremities (standing, walking, running).

A parallel process that contributes to the growth of the brain and especially to its functional maturation is the elaboration and refinement of synaptic connections between neuronal groups. In the earliest stages of development, axons that grow out from a group of neurons are led to the appropriate target neurons by genetically programmed molecular recognition. The tip of the growing axon, called the *growth cone,* is attracted to and able to recognize its target cells by this mechanism. After the growing axons recognize the target cell area, they sprout numerous small branches to produce synapses. The earliest pattern of synapses formed between functionally related neuronal groups may be imprecise and may not subserve normal function. As maturation proceeds, the synaptic pattern is modified and refined by the elaboration and strengthening of some connections and the atrophy and elimination of others. Although the mechanism of this anatomical refinement is not entirely known, there is evidence that it is related to the onset of electrical activity in the nervous system and to the pattern of action potentials that impinge on the synapses. This concept of synaptic remodeling through use has far-reaching implications, not only in normal processes, such as development of motor and sensory patterns and in learning, but in many pathologic situations, such as epilepsy and recovery processes after injury to the nervous system.

The increase in the mass of the brain as a whole is accompanied by a marked increase in the total surface area of the cerebral cortex, to about 2,300 cm^2 at maturity. If the surface remained smooth, the capacity of the cranial cavity would have to be increased several times to accommodate the brain. This is compensated for by the complex folding of the surface of the brain, which begins with the formation of the lateral sulcus (sylvian fissure) at about 50 days of gestation. The development of the normal pattern of fissures and of the secondary and tertiary gyri is nearly complete at 40 weeks of gestation. The sulci deepen and the gyri become more well defined throughout the growth period.

Differentiation of Peripheral Structures

The derivatives of the neural tube outlined in the previous sections become the central nervous system contained within the bony skull and spinal column. The peripheral nervous system is largely a derivative of the neural crest, and the peripheral neuromuscular structures of interest to us are derived from three sources: neural crest cells, somites, and outgrowths of the central nervous system. All these structures outside the spinal column and skull are at the *peripheral level.*

Neural Crest

As the neural tube closes, cells split from the neural tube and ectoderm, forming two columns of cells along the junction between the surface ectoderm and the neural tube (Figs. 11 and 12). These are the *neural crest.* As the neural tube separates from the overlying ectoderm, the cells of the neural crest proliferate and migrate laterally. As they differentiate, they form three of the four major components of the peripheral nervous system: dorsal root ganglia, visceral (autonomic) ganglia, and Schwann cells. The fourth component is an outgrowth of the neural tube, the motor axons.

Dorsal root ganglia are collections of cell bodies of sensory neurons. These neurons send axons peripherally to all areas of the body to gather sensory information and centrally into the alar plate to carry the sensory information into the central nervous system. Therefore, these neurons are the initial transmitters of sensory information; they are *primary sensory neurons.*

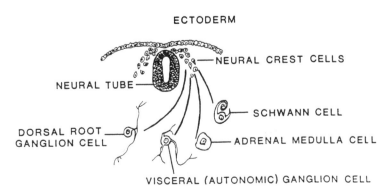

FIG. 11. Derivatives of neural crest cells formed at the junction of the neural tube and covering ectoderm.

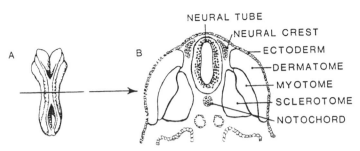

FIG. 12. Formation of myotome, sclerotome, and dermatome from somites in an embryo of 4 weeks, in whole embryo **(A)** and transverse section **(B)**.

The *autonomic ganglia* are collections of cell bodies of visceral neurons in the trunk and head that send out axons to innervate all the internal organs. They receive connections from axons of visceral neurons in the central nervous system and from sensory neurons in the internal organs. These ganglia mediate motor and sensory activities of the visceral organs.

Schwann cells form the myelin, or insulation, surrounding the axons in the peripheral nervous system, just as the oligodendroglia do in the central nervous system (Fig. 13). Schwann cells are located serially along the length of all peripheral axons and envelop them. Neural crest cells also give rise to an endocrine organ, the adrenal medulla.

Somites

As the neural tube closes, the embryonic mesoderm lateral to the tube becomes seg- mented into cell masses known as *somites* (Fig. 12). These masses differentiate into three components: the sclerotome, myotome, and dermatome. The ventromedial portion of the somite forms the *sclerotome,* which differentiates into the cartilage and bone forming the vertebrae of the spinal column and base of the skull surrounding the central nervous system. The notochord becomes incorporated into the ventromedial extensions of the sclerotome and thus remains ventral to the tube. The notochordal remnant within the vertebral column is the nucleus pulposus in the intervertebral disk. The dorsomedial portion of the somite forms the *myotome,* which gives rise to the striated skeletal muscle of the body, except for the striated muscle that forms from the branchial arches in the head and neck. The primordial muscle cells of the myotome migrate peripherally to form the muscles of the trunk and limbs. The lateral portion of the somite forms the *dermatome.*

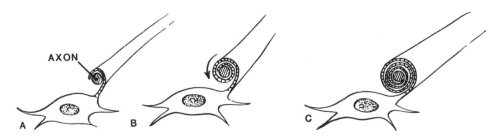

FIG. 13. Process of myelination of nerve fibers in the central and peripheral nervous systems. A layer of cytoplasm wraps around an axon **(A)** and then encircles it repeatedly **(B)**. Condensation of layers of cytoplasm forms myelin **(C)**.

Cells from the dermatome migrate peripherally to form the dermis, the connective tissue layer of the skin.

Peripheral Nerves

Connections between the central nervous system and the peripheral structures derived from the somites and the neural crest are established by the growth of axons from the dorsal root ganglia into the alar plate of the neural tube and by the outgrowth of axons from neurons in the basal plate. These distally growing motor axons join the peripherally growing sensory axons of the dorsal root ganglia to form a nerve that innervates the somite at the same level (Fig. 14). The nerves formed in this fashion at the spinal level are the *spinal nerves;* those formed at the posterior fossa level are the *cranial nerves.* Both types are composed of mixtures of sensory and motor axons. In these nerves, the motor axons from cells in the central nervous system innervate the myotomal derivatives and autonomic ganglia and the sensory axons innervate the dermatomes and endoderm derivatives. As the embryo develops and the cells forming the muscles, skin, and internal organs migrate to their adult locations, these neural processes are pulled along with them to establish the pattern of innervation of peripheral nerves.

The functions of the axons in peripheral nerves are classified into systems, just as are those in the central nervous system. *Afferent* fibers are those that conduct information toward the central nervous system (sensory), and *efferent* fibers are those that carry information away from the central nervous system. Axons are also subdivided on the basis of the type of structure they innervate. Fibers that innervate tissues derived from somites (muscles and skin) are designated *somatic;* fibers that innervate endodermal or other mesodermal derivatives (internal organs) are called *visceral.* Thus, afferent axons that carry sensations such as pain, temperature, touch, and joint movement from the body surface and supporting structures are *general somatic afferent* (GSA). Afferent axons that carry sensations such as pain, fullness, and blood chemical levels from the internal organs are *general visceral afferent* (GVA). Motor axons to skeletal muscle of somite origin are *general somatic efferent* (GSE). Motor axons that innervate smooth muscle of viscera, glands, and blood vessels are *general visceral efferent* (GVE).

Each of these types of fibers is found in the spinal and cranial nerves. The cranial nerves also have fibers that mediate special sensations and fibers that innervate branchial arch derivatives. Those to the branchial arch derivatives, especially facial muscles, are *special visceral efferent* (SVE); those mediating sensations of taste and smell are *special visceral afferent* (SVA). The fibers that carry the other special sensory information of vision, hearing, and balance are *special somatic afferent* (SSA). The somatic afferent fibers are considered in detail in the discussion of the sensory system; the somatic efferent fibers are considered in the discussion of the motor system; and the visceral afferent and efferent fibers are considered in the discussion of the visceral system. Other special functions are presented in the discussion of the posterior fossa and supratentorial levels. Table 2 summarizes the classification of the functional components of nerves on the basis of embryologic origin and destination.

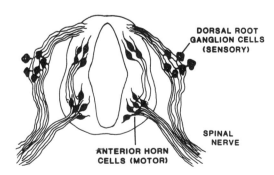

FIG. 14. Formation of spinal nerves by the combination of axons from the basal plate and dorsal root ganglia.

TABLE 2. *Classification of the functional components of nerves on the basis of embryologic origin and destination*

Type	Category	Tissue innervated	Tissue origin	Axon type
Afferent (sensory)	General	Skin, muscle, bone, joints	Somites	GSA
		Visceral organs	Endoderm	GVA
	Special	Ear, eye, balance	External receptors (ectoderm)	SSA
		Taste, smell	Visceral receptors (endoderm)	SVA
Efferent (motor)	General	Somatic striated muscle	Somites	GSE
		Glands, smooth muscle, visceral organs	Nonsomite (mesoderm and endoderm)	GVE
	Special	Head and neck muscle	Branchial arches	SVE

GSA, general somatic afferent; GSE, general somatic efferent; GVA, general visceral afferent; GVE, general visceral efferent; SSA, special somatic afferent; SVA, special visceral afferent; SVE, special visceral efferent.

Clinical Correlations ■

Although some developmental processes occur more or less simultaneously, they may be thought of as occurring in six stages, according to the process that is dominant at different stages of embryogenesis (Table 3).

The *first stage* is *neural tube formation,* sometimes called *dorsal induction* because of the important influence the notochord and other underlying mesodermal structures have on inducing the formation of the neural plate and its derivatives. This process dominates approximately the third and fourth weeks of embryogenesis. Injury (genetic or acquired) to the embryo during this stage produces defects in the dorsal midline, often obvious on the surface. The various degrees of severity of these defects in the caudal (lumbosacral) region are illustrated in Fig. 15. Thus, *spina bifida occulta,* a defect only in the vertebral arch (Fig. 15A); *meningocele,* protrusion of a meningeal sac through the bone defect (Fig. 15B); meningomyelocele, inclusion of herniated spinal cord in the sac (Fig. 15C); and myeloschisis, a completely open spinal cord through an overlying bone and skin defect (Fig. 15D), are viewed as increasingly severe manifestations of the same disorder. Similar defects occur at the rostral end of the neural tube and cause malformations, analogous to those at the caudal end, termed *cranium bifidum, cranial meningocele, meningoencephalocele,* and *cranioschisis* (or *anencephaly*). The most severe defect in this

TABLE 3. *Stage-development development defects*

Stage duration	Process	Defect
Dorsal induction (0–4 weeks)	Formation and closure of neural tube	Anencephaly Myeloschisis Meningocele Spina bifida
Ventral induction (5–6 weeks)	Formation of telencephalon and facial structures	Holoprosencephaly Agenesis of corpus callosum
Proliferation (8–16 weeks)	Increased number of neurons and glial cells	Microcephaly
Migration (12–20 weeks)	Neuronal migration into cerebral cortex, guided by radial glial cells	Heterotopy
Differentiation (6 months to maturity)	Axon growth Synaptic formation Synaptic stabilization	Mental retardation
Myelination (6 months to age 18)	Formation of central myelin by oligodendrocytes	Dysmyelinating disease (leukodystrophies)

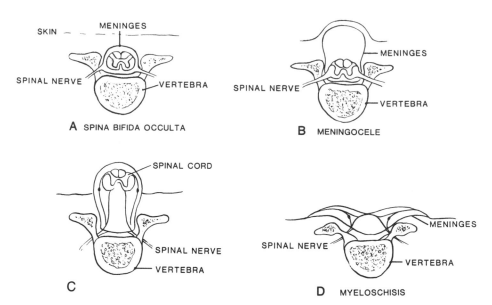

FIG. 15. Examples of failure of fusion at the spinal level. **A:** Spina bifida occulta with incomplete vertebral arch. **B:** Meningocele with outpouching of fluid-filled sac of meninges and skin. **C:** Meningomyelocele with sac containing abnormal neural tissue. **D:** Myeloschisis with no closure and a deformed neural plate open to the surface.

category is a completely open neural tube and dorsal midline, termed *craniorachischisis.*

The *second* stage occurs during the fifth and sixth weeks of development and relates to the formation of the telencephalon in conjunction with the cranial, facial, and neck structures derived from the branchial arches. This stage is sometimes called *ventral induction,* because of the relationship of the prechordal mesoderm to the cephalic end of the neural tube. Defects that occur during this stage can cause severe abnormalities in the formation of the telencephalon, such as *holoprosencephaly* (failure to form telencephalic vesicles), and craniofacial deformities.

The *third stage* is *proliferative activity* of the ventricular and subventricular zones, most active during the eighth to the 16th weeks of gestation. Because of injury (genetic, chemical, infectious) to the proliferating pool of neuroblasts during this stage, the number of neurons may not be sufficient to form a normal-sized brain, resulting in *microcephaly,* or, in less severe cases, to elaborate the proper number and type of synapses, which may account for some cases of mental retardation in persons with grossly normal brains.

The *fourth stage* is the period of most active *migration* of neurons and spongioblasts from the subventricular zone into the intermediate zone and, in the telencephalon, into the cortical plate. This process is most active from the 12th to the 20th week of gestation. Pathologic processes affecting the fetus during this period are likely to cause malformations attributable to disordered or arrested migration. The clearest example of this is *heterotopia,* collections of neurons and other gray matter components in areas where they do not occur normally, such as the subcortical white matter. Other malformations attributable to migratory disorders include formation of abnormal gyri, which may be larger (pachygyria) or smaller (microgyria) than normal. Migratory disorders may be either localized or generalized, depending on the nature of the pathologic process; they often occur in concert with disorders of proliferation, because the third and fourth stages overlap in time.

The process that dominates the *fifth stage* of development, which extends from the sixth gestational month to maturity, is *differentiation* of neurons and glia. This maturational process includes not only physical growth but also development of functional connections (synapses) and associated neurochemical mediators. Widespread disturbances of these processes do not usually lead to obvious gross malformations of the nervous system but rather to subtle functional disturbances, such as *learning disabilities* and *mental retardation.*

The *sixth stage* of development is associated with myelination of the nervous system. This process extends from the last half of gestation up to age 18 and is most evident from birth to age 2. Although myelination is defective in areas of the central nervous system affected by the processes mentioned above, damage that primarily affects this process does not produce obvious structural malformations, such as mentioned above. Instead, genetic or extrinsic damage to the process of myelination results in myelin either failing to form or, once formed, to degenerate due to faulty structure. Genetic disorders in this category are called *leukodystrophies,* which usually occur in the first 2 years of life.

Because the skin and nervous system are both derived from ectoderm, it is not surprising that genetically determined disorders may affect them together. A group of disorders known as *neurocutaneous syndromes,* or *neuroectodermal dysplasias,* is characterized by specific abnormalities in both the skin and the nervous system. Common manifestations of the three most commonly seen disorders of this type are outlined in Table 4.

The retina of the eye is also a derivative of the central nervous system. As with the skin, the retina may be affected by disorders that involve the nervous system, and observation of the retina with an ophthalmoscope may provide information about the disorder. An example of this association is *Tay-Sachs disease,* the lipid-storage disease in which neurons of the central nervous system accumulate large amounts of gangliosides. This accumulation is reflected in the retina by a cherry-red spot in the macula, due to the storage of lipids and the relative opacification of retinal ganglion cells surrounding the macula. Retinal tumors may also be seen in neuroectodermal dysplasias, and malformations of the eye sometimes accompany anomalies of the nervous system.

Clinical Problems

1. A newborn girl has a large bulging mass over the lower portion of the spinal column. There is no skin overlying this mass, and ill-defined neural structures can be seen through the glistening membranes of the fluid-filled mass. The infant does not move her legs.
   a. What embryologic process was not completed in this child?
   b. What primitive structure was involved and at what stage in the development?
   c. Which types of functions are probably absent in this child?

TABLE 4. *Examples of neuroectodermal dysplasias and some of their common skin and nervous system manifestations*

Disease	Skin	Nervous system
Von Recklinghausen disease	Neurofibromas Café-au-lait spots	Schwannomas Gliomas Meningeal angioma
Sturge-Weber syndrome	Port-wine nevus of face	Cortical calcification
Tuberous sclerosis	Adenoma sebaceum Subungual fibromas Depigmented patches	Periventricular tumors Cortical giant cell tumors Gliomas

    d. What is the origin of the structures involved in this defect?

    e. What primitive layers of the spinal cord might be involved?

    f. Name the disorder.

2. A 4-year-old boy has white spots (phakomas) in the retina of his eyes, as seen with an ophthalmoscope, and red lesions over his face. He also has convulsions and mental retardation.

    a. What is the congenital basis for all these findings?

    b. From what primitive structures do the eyes develop?

    c. What are the two primitive neural cell types from which tumors might arise?

    d. What is the functional embryologic classification of the nerve fibers from the eye?

    e. Name the disorder.

Additional Reading ▪

Brody, B. A., Kinney, H. C., Kloman, A. S., and Gilles, F. H. Sequence of central nervous system myelination in human infancy: I. An autopsy study of myelination. *J. Neuropathol. Exp. Neurol.* 46:283, 1987.

Cowan, W. M. The development of the brain. *Sci. Am.* 241(3):112, 1979.

Crelin, E. S., Netter, F. H., and Shapter, R. K. Development of the nervous system: A logical approach to neuroanatomy. *Clin. Symp.* 26(2):1, 1974.

Goodman, H. M. *Basic Medical Endocrinology.* New York: Raven Press, 1988.

Langman, J. *Langman's Medical Embryology* (6th ed.). Baltimore: Williams & Wilkins, 1990.

Levitan, I. B., and Kaczmarek, L. K. *The Neuron: Cell and Molecular Biology* (2nd ed.). New York: Oxford University Press, 1997.

Moore, K. L. *The Developing Human: Clinically Oriented Embryology* (4th ed.). Philadelphia: W. B. Saunders, 1988.

Purves, D., and Lichtman, J. W. *Principles of Neural Development.* Sunderland, MA: Sinauer Associates, 1985.

Shatz, C. J. The developing brain. *Sci. Am.* 267(3):61, 1992.

three

Diagnosis of Neurologic Disorders: Anatomical Localization

Objectives ■

1. Define the boundaries of the major anatomical levels (supratentorial, posterior fossa, spinal, and peripheral), and identify on gross specimen, photograph, or other reproduction the major anatomical structures contained in each level.

2. Given a cross-section specimen, drawing, or reproduction, identify the approximate area of the neuraxis to which the specimen belongs (that is, cerebral hemisphere, mesencephalon, pons, medulla, cerebellum, or spinal cord: cervical, thoracic, lumbar, or sacral segment).

3. Given a clinical problem, answer the following two questions:

   a. The signs and symptoms contained in the protocol are most likely the manifestation of disease at which of the following *levels* of the nervous system?
      i. Supratentorial level
      ii. Posterior fossa level
      iii. Spinal level
      iv. Peripheral level
      v. More than one level

   b. Within the level you have selected, the responsible lesion is most likely
      i. focal, on the *right* side of the nervous system.
      ii. focal, on the *left* side of the nervous system.
      iii. focal, but involving the *midline* and *contiguous* structures on both sides of the nervous system.
      iv. nonfocal and diffusely located.

Introduction ■

The diagnosis of neurologic disorders is a skill that requires the application of basic scientific information to a clinical problem. As knowledge of the nervous system grows, more complicated neurologic problems can be solved in more sophisticated ways; however, the basic approach to the solution of all neurologic problems remains unchanged. In arriving at a solution, three questions must be answered: (1) Is there a lesion involving the nervous system? (2) Where is the lesion located? (3) What is the (histopathologic) nature of the lesion?

Answering the first question is the most difficult, because it requires a familiarity not only with clinical neurology but also with other disciplines of medicine. In time, as the manifestations of neurologic disorders become better known, the neurologic origin of certain symptoms will be identified with increasing confidence.

To answer the question "Where is the location of the lesion that has caused the signs and symptoms?" requires an understanding of the organization of the nervous system and an ability to relate the patient's description and the physician's observations of dysfunction to a particular area or areas in the nervous system.

In addition to localizing a lesion in an area in the nervous system, the physician must determine the nature of the lesion. An infarct (stroke), tumor, or abscess may lead to similar signs and symptoms. The manner in which these symptoms evolve, the temporal profile, provides the clues to distinguish these disorders and to predict the histopathologic changes responsible for the observed abnormality.

A physician highly skilled in neurologic-anatomical diagnosis is capable of localizing a lesion in the nervous system to within millimeters of its actual site. Although this type of skill is laudable, it is often more than is required of even the practicing neurologist. In most clinical situations, for proper patient management it is sufficient to decide whether the responsible lesion is producing dysfunction in one or more longitudinal systems, to relate those abnormalities to one (or more) of several gross anatomical levels, and to determine whether the presumed lesion is on the right side, on the left side, or in the midline or is diffuse and involves homologous areas bilaterally. Neurologic disorders may affect one or more of the following systems:

1. Cerebrospinal fluid system
2. Sensory system
3. Motor system
4. Internal regulation system
5. Consciousness system
6. Vascular system

Neurologic disorders may occur at one or more of the following levels:

1. Supratentorial level
2. Posterior fossa level
3. Spinal level
4. Peripheral level

Familiarity with these major systems and levels will aid in the diagnosis of neurologic disorders. Each system and level will be discussed in further detail in subsequent chapters; this chapter discusses the anatomy of the levels.

Overview

The major structures of the central nervous system—the brain and the spinal cord—are surrounded by three fibrous connective tissue linings called *meninges* and are encased in a protective bony skeleton. The brain, consisting of derivatives of the primitive telencephalon, diencephalon, mesencephalon, metencephalon, and myelencephalon (Fig. 1), is enclosed in the *skull;* the spinal cord is situated in the spinal column. Cranial and peripheral nerves must pass through these surrounding investments to reach more peripheral structures.

The major anatomical levels to be discussed are defined by the meninges and bony structures to which they are related. The divisions between the anatomical levels used in this book are not exact, and there is some divergence from strict anatomical definitions found in other textbooks. However, as defined, the levels have boundaries that are clinically useful in understanding neurologic disorders.

Supratentorial Level

The floor of the human skull (Fig. 2) is divided into three distinct compartments *(fossae)* on each side: anterior, middle, and posterior. A rigid membrane, the *tentorium cerebelli,* separates the anterior and middle fossae from the posterior fossa (Fig. 3). The tentorium lies in a nearly horizontal plane and attaches laterally to the petrous ridges and posteriorly to the occipital bone. The portion of the nervous system located above the tentorium cerebelli constitutes the *supratentorial level.* The major anatomical structures of this level are derivatives of the telencephalon and diencephalon and consist primarily of the cerebral hemispheres, basal ganglia, thalamus, hypothalamus, and cranial nerves I (olfactory) and II (optic).

Posterior Fossa Level

Structures located within the skull below the tentorium cerebelli but above the *foramen magnum* (the opening of the skull to the spinal

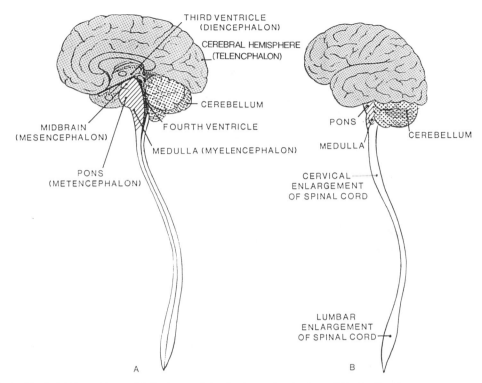

FIG. 1. Medial **(A)** and lateral **(B)** views of the brain and spinal cord illustrating the major levels: supratentorial *(dark shading)*, posterior fossa with brainstem *(lines)* and cerebellum *(dots)*, and spinal *(clear area)*. The peripheral level is not shown.

canal) constitute the *posterior fossa level.* These structures—the midbrain, pons, medulla, and cerebellum—are derivatives of the mesencephalon, metencephalon, and myelencephalon. Cranial nerves III through XII are located in the posterior fossa. Anatomically and physiologically, these nerves are analogous to other peripheral nerves; however, functionally they are intimately related to the mesencephalon, metencephalon, and myelencephalon and therefore are studied along with the structures of the posterior fossa. Those segments of cranial nerves contained in the bony skull are considered part of the posterior fossa level. After these nerves emerge from the skull, they are part of the peripheral level.

Spinal Level

The portion of the central nervous system located below the foramen magnum of the skull but contained in the vertebral column constitutes the *spinal level* (Fig. 4). This level has a considerable longitudinal extent, reaching from the skull to the sacrum. However, the spinal cord itself (the major structure at the spinal level) does not extend that entire length. A series of spinal nerves arise in the spinal canal and exit through the intervertebral foramina. Nerves contained in the bony vertebral column and in the intervertebral foramina are part of the spinal level. After these nerves leave the vertebral column, they become part of the peripheral level. The vertebral column itself is part of the spinal level.

Peripheral Level

The *peripheral level* includes all neuromuscular structures located outside the skull and vertebral column, including the cranial and peripheral nerves, their peripheral branches,

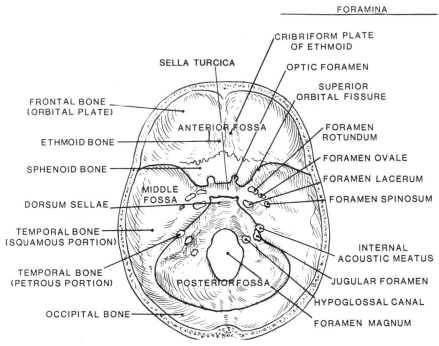

FIG. 2. Base of the cranial cavity viewed from above, illustrating the major cranial fossae, bones of the base of the skull, and the foramina.

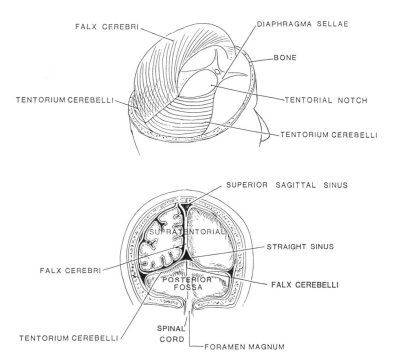

FIG. 3. Reflections of the dural mater forming the falx cerebri and the tentorium cerebelli **(top)**. Structures located above the tentorium are part of the supratentorial level; those below the tentorium but above the foramen magnum are part of the posterior fossa level **(bottom)**.

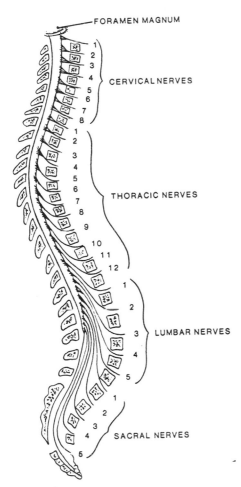

FIG. 4. Structures at the spinal level include the spinal cord, nerve roots contained in the vertebral column, and the vertebral column itself.

and the structures (including muscle) that are innervated by these nerves. The autonomic ganglia and nerves are also part of the peripheral level.

Gross Neuroanatomy—Introduction to Anatomical Levels

The major anatomical features of each of the major levels of the nervous system will be reviewed. Before doing so, however, it is useful to discuss individually certain structures

that may be related to more than one of the major levels previously defined.

The Skull

The skull (Fig. 5) is formed by the union of a number of bones and can be grossly subdivided into (1) the facial bones and orbits, (2) the sinus cavities within the bones that form the anterior aspect of the skull, and (3) the cranial bones. The cranial bones surround the brain in the cranial cavity and provide a nonyielding protective covering for the brain. In contrast to other protective structures in the body, the cranial bones severely limit the expansion of the brain, even when expansion becomes necessary in response to specific pathologic processes. The cranial cavity is formed by the *frontal, parietal, sphenoid, temporal,* and *occipital* bones. The bones forming the base of the cavity are shown in Fig. 2. Radiographs of the skull show the bones as lighter areas, and structures on the opposite sides of the skull are overlapped (Fig. 6).

When the base of the cranial cavity is viewed from above, three distinct areas are noted: the *anterior, middle,* and *posterior* fossae. In addition, there are symmetrically placed holes (foramina) in the base of the skull, through which the cranial nerves emerge to innervate peripheral structures (Table 1).

Meningeal Coverings

The meninges are an important supporting element of the central nervous system and include the dura mater, arachnoid, and pia mater (Fig. 7). The outermost fibrous membrane, the *dura mater,* consists of two layers of connective tissue that are fused, except in certain regions where they separate to form the *intracranial venous sinuses.* The dura mater is folded into the cranial cavity in two areas to form distinct fibrous barriers: the *falx cerebri,* which is located between the two cerebral hemispheres, and the *tentorium cerebelli,* which demarcates the superior limit of the posterior fossa. The delicate, filamentous *arachnoid* lies beneath the dura mater and appears to be loosely ap-

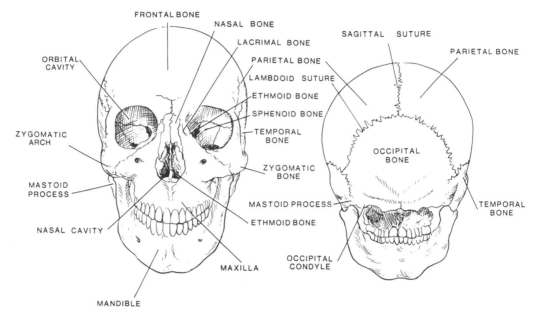

FIG. 5. Anterior **(left)** and posterior **(right)** views illustrating major bones of the skull. Hollow sinus cavities are located within frontal, ethmoid, sphenoid, and maxillary bones.

plied to the surface of the brain. *Pacchionian granulations* (arachnoid villi) are small tufts of arachnoid invaginated into dural venous sinuses, especially along the dorsal convexity of the cerebral hemispheres, superior to the longitudinal (interhemispheric) fissure. Many of the major arterial channels can be seen on the surface of the brain beneath the arachnoid. The in-

nermost layer, the *pia mater,* is composed of a very thin layer of mesoderm that is so closely attached to the brain surface that it cannot be seen in gross specimens.

Several important potential and actual spaces are found in association with these meningeal coverings (Fig. 7). Between the bone and the dura mater is the *epidural space,*

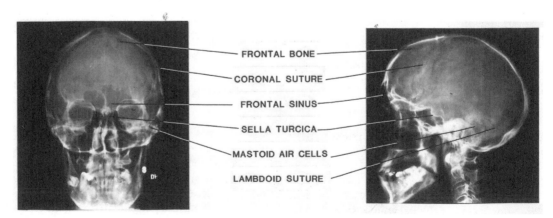

FIG. 6. Anterior **(left)** and lateral **(right)** views illustrating major bones of the skull. Air-filled sinuses and nasal cavities appear darker. Compare with Fig. 5.

TABLE 1. *Cranial foramina and associated structures*

Foramen	Associated structures
Cribriform plate of ethmoid bone	Olfactory nerves (CN I)
Optic foramen	Optic nerve (CN II)
	Ophthalmic artery
Superior orbital fissure	Oculomotor (CN III), trochlear (CN IV), abducens (CN VI) nerves and ophthalmic division of trigeminal nerve (CN V)
Foramen rotundum	Maxillary division of trigeminal nerve (CN V)
Foramen ovale	Mandibular division of trigeminal nerve (CN V)
Foramen lacerum	Sympathetic nerve
	Internal carotid artery
Foramen spinosum	Middle meningeal artery and vein
Internal acoustic meatus	Facial (CN VII) and vestibular and auditory nerves (CN VIII)
	Internal auditory artery
Jugular foramen	Glossopharyngeal (CN IX), vagus (CN X), and spinal accessory (CN XI) nerves
	Jugular vein
Hypoglossal canal	Hypoglossal nerve (CN XII)
Foramen magnum	Medulla, spinal accessory nerve (CN XI)
	Vertebral artery, anterior and posterior spinal arteries

CN, cranial nerve.

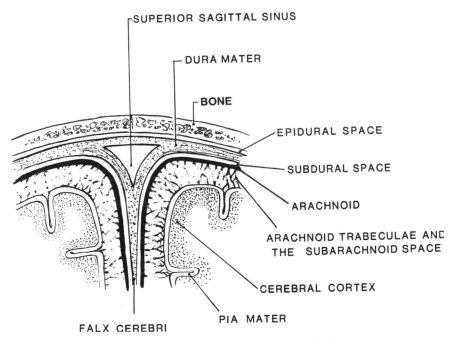

FIG. 7. Meninges and meningeal spaces. Coronal section through the paramedian region of the cerebral hemispheres.

and beneath the dura mater is the *subdural space.* The bone, dura, and arachnoid are normally closely applied to one another so that the epidural and subdural spaces are potential spaces in which blood or pus may accumulate. Beneath the arachnoid is the *subarachnoid space,* which surrounds the entire brain and spinal cord and is filled with cerebrospinal fluid. The subarachnoid space communicates with the interior of the brain via the ventricular system (Fig. 8).

The Ventricular System

Located within the depth of the brain is the ventricular system (Fig. 9), a derivative of the primitive embryonic neural canal. *Cerebrospinal fluid* is formed within the ventricles by the *choroid plexus* (located in each ventricle) and circulates throughout the ventricles and subarachnoid space.

The cavity contained within each cerebral hemisphere is the *lateral ventricle,* which communicates with the cavity of the diencephalon, the *third ventricle,* via the *foramen of Monro.* The caudal end of the third ventricle narrows into the cavity of the mesencephalon, the *aqueduct of Sylvius,* which leads into the *fourth ventricle.* Communication with the subarachnoid spaces is via the two lateral *foramina of Luschka* and the central *foramen of Magendie* (all located in the walls of the fourth ventricle). The portion of the primitive central canal of the spinal cord becomes obliterated in the mature human nervous system and is usually identified only as a cluster of ependymal and glial cells in the central regions of the spinal cord.

Blood Vessels

Blood enters the skull via two arterial systems (Fig. 10). The brain is supplied by the posteriorly located *vertebrobasilar system* and the anteriorly located *carotid system.* A series of anastomotic channels lying at the base of the

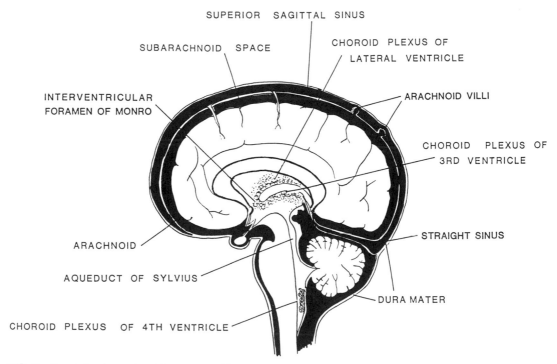

FIG. 8. Cranial subarachnoid space and its communication with both spinal subarachnoid space and ventricular system.

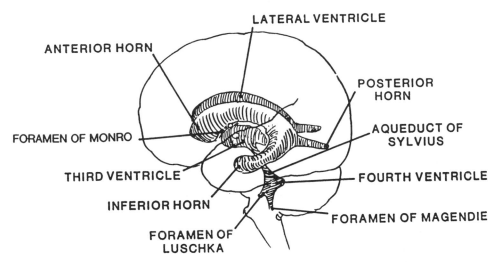

FIG. 9. Ventricular system. Cerebrospinal fluid is formed by choroid plexus in the ventricles. This fluid circulates and communicates with the subarachnoid space via the foramina of Luschka and Magendie.

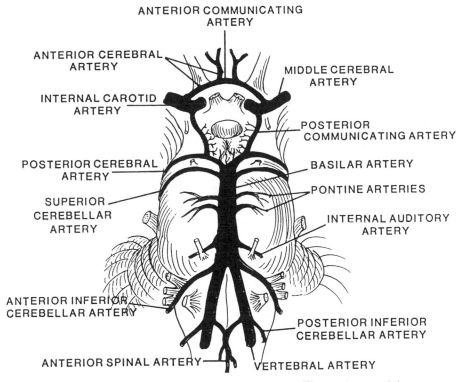

FIG. 10. Arterial supply to the brain as viewed from the base. The major arterial supply is via the internal carotid and vertebrobasilar systems, which communicate with each other via a series of anastomotic channels known as the circle of Willis.

brain, known as the *circle of Willis,* permits communication between these two systems.

The *internal carotid artery* and its major branches, the *anterior cerebral* and *middle cerebral* arteries, can be seen at the base of the brain (Fig. 10). The anterior cerebral arteries are connected to each other by the small *anterior communicating artery* and continue in the midline between the two hemispheres to supply blood to their medial surfaces. The middle cerebral artery courses laterally between the temporal and frontal lobes and emerges from the *insula* between the frontal and temporal lobes, where its branches spread over and supply blood to the lateral surface of the hemisphere (Fig. 11).

Additional blood is carried to the brain by the two *vertebral arteries,* which enter the skull via the foramen magnum and join at the caudal border of the pons to form the *basilar artery* (Fig. 10). Branches from these arteries normally provide the sole arterial supply to the occipital lobe, undersurface of the temporal lobe, thalamus, midbrain, pons, cerebellum, medulla, and portions of the cervical spinal cord. The *posterior inferior cerebellar arteries* are branches of the vertebral arteries, whereas the *anterior inferior cerebellar arteries* and *superior cerebellar arteries* are branches of the basilar artery.

The basilar artery continues cephalad until it divides into the *posterior cerebral arteries.* The *posterior communicating arteries* usually arise as branches of the posterior cerebral arteries and join those vessels with the internal carotid arteries to complete the circle of Willis.

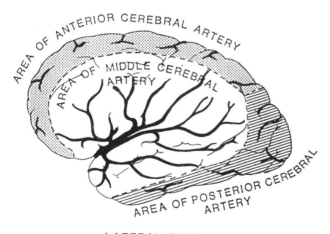

LATERAL SURFACE

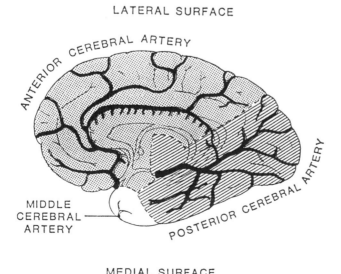

MEDIAL SURFACE

FIG. 11. Lateral and medial surfaces of the cerebral hemisphere illustrating the distribution of the major arteries. The anterior and middle cerebral arteries are branches of internal carotid arteries; posterior cerebral arteries are branches of the basilar artery. (**Right** modified from Pansky, B., and Allen, D. J. *Review of Neuroscience.* New York: Macmillan, 1980. With permission.)

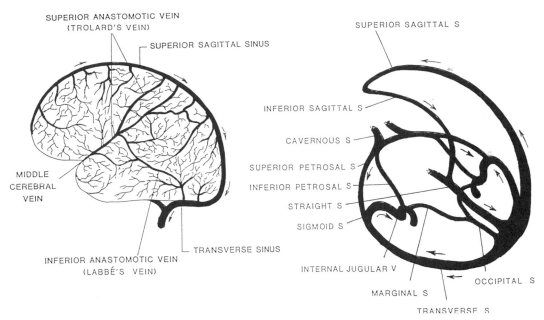

FIG. 12. Venous drainage of the cerebral hemispheres. Blood circulating over the cerebral cortex collects in the superior sagittal sinus **(left)**; blood from deeper structures enters other venous sinuses **(right)**. The direction of flow is toward the confluence of sinuses in the occipital region and then toward the internal jugular veins by way of the transverse and sigmoid sinuses. *S*, sinus; *V*, vein.) **(Left** modified from Pansky, B., and House, E. L. *Review of Gross Anatomy* [3rd ed.]. New York: Macmillan, 1975. With permission.)

Blood leaves the head by way of veins (Fig. 12) that course over the cerebral hemispheres to converge into large channels, the *venous sinuses,* contained within the layers of the dura mater. The most prominent of these sinuses are the *superior sagittal sinus* and *inferior sagittal sinus,* which run longitudinally from front to back in the falx cerebri between the hemispheres. The major venous channels merge in the occipital region and form the *transverse* and *sigmoid sinuses,* which exit through the skull via the jugular foramen as the *internal jugular veins.*

The Supratentorial Level

The major structures at the supratentorial level are the telencephalic derivatives (the cerebral hemispheres), the diencephalon, and cranial nerves I and II.

Cerebral Hemispheres

Through a process of growth and proliferation, the telencephalic structures differentiate into the cerebral hemispheres. The *longitudinal (interhemispheric) fissure* separates the cerebrum into two cerebral hemispheres. The surface of each hemisphere is convoluted: the folds are known as *gyri* and are separated from one another by grooves, or *sulci.* Certain grooves are more prominent, deeper, and more constant and are known as *fissures.* The fissures must be identified in order to locate the four major lobes into which each hemisphere is divided: *frontal, parietal, temporal,* and *occipital.* As shown in Fig. 13, the following serve as important landmarks in defining the limits of each lobe: *lateral fissure (fissure of Sylvius), central sulcus (fissure of Rolando), parieto-occipital fissure,* and *preoccipital notch.* The *calcarine fissure* divides the occipital lobe. Within the fissure of Sylvius is buried a portion of the cortex known as the *insula.* The central sulcus separates the *precentral gyrus* of the frontal lobe from the *postcentral gyrus* of the parietal lobe. A line drawn from the end of the fissure of Sylvius to the preoccipital notch serves to

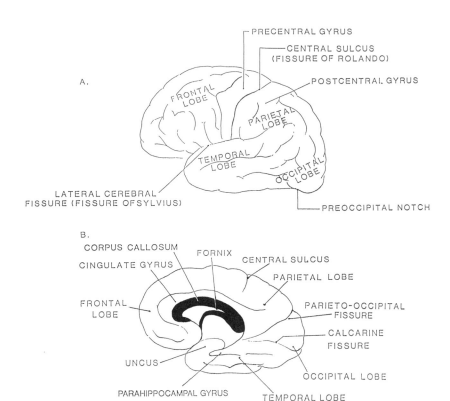

FIG. 13. Lateral **(A)** and medial **(B)** surfaces of the cerebral hemisphere illustrating the major gyri and sulci and division of the hemisphere into five major lobes: frontal, parietal, temporal, occipital, and limbic.

demarcate the limits of the temporal lobe, whereas a similar line from the preoccipital notch to the parieto-occipital fissure delineates the occipital lobe.

Certain structures, best seen on the medial surface of the hemispheres, are not included in the traditional division of the brain into four lobes. The *corpus callosum* represents a prominent fiber tract for transfer of information from one hemisphere to another. A number of the remaining prominent structures seen on the medial surface are related functionally and anatomically to the processing of memory and emotion. These structures have been grouped into a functional unit of the brain called the *limbic lobe* (Fig. 13). Some of the major structures visible on the medial surface of the brain are the *uncus* (located on the medial aspect of the temporal lobe), the *parahippocampal gyrus* (also on the medial temporal lobe), the *fornix* (a fiber bundle connecting the hypothalamus with the hippocampus), and the *cingulate gyrus* (located above the corpus callosum).

Coronal (Fig. 14), horizontal (Fig. 15), and sagittal (Fig. 16) sections through the cere-

FIG. 14. A: Coronal section through the cerebral hemispheres at the level of the anterior commissure. **Right,** diagram; **left,** magnetic resonance imaging (MRI) corresponding to the diagram. Note the relationships among the amygdala, basal forebrain, hypothalamus, and septal region. **B:** Coronal section through the brain at the level of the posterior commissure. Note the relationships between the caudate nucleus and anterior horn of the lateral ventricle, between the thalamus and third ventricle, the presence of the fornix limiting the connection between the lateral and third ventricles (that is, the foramen of Monro), the continuation of the internal capsule as the cerebral peduncles, and the relationships between the hippocampus and midbrain.

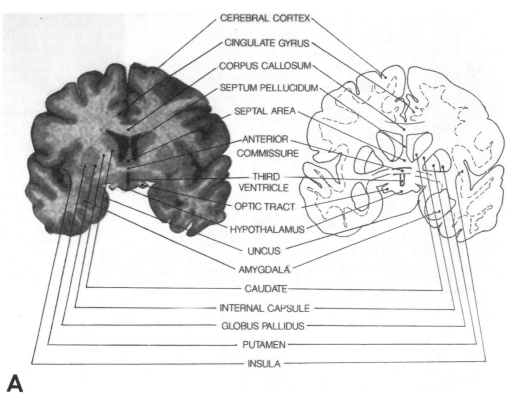

CEREBRAL CORTEX
CINGULATE GYRUS
CORPUS CALLOSUM
SEPTUM PELLUCIDUM
SEPTAL AREA
ANTERIOR COMMISSURE
THIRD VENTRICLE
OPTIC TRACT
HYPOTHALAMUS
UNCUS
AMYGDALA
CAUDATE
INTERNAL CAPSULE
GLOBUS PALLIDUS
PUTAMEN
INSULA

A

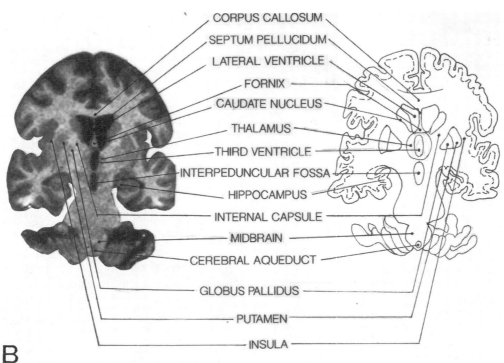

CORPUS CALLOSUM
SEPTUM PELLUCIDUM
LATERAL VENTRICLE
FORNIX
CAUDATE NUCLEUS
THALAMUS
THIRD VENTRICLE
INTERPEDUNCULAR FOSSA
HIPPOCAMPUS
INTERNAL CAPSULE
MIDBRAIN
CEREBRAL AQUEDUCT
GLOBUS PALLIDUS
PUTAMEN
INSULA

B

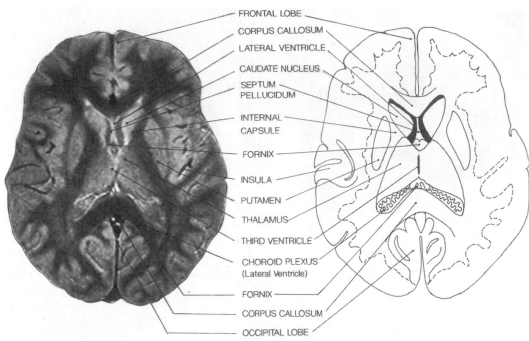

FRONTAL LOBE
CORPUS CALLOSUM
LATERAL VENTRICLE
CAUDATE NUCLEUS
SEPTUM PELLUCIDUM
INTERNAL CAPSULE
FORNIX
INSULA
PUTAMEN
THALAMUS
THIRD VENTRICLE
CHOROID PLEXUS (Lateral Ventricle)
FORNIX
CORPUS CALLOSUM
OCCIPITAL LOBE

FIG. 15. **Right:** Diagram of a horizontal section through the cerebral hemispheres at the level of the thalamus. **Left:** Magnetic resonance image obtained at the same level as the diagram. Magnetic resonance images reflect variations in composition of bound water in tissues. In this image sequence, the white matter is darker than the gray matter; this reflects the higher content of water in the gray matter (containing neuronal cell bodies) and of lipid in the white matter (containing myelinated axons). Note the relationship between the caudate nucleus and lateral ventricles and between the thalamus and the third ventricle. The internal capsule consists of an anterior limb (in relation with the caudate) and a posterior limb (in relation with the thalamus).

brum reveal several important structures within the substance of the brain. The anatomy of the brain can be visualized with neuroimaging techniques, particularly magnetic resonance imaging (MRI).

The two lateral ventricles and the third ventricle occupy a central position. The *gray matter* (mainly nuclear areas and cerebral cortex) and *white matter* (regions where fiber tracts are traveling) can be differentiated. Several distinct, large gray nuclear masses can be seen. The *thalamus* (an important relay area for the motor and sensory systems) is lateral to the third ventricle. The *basal ganglia,* composed of the *caudate nucleus, putamen,* and *globus pallidus,* are all part of the motor system. A

large and important area of white matter, the *internal capsule,* passes between these central nuclear masses and transfers information between the *cerebral cortex* and lower structures.

Diencephalon

The diencephalon represents a zone of transition between the cerebral hemisphere at the supratentorial level and the structures in the posterior fossa. The diencephalon consists of the *third ventricle* and those structures related to it, including the *thalamus, hypothalamus, optic pathways,* and *pineal body* (Fig. 16). At the base of the hypothalamus is an important neuroendocrine struc-

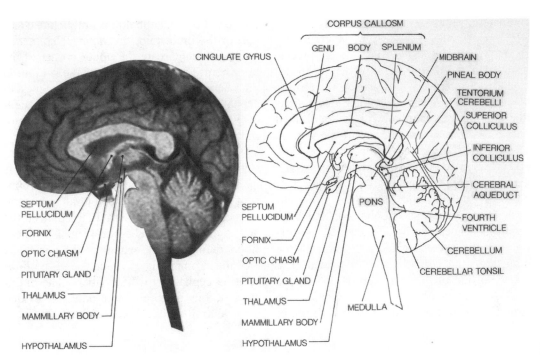

FIG. 16. A: Diagram of a median sagittal section through the cerebral hemispheres, diencephalon, brainstem, and cerebellum. B: The corresponding magnetic resonance image. The tentorium cerebelli and the upper border of the superior colliculus separate the supratentorial level from the posterior fossa level. The
genu, body, and splenium of the corpus callosum form the roof of the lateral ventricle. The diencephalic components include the thalamus, hypothalamus, and epithalamus (pineal body). The walls of the third ventricle are formed by the thalamus
rostrally and the hypothalamus caudally. The fornix courses over the thalamus and
terminates in the mamillary bodies of the posterior hypothalamus. The optic chiasm is located at the base of the brain, between the hypothalamus and pituitary
gland. The ventricular system consists of the lateral ventricles in the telencephalon, the third ventricle in the diencephalon, the cerebral aqueduct of Sylvius
in the midbrain, and the fourth ventricle in the pons and medulla. The superior and
inferior colliculi constitute the collicular plate, or tectum, of the midbrain. Note the
location of the cerebellar tonsil just above the level of the foramen magnum and
the close relationship of these structures with the medulla.

ture, the *hypophysis* or *pituitary gland.* It is
located in the middle of the skull in the bony
sella turcica. All these structures are at the
supratentorial level.

Cranial Nerves I and II

The *olfactory bulb* and *tract* (cranial nerve
I) are located at the base of each frontal lobe.
The olfactory nerves are axons passing from
the nasal cavity through the cribriform plate
to connect to the olfactory bulb. The *optic*

nerves (cranial nerve II) develop as an outgrowth from the primitive diencephalon. The
optic pathway from the orbit consists of the
optic nerve, optic chiasm, and *optic tract.* The
intracranial portions of these nerves are at the
supratentorial level.

The Posterior Fossa Level

The major structures contained in this level
are the *brainstem,* the cerebellum, and the origins of cranial nerves III through XII.

Brainstem

The term *brainstem* is not a precise anatomical term and therefore has been defined in different ways. However, the term is so commonly used in neurologic discussions that one must be familiar with it. As defined herein, the *brainstem* consists of the portion of the brain that remains after removal of the cerebral and cerebellar hemispheres (Fig. 1). Cephalad from the spinal cord, the brainstem includes the *medulla oblongata* (myelencephalon), *pons* (metencephalon), and *midbrain* (mesencephalon). Only the pontine portion of the metencephalon is part of the brainstem; the cerebellum is excluded. The upper portion of the brainstem is continuous with the diencephalon, where overlapping structures make precise definition difficult. In this text, the diencephalon is not included as a part of the brainstem; the *superior colliculus* is used to demarcate the upper border of the brainstem. The *red nucleus* and the *substantia nigra* are both present in the upper mesencephalon and extend into the posterior diencephalon, thereby overlapping the supratentorial and posterior fossa levels.

The longitudinal separation of the brainstem into midbrain, pons, and medulla is made primarily by a large bundle of prominent crossing fibers on the ventral and lateral surfaces of the brainstem that connect the brainstem to the cerebellum (Fig. 17). These fibers demarcate the extent of the pons. The medulla is immediately caudal and the midbrain is cephalad to these fibers. The brainstem at the midbrain and pons is divided dorsoventrally into three regions. The area

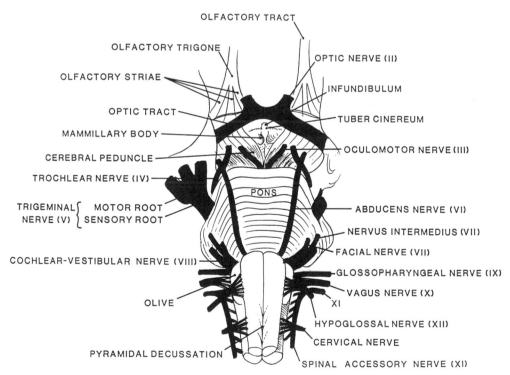

FIG. 17. Ventral aspect of the brainstem and cranial nerves. Cranial nerve I is not shown. It ends at the olfactory bulb, from which the olfactory tract arises. Cranial nerves I and II arise at the supratentorial level; cranial nerves III through XII arise in the posterior fossa.

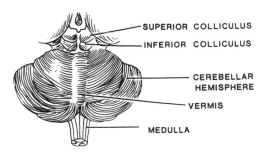

FIG. 18. Cerebellum as viewed from its dorsal surface.

dorsal to the aqueduct of Sylvius is the *tectum,* whose major structures are the superior and inferior colliculi (corpora quadrigemina). The area of numerous nuclei and intermingled pathways ventral to the aqueduct and fourth ventricle is the *tegmentum.* The large distinct cerebral and cerebellar white matter pathways in the most ventral regions below the tegmentum make up the *base,* or *basal region,* of the midbrain and pons.

Cerebellum

The cerebellum consists of two *hemispheres* and a midline *vermis* (Fig. 18). The cerebellar surface is more highly convoluted than the surface of the cerebral hemisphere, with folds known as *folia.* The cerebellum is metencephalic in derivation and therefore is associated structurally with the pons. The

cerebellum lies dorsal to the fourth ventricle, the pons, and the medulla.

Cranial Nerves III Through XII

Emerging from the brainstem are ten pairs of nerves, which can be identified in Fig. 17. (Cranial nerves I and II are *not* contained in the posterior fossa.) The names, location, and general function of all the cranial nerves are summarized in Table 2.

The Spinal Level

The major structures contained in this level are the spinal cord, the origins of the spinal nerves within the vertebral column, and the vertebral column itself.

The *spinal cord* is surrounded by meninges similar to those that surround the brain (Fig. 19). Outside the dura mater is the *epidural space,* an actual space that contains fat and venous plexuses. The *arachnoid* adjacent to the inner surface of the dura mater forms the subarachnoid space, which contains the cerebrospinal fluid. The spinal *pia mater* is closely applied to the surface of the spinal cord but is visible as the *dentate ligaments* extending on either side between the origins of the spinal nerve roots. These ligaments join the arachnoid at intervals and are inserted into the dura mater. The dural sac and *subarachnoid space* end at the level of the second sacral vertebra

TABLE 2. *Location and general function of the cranial nerves*

Nerve	Anatomical relationship	Function
I Olfactory	Cerebral hemispheres	Smell
II Optic	Diencephalon, cerebral hemispheres	Vision
III Oculomotor	Midbrain	Eye movement
IV Trochlear	Midbrain	Eye movement
V Trigeminal	Pons	Facial sensation, jaw movement
VI Abducens	Pons	Eye movement
VII Facial	Pons	Facial movement
VIII Cochlear-vestibular	Pons, medulla	Hearing and balance
IX Glossopharyngeal	Medulla	Throat movement
X Vagus	Medulla	Throat and larynx movement and control of visceral organs
XI Spinal accessory	Medulla, spinal cord	Shoulder and neck movement
XII Hypoglossal	Medulla	Tongue movement

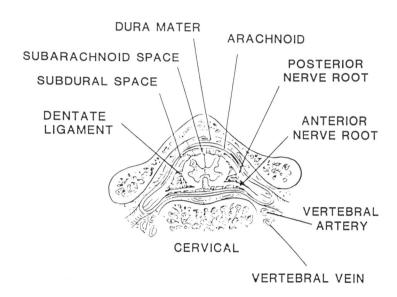

DURA MATER

ARACHNOID

SUBARACHNOID SPACE

POSTERIOR
NERVE ROOT

SUBDURAL SPACE

DENTATE
LIGAMENT

ANTERIOR
NERVE ROOT

VERTEBRAL
ARTERY

CERVICAL

VERTEBRAL VEIN

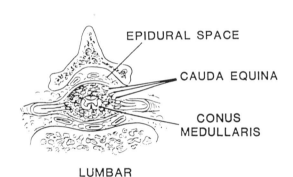

EPIDURAL SPACE

CAUDA EQUINA

CONUS
MEDULLARIS

LUMBAR

FIG. 19. Cross sections of the vertebral column at cervical and lumbar vertebral levels.

(Fig. 20). The pia mater continues caudally as a filamentous membrane (the *filum terminale*) from the end of the spinal cord (the *conus medullaris*). It fuses with the dural sac at the second sacral vertebral level and is attached to the dorsal surface of the coccyx as the *sacro-coccygeal ligament.*

The adult spinal cord begins rostrally from the caudal margin of the medulla at the level of the foramen magnum and terminates opposite the caudal margin of the first lumbar vertebra. The spinal cord, therefore, does *not* extend the entire length of the spinal canal. Throughout much of the length of the cord a spinal segment is *not* adjacent to its corresponding vertebral segment.

The spinal cord exhibits *cervical* and *lumbosacral enlargements.* Cross sections show a relative increase in gray matter in these two regions, to account for the relative enlargement in these areas. Thirty-one pairs of *spinal nerves* are attached to the spinal cord via *dorsal* (posterior) and *ventral* (anterior) *nerve roots.* Segmentally there are 8 cervical, 12 thoracic, 5 lumbar, 5 sacral, and 1 coccygeal spinal nerve on each side. At their origins, the nerve roots consist of multiple filaments, which, on the posterior (dorsal) surface of the

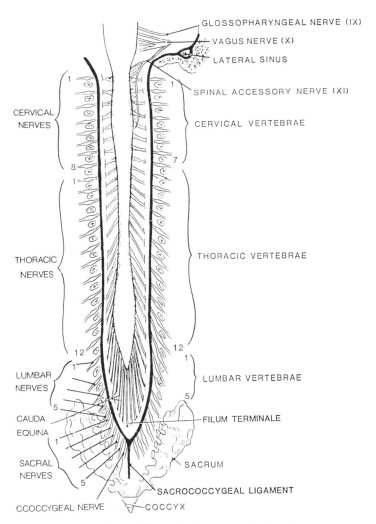

GLOSSOPHARYNGEAL NERVE (IX)

VAGUS NERVE (X)

LATERAL SINUS

SPINAL ACCESSORY NERVE (XI)

CERVICAL VERTEBRAE

CERVICAL NERVES

THORACIC VERTEBRAE

THORACIC NERVES

LUMBAR NERVES

LUMBAR VERTEBRAE

CAUDA EQUINA

FILUM TERMINALE

SACRAL NERVES

SACRUM

SACROCOCCYGEAL LIGAMENT

CCOCCYGEAL NERVE   COCCYX

FIG. 20. Dorsal view of the spinal level. The spinal cord terminates between vertebrae L-1 and L-2 and is enlarged at the cervical and lumbosacral levels. These enlargements correspond to the segments that innervate the upper (cervical enlargement) and lower (lumbosacral enlargement) limbs. The roots form the spinal nerves that exit through the intervertebral foramina. The cervical roots exit above the corresponding vertebra, and the eighth cervical root exits between vertebrae C-7 and T-1. The rest of the roots exit below the corresponding vertebra. Because of the difference in length between the spinal cord and the spinal canal, the lumbar and sacral roots of the conus medullaris travel a relatively long distance in the subarachnoid space before exiting through their corresponding foramen. These roots form the cauda equina.

cord, exit from a relatively constant groove, the *posterior lateral sulcus*. The dorsal and ventral roots of each spinal nerve join as they enter the intervertebral foramen of the spine. After leaving the spinal cord, the roots of the lumbar and sacral spinal nerves run caudally a number of segments toward their exit. The collection of spinal nerve roots contained in the lumbosacral spinal canal is known as the *cauda equina* (Fig. 19). Although most of the spinal nerves have both a ventral (motor) and a dorsal (sensory) root, often the first cervical nerve has only a motor root, and the first coccygeal nerve and the fifth sacral nerve have only a sensory root. Surrounding the spinal cord is the *vertebral column,* consisting of 7 cervical, 12 thoracic, and 5 lumbar vertebrae, the fused sacrum, and the coccyx (Fig. 20).

The Peripheral Level

The major structures of the peripheral level are the somatic nerves, the autonomic nerves and ganglia, the neuromuscular junction, the muscles of the skeleton, and the peripheral sensory receptors. The spinal nerves, as they emerge from the vertebral column, enter the peripheral level. Spinal nerves are formed by the joining of dorsal and ventral roots and thus contain somatic and autonomic motor and sensory nerve fibers. Spinal nerves branch into posterior and anterior divisions as they enter the peripheral level. Fibers of the anterior divisions en route to the limbs come together and are rearranged in plexuses. The *brachial plexus,* located in the axillary region, redistributes the fibers to the major nerves of the upper extremities: median, ulnar, radial, axillary, and musculocutaneous The *lumbosacral plexus,* located in the lower abdominal cavity and pelvis, redistributes the fibers to the major nerves in the lower extremities—femoral, obturator, and sciatic, which divides into the tibial and peroneal nerves.

Gross Neuroanatomy—Introduction to the Longitudinal Systems   ■

The gross anatomical features of each of the major levels have been reviewed. At this point, some of these same structures should be related to the major longitudinal systems, which will be studied in further detail in subsequent chapters.

The Cerebrospinal Fluid System

Structures included in the cerebrospinal fluid system are the meninges (the dura mater, arachnoid, and pia mater), the meningeal spaces (epidural, subdural, and subarachnoid), the ventricular system, and the cerebrospinal fluid. This system, present at the supratentorial, posterior fossa, and spinal levels, provides both cushioning and buffering for the central nervous system and helps maintain a stable environment for neural function.

The Sensory System

This system receives somatosensory information from the external environment and transmits it to the central nervous system (afferent), where it can be processed and used for adaptive behavior. Elements of the somatosensory system are found at all major levels and include the peripheral receptor organs; afferent fibers traveling in cranial, peripheral, and spinal nerves; dorsal root ganglia; ascending pathways in the spinal cord and brainstem; portions of the thalamus; and the thalamocortical radiations that terminate primarily in the sensory cortex of the parietal lobe. In addition, structures related to the special sensory systems (vision, taste, smell, hearing, and balance) are located at the supratentorial, posterior fossa, and peripheral levels.

The Motor System

The motor system initiates and controls activity in the somatic muscles. Components of this system include motor cortex and other areas of the frontal lobes; descending pathways that traverse the internal capsule, cerebral peduncles, medullary pyramids, and other areas of the brainstem; portions of the spinal cord, including the ventral horns; ventral roots; efferent fibers traveling in both peripheral and cranial nerves; and muscle, the major effector organ of the motor system. Also included in this system are the cerebellum and basal ganglia and related pathways. Thus, the motor system is present at all major levels and is directly involved in the performance of all motor activity mediated by striated musculature.

The Internal Regulation System

The internal regulation system is composed of the structures in the nervous system that monitor and control the function of visceral glands and organs. It contains both afferent and efferent components, which interact to maintain the internal environment (homeostasis). The system has major representation at all levels of the nervous system. Important structures include areas of the limbic lobe and hypothalamus (supratentorial); the reticular formation and fibers traveling in cranial nerves (posterior fossa); longitudinal pathways in the spinal cord and brainstem; and numerous ganglia, receptors, and effectors found at the peripheral level.

The Consciousness System

Functioning as an additional afferent system, the consciousness system allows a person to attend selectively to and perceive isolated stimuli. This system maintains various levels of wakefulness, awareness, and consciousness. Structures contained within this system are found only at the posterior fossa and supratentorial levels and include portions of the central core of the brainstem and diencephalon (reticular formation and ascending projectional pathways), portions of the thalamus, basal forebrain, and pathways that project diffusely to the cerebral cortex. All lobes of the brain are part of this system.

The Vascular System

Each organ in the body must have blood vessels to provide a relatively constant supply of oxygen and other nutrients and to remove metabolic waste. The vascular system is found at all major levels of the nervous system and includes the arteries, arterioles, capillaries, veins, and dural sinuses. These supply supratentorial, posterior fossa, spinal, and peripheral nervous system structures.

As noted in Chapter 2, a transverse organization is imposed on the neural tube. Structures located near the core, or inner tube, represent phylogenetically older pathways with indirect, diffuse, and nonspecific relay functions related largely to the consciousness and internal regulation systems. Structures located near the outer surface represent newer pathways that have more direct, relatively specific relay functions related to the sensory and motor systems.

At this point in the study of gross neuroanatomy, a precise distinction is not made between the structures of the inner and outer core. However, as the student progresses through the study of the longitudinal systems, further reference will be made to these areas. Further details about the anatomical structures associated with these areas are given in Chapter 12.

Clinical Correlations

Neurologic diagnosis includes identification of the anatomical location and pathology of the disorder. Through the use of problem-solving skills that are already familiar and the assignment of some functional significance to the anatomical structures discussed in this chapter, the reader can begin to solve clinical neurologic problems by identifying the anatomical location.

In certain respects, an analogy may be drawn between the nervous system and an electrical circuit. The nervous system can be considered as a series of electrical cables laid out in a specific plan (Fig. 21). Leading to and from the cerebral hemispheres are two parallel cables (representing a longitudinal system) that conduct impulses from one segment to another. Scattered along these *intersegmental* cables are several smaller branching *segmental* wires. As in basic electricity, damage (a lesion) anywhere along the course of the main intersegmental cables causes malfunction in all areas beyond that point, whereas damage to the segmental wires causes malfunction only within that specific segment. In applying this analogy to humans, we note that the higher centers exert control or receive information from the body segments through long *intersegmental pathways* and that one side of

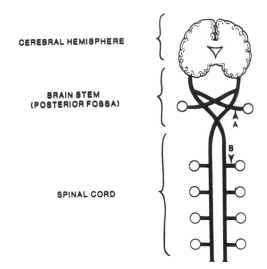

CEREBRAL HEMISPHERE

BRAIN STEM
(POSTERIOR FOSSA)

SPINAL CORD

FIG. 21. Major nervous system connections. *A,* cranial nerves; *B,* peripheral nerves. Note long intersegmental pathways leading to and from higher centers and multiple, short segmental pathways (cranial and peripheral nerves) to the peripheral level.

the brain is associated with function on the *opposite* side of the body.

Anatomical diagnosis first requires the ability to relate the patient's signs and symptoms to specific longitudinal systems within the nervous system. Neurologic diagnosis relies mainly on the symptoms of dysfunction in the sensory, motor, and consciousness systems, whose organization is similar to the schematic pathways seen in Fig. 21. Symptoms of dysfunction in the sensory system consist of altered sensation, described by the patient as pain, numbness, tingling, or loss of sensation. Symptoms of dysfunction in the motor system consist primarily of weakness, paralysis, incoordination, shaking, or jerking. Lesions of the consciousness system, which is located only at the supratentorial and posterior fossa levels, are expressed as altered states of consciousness and coma. The presence of any of these or related symptoms identifies the longitudinal system involved in a disease.

Localization is determined by the level of the nervous system in which the pathway function is interrupted. To aid in localization, the functions of each of the major anatomical

levels are described in the following sections and are schematically represented in Fig. 22 and summarized in Table 3.

Peripheral Level

The spinal and cranial nerves, after they emerge from the vertebral column and skull, and the structures they innervate, constitute the major components of the peripheral level. Each emerging nerve defines a specific *segment.* A lesion in one of these pathways alters all function within that segment but has no effect on functions carried to and from other segments. Thus, in the presence of a peripheral lesion, *loss of sensation and muscle weakness* in a focal area are common. Often, peripheral nerve damage is not complete and the sensation of *pain* is produced. Therefore, in addition to sensory loss and weakness, pain in a segmental distribution is an important clue to a lesion at the peripheral level.

Spinal Level

The spinal cord has two functions. It is the structure from which individual segments of the limbs and trunk originate, and it transmits information to and from higher centers. Therefore, lesions at the spinal level may alter *segmental* functions in the region of the abnormality and alter *intersegmental* function below the lesion. Except in complete transections of the spinal cord, all functions are not altered equally; however, even under those circumstances, the characteristic combination of segmental loss of function at the site of the lesion and intersegmental loss below it usually can be identified.

The spinal cord is a narrow structure that contains the major intersegmental pathways for both sides of the neuraxis (nervous system). Therefore, in spinal lesions, bilateral involvement from a single focal lesion is not uncommon. Furthermore, because of the length of the spinal column, specific segmental functions can be assigned to certain areas of it. The upper portion (cervical) is related primarily to arm function, the midportion

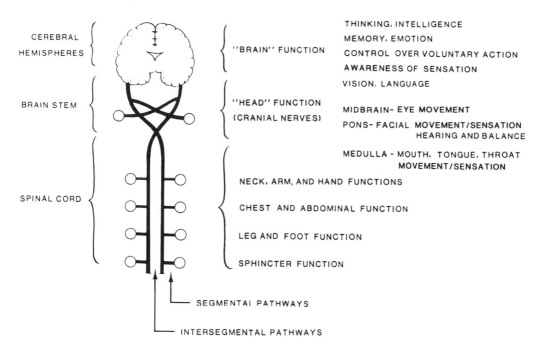

FIG. 22. Summary of the functions associated with the major anatomical levels.

TABLE 3. *Summary of clinical findings by level*

Level	Clinical finding	Side of lesion	Segmental signs of the level
Supratentorial	Loss of sensation and/or weakness on the *same* side of the body and face	Contralateral to deficit	Vision Olfaction Cognition Memory Intelligence Behavior Seizures
Posterior fossa	Loss of sensation and/or weakness on *one* side of the face and *opposite* side of body	Ipsilateral to side of the face	Hearing Tinnitus Vertigo Diplopia Dysarthria Dysphagia
	Cranial nerve deficit	Ipsilateral to cranial nerve	
	Cerebellar deficit	Ipsilateral to cerebellar deficit, cerebellar signs (incoordination)	
Spinal	Sensory level		Neck/back pain
	Loss of pain and temperature on *one* side and weakness and loss of position sense on *opposite* side of the body	Ipsilateral to loss of position sense and weakness	Findings related to specific level—cervical, lumbar, etc. Meningeal signs (stiff neck)
Peripheral	Loss of sensations to all modalities in distribution of nerve or sensory loss in glove-and-stocking distribution	Ipsilateral to sensory loss	Limb pain without back pain Loss of sensation and muscle weakness in distribution of a nerve
	Muscle weakness in distribution of nerve		

(thoracic) to the trunk, the lower portion (lumbar) to the legs, and the lowermost area (sacral) to anal-genital-urinary functions.

Posterior Fossa Level

The cranial nerves mediate segmental function for the head and arise in the posterior fossa. Lesions at the posterior fossa level therefore produce segmental and intersegmental disturbances, just as occur at the spinal level. The *segmental* nerves of the brainstem are the cranial nerves, which control movement and sensation in the head (Table 2). Brainstem lesions often alter these segmental functions. In addition, because the brainstem is also an area where intersegmental pathways cross, or have crossed, to the opposite side of the brain, a characteristic pattern is often seen with focal lesions. Lesions of the posterior fossa cause loss of segmental head function *ipsilateral* (same side) to the lesion; if the lesion also involves intersegmental pathways, it causes loss of intersegmental function on the side of the body *contralateral* (opposite) to the lesion (Fig. 22). Extensive lesions in the brainstem may affect the consciousness system and produce coma.

Supratentorial Level

Each cerebral hemisphere exerts its control over the opposite side of the body. Therefore, supratentorial lesions are associated with loss of intersegmental sensory or motor function on the opposite side of the body. In addition, some functions are associated almost exclusively with the supratentorial level and may be considered segmental functions of this level. These functions are language (almost always localized to the left side of the brain), memory, intelligence, cognition, olfaction, and vision. When abnormal, they serve to further localize the disorder to the supratentorial level (Fig. 22). Extensive lesions involving the structures of the supratentorial level may alter consciousness and produce coma.

Precise localization is possible when an area can be identified where both segmental and intersegmental functions are altered in one or more systems.

The major features to be determined in the anatomical diagnosis of neurologic disorders are the following:

1. Is the responsible lesion *focal,* strictly confined to a single well-circumscribed area? If the lesion is focal, the *anatomical level* and whether the abnormality is located on the right or left or in the midline of the nervous system must be defined.
2. Is the responsible lesion *diffuse* and nonfocal? A diffuse lesion may involve only a single level or may involve multiple levels. In general, a lesion is considered to be diffuse it if involves bilateral regions in the nervous system without extending across the midline as a single, circumscribed lesion.

Clinical Problems   ■

The following is a series of case histories of neurologic disorders. The problems were selected to illustrate examples of involvement in different regions of the nervous system. Read each history carefully. On the basis of the information presented, try to localize the lesion in accordance with the objectives above. When you have arrived at a conclusion for each case, review the pertinent anatomical structures in that area.

1. A 19-year-old man was involved in an automobile accident 4 months earlier. He sustained only minor bruises about the head and face. When he returned to school in the fall, he seemed to be uninterested in his schoolwork and began to complain of headaches. He dragged his right foot when he walked and used his right hand clumsily. He had a slight droop to the right side of his face. (Answers refer to items *a* and *b* of objective 3.)
2. A 68-year-old man awakened one morning and noted that he was unable to speak clearly. He wanted to ask for help but

could utter only the words go now. His wife noted some weakness of the right side of his face and right arm and leg. He seemed unable to answer the questions that his wife posed to him.

3. A 26-year-old man awoke and noted that all the muscle on the left side of his face seemed to be paralyzed. Sensation was normal, although he was aware of an inability to taste on the left side of his tongue. He had no other difficulties. Six weeks later, he noted gradual and continued improvement.

4. A 42-year-old man noted, over a period of several years, the onset of ringing in his right ear and loss of hearing in that ear. In addition, he experienced right facial weakness and decreased sensation. In the weeks before his examination, he noted stiffness and weakness of his left arm and leg.

5. A 24-year-old woman was involved in an automobile accident. When examined, she had complete loss of sensation from the arms downward. She could not move her hands or legs and had no sensation below the armpits. She was incontinent.

6. For no apparent reason, a 64-year-old woman began to experience pain beginning in her back and encircling the right side of her chest about the level of her breast. A rash later appeared in the same distribution. She continued to have pain in that region, and sensation in that region was greatly diminished.

7. The patient, a 46-year-old woman, described a pain that was similar to the one noted in problem 6. The pain involved the left side of her chest. (No rash was present.) Her symptoms increased over several months but remained localized in a rather circumscribed region of her chest. She was concerned about heart trouble. In addition, she complained of difficulty in walking. Her left leg seemed to be weak and stiff, and at times the left leg felt numb.

Additional Reading

Brodal, P. *The Central Nervous System: Structure and Function.* New York: Oxford University Press, 1992.

Carpenter, M. B. *Core Text of Neuroanatomy* (4th ed.). Baltimore: Williams & Wilkins, 1991.

Gilman, S., and Winans Newman, S. (eds.). *Manter and Gatz's Essentials of Clinical Neuroanatomy and Neurophysiology* (8th ed.). Philadelphia: F. A. Davis, 1992.

Haines, D. E. *Neuroanatomy: An Atlas of Structures, Sections, and Systems* (3rd ed.). Baltimore: Urban & Schwarzenberg, 1991.

Netter, F. H. *The Ciba Collection of Medical Illustrations. Vol. 1: Nervous System.* Part I: Anatomy and Physiology. West Caldwell, N. J.: CIBA Pharmaceutical, 1983.

Watson, C. *Basic Human Neuroanatomy: An Introductory Atlas* (4th ed.). Boston: Little, Brown, 1991.

Diagnosis of Neurologic Disorders: Neurocytology and the Pathologic Reactions of the Nervous System

Objectives

1. Define the general functional role and embryonic origin of neuron, astrocyte, oligodendroglia, microglial cell, ependymal cell, and Schwann cell.
2. Describe ischemic cell change, neurofibrillary degeneration, inclusion body formation, central chromatolysis, wallerian degeneration, astrocytosis, demyelination, and cerebral edema.
3. Describe the clinical and pathologic features of degenerative disease, neoplastic disease, vascular disease, inflammatory disease, toxic-metabolic disease, and traumatic disease.
4. On a photograph, be able to recognize neuron, astrocyte, oligodendroglia, microglial cell, ependymal cell, ischemia and infarction, neoplasia, diffuse inflammation, abscess formation, and degenerative disease.
5. In a clinical situation, be able to answer the following four questions:
   a. The signs and symptoms contained in the protocol are most likely the manifestation of disease at which of the following *levels* of the nervous system?
      i. Supratentorial level
      ii. Posterior fossa level
      iii. Spinal level
      iv. Peripheral level
      v. More than one level
   b. Within the level you have selected, the responsible lesion is most likely
      i. focal, on the *right* side of the nervous system.
      ii. focal, on the *left* side of the nervous system.
      iii. focal, but involving *midline* and *contiguous structures* on both sides of the nervous system.
      iv. nonfocal and diffusely located.
   c. The principal pathologic lesion responsible for the symptoms is most likely
      i. some form of *mass* lesion.
      ii. some form of *nonmass* lesion.
   d. The cause of the responsible lesion is most likely
      i. vascular.
      ii. degenerative.
      iii. inflammatory.
      iv. immunologic.
      v. neoplastic.
      vi. toxic-metabolic.
      vii. traumatic.

Introduction

The principles of anatomical localization are introduced in Chapter 3. Anatomical localization, however, is but one part of the diagnosis of neurologic disorders; it is also necessary to determine the pathologic features of the lesion involved. Identification of the pathologic condition requires knowledge of the cellular elements of the nervous system (neurocytology) and the ways in which these cells react to noxious stimuli (pathologic reactions).

Two major factors must be considered in describing lesions of the nervous system:

1. The topography of the lesion—the anatomical location of the pathologic process and a judgment as to whether the abnormality is
   a. *focal:* strictly confined to a single circumscribed anatomical area.
   b. *diffuse:* distributed over wide areas of the nervous system. A diffuse lesion may involve only a single level (for example, supratentorial or spinal level), or it may be distributed over multiple levels. A diffuse lesion involves bilaterally symmetrical areas in the nervous system, without extending across the midline as a single, circumscribed lesion.
2. The morphology of the lesion—the gross and histologic appearance of the abnormal area and a judgment as to whether the pathologic process is a
   a. *nonmass:* one that is altering cellular function in the area of the lesion but is not significantly interfering with neighboring cell performance. In this type of lesion, the pathologic process is not, by virtue of its size or volume, compressing, destroying, or damaging nearby structures.
   b. *mass:* one that not only alters cellular function in the area of the lesion but also is of sufficient size and volume to interfere with neighboring cell functions by compressing, destroying, or altering nearby cells.

Integration of the *topographic* and *morphologic* descriptions provides a precise pathologic diagnosis. When patients are examined clinically, tissue is not available for study, yet on the basis of the signs and symptoms and their evolution, the nature of the responsible pathologic lesion can be deduced. This chapter provides the information necessary to accomplish that task.

Overview

The nervous system is composed of neurons, supporting cells of neuroectodermal origin, and supporting cells of mesodermal origin. *Neurons* are derived solely from ectoderm and are the functional units of the nervous system, capable of generating and conducting the electrical activity that underlies nervous system performance. Mature neurons do not undergo proliferation; therefore, most disease processes that affect neurons produce only neuronal degeneration and loss.

The *supporting cells of neuroectodermal origin* are the oligodendroglia, Schwann cells, astrocytes, and ependymal cells. *Oligodendroglial cells* are responsible for the formation of the myelin sheaths that invest and surround axons in the central nervous system, and *Schwann cells* serve a similar function in the peripheral nervous system. Disease processes affecting these cells are associated with myelin breakdown and loss (demyelination). *Astrocytes* are widely distributed throughout the central nervous system, lie near both the neurons and the blood vessels, and thus help to provide much of the metabolic support of neural elements. Disease processes are often associated with astrocytic proliferation, which results in gliosis, the scar tissue of the central nervous system. Astrocytes also may react to metabolic disturbances in more specific ways. *Ependymal cells* line the entire ventricular system and provide a selective barrier between the ventricular fluid and the brain substance. Noxious stimuli may produce a loss of ependymal cells. Epithelium of the choroid plexus is a derivative of ependyma and has an important role in the formation of cerebrospinal fluid.

The *supporting cells of mesodermal origin* are microglia and connective tissue cells. *Microglia* migrate into the central nervous system, and although normally present in small numbers, they can proliferate rapidly to become scavenger cells, or *macrophages,* which remove damaged tissue. With the exception of vascular structures, the parenchyma of the brain is almost devoid of elements of *connective tissue;* however, the nervous system is surrounded by the meninges, which are of mesodermal, connective tissue origin.

Disease processes may affect one or more of these cytologic elements, and differences in their histologic features form the morphologic basis for the various clinical features of neurologic diseases. The signs and symptoms produced by these disorders reflect the anatomical location and histologic evolution (temporal profile) of the underlying pathologic lesion.

Degenerative disorders are characterized by gradual neuronal damage in widespread areas of the nervous system and therefore are seen clinically as chronic, progressive, and diffuse diseases. *Neoplastic disorders* present clinically as chronic, focal, progressive disorders. Any cell type in the nervous system can undergo neoplastic change to form a gradually enlarging, localized mass of proliferating cells (a neoplasm).

Vascular diseases may be of several pathologic types, but they are all associated with sudden alteration in structure and function. Therefore, disorders of this etiologic category are always acute in onset, but they may be either focal (infarct, intracerebral hemorrhage) or diffuse (subarachnoid hemorrhage, anoxic encephalopathy) in distribution. Because foreign pathogens invading the nervous system generally produce a rapid but not immediate cellular response, *inflammatory disease,* which may be either focal (abscess) or diffuse (meningitis, encephalitis), commonly presents as a progressive, subacute disorder. The temporal profile of *immunologic diseases* is variable, but it generally takes the form of a multifocal or diffuse disorder, with subacute or chronic progression.

Toxic or metabolic diseases alter neural function over widespread areas and therefore present with diffuse signs and symptoms. However, depending on the responsible agent, the resultant symptoms may make their appearance as acute, subacute, or chronic disorders. *Traumatic lesions* of the nervous system usually are focal and of acute onset, reflecting the effects of the immediate damage of tissue produced by the offending agent. At times, however, delayed effects of a traumatic lesion may produce clinical symptoms and present a pattern of a chronic, progressive lesion.

Structural Elements of the Nervous System

The nervous system is composed of three basic categories of cells: (1) nerve cells, called *neurons,* which are the major functional units of the nervous system; (2) supporting cells of neuroectodermal origin (oligodendroglia, Schwann cells, astrocytes, and ependymal cells); and (3) supporting cells of mesodermal origin (microglia and connective tissue elements).

The first two categories of cells, the neurons and the supporting cells of neuroectodermal origin, are derived from the primitive neuroepithelium that lines the neural tube and from the cells of the neural crest. The processes of differentiation and migration followed by these cells are outlined in Chapter 2. The third category, mesodermal supporting tissue, is derived from the mesoderm that surrounds the neural tube during development.

The structure of all these cell types and their interrelationships have been studied extensively at the light microscopic and electron microscopic levels. Any description of their microscopic appearance, therefore, must include a statement of the method on which the description is based. Nerve tissue is routinely studied at the light microscopic level by using thin sections of tissue to which stains are applied. Stains have been developed that emphasize certain features of cells while obscuring others. Some of these stains are dyes that react with and bind to certain chemical groups in the tissue, coloring them. Other stains are salts of heavy metals, especially silver salts, which undergo a physiochemical reaction with and "impregnate" certain structural elements in the tissue.

Neurons

The neuron is the most important structural element of the nervous system because it generates and conducts the electrical activity that is associated with the function of the nervous system.

Unlike most other cells of the body, normal nerve cells in a fully developed human do not undergo division and replication. Neurons vary greatly in size and shape from one region of the nervous system to another (Fig. 1). However, they possess certain common features that are most readily demonstrated in the largest neurons, for example, the large motor neurons of the ventral horn of the spinal cord (Fig. 2 and 3). In routine preparations, the cell bodies of these neurons, which may be 100 μm in diameter, are irregular in outline because of the numerous processes that extend outward from the cell body at irregular intervals. Neurons possess a large nucleus within which is a conspicuous nucleolus. Otherwise, the nucleus appears to be relatively clear, or vesicular, because of the dispersion of the nuclear chromatin. The cytoplasm surrounding the nucleus constitutes the main cell body, or *perikaryon,* and contains the same types of organelles for metabolism as do other cells in the body, for example, mitochondria, Golgi apparatus, lysosomes, and endoplasmic reticulum. However, two types of organelles are unusually conspicuous in neurons and distinguish them from other cells in the body.

The endoplasmic reticulum is heavily laden with ribonucleoprotein granules (rough endoplasmic reticulum). Concentrations of these rough endoplasmic reticulum membranes

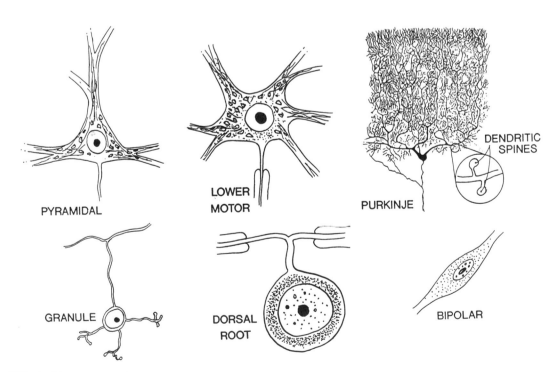

FIG. 1. Neurons of different sizes and configurations from various areas of the nervous system.

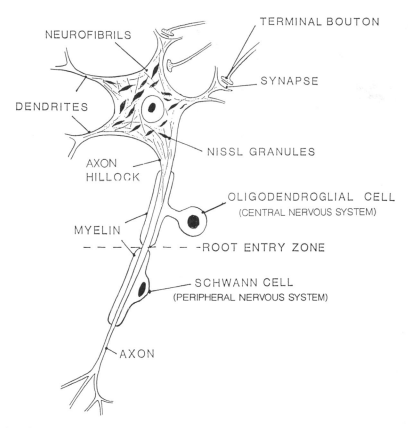

FIG. 2. Spinal motor neuron.

produce the appearance, at the light microscopic level, of dense basophilic bodies (Fig. 3). These structures are called *Nissl granules* (named after the German pathologist, Franz Nissl, who first described them). Various basic blue dyes, which stain Nissl granules as the most conspicuous element in brain tissue, are called Nissl stains; the Nissl granules also are well seen in routine preparations stained with hematoxylin and eosin.

The second type of organelle that is conspicuous in neurons is the fibrillar component of the cytoplasm. With the light microscope, neurofibrils can be demonstrated with silver impregnation stains (Fig. 4). The fibrils demonstrated in this way correspond to three ultrastructural components of the cell:

1. Neurofilaments, which are 10-nm-diameter intermediate cytoskeletal filaments and immunologically unique to nerve cells. They are distributed throughout the cell body and all the processes of the neuron.

2. Neurotubules, which are 20 to 30 nm in diameter and indistinguishable from the microtubules of other cells. They are

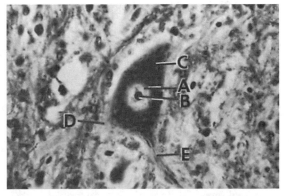

FIG. 3. Spinal motor neuron: nucleus (A), nucleolus (B), cytoplasm filled with Nissl granules (C), axon hillock (D), and dendrite (E). (Nissl stain; ×400.)

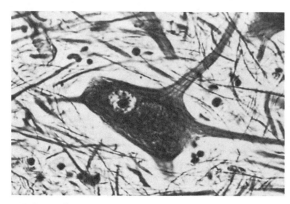

FIG. 4. Spinal motor neuron showing numerous fibrils streaming through the cytoplasm of the cell body and processes. The background contains processes of other neurons. (Bodian stain; ×400.)

more numerous in dendrites than axons and function in cytoplasmic transport mechanisms.

3. Microfilaments, which are 5 nm in diameter and identical to those found in all animal cells.

Processes of nerve cells extend outward from the cell body into the surrounding tissue. These processes are called either *dendrites* or *axons,* and the number, length, and branching of these processes vary markedly from one type of neuron to another. Neurons possess only one axon; the remaining processes are dendrites. The region of the cell body that forms the root of the axon, the *axon hillock,* does not have Nissl granules and appears to be relatively pale on Nissl and hematoxylin and eosin staining (Fig. 3). From this region, the axon extends outward for distances that vary from a few millimeters to several feet. In general, the diameter of an axon varies with its length. Functionally, the axon is the portion of the neuron that conducts electrical activity away from the cell body, toward an effector organ (muscle, glands) or toward the next neuron in a chain or circuit.

Axons are unable to synthesize proteins. Axonal survival depends on transport of substances from the cell bodies. This is called *axonal transport.* There are three types of ax-onal transport: (1) fast anterograde transport, which transports proteins for synaptic function; (2) slow anterograde transport, which transports proteins of the cytoskeleton; and (3) retrograde transport, which transports growth factors and other substances from the periphery to the cell body. Axonal transport requires adenosine triphosphate (ATP) and is impaired during energy failure.

Neurons of the central nervous system have one or, usually, many dendrites. Nissl granules in at least the proximal portions of the dendrites make them visible in routine preparations. The dendrites extend a relatively short distance from the cell body and usually branch repeatedly. Dendrites are, in a sense, the antennae of the nerve cell, and they transmit incoming signals toward the cell body.

Communication between neurons is accomplished at specialized regions of these cells called *synapses* (Fig. 2). Synapses are the anatomical basis for the transfer of a signal from one neuron to another. The axon of a nerve cell usually terminates on and forms a synapse with the dendrites or cell body of another. At the region of the synapse, the axon terminal may be enlarged *(terminal bouton).* At some synapses, the dendrite presents a small projection, the dendritic spine, on which the axon terminates. Synapses do not always occur at the terminal end of an axon but may form in places where an axon passes by a dendrite or cell body. These are called *en passant synapses.* Electron micrographs show that the axonal (presynaptic) and dendritic (postsynaptic) membranes are thickened. They do not actually touch but are separated by a space, the *synaptic cleft,* which is 200 to 300 Å wide. Rare synapses in the human brain have bridges across the synaptic cleft, providing the opportunity for direct electrical contact. In the axon terminal are tiny vesicles (synaptic vesicles) that contain the chemical neurotransmitters responsible for the transfer of the signal from the presynaptic to the postsynaptic cell. The dendritic tree and cell body of the neuron may be covered by hundreds of synapses from numerous sources. Its axon may branch repeatedly and form synapses on many other neurons. This is partly the basis for the complexity and the flexibility of the function of the nervous system. In the periphery, axons may terminate not only on other nerve cells but also on gland or muscle cells where synapse-like structures are also found.

Certain neurons have characteristic appearances that bear the names of the neuroanatomists who originally described them. Examples include the Betz cells of the inner pyramidal layer of the cerebral cortex and the Purkinje cells in the middle layer of the cerebellar cortex. In addition, Golgi recognized two distinct types of neurons. Axons of type I neurons project well outside the dendritic field of the cells and travel some distance away from the cell body of origin. These cells can conduct information for long distances within the central nervous system. Type II neurons have very short axons that terminate on cells near (and often within) the dendritic field of the cell body of origin. These cells are probably more involved in data processing than in data conduction.

Supporting Cells of Neuroectodermal Origin

Oligodendroglia and Schwann Cells

These two cell types are discussed together because they share a very important function: they form the insulating sheaths (called myelin) that surround the axons in the central and peripheral nervous systems (Fig. 2). The myelin sheath around peripheral axons is formed by Schwann cells. In routine histologic sections of the axons in peripheral nerves, nuclei of Schwann cells are recognized as elongated structures oriented in the direction of the axis cylinders (Fig. 5). In transverse sections of peripheral nerves, most of the axons are surrounded by a myelin sheath (Fig. 6), but the relationship among the myelin sheath, Schwann cell, and axon is not obvious with the light microscope. In transverse sections of a peripheral myelinated axon viewed in the electron microscope, the relationship becomes more apparent (Fig. 7). The plasma membrane of the Schwann cell invests

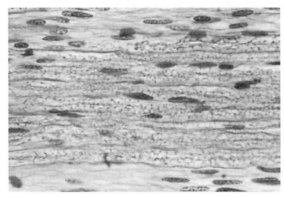

FIG. 5. Longitudinal section of a peripheral nerve showing Schwann cell nuclei oriented in parallel with the long axis of nerve fibers. (H&E; ×250.)

the axon and is wound around it (Fig. 8). The cytoplasm is squeezed out, and the internal surfaces of the cell membranes are fused. In each successive turn, the outer surfaces of adjacent turns also fuse. Thus, a spiral of fused Schwann cell cytoplasmic membrane is

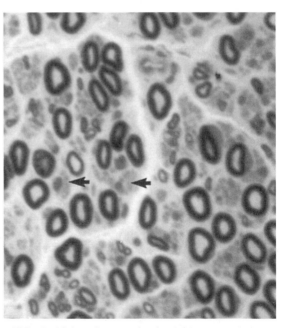

FIG. 6. Light micrograph of a transverse 1-μm-thick section of a normal human sensory (sural) nerve showing the spectrum of myelinated fiber diameters and less distinct profiles of Schwann cells *(arrows)* containing unmyelinated fibers. (Original magnification ×400.)

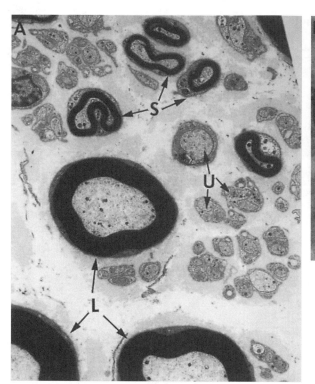

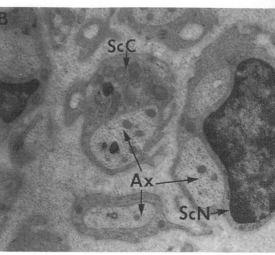

FIG. 7. A: Electron micrograph (×3,600) of a human sural nerve showing a mixture of large myelinated *(L)*, small myelinated *(S)*, and unmyelinated *(U)* fibers. **B:** Higher power view of unmyelinated fibers. (×10,000.) *ScC,* Schwann cell cytoplasm; *Ax,* axon; *ScN,* Schwann cell nucleus.

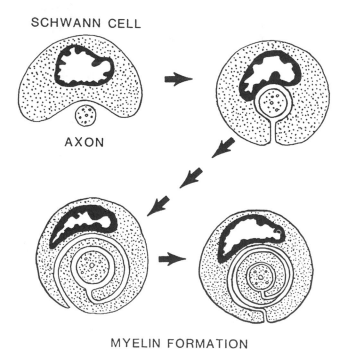

MYELIN FORMATION

FIG. 8. Progressive steps in myelination of an axon by a Schwann cell.

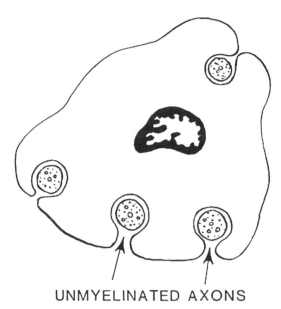

UNMYELINATED AXONS

FIG. 9. Relationship between a Schwann cell and unmyelinated axons. Many unmyelinated axons may be invested by a single Schwann cell.

formed. The resulting multilayered protein-lipid substance is called *myelin.* The number of spirals that the Schwann cell process makes around the axon determines the thickness of the myelin sheath. In very small axons, the Schwann cell membrane may simply invest them once and make no turns at all. These axons are considered unmyelinated fibers. A single Schwann cell may invest a segment of several unmyelinated fibers in this way (Fig. 9). However, in myelinated fibers, a Schwann cell is related to a segment of only one axon. The physiologic significance of the thickness of the myelin sheath and of unmyelinated fibers is discussed in later chapters.

If myelinated axons of a peripheral nerve are teased apart so that a single fiber may be studied, there are numerous Schwann cells along its length, each forming the myelin sheath over a short segment of the axon (Fig. 10). Each segment of myelin belongs to a single Schwann cell along a given axon. There is a minute gap between each myelin segment, where the fiber appears to be constricted. These gaps are the *nodes of Ranvier.* Therefore, the myelin segment is often referred to as an internode, and the distance between the nodes of Ranvier as the internodal length. The internodal length varies directly with the thickness of the myelin sheath along any given fiber, approaching 1 mm in length in the largest fibers.

In routine preparations of the central nervous system, oligodendroglial cells are recognized as small, round nuclei with a dense chromatin network (Fig. 11). With no cytoplasm being stained, the nuclei seem to be surrounded by a clear halo. Oligodendroglial cells lie in both gray and white matter. In gray matter, they lie near neurons (perineuronal satellites) and their function is unknown. In white matter, the oligodendroglia lie among the myelinated fibers, but their precise relationship to myelin is not apparent at the light microscopic level. With the electron microscope, the same relationship of oligodendroglial cell to myelin that is present between Schwann cell and peripheral myelin can be demonstrated. The oligodendroglial cell sends out cytoplasmic extensions that wrap themselves around an axon and fuse (Figs. 2 and 8).

A major difference between the central and the peripheral nervous system is that a single oligodendroglial cell may myelinate a segment

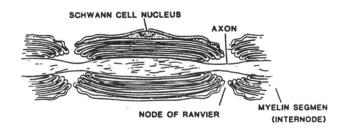

SCHWANN CELL NUCLEUS

AXON

NODE OF RANVIER

MYELIN SEGMEN (INTERNODE)

FIG. 10. Schwann cell–myelin-axon relationship in longitudinal section. Portions of three myelin segments (internodes) separated by two nodes of Ranvier are represented.

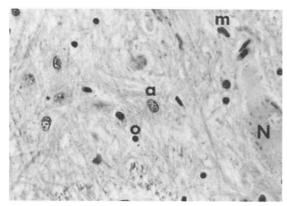

FIG. 11. Section of brain tissue in which nuclei belonging to various types of glial cells are seen, including oligodendroglia *(o)*, astrocytes *(a)*, and microglia *(m)*. A portion of a neuron *(N)* is seen at the lower right. (H&E; ×250.)

of several axons in its vicinity, whereas a Schwann cell myelinates a segment of only one axon. A second major difference is that each nerve fiber in a peripheral nerve is invested by a *basement membrane* that is continuous over each Schwann cell that contributes a myelin segment to that fiber. No basement membranes occur around oligodendroglial cells or central axons. These two differences are among the more significant factors in the different abilities of central and peripheral axons to regenerate after axonal injury.

Astrocytes

Astrocytes are easily recognized in sections of central nervous system tissue stained with hematoxylin and eosin; they have oval nuclei, slightly larger and less densely stained than oligodendroglial nuclei (Fig. 11). Cytoplasm and processes of normal astrocytes are not seen with these methods. However, with metallic impregnation stains, notably the gold sublimate stains of Cajal, astrocytes show an elaborate radiating system of processes from which their name is derived (Fig. 12). There are minor anatomical variations by which astrocytes may be separated into different types, for example, protoplasmic astrocytes, which predominate in gray matter, and fibrous astro-

cytes, which predominate in white matter. These minor morphologic differences have no known functional significance.

Astrocytes traditionally have been assigned a largely passive function in the central nervous system because of the historical concept of glial cells as the "glue" and as cells that form the framework on which neurons and their processes are organized and held together. This function is most evident during embryogenesis, in which the migration of neurons from the ventricular layer to the outer layers of the neural tube is directed and guided by the radiating processes of astrocytes. There is, however, substantial evidence that astrocytes have a more active role in the physiology of the central nervous system. One or more expanded processes of each astrocyte abuts on the wall of a capillary, forming part of the nearly continuous sheath of astrocytic foot processes that surround the capillary network in the brain and spinal cord (Fig. 12). The remaining processes terminate in relationship to the nonsynaptic regions of neurons and to other glial cells. This arrangement suggests that astrocytes function as a conduit for the transport of ions and molecules between the extracellular environment of these cells and the capillary wall. The relationship of this function to the phenomenon called the *blood–brain barrier* is described below. Finally, astrocytes play a critical role in

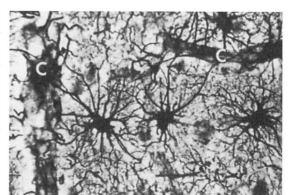

FIG. 12. Astrocytes as seen with a gold sublimate stain. Note the many processes ending on walls of capillaries *(C)*. (Cajal stain; ×400.)

almost all pathologic reactions of the nervous system, as described in the following section.

Ependymal Cells

After the epithelium of the neural tube has proliferated in the ventricular zone and the major portion of its cells have differentiated and migrated, a single layer of ciliated columnar epithelial cells (the *ependyma*) is left lining the cavity of the neural tube (Fig. 13).

In the cerebral hemispheres and brainstem of the mature brain, the ependyma lines the entire ventricular system. The central canal of the spinal cord is usually obliterated as an open cavity when development is complete, and the central region of the adult cord is represented by a nest of ependymal cells with a disorganized appearance. The ependymal lining of the ventricular system forms a selective barrier between the ventricular fluid and the brain substance, because tight junctions between the plasma membranes of adjacent ependymal cells serve to inhibit the passage of certain substances.

The choroid plexus is formed when the thinned roof plate, consisting of a layer of ependymal cells, invaginates the ventricular cavity ahead of a vascular-connective tissue component derived from the pia mater. Enormous elaboration of these evaginations leads to the formation of many small tufts, each of which has essentially the same structure (Fig. 14). The ventricular surface of a choroidal tuft

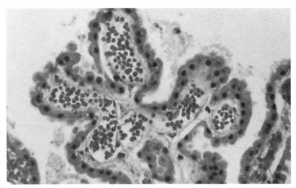

FIG. 14. Choroid plexus. Each tuft consists of a core containing a dilated capillary surrounded by a small amount of connective tissue and covered by choroidal epithelial cells. (H&E; ×100.)

is lined by cuboidal epithelial cells, which are modified ependymal cells. The free surface of a choroidal cell displays numerous microvilli on electron microscopic examination. Beneath the surface epithelium is a core of richly vascular connective tissue.

The function of the choroid plexus is to form the cerebrospinal fluid. It does this by filtering water and selected molecules out of the blood that passes through its capillaries and by passing this solution through its epithelial cells into the ventricular system.

Supporting Cells of Mesodermal Origin

Capillaries and the Blood–Brain Barrier

The anatomy and physiology of the arterial supply and venous drainage of the central nervous system are described in Chapter 11. Cerebral arteries, arterioles, venules, and veins do not differ structurally from vessels of similar size and function in other organs. However, capillaries of the nervous system are unique in their ultrastructure and physiology. Capillaries are composed of a single layer of endothelial cells surrounded by a basement membrane. In the central nervous system, capillaries are invested by a nearly continuous layer of *astrocytic extensions* called *foot processes* (Fig. 15). Only the capillary basement membrane intervenes be-

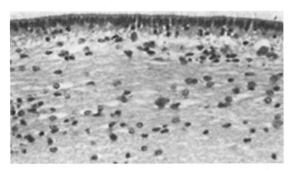

FIG. 13. Ependyma lining the ventricle of an infant. Note the continuous layer of columnar cells with cilia on their free (ventricular) border. (H&E; ×100.)

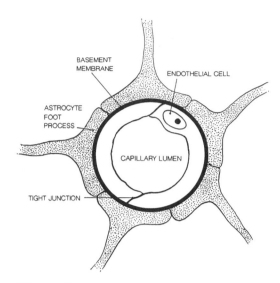

FIG. 15. Nonfenestrated capillary in the central nervous system. Endothelial cells are joined by tight junctions and surrounded by a basement membrane and sheath of astrocytic foot processes.

tween the plasma membrane of the astrocyte and the endothelial cell plasma membrane. In the capillaries of all other organs, there are pores and channels between individual endothelial cells through which water and solutes can pass from the blood to the extracellular space. In most of the central nervous system, however, adjacent endothelial cells are joined by continuous tight junctions formed by the fusion of the external layers of the plasma membranes. Thus, for substances to enter the extracellular space of the brain, they must pass through rather than between endothelial cells. This is the anatomical basis of the *blood–brain barrier.*

The barrier is not absolute, and its efficiency in preventing the entry of substances into the central nervous system varies widely with different classes of molecules. Small, highly lipid-soluble molecules such as volatile anesthetics and alcohol pass through the blood–brain barrier easily because of their solubility in the lipid bilayer of the endothelial cell membrane. Large, complex molecules, including most proteins and many drugs, are completely excluded from the brain

under normal circumstances. Between the two extremes of uninhibited access and total exclusion are many other substances such as electrolytes, glucose, and amino acids that enter the brain by highly selective transport mechanisms. Specific transport proteins move these molecules across the luminal cytoplasmic membrane of the endothelial cell, through the cytoplasm, and out of the endothelial cell across the antiluminal cell membrane. The layer of astrocytic foot processes that ensheathes the capillaries of the central nervous system was once thought to contribute to blood–brain barrier function. However, it appears that it does not exclude substances from entering the extracellular space of the brain, but rather that its main function is the rapid transfer of ions such as potassium from the extracellular environment of neurons, where they might be harmful, to the region of the capillary wall where they can be transported out of the central nervous system. The barrier function is usually absent from a few small regions of the central nervous system such as the anterior third ventricle, tuber cinereum of the hypothalamus, the pineal gland, and the area postrema of the caudal fourth ventricle. Through these selected areas, the brain is able to monitor the composition of the blood, which is important for certain critical homeostatic functions.

The tight junctions that join the capillary endothelial cells in the central nervous system are quite fragile. Also, the active transport mechanisms that are critical to the function of the blood–brain barrier are highly energy-dependent and require a constant supply of ATP generated by oxidative metabolism. It is not surprising, then, that breakdown of the barrier is a common and early pathologic response to almost any form of injury to the central nervous system, including trauma, ischemia, inflammation, and pressure from mass lesions. The most conspicuous result of this breakdown is the influx of excessive water into the extracellular space of the brain, which produces cerebral edema (see Chapter 6, Fig. 12A).

In the later subacute and chronic stages of cerebral injury, endothelial cells participate in the reparative process by proliferation and formation of new capillaries, which again acquire the barrier mechanism. The mechanism of this process is not fully understood, but it clearly requires contact between endothelial cells and neural tissue.

The capillaries of peripheral nerves (endoneural capillaries) are also nonfenestrated and joined by tight junctions, providing the *blood-nerve barrier,* which is similar in function to the blood–brain barrier. Ganglia, in contrast, have fenestrated capillaries, theoretically making them more susceptible to blood-borne disorders.

Microglia

Microglia are not derived from the neuroepithelium; they are mesodermal cells that migrate into the central nervous system along with blood vessels from the mesoderm that surround the neural tube. They are seen as small, elongated, darkly staining nuclei in hematoxylin and eosin–stained sections (Fig. 11). Normally they are present only in small numbers and are widely scattered in the nervous system. Their major function becomes manifest only when a destructive process affects the central nervous system, at which time the cells proliferate rapidly and become scavenger cells, or macrophages, ingesting and removing damaged tissue.

Connective Tissue

The brain and spinal cord are permeated by a rich network of blood vessels, which, except at the capillary level, have a thin collagenous investment making up the adventitia. Other than the vascular structures, the parenchyma of the central nervous system is almost devoid of fibrous connective tissue elements, which accounts for its extremely soft consistency. Thus, fibroblasts rarely participate in reactive or reparative processes (scar formation) in diseases of the central nervous system.

The central nervous system is surrounded by three connective tissue membranes called *meninges.* The two inner membranes, the pia mater and arachnoid, are the *leptomeninges* and are very thin and delicate. The outer membrane, the *dura mater* (or pachymeninx), is thick and tough.

The peripheral nerves are rich in fibrous connective tissue. Each myelinated nerve fiber in a peripheral nerve is invested by a thin layer of collagen, the *endoneurium.* Groups of nerve fibers are bound together in fascicles by a *perineurium.* Finally, the fascicles that comprise a nerve trunk are surrounded by a thick sheath, the *epineurium.* The three connective tissue sheaths of a peripheral nerve are analogous to the three layers of the meninges (pia mater, arachnoid, and dura mater) and are continuous with them at the spinal nerve level.

Pathologic Reactions of the Structural Elements ▪

Each of the cellular elements of the nervous system may undergo physical change in response to disease states. In some disorders, the pathologic alteration may be primarily functional (physiologic)—there may be little change in the physical appearance of the cell, yet the cell cannot function normally. In many diseases of the nervous system, however, the physical appearance of the cell is altered. When the nervous system is affected by disease, the cells undergo changes that reflect either the damage done to them by the pathologic process or their reaction to it. Some of these morphologic changes are nonspecific and may be seen in many entirely different types of diseases. Other changes may be specific and indicate a particular type of disease or even a specific disease entity. In this section, we review some of the more common and important pathologic changes seen in the individual cell types studied above. In most pathologic conditions, the various cell types react in concert, and the pathologic diagnosis is derived from analysis of the total tissue reaction.

The pathologic appearance of cells revealed under the light microscope or electron microscope, as described in this section, ultimately reflects changes in the structure and arrangement of molecules in the cell. The molecular species that are most affected and the manner in which they are affected depend on the mechanism of the injury. In some diseases, the mechanism of cell injury or death is programmed into the genetic material of the cell. The defective DNA template results in faulty structure and function of the gene product, often an enzyme or an important structural protein. Defects of this type may be compatible with normal cell function for long periods of time, but ultimately they cause damage to the metabolic machinery or structural integrity of the cell, with eventual loss of function. In most disease processes, damage to cells results from extrinsic factors, such as loss of availability of essential nutrients, entry of toxic substances into the cell, or attachment of antibodies to the cell membrane. Any of these mechanisms can initiate a cascade of events that finally produces cell damage and death. Some of these mechanisms are discussed in more detail in the following paragraphs dealing with specific pathologic changes.

Pathologic Reactions of Neurons

Nonspecific Reactions

Almost any disease leading to the death of a patient is associated with changes in body chemistry and physiology that may affect the appearance of neurons. In addition, catabolic processes that proceed after death (autolysis) and the mechanical procedures involved in obtaining and processing tissue can distort the appearance of neurons. It is not surprising, then, that almost any histologic section of brain tissue contains some neurons that deviate from normal in size, shape, and affinity for stains. Shrunken, dark-staining neurons, as well as swollen, pale-staining cells, are often encountered. Although these neurons are not normal in the strict sense, the factors responsible for their nonspecific change are usually not identifiable. Neuronal loss is another nonspecific change that may result from any form of severe damage to a neuron. Under pathologic circumstances, neuronal loss is usually accompanied by a reaction of other tissue elements (astrocytes, microglia), which marks the site of damage. Neuronal changes of a more specific type can accompany certain pathologic processes and, when present, can help to define the pathophysiologic basis for those disorders.

Cell Death

The death of cells and the removal of cellular debris are important in both the normal function of the nervous system and the pathogenesis of diseases of the nervous system. Conceptually, two fundamental types of processes lead to cell death, necrosis and programmed cell death, which might be likened to murder and suicide, respectively (Table 1).

Necrosis is thought of as a process of cell death that is initiated by an external pathologic event. Generally, it is an acute process that is initiated by damage to the integrity of

TABLE 1. *Characteristics of necrosis and apoptosis*

Feature	Necrosis ("murder")	Apoptosis ("suicide")
DNA damage	Degradation	Internucleosomal cleavage
Nucleus	Pyknosis	Chromatin margination
Membrane integrity	Compromised early	Persists until late
Mitochondria	Swollen	Appear normal
Cell volume	Increased early (swollen neuron), then shrinkage (dead red cell)	Decreased
Pattern	Foci of numerous cells affected	Individual cells affected
Inflammatory changes	Yes	No
Normal during development	No	Yes
Response to injury	Acute, severe	Slow, delayed

the plasma membrane, which allows the influx of sodium and calcium ions and water. Thus, the early morphologic features of necrosis include swelling of the cell. The cascade of cellular events initiated by the influx of calcium, especially the activation of autolytic enzymes, ultimately leads to dissolution of the cell. This relatively acute process may initiate an inflammatory response, an additional histopathologic feature that distinguishes necrosis from programmed cell death.

Programmed cell death is an important feature of normal development and other biologic processes in which cell proliferation is controlled and an excess number of cells is removed. The term *apoptosis* refers to one of the morphologic consequences of programmed cell death, and the two terms are often used interchangeably. In programmed cell death, enzymatic activity normally inhibited by protective molecules is activated and proceeds to degrade the cellular machinery. Endonucleases are activated, and nuclear chromatin is cleaved and compacted into sharply circumscribed clumps that abut the nuclear envelope. As the process continues, the nucleus shrinks, the cytoplasm condenses, and the nucleus and cytoplasm fragment into membrane-bound bodies containing relatively intact organelles *(apoptotic bodies)* that are phagocytosed without evidence of activation of an inflammatory response. The molecular machinery for programmed cell death is programmed in the genetic code of all cells and is kept in check by inhibitory proteins. The internal mechanisms of the cell that promote or inhibit apoptosis may, in turn, be activated or inhibited by various extracellular influences, including cytokines such as tumor necrosis factor and growth factors such as brain-derived neurotropic factor.

During normal development of the nervous system, programmed cell death is critical for the elimination of the large number of extraneous neuroblasts created during the proliferative phase. In this case, the apoptotic cascade is probably activated by the absence of target cell–derived neurotropic factors. Many neuronal degenerative diseases and even some infectious diseases (for example, human immunodeficiency virus–induced neuronal damage) appear to involve the activation of the apoptotic cascade through various mechanisms, such as genetic mutation of an inhibitory protein or cytokine-induced inhibition of an inhibitory protein. Uninhibited cell proliferation in neoplasms may often be the result of the mutation of genes, such as the *p53* tumor suppressor gene, that normally transcribe proteins that mediate programmed cell death in precancerous cells.

Despite the differences cited above, programmed cell death and necrosis are not mutually exclusive. The cascade of biochemical events that lead to dissolution of the cell broadly overlap in the two processes. The distinction is clear in comparing a normal biologic form of programmed cell death (such as removal of excess neuroblasts during development), with an acute necrotizing process (such as a stroke). However, the distinction between the two processes is blurred in slowly evolving neuronal loss, as in degenerative diseases. Neuronal damage in degenerative disorders might begin with compromise of the electrochemical stability of the plasma membrane. Acute or severe changes in membrane integrity typically activate the processes involved in necrosis. However, if the injury evolves slowly, the electrolyte shifts, especially increased cytosolic calcium, may be insufficient to induce necrosis but sufficient to trigger the programmed cell death cascade leading to apoptosis. There are many mechanisms that may produce this type of chronic membrane dysfunction. A widely recognized and extensively studied mechanism is *excitotoxicity,* which refers to excessive depolarization of the neuronal plasma membrane by excitatory neurotransmitters, especially glutamate (the major excitatory neurotransmitter in the central nervous system).

Specific Pathologic Reactions

Ischemic cell change (Fig. 16) occurs in response to deprivation of oxygen and cessation of oxidative metabolism; neurons undergo a

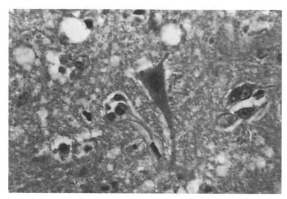

FIG. 16. Ischemic cell change. The neuron is shrunken, the nucleus is pyknotic, and the cytoplasm is diffusely eosinophilic. (H&E; ×400.)

readily recognized morphologic change. Eight to 12 hours after the insult, the neuron becomes smaller and its outline becomes more sharply angular. The cytoplasm becomes distinctly eosinophilic. The nucleus shrinks and becomes homogeneously darkly stained. This is an irreversible change, and the end result is complete dissolution of the cell. Ischemic cell change may be brought about by any condition that deprives the neuron of oxygen, including loss of blood flow, lack of oxygen in the blood, lack of substrates necessary for oxidative metabolism, or the presence of a poison such as cyanide, which blocks oxidative metabolism. The typical morphologic change of ischemic damage may be preceded briefly by certain nonspecific changes, such as acute swelling of the neuron.

The biochemical and molecular events that result in ischemic damage to neurons are complex. The exact point at which these events become irreversible and produce necrosis is uncertain. It generally is accepted that several (2 to 5) minutes of complete oxygen deprivation result in irreversible neuronal damage, although under certain circumstances, such as extreme hypothermia, this period of time may be significantly increased. Without oxygen, the respiratory chain process on the inner mitochondrial membrane—the most important source of ATP for energy-dependent cell functions—comes to a rapid halt. ATP stores are

quickly depleted, and these functions, including maintenance of transmembrane ion channels, become impaired. With the mitochondrial respiratory chain impaired, glycolysis of the remaining stores of glucose is anaerobic and proceeds only to pyruvate, which is then reduced to lactate. The accumulation of lactic acid and free fatty acids (resulting from impaired ATP-dependent lipid metabolism) produces *intracellular acidosis,* which further inhibits mitochondrial function.

At least three other processes occur more or less in concert and ultimately lead to cell death and destruction. These are excitotoxicity, accumulation of intracellular calcium, and generation of free radicals.

Much attention has been focused on the role of *excitatory neurotransmitters,* especially glutamate, in both acute and chronic nerve cell damage. Hypoxia affects the presynaptic membranes at excitatory synapses in a manner that impairs reuptake of glutamate and perhaps enhances its release. The excess extracellular glutamate has several damaging effects due to the opening of ion channels associated with glutamate receptors *(excitotoxicity).* The opening of sodium and chloride channels leads to the influx of these ions along with water. In extreme situations, this can lead to acute swelling and lysis of the cell. The opening of voltage-dependent calcium channels, allowing influx of calcium into the cytosol, as discussed below, is an additional harmful effect of excitotoxicity.

Intracellular calcium ion concentration is normally maintained at a low level by its relative impermeability at resting membrane potential and by active transport mechanisms that favor the extrusion of calcium from the cell. In addition, calcium concentration in the cytosol is particularly low, because normally it is sequestered by active transport mechanisms in the endoplasmic reticulum and mitochondria. In hypoxic conditions, all the processes cited above (loss of energy-dependent transport mechanisms, excitotoxic membrane depolarization) and other processes combine to increase cytosolic calcium concentration, producing several adverse effects on the cell. The most important is the activation of calcium-dependent degradative enzymes (proteases, phospholipases, and endonucleases) that attack the cytoskeleton, cell membranes, and nuclear DNA. Also, high calcium concentration further inhibits mitochondrial function (Fig. 17).

The generation of free radicals, especially oxygen free radicals such as superoxide and hydroxyl ions, is another mechanism of hypoxic cell injury. Like excitatory transmitter release and intracellular calcium accumulation, it can be the result of tissue hypoxia as well as the mediator of further tissue damage. Free radical generation seems to occur pri-

marily during reperfusion after a period of ischemia. Among the direct effects of free radicals are the peroxidation of fatty acids, which leads ultimately to the destruction of lipid molecules, and further disruption of calcium homeostasis, which leads to aggravation of the sequence of events described above.

Although the above mechanisms of cell injury and death have been described in the context of acute hypoxic injury, it should be emphasized that one or several of them, evolving much more slowly, may be the ultimate mechanism of cell death in chronic neurologic diseases. As examples, one could cite the pro-

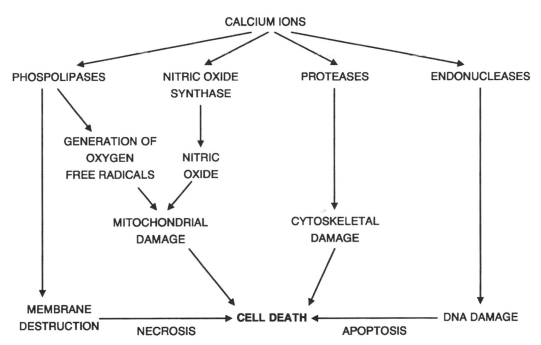

FIG. 17. Metabolic cascades triggered by increased free cytosolic calcium, as in ischemia, hypoglycemia, seizures, or other conditions causing energy failure. The impairment of adenosine triphosphate (ATP)-driven pumps produces membrane depolarization (allowing calcium influx through voltage- and glutamate-gated channels), increased release of calcium from intracellular stores, and failure of calcium reuptake in organelles and its extrusion from the cells. Activation of phospholipase A produces oxygen free radicals, which damage the cell membranes through fatty acid peroxidation. Nitric oxide synthase produces nitric oxide, which in combination with oxygen free radicals causes mitochondrial damage, further decreasing ATP production and increasing the generation of free radicals. Proteases destroy cytoskeletal proteins, thus impairing intracellular and axonal transport. Damage of the cell membrane and organelles leads to necrosis. Endonucleases in conjunction with free radicals damage DNA and trigger the cascades for apoptosis.

posed excitotoxic damage to motor neurons in amyotrophic lateral sclerosis and the oxygen free radical–mediated damage to the substantia nigra in Parkinson's disease.

Central chromatolysis (Fig. 18) is a change in neuron cell bodies after severe injury to their axons. Thus, it is sometimes called the *axonal reaction*. In human pathology, this change is usually recognized only in large motor neurons in the spinal ventral horn or motor nuclei of cranial nerves when their axons are injured close to the central nervous system. The reaction consists of swelling of the cell body and dissolution of the Nissl granules, beginning close to the nucleus and spreading to the periphery of the cell, where a rim of Nissl granules may be found intact. The nucleus migrates to the periphery of the cell body. These changes usually begin 2 to 3 days after injury and reach a maximum in 2 to 3 weeks. Unlike ischemic cell change, central chromatolysis is reversible and the neuron may revert to a normal appearance in a few months.

The process of degeneration of the axon and its myelin sheath is called *wallerian degeneration* (after Waller, who in 1850 first described it in peripheral nerves). *Wallerian degeneration* occurs in the distal part of an axon, when the parent cell body is destroyed or separated from the axon by disease or injury along the axon. In both the central and peripheral nervous systems, an axon cannot survive when it is separated from its cell body.

The changes seen in the degenerating axon are impairment of axonal transport and the rapid disappearance of neurofibrils, followed by breaking up of the axon into short fragments that eventually disappear completely (Fig. 19). As axonal fragmentation proceeds, the myelin sheath begins to fragment in a similar manner into oval segments (ovoids). Each oval segment of myelin, containing a fragment of axon, is called a *digestive chamber,* because the axon seems to be digested within it. At this same time, the myelin fragment undergoes biochemical changes, including breakdown into its component lipids. These lipids are eventually removed by phagocytosis.

Some notable differences exist between this process in the central and peripheral nervous systems. Wallerian degeneration proceeds more rapidly in peripheral nerves, where degenerative changes are completed in a few weeks. In the central nervous system, the degeneration proceeds over several months. More importantly, in the peripheral nervous system, regeneration of the nerve is possible if the parent cell body survives; this regeneration does not occur in the central nervous system. Each axon and myelin sheath in a peripheral nerve is surrounded by a basement membrane, which belongs to the Schwann cell, and by a delicate connective tissue sheath, the *endoneurium*. These structures maintain their integrity even as the axon and myelin degenerate. In addition, Schwann cells, with the potential of forming new myelin, proliferate along the length of the degenerating fiber. Thus, the distal portion of a damaged nerve provides a superstructure that is ready to receive and myelinate new axonal sprouts growing from the proximal portion. If these axonal sprouts can find their way into one of these "tubes," they will continue to grow at a rate of about 3 mm per day, and function may eventually be restored. In the central nervous system, no basement membranes or collagen sheaths surround nerve fibers, and oligodendroglia are incapable of proliferation. Thus, new axonal growth, even if it should begin, has no path to

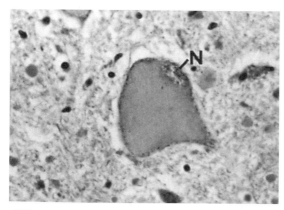

FIG. 18. Central chromatolysis. The neuron is swollen, the nucleus *(N)* is eccentric, and the Nissl granules have disappeared except at the periphery. (H&E; ×400.)

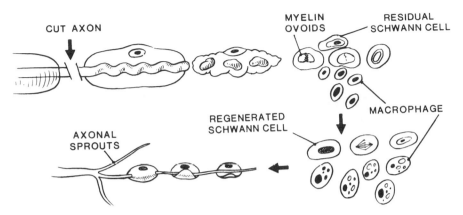

FIG. 19. Sequence of events in wallerian degeneration and early peripheral nerve regeneration. After degeneration and removal of myelin and axonal debris, sprouts from the severed end of an axon may find their way into a tube of regenerated Schwann cells.

follow. Functionally significant regeneration of tracts does not occur after damage to the central nervous system.

Injury of an axon generally results in no change in the postsynaptic cell. There are exceptions; for example, when the motor innervation of a muscle is destroyed, the muscle becomes atrophic. A similar phenomenon, *transneuronal degeneration,* has been observed in certain pathways in the central nervous system. The process apparently depends on the removal of some trophic influence by which the axon maintains the condition of the postsynaptic element. The nature of such trophic influences is unknown.

The processes of chromatolysis and wallerian degeneration were used in the past to trace neuroanatomical pathways. When the axons of a functional group of neurons are sectioned or otherwise damaged, the cell bodies of the neurons from which the axons originate can be located by finding which neurons undergo chromatolysis. Conversely, a neuroanatomist may destroy a group of neuronal cell bodies within a particular nucleus of the central nervous system and then trace the route taken by the axons by staining the degenerating fibers with techniques designed to demonstrate either degenerating myelin or degenerating axons.

Neurofibrillary degeneration is the formation of clumped masses of neurofibrils within the cytoplasm (Fig. 20) and is a common, readily recognized change in neurons of the central nervous system. This change, *Alzheimer's neurofibrillary degeneration,* is best seen with silver-impregnation stains. It is a neuronal degeneration that is most closely associated with clinical dementia. The change is seen to some extent in hippocampal neurons of many normal older people and is found throughout the cerebral cortex and in other parts of the brain in a severe dementing process known as Alzheimer's disease. Alzheimer's degeneration is also a prominent

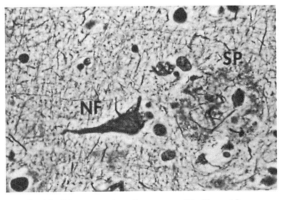

FIG. 20. Neuron showing neurofibrillary degeneration *(NF)*. Note the tangle of thickened neurofibrils in the cell body and axon. A senile plaque *(SP)* is seen on the *right*. (Bodian stain; ×400.)

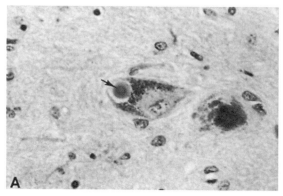

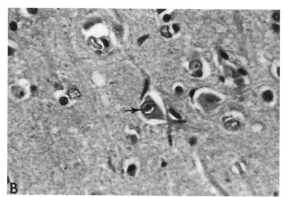

FIG. 21. A: Lewy body *(arrow)* in the cytoplasm of a pigmented neuron in Parkinson's disease. **B:** Cowdry type A intranuclear inclusion *(arrow)* in subacute sclerosing panencephalitis. (H&E; ×400.)

change found in a few other conditions classed as degenerative diseases. The senile plaque is a closely associated pathologic change noted primarily in senile dementia and Alzheimer's disease. Typical senile plaques consist of a central deposit of amyloid (the core) surrounded by a halo of degenerated nerve processes and reactive elements, such as astrocytic fibers and microglia.

Inclusion body formation refers to abnormal, discrete deposits in nerve cells (Fig. 21) and, when present, often identifies the type of disease and sometimes the specific disease. Inclusion bodies can be divided into intranuclear and intracytoplasmic types. The appearance and significance of the most important types of neuronal inclusions are outlined in Table 2.

Storage cells refer to the accumulation of metabolic products within nerve cells. Several metabolic diseases of the nervous system are associated with this accumulation. Most of these disorders involve the storage of lipids. As these lipid products accumulate, the cell body swells so much that it is referred to as a balloon cell (Fig. 22). Identification of the specific disease requires biochemical identification of the stored material.

Pathologic Reactions of Oligodendroglia

Oligodendroglial cells, as identified in routine preparations, undergo few reactions of pathognomonic importance. They seem to be extremely sensitive to injury and, when affected by a pathologic process, oligodendroglial nuclei shrink or break up and vanish. The myelin that they form, however, is an extremely important indicator of disease of the central nervous system. Just as the oligodendroglial cell is readily damaged by most pathologic processes, the myelin sheaths are also extremely sensitive to injury. Partial or complete loss of myelin in an area of injury is easily seen

TABLE 2. *Inclusion bodies*

Location	Name	Staining characteristics	Disease association
Cytoplasm	Lewy body	Eosinophilic with concentric lamination	Parkinson's disease
Cytoplasm	Pick body	Metallophilic (silver, gold)	Pick's disease
Cytoplasm	Lafora body	Basophilic	Myoclonus epilepsy
Cytoplasm	Negri body	Eosinophilic	Rabies
Nucleus	Cowdry type A inclusion	Eosinophilic	Viral infections: herpes simplex, subacute sclerosing panencephalitis, cytomegalic inclusion disease

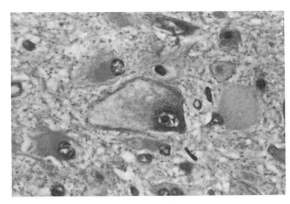

FIG. 22. Neuron in Tay-Sachs disease (lipid-storage disease). Note ballooning of the cytoplasm with stored material, forcing the nucleus and Nissl granules to one corner of the cell body. (H&E; ×400.)

in myelin stains such as the Luxol-fast blue stain (Fig. 23A). Sections stained in this way provide the most reliable method of studying the topography of most disease processes.

In addition to the nonspecific injury to myelin associated with most kinds of disease, there are two groups of diseases that specifically affect myelin sheaths. The first group is called the *demyelinating,* or *myelinoclastic,* diseases. In these disorders, normal myelin is attacked by some exogenous agent, usually unknown, and broken down into its component lipids (as in wallerian degeneration) and absorbed. The axons that the myelin surrounds are left relatively intact. The most common and important disease in this group is multiple sclerosis.

The process of demyelination in multiple sclerosis and some other diseases of the central and peripheral nervous system, such as postvaccinal encephalomyelitis and Guillain-Barré syndrome, involves immunologic mechanisms. Although the details of the pathogenesis of these disorders remain to be clarified, humoral- and cell-mediated immunologic reactions involving myelin components set in motion the cytotoxic and inflammatory processes that lead to demyelination.

The second group of diseases are the *leukodystrophies,* or *dysmyelinating,* diseases. In these disorders, myelin is abnormally formed because of a genetically determined error in metabolism. The abnormally constituted myelin is unstable and breaks down. The type of metabolic defect often can be determined by histochemical staining reactions and biochemical analysis of the tissue.

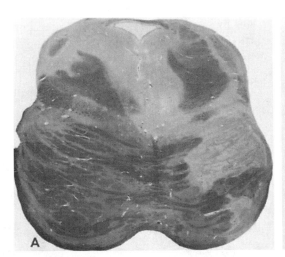
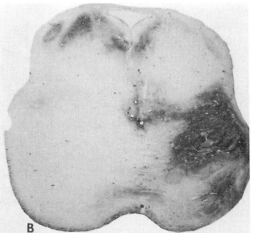

FIG. 23. Transverse section of the pons of a patient with multiple sclerosis. **A:** Myelin stain showing plaques of demyelination *(light areas).* (Luxol-fast blue; ×4.) **B:** Glial fiber stain showing gliosis of demyelinated areas *(dark areas).* (Holzer stain; ×4.)

Pathologic Reactions of Schwann Cells

Disease processes affecting the Schwann cells that surround peripheral axons produce segmental loss of myelin (segmental demyelination). If the disease is severe, there also may be associated secondary axonal destruction and wallerian degeneration. In certain genetic disorders affecting peripheral nerve (hypertrophic neuropathies), there is repeated demyelination and remyelination of nerve fibers. Each episode leaves a layer of Schwann cells and collagen, forming concentric layers around the axon. Such nerves become large and firm; the axons may finally be lost, leaving only the stroma of the connective tissue.

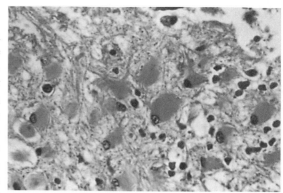

FIG. 24. Reactive astrocytes at the border of an infarct. Note the expansion of cytoplasm, producing a plump appearance, and the dense tangle of fibers in the background. (H&E; ×250.)

Pathologic Reactions of Astrocytes

Almost any injury to central nervous system tissue can produce a reaction of astrocytes. The terms *astrocytosis, astrogliosis,* and *gliosis* refer to this nonspecific response, whereby astrocytes form "scars" in injured neural tissue. Strictly speaking, astrocytosis refers to the early stages of the reaction in which astrocytes proliferate and increase greatly in number. As this occurs, their cytoplasm becomes visible with hematoxylin and eosin stains as an eosinophilic apron of cytoplasm with somewhat irregular margins. At this stage, they are known as "plump" or *gemistocytic* (from the German *gemaste,* meaning "stuffed") astrocytes (Fig. 24). These plump astrocytes then form progressively longer and thicker processes, which create a dense network in the damaged tissue. This network of tissue is the equivalent of a scar formed by fibroblasts in other body tissues. The fibers of reactive astrocytes, although readily visible in hematoxylin and eosin stains, are seen even more clearly with special stains like Mallory's phosphotungstic acid-hematoxylin or Holzer stain. With the latter techniques, an area of gliosis can be seen in a section even without the aid of a microscope, which is of advantage in mapping the topography of a large lesion (Fig. 23B).

Astrocytes also may react in more specific ways to certain injuries, especially metabolic disturbances. The most notable example is the presence of acutely swollen astrocytic nuclei, called Alzheimer's type 2 astrocytes, in hepatic failure. Astrocytes may also form intranuclear inclusion bodies in certain viral infections.

Pathologic Reactions of Microglia

Microglial cells react in a stereotyped way to most diseases that affect the central nervous system. Injury to other cellular constituents of the central nervous system usually leads to multiplication of nearby microglial cells (Fig. 25). The nuclei of these microglial cells become elongated and form *rod* cells. If

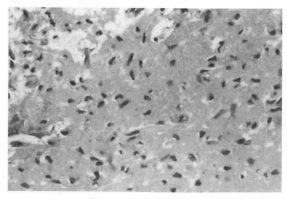

FIG. 25. Margin of a recent infarct, showing proliferating microglial cells. (H&E; ×100.)

actual tissue necrosis does not occur, the re-action may progress no further. The presence of many rod cells usually indicates the presence of low-grade chronic irritation of the tissue. An example of such a condition is the chronic encephalitis associated with syphilis (general paresis).

If tissue necrosis occurs, microglial cells continue to proliferate and their nuclei become rounded. Their cytoplasm becomes evident as it begins to engulf the debris of the necrotic tissue. Because of the high fat content of central nervous system tissue, most of the engulfed material is lipid, and the cytoplasm assumes a foamy appearance. At this stage, the cells are referred to as *lipid-laden macrophages,* or gitter cells (Fig. 26). In large lesions, many, perhaps even most, of the gitter cells probably were not microglial cells originally but blood-borne macrophages that migrated into the lesion. Eventually, most of the macrophages in a destructive lesion of the central nervous system are reabsorbed into the blood stream. At times, microglia attack isolated, damaged neurons. This process is called *neuronophagia* (Fig. 27). After the neuron has been engulfed, the cluster of microglia remaining in its place is a *microglial nodule.*

Cerebral Edema

In the discussion of the blood–brain barrier, it was noted that almost any pathologic

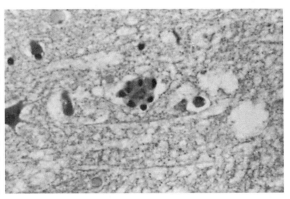

FIG. 27. Damaged neuron undergoing neuronophagia by a cluster of microglial cells. (H&E; ×250.)

process that affects the brain can result in cerebral edema by virtue of its effect on cerebral capillaries. The loss of integrity of the blood–brain barrier allows excessive water accompanied by solutes (such as serum proteins) normally excluded from the extracellular space of the brain to enter this compartment. This is the most common variety of cerebral edema, called *vasogenic edema.* The fluid collects in the extracellular space, predominantly in the white matter. The resulting mass effect can produce a clinically significant increase in intracranial pressure, as described in Chapter 6 (Fig. 12A).

Another commonly recognized form of cerebral edema is *cytotoxic edema.* It results from pathologic processes, usually toxic or metabolic, that affect the cell membranes of neurons and glial cells so they are unable to maintain normal pump mechanisms. The loss of membrane integrity results in the intracellular accumulation of water. This type of edema is more likely to affect gray matter. Although it may cause severe functional abnormalities, it is rarely sufficient to produce a clinically significant mass effect. The two types of cerebral edema are not mutually exclusive and often occur together in pathologic processes such as infarction, which affects both the blood–brain barrier and neuronal and glial cell membranes.

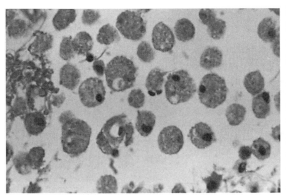

FIG. 26. Lipid-laden macrophages (gitter cells) in an area of necrosis. Note the small eccentric nuclei and foamy cytoplasm. (H&E; ×250.)

Other Pathologic Reactions

Ependymal cells react in a very limited way to noxious stimuli (which most often are infectious). There is often loss of ependymal cells; however, the proliferation of subependymal astrocytes that is frequently associated with this loss forms *ependymal granulations* that may be seen along certain areas of the ventricular system.

In response to injury, blood vessels may respond by capillary proliferation, and when inflammation is present, infiltration of leukocytes occurs, as it does in other tissues.

Uncontrolled cellular proliferation of any of the cellular elements results in a *neoplasm* (a localized accumulation of abnormal tissue, a mass lesion). The type of neoplasm is named after the predominant cell type (such as astrocytoma, oligodendroglioma, or schwannoma).

Clinicopathologic Correlations

Clinical diagnosis in neurology requires the analysis of two types of data. The first type is obtained from both the history and the neurologic examination and enables localization of the disease process within the nervous system. On this basis, neurologic disease may be classified as *focal,* involving a single circumscribed area or group of contiguous structures in the nervous system; *multifocal,* involving more than one circumscribed area or several noncontiguous structures; and *diffuse,* involving portions of the nervous system in a bilateral, symmetrical fashion.

The localization of the pathologic process depends partly on knowledge of the functional anatomy of the nervous system, outlined in Chapter 3. Vastly different types of pathologic processes located in the same anatomical structure may produce similar symptoms and signs. Because the manifestations of disease are dependent on where a lesion is located and not on its pathologic nature, the pathologic diagnosis must use a second type of data—information obtained from the patient's history that relates to the onset and evolution (temporal profile) of the disease. The development of symptoms can be classified in the following terms: *acute,* within minutes; *subacute,* within days; and *chronic,* within weeks or months. The evolution (course of symptoms after the onset) may be categorized as *transient,* when symptoms have resolved completely after onset; *improving,* when symptoms have decreased from their maximum but have not completely resolved; *progressive,* when symptoms continue to increase in severity or when new symptoms make their appearance; and *stationary,* when symptoms remain unchanged after reaching maximal severity and show no significant change during a period of observation.

Combining the above terms allows clinical differentiation between mass and nonmass lesions. Although other clues for differentiation are discussed in later chapters, the presence of a *mass lesion* should be considered when the signs and symptoms, whether acute, subacute, or chronic in onset, suggest progression of a focal lesion. A *nonmass* lesion should be considered when the lesion is diffuse in location or when the symptoms and signs suggest a nonprogressive focal abnormality.

As the text proceeds, qualification of these definitions will be required, and there will be exceptions to these general statements.

Interpretation of the temporal profile of disease depends on an understanding of the way in which pathologic processes affect nerve tissue and the rates at which various destructive and reparative processes proceed. Knowledge of the basic types of cellular and tissue reactions is a prerequisite to making this type of analysis. For the purposes of recognizing and understanding clinical neurologic disease, it is sufficient to become familiar with six types of pathologic changes that occur within the nervous system: (1) degenerative disease, (2) neoplastic disease, (3) vascular disease, (4) inflammatory disease, (5) toxic-metabolic disease, and (6) traumatic disease. In the following sections, the temporal and spatial characteristics of these major disease categories are outlined.

Degenerative Disease

The term *degenerative* is applied to a large group of neurologic diseases that have no apparent cause. As causes of these diseases are found (for example, viral infection or metabolic error), they are moved to another more appropriate disease category; many conditions in this group are genetically determined biochemical disorders. Degenerative disorders are characterized by a gradual decrease in neuronal function. Sometimes the pathologically altered neurons show specific changes, such as neurofibrillary tangles or inclusion body formation; more often, the neurons merely atrophy and disappear. In the central nervous system, the degeneration is usually accompanied by astrocytic proliferation.

Although much is still to be learned, the mechanisms of neuronal loss in degenerative diseases are gradually becoming clarified. The fundamental mechanisms leading to neuronal death appear to be the same in all degenerative diseases. These mechanisms are discussed to some extent above and include (1) excitotoxicity due to activation of glutamate receptors, (2) accumulation of cytosolic calcium and activation of calcium-triggered cascades, (3) *oxidative stress* due to the generation of free radicals (including superoxide, hydroxyl radicals, and nitric oxide), and (4) mitochondrial energy failure. As noted above, any of these components may initiate the process, but all of them usually contribute to a greater or lesser degree because of their interrelationships.

As an example, consider a primary mitochondrial disorder due to an inherited defect in one of the mitochondrial respiratory chain enzymes. The resulting inefficient utilization of molecular oxygen by the respiratory chain leads to excessive production of oxygen free radicals. These in turn can cause further damage to the mitochondria and the plasma membrane through lipid peroxidation. Further mitochondrial failure leads to a decrease in the ATP available to supply the energy needed to maintain membrane polarization,

which decreases. This in combination with free radical–induced membrane damage leads to the opening of voltage-dependent membrane channels and other adverse effects on the membrane. The result is an increase in intracellular calcium. At the same time, the ATP-dependent mechanisms for sequestering cytosolic calcium fail. Excitotoxicity becomes a factor when the low resting membrane potential exposes the membrane to depolarization by what might otherwise be nondepolarizing ("background") levels of glutamate, further opening calcium channels. The high level of cytosolic calcium activates the enzymatic cascades that lead to necrosis or apoptosis (or both), depending on the rate and severity of calcium accumulation and on other unknown variables. Thus, the four mechanisms cited here are interrelated and self-perpetuating, and when one of them is activated, all the others may eventually be activated. Thus, treatments for all degenerative diseases have certain common themes, including inhibiting the formation of (or scavenging) free radicals, blocking glutamate receptors, and blocking calcium channels.

The clinical differences among the degenerative diseases are related to the neuronal populations involved, the order in which the cell-damaging mechanisms are activated, and the pace at which they proceed. The determinants of these factors have not been defined for most degenerative diseases. Typically, degenerative diseases are bilateral and symmetrical and affect several levels of the nervous system. The clinical correlate of degenerative diseases can be labeled *chronic, progressive,* or *diffuse.*

Neoplastic Disease

Any cell type in the nervous system can undergo neoplastic change and proliferate in an unrestrained manner to produce tumor formation. The fundamental causes of neoplasia are obscure, but certain genetic, infectious, physical, and chemical factors that can alter nuclear DNA have been implicated in many neoplasms. The stimuli for cells to progress through the cell cycle and to undergo division under the genetic control of oncogenes are normally balanced by the tendency to restrain this activity and, especially for cells with altered DNA, to self-destruct (programmed cell death) under the influence of tumor suppressor genes. If this balance is upset by mutagenic stimuli and there is overexpression of oncogenes or failure of expression of tumor suppressor genes, unrestrained cell proliferation may result. Examples of this are found in the most common primary neoplasm of the central nervous system, malignant astrocytoma. In a large percentage of these tumors, mutations of the *p53* tumor suppressor gene occur. Another subset of tumors of the same type features overexpression of a proto-oncogene, the *epidermal growth factor receptor (EGFR)* gene. A dominantly inherited genetic mutation of the tumor suppressor gene *NF-1* underlies the tendency to develop neoplasms in neurofibromatosis.

Cells of the nervous system vary greatly in their apparent potential to undergo neoplasia. There is a general correlation between the normal capacity of a cell to undergo cell division and its tendency to undergo neoplasia. Nerve cells normally are incapable of cell division after differentiation is complete, and neoplasms of nerve cells (neurocytomas) are extremely rare. Astrocytes are the most reactive cells of the central nervous system, and astrocytomas are the most common primary tumors of the central nervous system. Oligodendrogliomas and ependymomas occur less frequently. Because of the lymphoreticular lineage of microglial cells, tumors thought to be derived from them are no longer classified as a separate category but as lymphomas, according to the same scheme used for systemic lymphomas. The cells of the leptomeninges and the Schwann cells of nerve roots and peripheral nerves give rise to meningiomas and Schwannomas, respectively.

All these tumor types are believed to arise from relatively mature cell types that are normally present in the nervous system. For each cell type, however, tumors vary in the rapidity of growth, the likelihood of recurrence after surgery, and the length of patient survival. These factors correspond fairly well to the histologic malignancy of the tumor. Tumors of the central nervous system, except in extremely rare instances, do not metastasize outside the central nervous system; thus, one of the major criteria of malignancy in other forms of neoplasia does not apply to tumors of the central nervous system. The degree of malignancy of these tumors may be graded by considering the degree of pleomorphism (lack of uniformity of appearance and nuclear-cytoplasmic ratio) of tumor cells, frequency of mitotic figures, proliferation of tumor vessels, and necrosis of tumor tissue. Especially in infants and children, tumors of immature cellular elements (primitive neuroectodermal tumors) or tumors of cells not normally present in the nervous system (teratomas) are often seen. In children, one type of primitive neuroectodermal tumor, medulloblastoma of the cerebellum, is especially common and probably derived from immature cerebellar stem cells, with both neuroblastic and spongioblastic potential. In addition, systemic cancer can spread as secondary growth (metastasize) to the central nervous system.

A neoplastic mass progressively increases in size and alters the function of the region in which it lies. It may also alter the function of adjacent structures by compression or by the formation of edema around the primary mass. The cardinal topographic feature of a neoplasm, therefore, is its focal character. The clinical correlate of neoplastic disease may be labeled *chronic, progressive,* or *focal.* Not all progressively expanding (mass) lesions in the nervous system are composed of neoplastic cells. Blood clots (hematomas) and edema may be produced by different basic disease processes, and they represent common examples of nonneoplastic mass lesions.

Vascular Disease

Neurons deprived of metabolic support from the blood in the form of oxygen and glucose cease functioning in seconds and undergo pathologic change in minutes. Therefore, the hallmark of a vascular disease process is its *sudden onset.* Neurologic function is altered abruptly and usually maximally at the time of the initial insult. However, vascular disease is of several types, and although this is considered more fully in the section on the vascular system, certain general distinctions must be drawn here. The most common type of vascular disease is *infarct.* The chronologic, microscopic events that occur in a region of an infarct are as follows:

6 to 12 hours	Nerve cells may show acute swelling with staining pallor; as the process progresses, the neurons show the typical ischemic change described earlier in this chapter.
24 to 48 hours	Leukocytes appear from the blood vessels and begin migrating into the brain substance.
48 to 72 hours	Microglia proliferate and macrophages begin to appear and steadily increase in number up to the third week, after which they gradually diminish in number; the early stage corresponds only to the gross softening of the lesion (encephalomalacia) and then later to cyst formation.
4 to 5 days	In the region of astrocyte survival, the astrocytes begin to proliferate and show the changes described on page 76; this process goes on, reaching a peak at about 6 weeks, and a glial scar is formed.
2 weeks	During the second week, surviving capillaries also proliferate and take part in the attempted repair process.

The characteristic ischemic cell change is the hallmark of infarction. Although diffuse anoxic insults may occur, infarcts usually result from the cessation of the blood supply to a specific area of the nervous system and are generally *well localized.* The histologic events are primarily attempts at repair, and therefore the course of a patient's symptoms is generally one of stabilization or improvement. Clinical progression of symptoms, when it occurs, usually indicates cerebral edema or, more rarely, continuing infarction of adjacent tissue after the initial event (progressing stroke).

The second type of vascular disorder is *cerebral hemorrhage.* Instead of an interruption of vascular supply to an area, a blood vessel may rupture within the brain tissue, with localized accumulation of a blood clot in the neural tissue (an intraparenchymal hemorrhage). In this situation, both the symptoms and the pathologic changes would be expected to appear abruptly and to be focal, but because of the continuing pathologic changes that occur in response to a localized hemorrhage compressing neighboring tissue, progression might be seen.

A third type of vascular change occurs when a blood vessel, usually on the surface of the brain, suddenly ruptures and blood is spread over the surface of the brain and throughout the subarachnoid space (a subarachnoid hemorrhage). In this situation, the symptoms and pathologic changes are of abrupt onset but are diffusely distributed in the nervous system.

Although seemingly complex, the clinical correlates of vascular disease can be summarized as follows: (1) vascular disease is always acute in onset; (2) vascular disease may be focal or diffuse in distribution; (3) if diffuse in distribution, a condition such as a subarachnoid hemorrhage or a diffuse anoxic process is considered; and (4) if distribution is focal, the lesion is likely to be an infarct or a hemorrhage, and if it shows features of progression, it is likely to be a hemorrhage.

Inflammatory Disease

In response to microorganisms, immunologic reactions, and toxic chemicals, a complex series of events called the *inflammatory response* occurs in any system or organ of the body, including the nervous system. This response usually occurs rapidly but not suddenly and thus may be *subacute* in its temporal profile. The pathologic hallmark of the inflammatory response is the outpouring of white blood cells. In certain types of infections, especially bacterial, the major component of the exudate is polymorphonuclear leukocytes. In immunologic reactions and indolent infections, the predominant cells are mononuclear cells, especially lymphocytes.

Most inflammatory diseases of the central nervous system, particularly infections, are diffusely distributed either in the leptomeninges and cerebrospinal fluid (meningitis) or in the parenchyma of the brain (encephalitis). Other inflammatory diseases in the central nervous system are more likely to be focal, such as inflammation in the spinal cord, which occurs in multiple sclerosis. Inflammation also may occur in the peripheral nervous system, either in single nerves (mononeuritis) or in multiple nerves (polyneuritis). Infections sometimes localize in a specific area of the brain. In response to this localized area of inflammation, astrocytes proliferate in the surrounding tissue, and a wall of glial fibers is formed that limits the spread of the infection. The inflamed brain becomes softened and liquefied, and eventually there may be a cavity. This process is called *abscess formation.* A brain abscess can exert a mass effect and progressively expand and compress neighboring structures.

The clinical correlates of inflammatory disease may be summarized as follows: (1) the course is usually subacute and progressive; and (2) it may be diffuse in distribution, as in meningitis or encephalitis, or focal, as in an abscess, myelitis, or mononeuritis.

Immunologic Disease

The body may defend itself against various pathogens by developing an immunologic response to targeted proteins. These are usually agents foreign to the body, such as microorganisms; however, because of faulty recognition mechanisms, they may be a normal constituent of the body. The response may be mediated by humoral or cellular mechanisms or by both. The humoral mechanism involves the activation of B lymphocytes and the production of antibodies. Antibodies may affect neuronal function by binding to neurotransmitter receptor sites or to ion channels in the cell membrane of neurons. Cellular mechanisms involve the activation of T lymphocytes, which feature a variety of the functional classes, including cytotoxic T cells that may bind to the antigen-presenting target cell and destroy it. T lymphocytes also produce a group of soluble substances called *cytokines,* which include interleukins, interferons, and tumor necrosis factor. Cytokines may have a direct toxic effect on neurons, oligodendrocytes, and astrocytes and cause altered function in the nervous system.

The demyelination that occurs in multiple sclerosis and the failure of neuromuscular transmission that occurs in myasthenia gravis are examples of immunologic processes that result in neurologic disease. In acquired immunodeficiency syndrome (AIDS), nervous system macrophages are infected with the human immunodeficiency virus. These cells respond by releasing cytokines that indirectly attack neurons, producing some of the neurologic symptoms observed in patients with AIDS.

The scope of immunologic disease is undefined, but it is quite broad. Therefore, the clinical correlates of immunologic disease are variable. The symptoms produced are usually diffuse, but their pathophysiology may involve only selected cells or portions of cells in the nervous system or elsewhere in the body. Suppression or failure of normal immunologic mechanisms also predisposes the body to clinical infection by organisms ordinarily not pathogenic under conditions in which there is an intact immunologic system. The course of immunologic disease is usually one of subacute or chronic progression.

Toxic-Metabolic Disease

Various chemical agents, both endogenous and exogenous, may alter neuronal function. Vitamin deficiencies, genetic biochemical disorders, and the encephalopathies of kidney and liver disease are examples. When function is altered, the manifestations are almost always diffusely distributed throughout the nervous system. Depending on the nature of the specific toxin or metabolic abnormality, the effect may be exerted on the nervous system *acutely, subacutely,* or *chronically.* Pathologic changes vary with the noxious agent but may include such reactions as ischemia, edema, demyelination, and cell death.

Traumatic Disease

Trauma to the nervous system is almost always acute in onset, with a clearly identifiable precipitating event (automobile accident, fall, missile wound). Injuries to the peripheral nervous system are focal. Injuries to the central nervous system are frequently diffuse in their initial manifestations, presenting as the syndrome of concussion, which reflects widespread physiologic damage to the central nervous system. Traumatic damage is usually maximum at onset, and the natural course is one of resolution or improvement. This type of disturbance usually improves, until only the areas of severe anatomical damage (contusions, lacerations, hematomas) become clinically manifest, and the symptoms therefore become focal.

An important exception to the rule of trauma being maximal at onset and improving thereafter is that of delayed intracranial hemorrhage. The two most common forms are epidural and subdural hemorrhages. Epidural hematoma usually results from fracture of the temporal bone and a tear in the middle meningeal artery, which runs in a groove in the inner table of the skull. Bleeding occurs between the temporal bone and the dura mater. The bleeding is arterial and therefore brisk, and a significant hematoma accumulates within minutes to hours after the injury. Symptoms progress rapidly. Subdural hematomas result from tears in the veins that cross the subdural space in passing from the brain surface to the dural sinuses. The bleeding is venous and therefore under low pressure. The slow accumulation of blood with progression of symptoms may not manifest itself for days, weeks, or even months after the trauma.

The clinical correlates of traumatic disease may be summarized as follows: (1) in the peripheral nervous system, the symptoms are focal; in the central nervous system, they may be focal but are often diffuse at onset and later become focal; (2) the onset is usually acute; and (3) the usual course is one of improvement or stabilization, but the symptoms may be subacutely or chronically progressive.

The most important temporal and spatial features of the major disease categories are summarized in Table 3.

TABLE 3. *Summary of the most important temporal and spatial features of the major disease categories[a]*

	Acute	Subacute	Chronic
Focal	Vascular (infarct or intraparenchymal hemorrhage)	Inflammatory (abscess, myelitis)	Neoplasm
Diffuse	Vascular (subarachnoid hemorrhage, anoxia)	Inflammatory (meningitis, encephalitis)	Degenerative

[a]Metabolic and toxic disorders are usually diffuse and may follow any temporal profile, depending on the toxin or metabolite involved. Traumatic disorders are usually acute in onset, but their localization and course depend on the site of trauma, severity of trauma, and delayed complications. Immunologic disorders are usually diffuse but may involve selected cells or portions of cells. They are usually subacute or chronic and progressive. Almost all focal, progressive disorders are mass lesions; in general, the type of mass determines the course. For example, hemorrhages are acute, abscesses subacute, and neoplasms chronic. The basic distinction between *mass* and *nonmass* lesions carries extremely important therapeutic as well as diagnostic implications.

Clinical Problems ▪

For each of the following problems, identify the level, lateralization, presence of mass, and cause, as outlined in objective 5.

1. A 68-year-old, right-handed man noted heaviness in his left arm while reading a newspaper. He tried to stand up but could not support his weight on his left leg. He was able to call for help. When his wife came to the room, she noted that the left side of his face was sagging.

2. A 6-year-old, right-handed girl with known congenital heart disease began to complain of headaches. Several days later, the severity of the headaches increased, and she was noted to have a left hemiparesis and a left homonymous hemianopia.

3. A 54-year-old, right-handed woman noted some difficulty in expressing her thoughts. This difficulty was mild, and she paid little attention to it. Weeks later, she complained of clumsiness and weakness in her right arm and leg, but the results of an examination by her physician were considered to be normal. Headaches appeared several months later, along with increasing right-sided weakness. She was also aware of an inability to see the right half of the visual field with either eye.

4. A 46-year-old, left-handed woman suddenly noted the onset of a severe bitemporal-occipital headache. On lying down, she became violently ill, with nausea and vomiting. She complained of a stiff neck. She was taken immediately to the hospital, where she was noted to be somnolent but to respond appropriately when stimulated. She could move all four extremities with equal facility. Her level of consciousness deteriorated, and she became deeply comatose.

5. A 4-year-old, right-handed boy complained of a sore throat, chills, and fever. He was put to bed and given aspirin and fluids. The next morning, he complained of headache and an increasingly stiff neck. His temperature was 105°F (40.5°C). When seen at a physician's office later that afternoon, he was difficult to arouse. He was confused and delirious when stimulated. He held his neck rigid but moved his extremities on command.

6. A 50-year-old, right-handed woman, formerly an executive secretary for a local banker, underwent neurologic evaluation because she had had a marked personality change during the last several months. Her memory was poor. She could no longer do even simple calculations, and she had difficulty in following commands. She seemed ill informed about current events and no longer seemed interested in her personal appearance. Results of the rest of the examination were unremarkable.

7. A 54-year-old, right-handed woman suddenly became dizzy, with nausea and vomiting. Examination revealed dysarthria, difficulty in swallowing (with weakness of the left palate), loss of pinprick sensation over the left side of the face and the right side of the body, and marked ataxia on using the left extremities.

8. A 62-year-old, right-handed man began to note generalized muscle cramps, which he attributed to a charley horse. In the ensuing months, he became aware of weakness in his arms and legs and some difficulty in speaking and swallowing. Examination revealed weakness and atrophy and fasciculations of nearly all muscle groups, with no sensory changes. The sign of Babinski was present bilaterally.

9. A 68-year-old, right-handed man noted the sudden onset of severe pain in the chest and abdomen. Almost immediately after the pain, he became weak and was unable to support any weight on his right leg. Examination revealed marked weak-

ness of the right lower extremity, with a decrease in the perception of pinprick in the left leg to about the level of the umbilicus.

10. A 46-year-old, right-handed woman noted (in the absence of back pain) gradually increasing pain and numbness extending down her right leg. After these symptoms had been present for 12 months, she consulted her physician, who found slight weakness of the plantar-flexor muscles, absent ankle reflex, and decreased sensation in the posterior aspect of the calf—all on the right side.

Additional Reading ■

Adams, J. H., and Duchen, L. W. (eds.). *Greenfield's Neuropathology* (5th ed.). New York: Oxford University Press, 1992.

Goldstein, G. W., and Betz, A. L. The blood–brain barrier. *Sci. Am.* 255:74, Sept. 1986.

Haymaker, W., and Adams, R. D. *Histology and Histopathology of the Nervous System.* Springfield, Ill.: Charles C Thomas, 1982.

Hirano, A. (ed.). *Color Atlas of Pathology of the Nervous System* (2nd ed.). New York: Igaku-Shoin, 1988.

Hirano, A. *A Guide to Neuropathology.* New York: Igaku-Shoin, 1981.

Okazaki, H. *Fundamentals of Neuropathology: Morphologic Basis of Neurologic Disorders* (2nd ed.). New York: Igaku-Shoin, 1989.

Poirier, J., Gray, F., and Escourolle, R. *Manual of Basic Neuropathology* (3rd ed.). Philadelphia: W. B. Saunders, 1990.

Diagnosis of Neurologic Disorders: Transient Disorders and Neurophysiology

Objectives

1. Describe cell membrane and ion channel structure.
2. Describe and distinguish between neurotransmitters and neuromodulators in their interactions with ion channels.
3. Describe the mechanism by which the resting potential is generated and maintained.
4. List the characteristics of a local potential, and name three examples.
5. Describe the features of an action potential and the associated ionic changes.
6. Describe the events in synaptic transmission.
7. Define the following terms: depolarization, steady state, equilibrium potential, sodium pump, threshold, afterpotential, accommodation, refractory period, saltatory conduction, excitatory postsynaptic potential, end-plate potential, conductance, active transport, spatial summation, presynaptic inhibition, and denervation hypersensitivity.
8. Describe the effect of anoxia and of an alteration in extracellular sodium, potassium, or calcium on the resting and action potentials. List which of these conditions could result in excessive electrical discharges.

Introduction

Knowing the location and function of the structural components of the nervous system presented in Chapter 3 permits localization of the site of a lesion. The temporal profile of the major types of disease, as presented in Chapter 4, assists in identifying the cause of the disorder. However, one temporal profile has not yet been considered, that of the *transient* or rapidly reversible abnormality. Many diseases that produce signs or symptoms of brief duration may not produce destructive changes in cells and may occur without demonstrable histologic abnormality of the involved structures. To understand transient manifestations of disease, it is necessary to understand the mechanism by which the cells of the nervous system process information and to understand their physiology. Transient alterations in the physiology of the cells cause transient symptoms and signs. This chapter provides an introduction to the physiology of neurons, axons, and muscle fibers, which is the basis for information transmission in the central and peripheral neural structures and for the transient symptoms and signs that accompany disease states.

The major function of the nervous system is the transmission, storage, and processing of information. This function is accomplished by the generation, conduction, and integration of electrical activity and by the synthesis and release of chemical agents.

Information is conducted from one region to another as electrical activity, commonly known as nerve impulses, which are *generated* by neuronal cell bodies or axons and *conducted* by axons. Information is *transmitted* between cells by neurochemical agents that convey the signals from one cell to the next. Information is *integrated* by the interaction of electrical activity in single cells and in groups of cells. Although this chapter discusses only the physiology of single cells, it must be remembered that the activity of the central and peripheral nervous systems never depends on the activity of a single neuron or axon but is always mediated by a group of cells or nerve fibers. Information is represented in the nervous system by a change in activity in a group of cells or fibers as they respond to some change in their input. The interactions of neurons in large groups are considered in later sections.

Overview   ■

Normal function in a single neuron as it participates in the processing of information is manifested as electrical potentials. These potentials are called membrane potentials. The *membrane potential* is the difference in electrical potential between the inside and the outside of a cell. All neurons, axons, and muscle fibers have a membrane potential. Membrane potentials include resting potentials, action potentials, and local potentials such as synaptic potentials, generator (or receptor) potentials, and electrotonic potentials. All membrane potentials result from ion flow through channels in the membrane.

Cell membranes separate ions into different concentrations on the exterior and interior of the cell. These concentration differences produce an electrical potential across the membrane, the *membrane potential.*

The concentration gradients are maintained by the cell membrane, a lipid bilayer that is relatively impermeable to sodium, potassium, chloride, and calcium ions, the ions involved in electrophysiologic activity and signal transmission. The concentration of sodium, calcium, and chloride ions is higher extracellularly and that of potassium ions and impermeable anions (A^-) is higher intracellularly (Table 1). The *equilibrium potential* of each ion is the voltage difference across the membrane that exactly offsets the tendency of the ion to move down its concentration gradient.

Ions can move across the cell membrane passively through *ion channels* or by adenosine triphosphate (ATP)-dependent binding to carrier molecules. Some ion channels are open at rest, but most open (or close) in response to stimuli, including changes in membrane potential (*voltage-gated* ion channels), binding of a neurotransmitter to a postsynaptic receptor (*ligand-gated* channels), or chemical changes in the cytoplasm (*chemical-gated* ion channels). The opening of a channel for a particular ion brings the membrane potential toward the equilibrium potential of that ion.

Thus, at a given time, the membrane potential is determined by the concentration gradient of the ions (which determines their respective equilibrium potentials) and by any changes in the permeability to individual ions across the membrane (Fig. 1). The survival and excitability of the cell depend on the membrane potential. Maintaining this potential requires energy metabolism for the ATP-dependent *sodium-potassium pump.*

TABLE 1. *Relative ionic concentrations in mammalian neurons*

	Sodium	Potassium	Chloride	Calcium
Internal concentration	Low	High	Low	High
External concentration	High	Low	High	Low
Resting permeability	Low	High	Moderate	Low

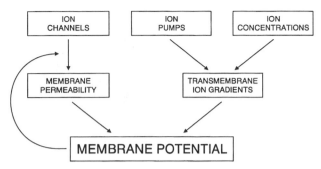

FIG. 1. Variables that determine the membrane potential. Transmembrane ion gradients determine the equilibrium potential of a particular ion. The transmembrane gradients depend on the activity of adenosine triphosphate (ATP)-driven ion pumps and the buffering effects of the astrocytes on extracellular fluid composition. Membrane permeability to a particular ion depends on the opening of specific ion channels. This opening can be triggered by voltage (voltage-gated channels), neurotransmitters (ligand-gated channels), or intracellular chemicals such as calcium, ATP, or cyclic nucleotides (chemically gated channels). Increased membrane permeability to a given ion (the opening of the ion channel) brings the membrane potential toward the equilibrium potential of this ion.

The *resting potential* is the baseline level of the membrane potential when the cell is at rest and not processing information. This potential depends primarily on the potassium channel. When a cell is active in the processing of information, the membrane potential varies. These variations are either local potentials or action potentials (Table 2).

Action potentials are the electrical signals, or nerve impulses, by which information is conducted from one area to another within a single cell. The action potential is an all-or-none change in membrane potential in the body or axon of a neuron or within a muscle fiber. It either occurs fully or not at all and depends on the sodium channel. The function of action potentials is to conduct bits of information from one place to another. The action potential is initiated by one form of local potential, the electrotonic potential.

Local potentials are localized changes in a number of ion channels that change the membrane potential in response to stimuli. They are graded signals whose size varies in proportion to the size of the stimulus. They remain localized in the area of the cell in which they are generated; that is, they do not spread to involve the entire cell. Local potentials can

TABLE 2. *Characteristics of different membrane potentials*

	Local potentials			
Characteristic	Generator potential	Synaptic potential	Electrotonic potential	Action potential
Graded and localized	+	+	+	−
All-or-none spread	−	−	−	+
Active membrane channel	Na$^+$, K$^+$	Na$^+$, Ca^{2+}, K$^+$, Cl$^-$	None	Na$^+$, K$^+$, sometimes Ca^{2+}
Initiated by	Sensory stimulus	Neurotransmitter	Generator, synaptic, or action potentials	Electrotonic potential

be summated and integrated by single cells and are an integral part of the processing of information by the nervous system. Changes in ion channels underlying local potentials are generated (1) by a neurochemical transmitter; (2) by synaptic potentials and generator potentials; or (3) by the flow of electrical current, the electrotonic potentials.

Generator, or receptor, potentials occur in receptors—those neural structures in the body, such as the touch receptors in the skin or the light receptors in the eye, that respond to specific stimuli. Receptor potentials are also local potentials caused by opening of ion channels and are localized and graded. They can generate electrotonic potentials and thereby initiate action potentials (Fig. 2).

A localized change in membrane potential results in current flow to surrounding areas of membrane. This current flow produces a small change in the membrane potential of adjacent areas. This change is called an *electrotonic potential.*

Synaptic potentials are variations of the membrane potential that occur at *synapses,* the specialized areas where adjacent neurons are in intimate contact. Synaptic potentials are local potentials arising from postsynaptic ion channels opening in response to the action of a neurotransmitter released by presynaptic cells. Neurotransmitters transmit information from one cell to another by converting the electrical signal (action potential) into a chemical signal (neurotransmitter release) and then back into an electrical signal (synaptic potential or membrane potential change). In turn, synaptic potentials produce electrotonic potentials, which can then initiate another action potential.

Chemical synapses are the most common form of communication between neurons. They consist of a presynaptic axon terminal and a postsynaptic element, which can be a dendrite, cell body, or axon of the target neuron. The presynaptic terminal contains the chemical transmitter, which is stored in synaptic vesicles. The arrival of an action potential produces an influx of calcium ions into the presynaptic terminal, and this triggers the vesicular release of the chemical transmitter, an example of the process known as *exocytosis.* Neurochemical transmitters act on different types of postsynaptic receptors to produce two different types of responses: (1) The classic responses (referred to as classic neurotransmission) are the postsynaptic potentials described above. (2) Neurochemicals may also produce changes in the excitability and responses of the postsynaptic neuron to other neurotransmitters, a process called *neuromodulation.*

Transient alterations in function are the result of reversible disturbances in neuronal excitability, the ability to propagate action potentials, or communication via chemical synapses. Transient disorders reflect abnor-

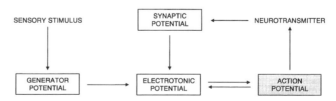

FIG. 2. Local potentials and triggering of the action potential. Three types of local potentials are (1) receptor (or generator) potential, triggered by the action of a sensory stimulus on a sensory receptor; (2) synaptic potential, triggered by the action of a neurotransmitter; and (3) electrotonic potential, which consists of the passive movement of charges according to the cable properties of a membrane. Both the generator and synaptic potentials give rise to electrotonic potentials, which depolarize the membrane to threshold for triggering an action potential. The action potential is a regenerating depolarizing stimulus that, via electrotonic potentials, propagates over a distance without decrement in its amplitude.

malities in resting, local, or action potentials due to the failure of ion pumps to maintain electrochemical gradients, impaired function of ion channels, or alterations in the ionic composition of the extracellular fluid. Transient disorders may be generalized or focal and be manifested by excessive activity, decreased activity, or both.

Cell Membrane ■

Transmembrane Ion Gradients

The plasma membrane is a lipid bilayer with the polar (hydrophilic) heads facing outward and the nonpolar (hydrophobic) tails extending to the middle of the bilayer. Embedded in this lipid bilayer are protein macromolecules, including ion channels, receptors, and ionic pumps, that are in contact with both the extracellular fluid and the cytoplasm.

The lipid bilayer is relatively impermeable to water-soluble molecules, including ions such as sodium (Na^+), potassium (K^+), chloride (Cl^-), and calcium (Ca^{2+}). These ions are involved in electrophysiologic activity and signal transmission. The concentrations of sodium, chloride, and calcium are higher extracellularly, and the concentrations of potassium and impermeable anions (A^-) are higher intracellularly (Fig. 3). Maintenance of transmembrane ion concentration depends on the balance between (1) *passive* diffusion of ions across *ion channels*, or "pores," of the membrane, driven by their concentration gradient; and (2) *active*, energy (ATP)-dependent trans-

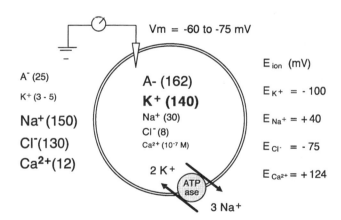

FIG. 3. Transmembrane ion concentrations, equilibrium potential, and resting membrane potential. The semipermeable cell membrane determines a differential distribution of ions in the intracellular and extracellular compartments. Sodium and chloride predominate extracellularly, and potassium and nondiffusible ions (A^-) predominate intracellularly. Transmembrane ion composition is maintained by the activity of ATP-dependent pumps, particularly sodium-potassium adenosine triphosphatase (ATPase). The different transmembrane concentrations of diffusible ions determine the equilibrium potential of each ion (E_{ion}). The contribution of each ion to the membrane potential depends on the permeability of the membrane for that particular ion. Increased permeability to an ion brings the membrane potential toward the equilibrium potential of that ion. At rest, the membrane is predominantly, but not exclusively, permeable to potassium. There is continuous leakage of potassium out of the cell and of sodium into the cell, driven by both their concentration gradient and electrical gradient. The ion gradient is restituted by the activity of sodium-potassium ATPase, which is electrogenic (as it exchanges two potassium for three sodium ions) and contributes to the maintenance of the resting potential.

port of ions against their concentration gradient, via ATP-driven *ion pumps.* In the central nervous system, astrocytes provide a buffer system to prevent excessive accumulation of extracellular potassium ions.

Active Transport

Nerve and muscle cells obtain energy from glucose and oxygen via the glycolytic pathways, the Krebs cycle, and the electron transport system. These pathways provide the energy for normal cell function in the form of ATP. ATP is partly consumed in generating the resting potential by a mechanism in the membrane, which moves potassium in and sodium out of the cell, with slightly more sodium being moved than potassium. This movement is referred to as *active transport,* and the system through which it occurs is the *sodium pump.* The sodium pump moves sodium out of the cell and potassium into the cell against their concentration gradients. Chloride moves out of the cell passively with sodium.

Equilibrium Potential

The diffusible ions (sodium, potassium, and chloride, but not calcium) tend to move across the cell membrane according to their concentration gradient. The molecular motion of ions is a source of energy known as the *diffusion pressure.* For example, the intracellular concentration of potassium is 30 times higher than the extracellular concentration, $[K^+]_o$; therefore, potassium tends to diffuse from intracellular to extracellular fluid. The opposite occurs with sodium. As ions diffuse across the cell membrane, a separation of charges develops because the nondiffusible negatively charged intracellular ions (principally proteins) have a charge opposite that of the diffusible ions. Two regions that accumulate different charges have an electrical potential difference. The voltage that develops as a diffusible ion moves across the membrane produces an *electrical pressure* that opposes the movement of the ion. The net ionic movement continues until *the electrical pressure equals the diffusion pressure.* At this time, the system is in equilibrium. At equilibrium, random ionic movement continues, but no net movement of ions occurs.

The electrical potential that develops across the membrane at equilibrium is called the *equilibrium potential,* and this potential is different for each ion. The equilibrium potential of a ion (E_{ion}) is the voltage difference across the membrane that exactly offsets the diffusion pressure of an ion to move down its concentration gradient. Therefore, the equilibrium potential is proportional to the difference between the concentration of the ion in the extracellular fluid and the concentration in the intracellular fluid. An algebraic representation of the equilibrium potential can be derived because the physical determinants of the diffusion pressure and electrical pressure expressed are known. The final equation is the *Nernst equation.*

Electrical pressure is defined by:

$$W_e = E_m \cdot Z_i \cdot F$$

in which W_e = electrical pressure (work required to move an ion against a voltage)

E_m = absolute membrane potential

Z_i = valence (number of charges on the ion)

F = faraday (number of coulombs per mol of ion)

Diffusion pressure is defined by:

$$W_d = R \cdot T \cdot (\ln[C]_{hi} - \ln[C]_{lo})$$

in which W_d = diffusion pressure (work required to move an ion against a concentration gradient)

R = universal gas constant

T = absolute temperature

$\ln$ = natural logarithm

$[C]_{hi}$ = ion concentration on the more concentrated side of the membrane

$[C]_{lo}$ = ion concentration on the less concentrated side

At equilibrium:

$$W_e = W_d$$

and therefore

$$E_m \cdot Z_i \cdot F = R \cdot T \cdot (\ln[C]_{hi} - \ln[C]_{lo})$$

By rearrangement, the equilibrium potential is:

$$E_m = \frac{R \cdot T}{F \cdot Z_i} \cdot \ln \left(\frac{[C]_{hi}}{[C]_{lo}} \right)$$

The *Nernst equation* is an important relationship that defines the equilibrium potential, E_m, inside the cell for any ion in terms of its concentration on the two sides of a membrane. From the Nernst equation, the polarity of the potential depends on whether the ion is an anion or a cation: E_m for a cation will be (+) on the low concentration side, and E_m for an anion will be (−) on the low concentration side. By substituting for the constants at room temperature, converting to a base 10 logarithm, and converting to millivolts, we get a useful form of the equation:

$$E_m = 58 \log_{10} \frac{[C]_{hi}}{[C]_{lo}} \text{ for cations}$$

For example:

$$E_{na} = 58 \log_{10} \frac{[140]}{[25]} = 43.3$$

$$E_m = 58 \log_{10} \frac{[C]_{hi}}{[C]_{lo}} \text{ for anions}$$

We may use these equations to calculate the equilibrium potential for any ion if we know the concentrations of that ion on the two sides of the membrane. This potential only develops if the membrane is permeable to the ion.

The approximate neuronal equilibrium potentials of the major ions are $K^+ = -100$ mV, $Na^+ = +40$ mV, $Cl^- = -75$ mV, $Ca^{2+} = +124$ mV (Fig. 3).

Membrane Potential

The contribution of a given ion to the actual voltage developed across the membrane with unequal concentrations of that ion depends not only on its concentration gradient but also on the *permeability* (P) of the membrane to that ion. Permeability is the ease with which

an ion diffuses across the membrane and is a reflection of the probability that the membrane channel that conducts the ion will open. For example, an ion with a high concentration gradient that has very low permeability (for example, calcium) does not contribute to the resting membrane potential. Algebraically, for potassium in which P_K = potassium permeability:

$$E_k = \frac{R \cdot T}{F \cdot Z_i} \cdot \ln \frac{P_K \cdot [K+]_o}{P_K \cdot [K+]_i}$$

If a membrane is permeable to multiple ions that are present in differing concentrations on either side of the membrane, the resultant membrane potential is a function of the concentrations of each of the ions and of their relative permeabilities. The *Goldman equation* combines these factors for the major ions that influence the membrane potential in nerve and muscle cells:

$$E_m = \frac{R \cdot T}{F \cdot Z_i} \cdot$$

$$\ln \frac{P_K \cdot [K+]_o + P_{Na} \cdot [Na^+]_o + P_{Cl} \cdot [Cl^-]_i}{P_K \cdot [K+]_i + P_{Na} \cdot [Na^+]_i + P_{Cl} \cdot [Cl^-]_o}$$

The Goldman equation permits the calculation of the membrane potential for various neurons or muscle fibers. Such calculations, on the basis of the actual ionic concentrations and ionic permeabilities, agree with measurements of these values in living cells.

These equations also show that a change in either ionic permeability or ionic concentrations can alter membrane potential. If the *concentration gradient* of an ion is reduced, there will be a lower equilibrium potential for that ion. If the resting membrane potential is determined by the equilibrium potential of that ion, the resting potential will decrease. In contrast, if the *permeability* for an ion is increased by opening of channels for that ion, the membrane potential will approach the equilibrium potential of that ion, and it may increase or decrease, depending on whether the membrane potential is above or below the equilibrium potential. The movements of ions that occur with normal cellular activity are not sufficient to produce significant concentration changes; therefore, membrane potential fluctuations are normally due to permeability changes caused by channel opening and closing.

Increased permeability (that is, opening of the channel) to a particular ion brings the membrane potential toward the equilibrium potential of that ion.

In an electrical model of the membrane, the concentration ratios of the different ions are represented by their respective *equilibrium potentials* (E_{Na}, E_k, E_{cl}); their ionic permeabilities are represented by their respective *conductances* (G). The conductance (that is, the reciprocal of the resistance) for a particular ion is the sum of the conductances of all the open channels permeable to that ion. The movement of ions across the membrane is expressed as an *ion current*. By Ohm's law, this current depends on two factors: the conductance of the ion and the *driving force* for the ion. The driving force is the difference between the membrane potential and the equilibrium potential of that ion.

Ion Channels

Ion channels are intrinsic membrane proteins that form hydrophilic pores (aqueous pathways) through the lipid bilayer membrane. They allow the passive flow of selected ions across the membrane on the basis of the electrochemical gradients of the ion and the physical properties of the ion channel. Most channels belong to one of several superfamilies of homologous proteins with great heterogeneity in amino acid composition. They are defined on the basis of their ion selectivity, conductance, gating, kinetics, and pharmacology. In general, the transmembrane portion of the protein forms the "pore," and the specific amino acids in the region of the pore determine ion selectivity, conductance, and voltage sensitivity of the channel. Amino acids in the extracellular or intracellular portion (or both) of the channel protein determine the gating mechanism and the kinetics of inactivation.

Ion channels vary in their selectivity; some are permeable to cations (sodium, potassium, and calcium) and others to anions (primarily chloride). The open state predominates in the resting membrane for a few channels; these are mostly the potassium channels responsible for the resting membrane potential (see below). Most ion channels are *gated;* that is, they open in response to specific stimuli. According to their gating stimuli, ion channels can be subdivided into (1) *voltage-gated* channels, which respond to changes in membrane potential; (2) *ligand-gated* channels, which respond to the binding of a neurotransmitter to the channel molecular complex; and (3) *chemically gated* channels, which respond to intracellular molecules such as ATP, ions (particularly calcium), and cyclic nucleotides. Important examples of chemically gated channels include the *cyclic nucleotide-gated* channels found in many sensory receptors (for example, photoreceptors in the retina). Mechanoreceptors are activated by mechanical distortion of the cell membrane and are sometimes referred to as *stretch-activated* channels. Gating stimuli may interact in some channels. For example, the ion permeability of some ligand-gated channels is affected by membrane voltage or intracellular factors (or both).

Voltage-gated channels are critical for neuronal function. They control excitability, spontaneous neuronal activity, generation and conduction of action potentials, and neurotransmitter release. Sensitivity to voltage is due to a voltage sensor at the pore. A region of the pore acts as a selectivity filter, which regulates ion permeability according to the size and molecular structure of the ion. The range of voltage for activation and the rate of activation (opening) and inactivation (closing) are important variables in voltage-gated channels.

Voltage-gated cation channels are responsible for the maintenance of neuronal excitability, generation of action potentials, and neurotransmitter release (Table 3). They are members of a superfamily of proteins with a common basic structure consisting of a principal subunit (α) and one or more auxiliary

TABLE 3. *Examples of ion channels*

Ion channel	Equilibrium potential	Location	Function
Voltage-gated			
Na+	+35	Node of Ranvier	Initiation and conduction of action potential
		Axon hillock	
K+	−90	Diffuse along internode	Repolarization of action potential
		Diffuse in neurons	Decrease neuronal excitability and discharge
Ca2+	+200	Dendrite	Slow depolarization
		Soma	Burst firing
			Oscillatory firing
		Axon terminal	Neurotransmitter release
Chemical-gated	−75	Dendrite	Synaptic inhibition
Cl− (GABA)		Soma	
Cation channel (L-glutamate, acetylcholine)	0	Dendrite	Synaptic excitation

GABA, γ-aminobutyric acid.

subunits. The amino acid composition of the α subunit determines ion selectivity, voltage sensitivity, and inactivation kinetics of the channel.

Voltage-gated sodium channels are critical for the generation and transmission of information in the nervous system by action potentials. In neurons, sodium channels are concentrated in the initial segment of the axon (the site of generation of action potentials) and in the nodes of Ranvier (involved in rapid conduction of action potentials). In muscle, these channels participate in excitation-contraction coupling.

There are several varieties of voltage-gated calcium channels, and they have different distributions, physiology, pharmacology, and functions (Table 4). Calcium influx occurs not only through voltage-gated channels but also through ligand-gated and cyclic nucleotide-gated channels. Calcium ions are important in the regulation of numerous processes in neurons, including modulation of neuronal firing pattern, neurotransmitter release, signal transduction, enzyme activation, intracellular transport, intermediate metabolism, and gene expression. Intracellular calcium is also necessary for muscle contraction and glandular secretion. These functions depend on levels of calcium in the cytosol that are determined by the calcium influx through various channels, release from intracellular stores (particularly the endoplasmic reticulum), and counterbalancing active mechanisms of reuptake and extrusion.

Large numbers of voltage-gated potassium channels determine much of the pattern of activity generated by neurons. They are responsible primarily for the resting membrane potential, repolarization of the action potential, and control of the probability of generation of repetitive action potentials.

Ligand-gated channels open in response to the binding of neurotransmitters (Fig. 4). They include (1) nonselective cation channels permeable to sodium, potassium, and, in some cases, calcium; and (2) anion channels permeable to chloride. These channels are discussed in relation to synaptic transmission.

Neuronal Excitability

Neuronal excitability is defined as the ability of the neuron to generate and transmit *action potentials*. It depends on the membrane potential, which determines the gating of the sodium channels. The membrane potential depends on the transmembrane ion concentration (which determines the equilibrium potential)

TABLE 4. *Voltage-gated calcium channels*

Channel type	Location	Function
T	Apical dendrites	Rhythmic firing
L	Soma, dendritic shafts, and spines	Slow action potentials
	Skeletal muscle	Excitation-contraction coupling
N	Synaptic terminals	Neurotransmitter release
P/Q	Synaptic terminals	Neurotransmitter release
	Dendritic shafts and spines	Persistent depolarization

and ion permeability. Increased permeability to an ion moves the membrane potential toward the equilibrium potential of that ion. In the absence of a stimulus, the membrane potential of the neuron, or *resting membrane potential,* is dominated by its permeability to potassium, whose channels are open; therefore, this potential varies between −60 and −80 mV. Because the threshold for opening voltage-gated sodium channels that are needed to trigger and propagate action potentials is approximately −50 to −55 mV, any change of the membrane potential in this direction will increase the probability of triggering an action potential. An

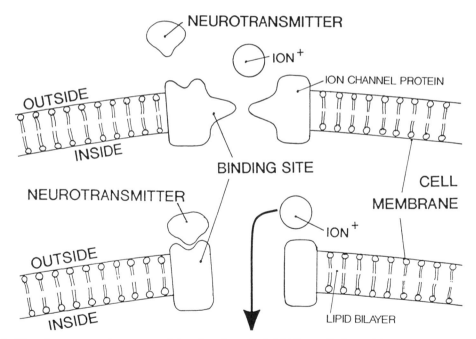

FIG. 4. The plasma membrane consists of a phospholipid bilayer that provides a barrier to the passage of water-soluble molecules, including ions. Passage of ions across the membrane depends on the presence of transmembrane proteins, including ion channels and ion pumps. Ion channels provide an aqueous pore for the passage of ions across the membrane, according to their concentration gradients. The opening of an ion channel, or pore, may be triggered, or gated, by several stimuli, such as voltage (voltage-gated channel) or neurotransmitters (ligand-gated channel). In the example shown here, a neurotransmitter (such as glutamate) binds to a specific ligand-gated cation channel, and this produces a change in the spatial configuration of the channel protein, allowing the pore to open and the cation to pass through the membrane. Changes in the amino acid composition of the ion channel protein affects its ion selectivity, gating mechanism, and kinetics of channel opening (activation) and closing (inactivation).

TABLE 5. *Ionic basis of local potentials*

Ion	Equilibrium potential, mV	Effect of increased permeability on membrane potential	Examples of local potentials
Na^+	+40	Depolarization	Generator potentials Excitatory postsynaptic potential
Ca^{2+}	+200	Depolarization	Excitatory postsynaptic potential
K^+	−90	Hyperpolarization	Inhibitory postsynaptic potential
Cl^-	−75	Hyperpolarization, depolarization, or no change	Inhibitory postsynaptic potential

increase in membrane permeability to sodium or calcium increases excitability, and an increase in permeability to potassium or chloride will decrease excitability (Table 5).

Resting Potential

The resting potential is the *absolute difference* in electrical potential between the inside and the outside of an inactive neuron, axon, or muscle fiber. If an electrical connection is made between the inside and the outside of a neuron, the cell acts as a battery and an electrical current will flow. The potential is generally between 60 and 80 mV, with the inside of the cell *negative* with respect to the outside. The resting potential can be measured directly by using a microelectrode. The tip of such an electrode must be less than 1 μm in diameter to be inserted into a nerve or muscle cell. By connecting the microelectrode to an appropriate amplifier, the membrane potential can be recorded and displayed on an oscilloscope (Fig. 5).

The oscilloscope registers the potential difference between the two electrical inputs and is displayed as a vertical deflection of a spot of light that moves continuously from left to right across the cathode ray tube of the oscil-

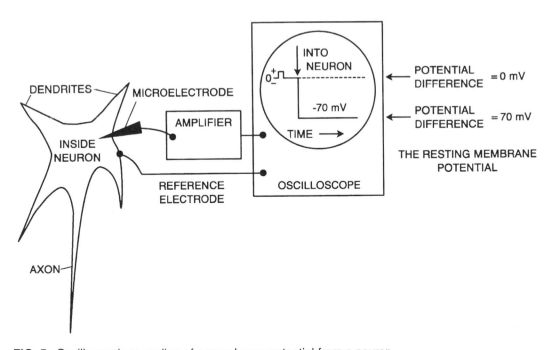

FIG. 5. Oscilloscopic recording of a membrane potential from a neuron.

loscope. A negative membrane potential is registered as a downward deflection; thus, when a microelectrode enters a neuron or muscle fiber, the oscilloscope beam moves down to a new position.

The resting membrane potential is the transmembrane voltage at which there is no net flow of current across the membrane. Its value determines spontaneous neuronal activity and neuronal activity in response to extrinsic input. Because the resting potential is the absolute difference in potential between the inside and the outside of the cell, it represents transmembrane polarity. A decrease in the value of the resting membrane potential means *less negativity* inside the cell and the membrane potential moves toward zero; this constitutes *depolarization*. When the membrane potential becomes more negative than the value of the resting potential, the potential moves away from zero; this is *hyperpolarization.*

The resting membrane potential depends on two factors: (1) the presence of *leak ion channels* open at rest with markedly different permeabilities to sodium and potassium, making the cell membrane a *semipermeable membrane;* and (2) the presence of *energy-dependent pumps,* particularly the sodium-potassium pump. At rest, there is a continuous "leak" of potassium outward and of sodium inward across the membrane. Cells at rest have a permeability to sodium ions that ranges from 1% to 10% of their permeability to potassium. Thus, in the absence of synaptic activity, the membrane potential is dominated by its high permeability to potassium, and the membrane potential is drawn toward the equilibrium potential of this ion (−100 mV). However, the membrane at rest is also permeable to sodium and chloride, so that the membrane potential is also pulled toward the equilibrium potential of these ions. The resting potential varies among different types of neurons, but it is typically −60 to −80 mV. The continuous leaking of potassium outward and sodium inward is balanced by the activity of the sodium-potassium pump.

Steady State

Potassium diffuses through the membrane most readily because potassium channels are more open and potassium conductance is much higher than that of other ions. Therefore, potassium is the largest source of separation of positive and negative charges (voltage) as it diffuses out and leaves the large anions behind. This is illustrated schematically in Fig. 6.

Small amounts of sodium entering the cells, driven by both electrical and chemical forces, tend to depolarize the membrane. As a result, potassium is no longer in equilibrium and leaves the cell. Thus, the cell is not in equilibrium but in a steady state dependent on metabolic energy. In this *steady state,* the small outward potassium leak must be exactly equal in magnitude to the rate at which potassium is transported into the cell. The same is true also for sodium. In this condition, the net movement of each ion across the membrane is zero, an exact description of the resting membrane potential.

Sodium Pump

The sodium pump (Na-K adenosine triphosphatase [ATPase]) maintains the intracellular concentrations of sodium and potassium despite their constant leaking through the membrane. The sodium-potassium pump transports three sodium ions out of the cell for every two potassium ions carried into the cell. Because the pump is not electrically neutral, it contributes directly to the resting potential; that is, it is *electrogenic.* The contribution of the sodium-potassium pump steady state to the resting potential is approximately −11 mV.

The cell membrane at rest is permeable also to chloride ions. In most membranes, chloride reaches an equilibrium simply by adjustment of its internal concentration to maintain electroneutrality, without affecting the steady-state membrane potential.

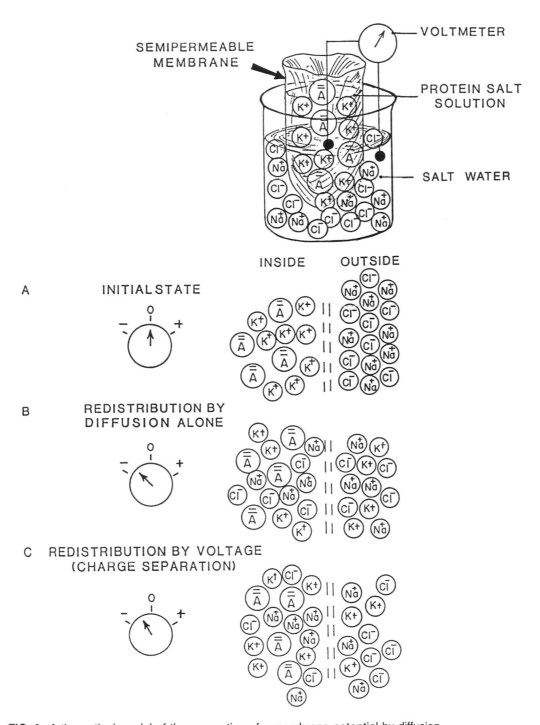

FIG. 6. A theoretical model of the generation of a membrane potential by diffusion across a semipermeable membrane. **A:** Equal amounts of anions and cations are dissolved on each side of the membrane—no voltage gradient. The membrane is permeable to all ions except large anions (A). **B:** K⁺, Na⁺, and Cl⁻ redistribute themselves solely by diffusion; this results in a charge separation, with greater negativity inside. **C:** Electrical pressure due to charge separation and diffusion pressure due to concentration differences are balanced at the resting membrane potential.

Role of Extracellular Calcium

The external surface of the cell membrane contains a high density of negative charges because of the presence of glycoprotein residues. This produces a local negative potential that contributes to the resting membrane potential. Divalent ions, such as extracellular calcium, alter the transmembrane potential by neutralizing this local, negative surface potential. Neutralizing the surface potential increases the contribution of the transmembrane potential to the resting potential, and this increases the threshold for opening voltage-gated sodium channels. This explains the stabilizing effect of extracellular calcium on membrane excitability and the presence of increased spontaneous activity (tetany) that occurs in patients with hypocalcemia or alkalosis.

Role of Glial Cells

Astrocytes are important in controlling the extracellular concentration of potassium. Astrocytes are highly permeable to potassium and are interconnected with each other by gap junctions. When the extracellular concentration of potassium increases because of neuronal activity, astrocytes incorporate potassium and transfer it from one cell to another through gap junctions. This prevents the extracellular accumulation of potassium and maintains neuronal excitability. This is referred to as *spatial buffering* of extracellular potassium.

Local Potentials

In a normal nerve cell or muscle cell with adequate sources of oxygen and glucose, the resting potential is maintained at a stable, relatively unchanging level. However, the resting potential readily changes in response to stimuli. The membrane potential can change from the resting state in only two ways. It can either become more negative inside, *hyperpolarization,* or less negative inside, *depolarization.* Even if the membrane potential reverses, so that the inside becomes positive with respect to the outside, it is still referred to as depolarization, because the potential is less negative than the resting potential.

The changes in the membrane potential that occur with anoxia or a change in the concentration of the ions on either side of the membrane are relatively long lasting (minutes to hours). In contrast, rapid changes (seconds or less) can occur in response to electrical, mechanical, or chemical stimuli. These changes occur as a result of current flow through the membrane. *Transient currents* in living tissues are due to the movement of charged ions and can flow through the membrane as a result of an applied voltage or of a change in membrane conductance.

A *local potential* is a transient depolarizing or hyperpolarizing shift of the membrane potential in a localized area of the cell. Local potentials result from the current flow due to localized change in ion channels that alter permeability to one or more ions. Ion channel opening or closing may result from (1) a chemical agent acting on the channel, a *synaptic potential;* (2) activation of a sensory receptor channel by a stimulus, a *receptor potential;* or (3) a current from an externally applied voltage, an *electrotonic potential.*

Synaptic potentials are the response to information carried by a neurotransmitter released by an adjacent neuron. Receptor potentials are the response to external stimuli. Electrotonic potentials participate in the transfer of information throughout a cell by action potentials.

Ionic Basis

Local potentials result from the flow of current through the membrane with a change in channels that are open or closed in response to a chemical agent, mechanical deformation, or an applied voltage.

Neurotransmitters and neuromodulators produce synaptic potentials by one of six mechanisms:

1. Opening of potassium channels increases potassium conductance, resulting in hyperpolarization, a relatively slow process.
2. Opening of sodium channels increases sodium conductance, resulting in depolarization, a relatively fast process.
3. Opening of both potassium and sodium channels increases the conductance of both ions, resulting in a depolarization but to a lesser degree than in item 2, above.
4. Opening of chloride channels increases chloride conductance, resulting in rapid stabilization or hyperpolarization of the membrane voltage.
5. Closing of potassium channels, resulting in a *slow* depolarization.
6. Opening of calcium channels, resulting in a *slow* depolarization.

Generator potentials occur primarily by opening of both sodium and potassium channels and increasing conductance of both ions. This produces depolarization. Generator potentials also occur in response to specific molecules that activate olfactory receptors and to photic stimuli that activate photoreceptors in the retina of the eye.

Electrotonic potentials occur in one of two ways:

1. Opening of sodium channels by a current arising from a voltage in an adjacent area of membrane. This produces depolarization.
2. Opening or closing of several different ion channels by an externally applied voltage. Application of a negative voltage to the outside of the membrane causes outward current flow and depolarization of the membrane. Application of a positive potential to the outside of the membrane causes inward current flow and hyperpolarization of the membrane.

When a voltage is applied to the outside of the axonal membrane, the negative pole is commonly referred to as the *cathode;* the positive pole is the *anode.* The current flow at the cathode depolarizes, whereas that at the anode hyperpolarizes a membrane.

Characteristics of Local Potentials

All local potentials have certain characteristics in common (Table 2). Importantly, the local potential is a *graded* potential; that is, its amplitude is proportional to the size of the stimulus (Fig. 7). Measurement of a local potential uses the resting potential as its baseline. If the membrane's resting potential is depolarized from 80 to 70 mV during the local potential, the local potential has an amplitude of 10 mV. This potential change is one of decreasing negativity (or of depolarization), but

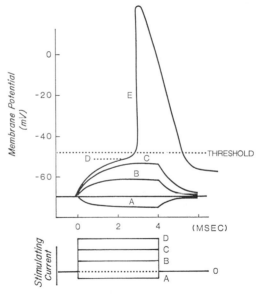

FIG. 7. Local potentials. These potentials are shown as an upward deflection if they are a depolarization and as a downward deflection if they are a hyperpolarization. Resting potential is 70 mV. At time zero, electrical currents of varied polarities and voltage are applied to the membrane **(bottom).** A is an anodal current; *B, C,* and *D* are cathodal currents. *A* produces a transient hyperpolarization; *B, C,* and *D* produce a transient depolarization that is graded and proportional to the size of the stimulus. All of these are local potentials. *D* produces an action potential, *E.*

it could also be one of increasing negativity (or of hyperpolarization).

Because the local potential is a graded response proportional to the size of the stimulus, the occurrence of a second stimulus before the first one subsides results in a larger local potential. Therefore, local potentials can be *summated*. They are summated algebraically, so that similar potentials are additive and hyperpolarizing and depolarizing potentials tend to cancel out each other. Summated potentials may reach threshold and produce an action potential when single potentials individually are subthreshold.

When a stimulus is applied in a localized area of the membrane, the change in membrane potential has both a temporal and a spatial distribution. A study of the temporal course of the local potential (Fig. 7) shows that the increase in the potential is not instantaneous but develops over a few milliseconds.

After the stimulus ends, the potential subsides over a few milliseconds as well. Therefore, local potentials have a temporal course that outlasts the stimulus. The occurrence of a second stimulus at the same site shortly after the first produces another local potential, which summates with any residual of the earlier one that has not yet subsided (Fig. 8). This summation of local potentials occurring near each other in time is called *temporal summation* (Fig. 8B).

Different synaptic potentials have different time courses. Most synaptic potentials range from 10 to 15 milliseconds in duration; however, some are very brief, lasting less than 1 millisecond, but others may last several seconds or several minutes. The longer the duration of the synaptic potential, the greater the chance for temporal summation to occur. By means of temporal summation, the cell can integrate signals that arrive at different times.

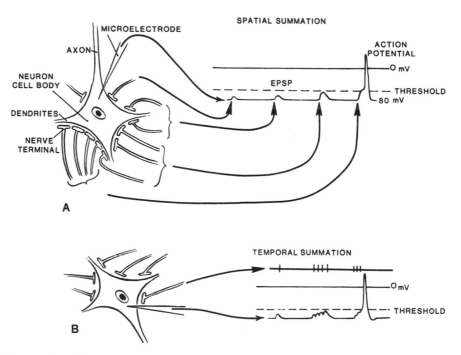

FIG. 8. Summation of local potentials in a neuron. **A:** Spatial summation occurs when increasing numbers of nerve terminals release more neurotransmitter to produce larger excitatory postsynaptic potentials (EPSPs). **B:** Temporal summation occurs when a single terminal discharges repetitively more rapidly to produce larger EPSPs.

Study of the spatial distribution of local potentials reveals another of their characteristics. As their name implies, they remain *localized* in the region where the stimulus is applied; they do not spread throughout the entire cell. However, the locally applied stimulus, because of local current flow, has an effect on the nearby membrane. The potential change is not sharply confined to the area of the stimulus but falls off over a finite distance along the membrane, usually a few millimeters. The application of a simultaneous second stimulus near the first (but not at the same site) results in summation of the potentials in the border zones—*spatial summation* (Fig. 8). Thus, the membrane of the cell can act as an integrator of stimuli that arrive from different sources and impinge on areas of membrane near one another. Spatial and temporal summation are important mechanisms in the processing of information by single neurons; when summated local potentials reach threshold, they initiate an action potential.

If a current or voltage is applied to a membrane for more than a few milliseconds, the ion channels revert to their resting state, changing ionic conductances of the membrane in a direction to restore the resting potential to baseline value. This phenomenon is known as *accommodation* (Fig. 9). Therefore, if an electrical stimulus is increased slowly, accommodation can occur and no change will be seen in the membrane potential. The changes in conductance during accommodation require several milliseconds, both to develop and to subside. As a result, if an electrical stimulus is applied gradually so that accommodation prevents a change in

resting potential, then when the stimulus is suddenly turned off, the residual change in conductance will produce a transient change in resting potential. Thus, accommodation can result in a cell responding to the cessation of a stimulus.

Action Potential

Action potentials have several advantages for the rapid transfer of information in the nervous system. Because action potentials are all-or-none—they either occur or do not occur—they can transfer information without loss over relatively long distances. Their all-or-none feature also allows coding of information as frequency rather than the less stable measure of amplitude. Also, their threshold eliminates the effects of small, random changes in membrane potential.

Threshold

The membranes of neurons, axons, and muscle cells have another characteristic that is basic to their ability to transmit information from one area to another—their *excitability*. If a membrane is depolarized by a stimulus, there is a point at which suddenly many sodium channels open. This point is known as the *threshold* for excitation (Fig. 7). If the depolarization does not reach threshold, the evoked activity is a local potential.

Threshold may be reached by a single local potential or by summated local potentials. When threshold is reached, there is a sudden increase in the membrane's permeability to sodium. This change in conductance results in the action potential.

Ionic Basis of Action Potential

In the resting state, many more potassium channels are open, the conductance of sodium is much less than that of potassium, and the resting potential is near the equilibrium potential of potassium. At threshold,

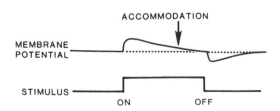

FIG. 9. Accommodation of the membrane potential to applied stimulus of constant strength. Note the response to sudden cessation of the stimulus.

many sodium channels open so that the conductance of sodium suddenly becomes greater than that of potassium, and the membrane potential shifts toward the equilibrium potential of sodium, which is approximately +60 mV. This depolarization reverses the polarity of the membrane, the inside becoming positive with respect to the outside. With the opening of the sodium channels and increased sodium conductance, there is a flow of current with the inward movement of sodium ions. The change in sodium conductance is usually transient, lasting only a few milliseconds, and is followed by opening of potassium channels, an increase in the potassium conductance, and an outward movement of potassium ions. These three changes overlap, and the potential of the membrane

during these changes is a function of the ratios of the conductances (Fig. 10). Sodium conductance increases several thousandfold early in the process, whereas potassium conductance increases less, does so later, and persists longer. The conductance changes for these two ions result in ionic shifts and current flows that are associated with a membrane potential change—the *action potential* (Fig. 10).

The action potential is a sudden, short-duration, all-or-none change in the membrane potential that occurs if the membrane potential reaches threshold (Table 6). Its components are shown in Fig. 11. The initial portion of the membrane potential change is the local potential. At threshold, the rising phase of the action potential suddenly changes be-

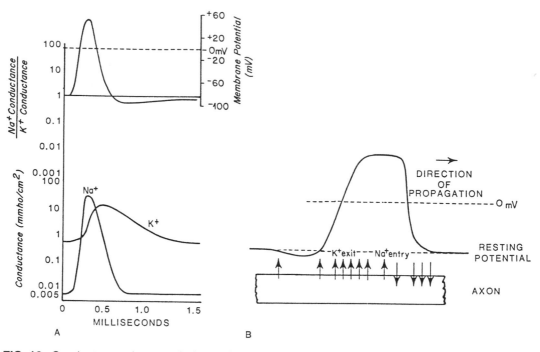

FIG. 10. Conductance changes during action potential. **A:** Temporal sequence at a single site along an axon. Changes in conductances (permeabilities) of sodium and potassium are plotted against time as they change with associated changes in membrane potential. Note that sodium conductance changes several thousandfold early in the process, whereas potassium conductance changes only about 30-fold during later stages and persists longer than sodium conductance changes. **B:** Spatial distribution of an action potential over a length of axon at a single instant.

TABLE 6. *Comparison of local potentials and action potentials*

Characteristic	Local potentials	Action potential
Example	Generator Synaptic Electrotonic	Nerve impulse
Duration, ms	5–100	1–10
Amplitude, mV	0.1–10	70–110
Ionic mechanism	Local changes in permeability to Na$^+$, K$^+$, Ca^{2+}, or Cl$^-$	Transient increase permeability to Na$^+$, followed by increase permeability to K$^+$
Threshold	No	Yes
Spatial and temporal summation	Yes	No (all-or-none)
Refractory period	No	Yes
Propagation	Passive and decremental	Active and nondecremental

cause of the influx of positive ions. In most nerve cells and skeletal muscle cells, the inward current during the rising phase of the action potential is carried by sodium ions, because sodium conductance is markedly increased. The action potential also could be carried by calcium ions if the calcium conductance increased sufficiently, as occurs in some dendrites. Repolarization begins as sodium conductance decreases or potassium conductance increases (or both). The decreased flow of sodium ions is followed by an efflux of potassium ions. The rate of return of the membrane potential to the baseline slows after sodium conductance has returned to baseline, producing a small residual on the negative component of the action potential, which is called the *negative afterpotential*. In some myelinated axons, repolarization occurs by a decrease in sodium conductance with no change in potassium conductance.

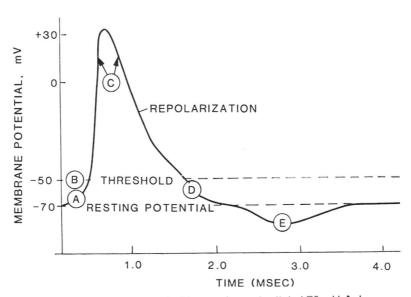

FIG. 11. Component of an action potential with a resting potential of 70 mV. **A:** Local electrotonic potential. **B:** Threshold level. **C:** Spike. **D:** Negative (depolarizing) afterpotential. **E:** Positive (hyperpolarizing) afterpotential.

The afterpotential is positive when the membrane potential is recorded with a microelectrode within the cell, but it is called negative because it is negative when recorded with an extracellular electrode. The increase in potassium conductance persists and results in a hyperpolarization after the spike component of the action potential, the *afterhyperpolarization*. The afterhyperpolarization is due to continued efflux of potassium ions, with a greater than resting difference in potential between the inside and outside of the cell. The afterhyperpolarization is positive when measured with extracellular electrodes and therefore is called a *positive afterpotential*. During the positive afterpotential, the membrane potential is near the potassium equilibrium potential, and oxygen consumption is increased with increased activity of the sodium pump.

The amounts of sodium and potassium that move across the membrane during the action potential are small, buffered by surrounding astrocytes, and do not change the concentration enough to result in a change in the resting potential. In addition, the sodium that moves in during the action potential is continually removed by the sodium pump during the rela-

tively long intervals between action potentials.

Excitability

The excitability of a membrane is the ease with which an action potential can be generated and is usually measured in terms of the voltage required to initiate an action potential. During increased sodium conductance, the membrane cannot be stimulated to discharge again. A second stimulus at this time is without effect; therefore, action potentials, unlike local potentials, cannot summate. This period of unresponsiveness is the *absolute refractory period* (Fig. 12). As sodium conductance returns to normal, the membrane again becomes excitable, but for a short period, the *relative refractory period*, it requires a larger stimulus to produce a smaller action potential. After the relative refractory period, while the negative afterpotential is subsiding, the membrane is partially depolarized, is closer to threshold, and has an increased excitability. This period is the *supernormal period*. Finally, during the positive afterpotential, the membrane is hyperpolarized, and stronger stimuli are required. This period is the *subnormal period*.

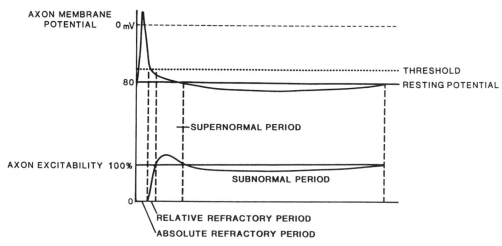

FIG. 12. Excitability changes during an action potential. The lower portion of the illustration shows the ease with which another action potential can be elicited (change in threshold). During absolute and relative refractory periods, the amplitude of the action potential evoked is low. Subsequently, it is normal.

Up to now, the term *threshold* has been used to refer to the membrane potential at which sodium channels open and an action potential is generated. The threshold of a membrane remains relatively constant. If the membrane potential becomes hyperpolarized, the membrane potential moves away from threshold, and the membrane is less excitable. If the membrane potential moves closer to threshold, the membrane becomes more excitable and will generate an action potential with a smaller stimulus. If the membrane potential is very near threshold, the cell may fire spontaneously. If the membrane potential remains more *depolarized* than threshold, however, the membrane cannot be stimulated to fire another action potential (Fig. 13).

The term *threshold* is also used to describe the voltage required to excite an action potential with an externally applied stimulus. When threshold is used in this sense, an axon with an increased excitability due to partial depolarization may be said to have a lower threshold for stimulation, even though the actual threshold is unchanged. The first meaning of threshold is used when intracellular recordings are considered, and the second is used in reference to extracellular stimulation and recording.

The threshold of the nerve membrane differs in different parts of the neuron: it is high in the dendrite and soma and lowest at the initial segment. Thus, an action potential is usually generated in the area of the axon hillock.

Propagation

Another important characteristic of action potentials is their propagation. If an action potential is initiated in an axon in the tip of the finger, for instance, the potential spreads along the entire length of that axon to its cell body in the dorsal root ganglion, and then along the central axon, ascending in the spinal cord to the brain stem. This characteristic permits the nervous system to transmit information from one area to another.

When an area of membrane is depolarized during an action potential, ionic currents flow (Fig. 14). In the area of depolarization, sodium ions carry positive charges inward. There is also a longitudinal flow of current both inside and outside the membrane. This flow of positive charges (current) toward nondepolarized regions internally and toward depolarized regions externally tends to depolarize the membrane in the areas that surround the region of the action potential. This depolarization is an electrotonic potential. In normal tissue, this depolarization is sufficient to shift the membrane potential to threshold and thereby generate an action potential in the immediately adjacent membrane. Thus, the action potential spreads away from its site of initiation along an axon or muscle fiber. Because of the refractory period, the potential cannot reverse and spread back into an area just depolarized.

The rate of conduction of the action potential along the membrane depends on the amount of longitudinal current flow and on the amount of current needed to produce depolarization in the adjacent membrane. The longitudinal current flow can be increased by increasing the diameter of an axon or muscle fiber, because this increase reduces the internal resis-

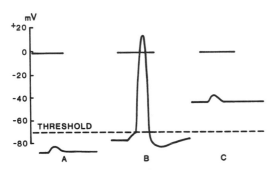

FIG. 13. The effect of stimulation of a neuron at different resting potentials as recorded with a microelectrode. **A:** The membrane is hyperpolarized, and a stimulus produces a subthreshold local potential. **B:** The membrane is normally polarized at -65 mV, and a stimulus produces a local potential that reaches threshold and results in an action potential. **C:** The membrane is depolarized beyond threshold, and a stimulus produces only a small local potential.

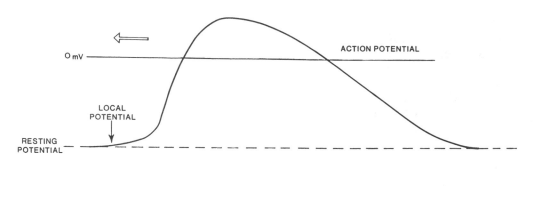

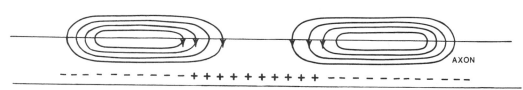

FIG. 14. Current flow and voltage changes in an axon in the region of an action potential. The voltage changes along the membrane are shown in the upper part of the figure and the spatial distribution of current flow is shown in the lower part as *arrows* through the axon membrane.

tance, just as a larger electrical wire has a lower electrical resistance. However, many axons in the central and peripheral nervous systems have an increased conduction velocity because they are insulated with a myelin sheath. A myelinated axon has its membrane bared only at the nodes of Ranvier, so that transmembrane current flow occurs almost exclusively at the nodal area. When current flow opens enough sodium channels to reach threshold in the nodal area, it results in many more sodium channels opening and an influx of sodium ions with a generation of an action potential. The nodal area in the mammalian nervous system is unique in that it consists almost exclusively of sodium channels, with an almost complete absence of potassium channels. The potassium channels are located at the paranodal regions (adjacent to the node), which are covered by myelin. The action potential generated at the node consists predominantly of inward sodium currents with little outward potassium currents, and repolarization is achieved by means of sodium inactivation and leakage currents. An action potential at one node of Ranvier pro-

duces sufficient longitudinal current flow to depolarize adjacent nodes to threshold, thereby propagating the action potential along the nerve in a skipping manner called *saltatory conduction* (Fig. 15).

Patterns of Activity

Information in the nervous system is coded by the number and type of axons that are active and by the firing pattern of action potentials. This activity is initiated in peripheral receptors or in neurons. Neuronal firing of action potentials may occur spontaneously or in response to external stimulation. *Beating,* or *pacing, neurons* fire repetitively at a constant frequency; their intrinsic firing rate may be increased or decreased by external stimulation. *Bursting neurons* generate regular bursts of action potentials separated by hyperpolarization of the membrane. Such neurons are important for rhythmic behavior such as breathing, walking, and chewing. Neurons that fire in response to external stimulation may do so in one of three ways. A *sustained*

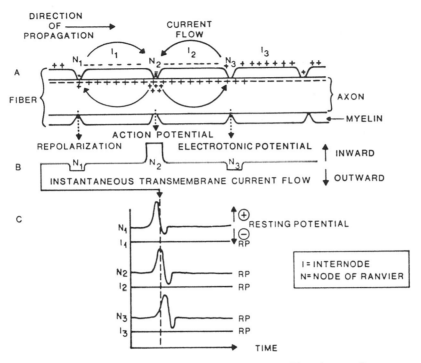

FIG. 15. Saltatory conduction along an axon from left to right. **A:** The charge distribution along the axon is shown with an action potential (depolarization) at the second node of Ranvier (N₂). Current flow spreads to the next node (*N₃*). **B:** Membrane current flow along the axon. **C:** The portion of the action potential found at each node is indicated by *dotted lines*.

response neuron shows repeated action potentials with a constant firing frequency that reflects the strength of the stimulus. A *delayed response neuron* fires action potentials only after stimulation of sufficient intensity. An *accommodation response neuron* fires only a single potential at the onset of stimulation and remains silent thereafter.

Some neurons (for example, in the thalamus) have the ability to discharge either in rhythmic bursts or with typical action potentials. The firing pattern depends on the level of the resting membrane potential. An important property of this type of neuron is the presence of a particular class of calcium channel, the *T channel*. This channel can be activated only if the membrane potential is relatively hyperpolarized (for example, −80 mV). Under this condition, a stimulus opens the T channel and calcium enters the cell and produces a small, brief calcium-based depolarizing potential change called the low-threshold calcium spike. This calcium spike triggers the opening of sodium channels, which produces a burst of repetitive action potentials. As calcium accumulates in the cell, it opens a *calcium-activated potassium channel* that allows the efflux of potassium. The resulting hyperpolarization (called *afterhyperpolarization*) allows reactivation of the T channel, the entry of sodium, and recurrence of the cycle. This sequence generates rhythmic burst firing of the neuron. Thus, T channels are an exception to the general rule of neuronal excitability: hyperpolarization "deinactivates" T channels and increases the likelihood that the neuron will discharge in rhythmic bursts of activity. Rhythmic burst firing in thalamic neurons that project to the cerebral cortex impairs the encoding of information by cortical neurons and interferes with the transmission of sensory information. Inactive states of the cerebral cortex occur during deep sleep and in some types of seizures (see Chapter 10).

Synaptic Transmission

A *synapse* is a specialized contact zone where one neuron communicates with another neu-ron. The contact zone between a neuron and a nonneural effector element (for example, a muscle fiber) is referred to as a *neuroeffector junction.* The two types of synapses are *chemical* and *electrical.*

The most common form of communication in the nervous system is through chemical synapses. A chemical synapse consists of a presynaptic component (containing synaptic vesicles), a postsynaptic component (dendrite, soma, or axon), and an intervening space called the synaptic cleft (Fig. 16).

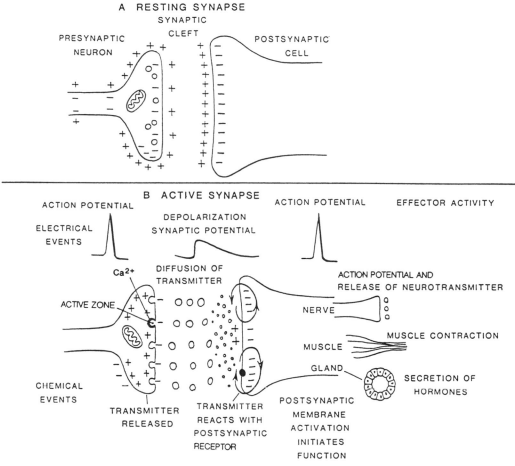

FIG. 16. Synaptic transmission. **A:** In a resting synapse, both the presynaptic axon terminal and the postsynaptic membrane are normally polarized. **B:** In an active synapse, an action potential invades the axon terminal (from *left* in the diagram) and depolarizes it. Depolarization of the axon terminal of a presynaptic neuron results in the release of neurotransmitter from the terminal. The neurotransmitter diffuses across the synaptic cleft and produces local current flow and a synaptic potential in the postsynaptic membrane, which initiates the effector activity (neuronal transmission, neurotransmitter release, hormonal secretion, or muscle contraction).

Many of the drugs used in clinical medicine have their pharmacologic site of action at the synapse.

The mechanism underlying chemical synaptic transmission should make it apparent that synaptic transmission has three unique characteristics. First, conduction at a synapse is delayed because of the brief interval of time required for the chemical events to occur. Second, because the two sides of the synapse are specialized to perform only one function, transmission can occur in only one direction across the synapse. Thus, neurons are polarized in the direction of impulse transmission. Third, because nerve impulses from many sources impinge on single cells in the central and peripheral nervous systems, synaptic potentials summate both temporally and spatially. The membrane of a cell is continually bombarded with neuromodulators and neurotransmitters, which produce either excitatory postsynaptic potentials (EPSPs) or inhibitory postsynaptic potentials (IPSPs) of varying du-

ration. When the membrane potential reaches threshold, an action potential is generated. Thus, a single neuron can integrate activity from many sources. A summary of the electrical events in a single cell underlying the transmission, integration, and conduction of information is shown in Fig. 17.

Biosynthesis, Storage, Release, and Reuptake of Neurochemical Transmitters

Neurochemical transmitters include amino acids, acetylcholine, monoamines (catecholamines, serotonin, histamine), neuropeptides, and purines (ATP and adenosine). Amino acids include *L-glutamate,* the most abundant excitatory neurotransmitter in the central nervous system, and *γ-aminobutyric acid (GABA),* the most abundant inhibitory neurotransmitter. Both of these neurotransmitters are synthesized from intermediate metabolites of the Krebs cycle. Acetylcholine and monoamines are synthesized by specific

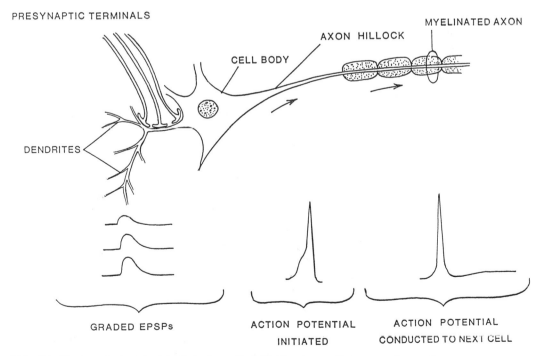

FIG. 17. Neuronal electrical activity from its initiation by excitatory postsynaptic potentials (EPSPs) to its transmission as an action potential to another area.

enzymes from precursors that are actively taken up by the presynaptic terminal (see Chapter 12). Neuropeptides are synthesized from messenger RNA in the cell body and transported to the synaptic terminal. Neurochemical transmitters are stored in special intracellular organelles called *synaptic vesicles.* Small clear synaptic vesicles store the classic neurotransmitters (amino acids, acetylcholine, monoamines), and large dense-core secretory granules store neuropeptides.

Neurotransmitter release is triggered by the influx of calcium through voltage-gated channels that open in response to the arrival of an action potential in the presynaptic terminal. These channels are clustered in specific regions of the presynaptic membrane called *active zones* (Fig. 16).

The synaptic vesicles are mobilized in the presynaptic terminal and dock close to the active zones. In response to the influx of calcium, the vesicle membrane fuses with the presynaptic membrane, which allows the release of the neurotransmitter into the synaptic cleft; this process is called *exocytosis.* The mobilization, docking, and fusion of synaptic vesicles depend on the interactions of various *synaptic vesicle proteins* with other components of the presynaptic terminal.

A neuron can produce and release different neurotransmitters. Neurons frequently contain a classic neurotransmitter (an amino acid or acetylcholine) and one or more neuropeptides. The neuron can release a variable mixture of these neurotransmitters according to its firing pattern, a process referred to as *frequency-dependent chemical coding.* Classic neurotransmitters can be released after a single action potential; neuropeptides are released in response to rapid, burst firing of a neuron.

Two other presynaptic mechanisms also regulate neurotransmitter release: (1) In many cases, the neurotransmitter inhibits its own release, acting via presynaptic inhibitory *autoreceptors.* (2) In other cases, inhibitory neurons (generally containing GABA) form axoaxonic synapses that inhibit the release of neurotransmitter from the postsynaptic axon, a process called *presynaptic inhibition* (Fig. 18).

The synaptic action of neurotransmitters is terminated by several mechanisms. Presynaptic reuptake, mediated by specific sodium-dependent and ATP-dependent neurotransmitter transporters, is the primary mechanism of inactivation of glutamate, GABA, and monoamines. Monoamines are metabolized after reuptake by monoamine oxidases and methyltransferases. Acetylcholine and neuropeptides do not undergo reuptake but are rapidly inactivated by enzymatic hydrolysis in the synaptic cleft.

Postsynaptic Effects of Neurochemical Transmitters

Postsynaptic effects are mediated by two main classes of receptors: (1) *Ligand-gated receptors* or *ion channels* mediate rapid changes in ionic conductance (ionotropic effect). (2) *G-protein–coupled receptors* produce slower changes in neuronal excitability and metabolism (metabotropic effect) (Table 7). These changes not only modify the electrical behavior of the neuron but they also may produce long-term effects, such as use-dependent modification of synaptic efficacy, cytoskeletal changes during development and repair, and control of genetic transcription.

Classic Neurotransmission

Classic neurotransmission is used for fast, precise, point-to-point transmission of excitatory or inhibitory signals. It involves rapid, brief opening of ligand-gated ion channel receptors. Neurotransmitters produce a transient increase or decrease in ion channel conductance to the passive flow of a specific ion current. These ionic currents produce local changes in the membrane potential called *postsynaptic potentials.* In most mammalian neurons, the resting membrane potential is approximately -60 to -80 mV. The threshold for opening voltage-gated sodium channels that trigger an action potential is reached when the postsynaptic potentials drive the membrane potential to a value that is about 10 mV less negative than the resting potential.

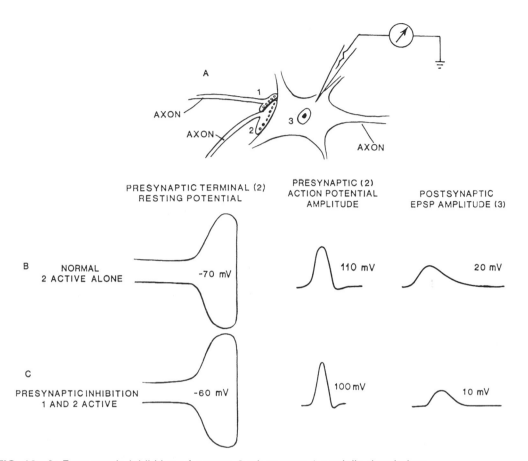

FIG. 18. **A:** Presynaptic inhibition of neuron 3 when axon 1 partially depolarizes axon 2. **B:** Response to axon 2 acting alone. **C:** Response to axon 2 after depolarization of axon 1. In the latter case, there is less neurotransmitter and a smaller excitatory postsynaptic potential (EPSP).

TABLE 7. *Comparison of classic neurotransmission and neuromodulation*

	Classic neurotransmission	Neuromodulation
Function	Rapid synaptic excitation or inhibition	Modulation of neural excitability
Receptor mechanism	Ion channel receptors	G-protein–coupled receptors
Ionic mechanism	Opening of either cation channel (fast EPSP) or Cl$^-$ channel (fast IPSP)	Opening or closing of voltage-gated K$^+$ or Ca^{2+} channels (slow IPSP and slow EPSP)
Example	L-Glutamate (ionotropic) GABA (GABA$_A$) Acetylcholine (nicotinic)	L-Glutamate (metabotropic) GABA (GABA$_B$) Acetylcholine (muscarinic) Monamines Neuropeptides Adenosine
Systems	Relay systems, direct Sensory Motor	Diffuse systems, indirect Internal regulation Consciousness

EPSP, excitatory postsynaptic potential; GABA, γ-aminobutyric acid; IPSP, inhibitory postsynaptic potential.

Ion currents that increase the net positive charge of the membrane produce depolarization EPSPs because they bring the membrane potential toward the threshold for triggering an action potential. In classic neurotransmission, *fast EPSPs* result from the *opening cation channels* (conducting sodium ions and, in some cases, calcium ions). Ligand-gated cation channel receptors that produce fast EPSPs include *nicotinic* acetylcholine receptors and several *ionotropic glutamate* receptors. Ion currents that increase the net negative charge of the membrane produce IPSPs. Fast IPSPs are produced by the opening of chloride channels. GABA (via $GABA_A$ receptors) and glycine act via this mechanism (Table 8 and Fig. 19).

Neuromodulation

Neurotransmitters acting through G-protein–coupled receptors, second messengers, and protein phosphorylation cascades control the excitability and responsiveness of neurons to rapid synaptic signals, a process called *neuromodulation.* G-protein–coupled receptors include metabotropic glutamate receptors, $GABA_B$ receptor, and receptors for catecholamines, serotonin and histamine, neuropeptides, and adenosine. Potassium channels are an important target of neuromodulatory signals. Potassium currents determine the pattern of activity generated by neurons through control of the resting membrane potential, repolarization of the action potential, and probability of generation of repetitive action potentials.

The opening of potassium channels brings the membrane potential toward the equilibrium potential of potassium (−100 mV) and thus away from the threshold for triggering an action potential. Closure of the potassium channels moves the membrane away from the equilibrium potential of potassium and thus closer to threshold. Neuromodulation involves the production of slow potentials. Activation of G-protein receptors that lead to closure of potassium channels produces slow depolarization and increased neuronal excitability. G-protein receptor mechanisms that increase potassium permeability lead to membrane hyperpolarization and reduce neuronal excitability.

The same neurotransmitter may act via different receptor subtypes, each coupled to a distinct transduction pathway. Also, different neurotransmitters, via their respective receptors, may activate a similar transduction pathway.

Electrical Synapses

Although most synapses in the nervous system use chemical transmitters, neurons with junctions that contain channels extending from the cytoplasm of the presynaptic neuron to that of the postsynaptic neuron interact electrically. In these electrical synapses, the bridging channels mediate ionic current flow from one cell to the other. Transmission across the electrical synapse is very rapid, without the synaptic delay of chemical synapses. Electrical synapses are also bidirectional, in contrast to chemical

TABLE 8. *Postsynaptic potentials*

Receptor	Ionic mechanism	Effect	Kinetics
Nicotinic Glutamate	Increased cation (Na^+, Ca^{2+}) conductance	Excitatory	Fast
$GABA_A$ Glycine	Increased Cl^- conductance	Inhibitory	Fast
G-protein–coupled receptors	Decreased K^+ conductance	Excitatory	Slow
	Increased K^+ conductance	Inhibitory	Slow

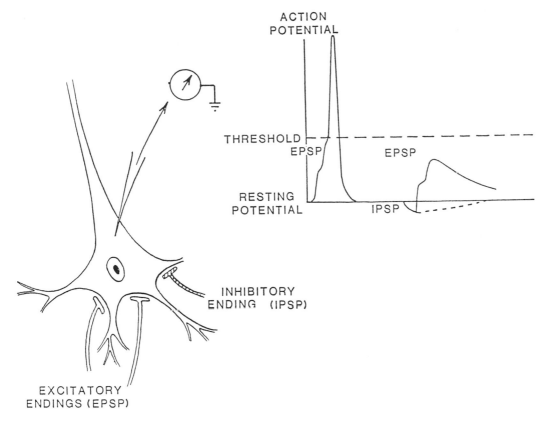

FIG. 19. Postsynaptic inhibition in the neuron on the left occurs when the inhibitory and excitatory endings are active simultaneously. On the right, a microelectrode recording shows two excitatory postsynaptic potentials (EPSPs) summating to initiate an action potential. When there is a simultaneous occurrence of an inhibitory postsynaptic potential (IPSP), depolarization is too low to reach threshold, and no action potential occurs.

synapses, which transmit signals in only one direction.

Clinical Correlations

Pathophysiologic Mechanisms

The mechanisms responsible for neuronal excitability, impulse conduction, and synaptic transmission in the central and peripheral nervous system may be altered transiently to produce either loss of activity or overactivity of neurons. A loss of activity results in a clinical deficit of relatively short duration (seconds to hours); overactivity results in extra movements or sensations. Both types of transient alteration are usually *reversible*. These transient disorders may be focal or generalized (Table 9) and may be due to different mechanisms (Table 10). Transient disorders reflect disturbances in neuronal excitability due to abnormalities in membrane potential.

Energy Failure

Energy metabolism is necessary for maintenance of the membrane potential by the ATP-coupled sodium-potassium pump. Most

TABLE 9. *Transient disorders of neuronal function*

Neuronal excitability	Focal disorder	Generalized disorder
Increased	Focal seizure Tonic spasms Muscle cramp Paresthesia Paroxysmal pain	Generalized seizure Tetany
Decreased	Transient ischemic attack Migraine Transient mononeuropathy	Syncope Concussion Cataplexy Periodic paralysis

of the ATP produced in the nervous system by aerobic metabolism of glucose is used to maintain the activity of the sodium pump. Conditions such as hypoxia, ischemia, hypoglycemia, or seizures affect the balance between energy production and energy consumption of neurons and cause energy failure and thus impaired activity of sodium-potassium ATPase. If the active transport process stops, the cell accumulates sodium and loses potassium and the membrane potential progressively decreases. This depolarization has two consequences. First, there may be a transient increase in neuronal excitability as the membrane potential moves closer to threshold for opening voltage-gated sodium channels and triggering the action potential. This may produce a paroxysmal discharge of the neuron or in an axon. Second, if depolarization persists, the sodium channel remains inactivated and the neuron becomes inexcitable. This is known as *depolarization blockade* and results in a focal deficit, such as focal paralysis or anesthesia, or a generalized deficit, such as paralysis or loss of consciousness (Fig. 20).

The neuron also uses ATP to maintain ion gradients that allow active presynaptic reuptake of neurotransmitters, such as the excitatory amino acid L-glutamate. Under conditions of energy failure, glutamate accumulates in the synapse and produces prolonged activation of its postsynaptic receptors, leading to neuronal depolarization and the accumulation of calcium in the cytosol. Because the lack of ATP also impairs active transport of calcium into the endoplasmic reticulum or toward the extracellular fluid, calcium accumulates.

Essentially all forms of neuronal injury involve to various extents (1) accumulation of glutamate and activation of glutamate receptors, (2) accumulation of cytosolic calcium and activation of calcium-triggered cascades, (3) generation of free radicals, and (4) mitochondrial failure. The consequences are functional and potentially reversible (for example, cell depolarization, pump failure, and accumulation of intracellular sodium). If the cause is not corrected, calcium accumulates and triggers irreversible changes, including destruction of cellular and mitochondrial membranes, disorganization of the cytoskeleton, and degradation of DNA by nucleases, and these effects lead to cell death by necrosis or apoptosis (see Chapter 4).

Ion Channel Blockade

Voltage-gated sodium channels mediate the initiation and conduction of action potentials.

TABLE 10. *Mechanisms of transient disorders*

Energy failure
  Hypoxia-ischemia
  Hypoglycemia
  Seizures
  Spreading cortical depression
  Trauma
Ion channel disorders
  Mutation of channel protein (channelopathies)
  Immune blockade
  Drugs
  Toxins
Electrolyte disorders
Demyelination

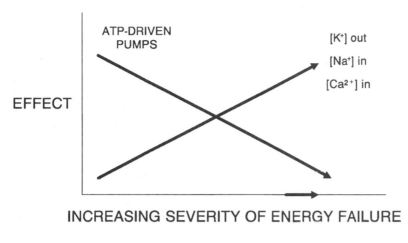

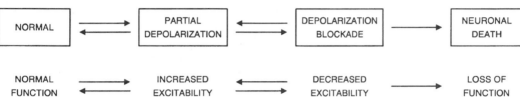

FIG. 20. Effects of increasing severity of energy failure (and ATP depletion) on activity of ATP-driven pumps, ionic concentrations in the intracellular and extracellular fluid, and neuronal electrical activity. With progressive failure of ATP-driven pumps, potassium accumulates in the extracellular fluid and sodium and calcium accumulate inside the neuron. This produces progressive neuronal depolarization. With partial depolarization, the resting potential moves closer to the threshold for triggering an action potential; this results in a transient increase in neuronal excitability, which may be manifested by paresthesias or seizures. With further depolarization, the membrane potential is at a level that maintains inactivation of the sodium channel, preventing further generation of action potentials and, thus, reducing neuronal excitability. This constitutes a depolarization block, which manifests with transient and reversible deficits such as paralysis or loss of consciousness. If the energy failure is severe and prolonged, the excessive accumulation of intracellular calcium triggers various enzymatic cascades that lead eventually to neuronal death and irreversible loss of function.

Voltage-gated calcium channels mediate neurotransmitter release, and ligand-gated cation (sodium and calcium) channels mediate excitatory postsynaptic potentials. All these channels may be blocked by autoantibodies, drugs, or toxins. Blockade of sodium channels at the node of Ranvier slows conduction velocity or causes conduction block; this produces a reversible focal deficit (weakness or anesthesia). For example, the blockade of sodium channels in sensory axons by local anesthetic agents produces anesthesia, and antibodies against ganglioside GM_1 (associated with sodium channels) in the nodes of Ranvier of motor axons produce focal paralysis. Autoantibodies may also block ion channels involved in neuromuscular transmission and produce reversible muscle fatigue or paralysis.

Specific Disorders

Electrolyte Disorders

Disorders affecting serum electrolyte levels may produce transient changes in the excitability of nerve and muscle. The changes in extracellular ionic concentration produce concomitant changes in the transmembrane ion gradient and, thus, the equilibrium potential of the ion. The impact of this change depends on the state of membrane permeability. An alteration in extracellular potassium affects mainly the resting membrane potential, whereas changes in extracellular sodium affect predominantly the magnitude of the action potential.

Changes in the serum concentration of potassium affect predominantly excitability in the periphery (peripheral axons and skeletal or cardiac muscle). A *decrease in extracellular potassium* increases the concentration gradient and the equilibrium potential of potassium; as at rest the membrane is predominantly permeable to potassium and the increased equilibrium potential will increase the resting potential (hyperpolarize the cell). This makes the cell less excitable and may result in severe weakness, as occurs when potassium is lost because of disease (vomiting or diarrhea) or medication (diuretics). An *increase in extracellular potassium* decreases the concentration gradient and the equilibrium potential of potassium, lowering the resting potential. The effects vary with the degree and duration of the increase in potassium. Small increases produce an initial depolarization that moves the resting membrane potential closer to the threshold for opening sodium channels and generating action potentials. The cell is more excitable and fires action potentials in response to weaker stimuli or even spontaneously. A large increase in extracellular potassium produces a persistently low resting membrane potential. Sodium channels remain inactive and the neuron is inexcitable (depolarization block). Therefore, an excess of extracellular potassium may produce either excessive activity or a loss of activity of neurons, axons, or muscle fibers.

An increase in extracellular sodium increases the sodium equilibrium potential, the size of the action potential, and the rate of rise of the action potential. Such increases do not have significant clinical effects. A decrease in extracellular sodium has the reverse effect; that is, it may lower the action potential amplitude and slow its rate of increase. If the action potential is low enough, it may not generate sufficient local current to discharge adjacent membrane, and action potential conduction may be blocked.

Calcium acts primarily as a membrane stabilizer; its absence results in a reduced concentration gradient for sodium and potassium. Thus, hypocalcemia reduces the resting potential, increases excitability, and may produce spontaneous activity. In addition, because the entry of calcium into the membrane is necessary for release of neurotransmitter, a low calcium level may block synaptic transmission. Therefore, hypocalcemia may have opposite effects; that is, it may impair synaptic transmission but produce spontaneous firing of a neuron or axon. An excess of calcium tends to block action potentials and to enhance synaptic transmission. Hypercalcemia does not produce demonstrable changes, except at very high calcium concentrations, whereas even moderate hypocalcemia may produce muscle twitching or tingling.

Channelopathies

Genetic disorders that alter the amino acid composition of ion channel subunits produce changes in the function of the channel. These disorders are called *channelopathies*. Several genetic disorders that affect sodium, potassium, or calcium channels have been described. For example, point mutations in the α subunit of the sodium channel in muscle prevent channel recovery after depolarization. This results in muscle weakness triggered by a transient increase in the serum level of potassium, a disorder called *hyperkalemic periodic paralysis*. Other congenital channelopathies increase the excitability of muscle membrane and produce *myotonia*. Mutations in some types of potassium or calcium channels produce *episodic ataxia*.

Immune Blockade or Impairment of Ion Channels

Several neuroimmunologic disorders produce abnormalities in voltage-gated or ligand-gated ion channels. For example, antibodies against *ganglioside GM₁* produce conduction block in motor axons by affecting the function of voltage-gated ion channels at nodes of Ranvier. Antibodies may affect neuromuscular transmission and cause transient and reversible muscle fatigue or weakness. Antibodies against voltage-gated calcium channels interfere with the release of acetylcholine from motor nerve endings, as in the *Lambert-Eaton myasthenic syndrome.* Antibodies against nicotinic acetylcholine receptors in muscle membrane at motor end plates are the hallmark of *myasthenia gravis.*

Seizures

Seizures are transient episodes of supratentorial origin in which there is abrupt and temporary alteration of cerebral function (see Chapter 10). They are produced by spontaneous, excessive discharge of cortical neurons that is caused by several pathophysiologic mechanisms. Excessive excitation or excessive inhibition may occur in focal areas of the cerebral cortex (focal seizures) or over the entire cerebral cortex (generalized seizures). A focal or generalized increase in neuronal excitability may result from energy failure producing transient depolarization or lack of local inhibition. Some seizures may result from excessive inhibition producing membrane hyperpolarization and activation of T-type calcium channels. The opening of T channels generates a burst discharge that may be transmitted to the neighboring neurons or, if arising in the thalamus, to the whole cerebral cortex. Thus, seizures may respond to drugs that block sodium channels, increase inhibitory neurotransmission, or block T channels.

Spreading Cortical Depression

Spreading cortical depression is a cortical phenomenon that has been associated with the induction of focal neurologic deficits during attacks of *migraine* (the migraine aura) and the progression of neurologic deficits during focal brain ischemia. It consists of a short-

lasting depolarization wave that moves across the cortex at a rate of 3 to 5 mm/min and produces a brief phase of excitation followed by prolonged neuronal depression. During spreading depression, there is an abrupt increase in the brain of extracellular potassium and release of excitatory amino acids. The spread of the depolarization may occur partly through the gap junctions of astrocytes.

Effect of Drugs and Toxins

The electrical activity of neurons can be altered by drugs or toxins acting on the cell membrane. Synaptic transmission is particularly susceptible to drugs that may act on presynaptic or postsynaptic membranes. Examples of the types of transmission block are illustrated in Fig. 21. There may be presynaptic block of transmitter release or postsynaptic block by competitive or noncompetitive inhibition of postsynaptic receptors or by depolarizing substances.

Several biologic toxins exert their actions by altering ion channels or synaptic transmission or both. For example, tetrodotoxin, a poison occurring in certain fish, blocks sodium channels and causes paralysis. Clostridial toxins, such as tetanus and botulinum toxin, prevent release of neurotransmitter by destroying a synaptic vesicle protein critical for docking.

Several drugs that act on ion channels or affect synaptic transmission have therapeutic applications. Drugs that block sodium channels (phenytoin, carbamazepine) or increase inhibitory synaptic transmission (benzodiazepines) are used for treatment of seizures and pain. The drug 3,4-diaminopyridine blocks voltage-gated potassium currents, delays repolarization, and thus increases the possibility of opening of voltage-gated calcium channels in presynaptic terminals.

Consequences of Demyelination

Demyelination is an important mechanism of neurologic disease. Myelin disorders may be caused by genetic defects in myelin composition or, more commonly, by acquired dis-

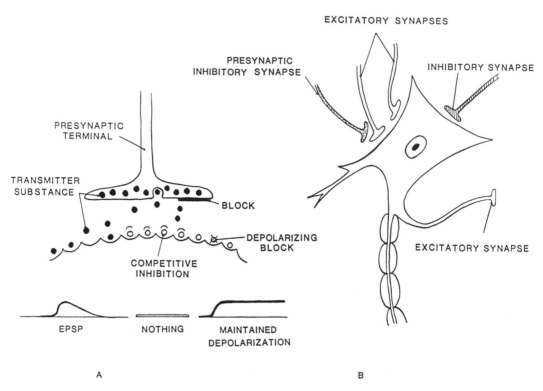

FIG. 21. Abnormalities of synaptic transmission may occur **(A)**. Types of transmission block include block of transmitter release (block), block of transmitter binding to postsynaptic membrane (competitive inhibition), and binding of another depolarizing agent to the membrane (depolarizing block). **B:** These types of abnormalities may occur at each neuronal synapse shown.

orders of myelin. Acquired disorders of myelin are frequently due to immune-mediated mechanisms. In the peripheral nervous system, these disorders include acute and chronic inflammatory demyelinating neuropathies. In the central nervous system, the most important example is multiple sclerosis.

In demyelinating diseases, there is not only loss of myelin but also a redistribution of sodium and potassium channels. The loss of myelin means that the insulation of the axon is lost and the electrical current is dissipated because of increased capacitance and decreased resistance of the membrane. The loss of myelin around the internodes and the loss of the concentration of sodium channels at the nodes of Ranvier interfere with saltatory conduction by slowing nerve conduction or, in severe cases, by causing *conduction block.* Conduction

block results in such deficits as paralysis and loss of sensation. Conduction block may also be caused by drugs (for example, local anesthetics) that block the sodium channels at nodes of Ranvier and by antibodies directed against ion channels. Conduction in demyelinated axons may be increased by blockade of the unmasked fast potassium channels with drugs such as 3,4-diaminopyridine.

In some cases, acquired disorders of myelin may result in spontaneous discharge of the axon or in abnormal electric currents generated between axons with different degrees of demyelination. These abnormal electrical impulses may produce positive symptoms such as paresthesias (pins-and-needles sensation), paroxysmal pain, or muscle spasms.

Longer duration action potentials are able to increase function in certain abnormal axons. Lambert-Eaton myasthenic syndrome is a paraneoplastic disorder due to antibodies formed by lung carcinoma cells. The antibodies block the calcium binding at nerve terminals that is necessary for the release of acetylcholine in neuromuscular and autonomic transmission. Thus, patients typically have muscle weakness, dry mouth, and other autonomic symptoms that are relieved by 3,4-diaminopyridine.

Patients with multiple sclerosis have an autoimmune disorder, with weakness and sensory loss due to demyelination of axons. Transmission of action potentials through partially demyelinated segments can be enhanced with 3,4-diaminopyridine. This can provide symptomatic relief. As might be expected, side effects associated with this drug are tingling sensation and seizures.

The membrane of a cell is also altered when it loses its synaptic input. Normal function of many neurons and muscle fibers depends on the release of a trophic factor from presynaptic nerve terminals. Loss of all or most of the input to a cell may result in cell atrophy and other structural changes in the appearance of the cell. A visceral organ that has lost its autonomic innervation becomes more sensitive to neurotransmitters, a phenomenon called *denervation hypersensitivity,* in which the cellular response to a constant stimulus increases after a cell has lost some of its normal input. This phenomenon is discussed further in subsequent chapters.

is moved from one area to another as action potentials conducted by single cells. The information is integrated in neurons by the interaction of local potentials generated in response to the neurotransmitters released from depolarized nerve terminals.

In this system, information can be coded either as the rate of discharge in individual cells or axons or as the number and combination of active cells. Both of these are important mechanisms, for although the activity of the nervous system can be conveniently described in terms of the electrical activity of single cells, the combined activity of large numbers of cells and axons determines the behavior of the organism.

Each type of alteration in neuronal or muscle cell physiology can produce symptoms or signs of short duration—transient disorders. The particular findings in a patient depend on which cells are altered. If the changes are in neurons that subserve sensation, there may be a loss of sensation or an abnormal sensation such as tingling, loss of vision, or "seeing stars." In other systems, there might be loss of strength, twitching in muscles, loss of intellect, or abnormal behavior.

In all these cases, the physiologic alterations are not specific and may be the result of any one of a number of diseases. Transient disorders do not permit a pathologic or etiologic diagnosis. Any type of disease (vascular, neoplastic, inflammatory) may be associated with transient changes. Therefore, the pathology of a disorder cannot be deduced when its temporal profile is solely that of transient episodes.

Summary ▪

The transmission of information in the nervous system depends on the generation of a resting potential that acts as a reserve of energy poised for release when the valve is turned on. Ionic channels act as the *valve,* controlling the *energy* in the ionic concentration gradient. The release of energy is seen either as local graded potentials or as propagated action potentials that arise when the local potentials reach threshold. Information

Clinical Problems ▪

1. A 64-year-old man had sudden occlusion of a blood vessel in an area of the brain that controls speech and was unable to speak for 10 minutes. His speech gradually returned to normal over a 15-minute period.

   How could anoxia of the involved cells result in loss of function?

By what mechanism could recovery occur?

2. A 55-year-old teacher with a brain tumor had severe right-sided paralysis and signs of brain swelling. When he was given a drug that reduced cerebral edema, his paralysis improved.
   a. If the edema resulted in extracellular sodium dilution, what would be the effect on the action potential amplitude and electrotonic potential amplitudes?
   b. If the osmotic pressure changes produced efflux of potassium from the cell and influx of water into the cell, what would be the effect of the edema on the resting potential?

3. A 36-year-old woman with multiple sclerosis with focal areas of myelin loss in the central nervous system had a 2-week loss of vision in one eye. How could loss of myelin in the optic nerve have affected her vision?

4. After sitting in a biochemistry lecture for 1½ hours and sleeping with your arm over a chair for 10 minutes, you awaken with a numb hand. As you rub it, it tingles. Which of the following could account for the tingling?
   a. The resting membrane potential moves closer to threshold.
   b. Hyperpolarization of the nerve membrane.
   c. Increased extracellular potassium concentration.
   d. Prolonged positive afterpotential.

5. Some poisons block the action of neurotransmitter at the postsynaptic membrane. What effect could this have on (a) end-plate potential, (b) generator potential, (c) excitatory postsynaptic potential, (d) accommodation?

6. A 28-year-old man has a focal seizure that starts with a twitching in the right corner of his mouth and spreads within 1 second to involve the right hand and leg and then leads to a generalized tonic-clonic seizure. After the seizure, he recovers over a 20-minute period, with residual weakness of the right side of the body that recovers after 1 hour.
   a. What mechanisms can cause increased excitability of neurons?
   b. What is the mechanism of the right-sided weakness after the seizure?
   c. What are the possible mechanisms by which drugs may prevent the initiation or spread of seizure activity?

7. A man named Nernst has a wooden boat with a hole in the bottom that he uses on Lake Sodium. When he wants to sit and fish, he lets the boat fill with water until no more comes in, and he keeps his feet up. This condition is one of (a) _____. If he wants to go elsewhere, he must lower the water level in the boat, so he turns on his Lake Sodium pump, which pumps water out. He then achieves a condition in which inflow equals outflow, with little water in the boat. This he calls (b) _____. It requires energy, so the pumping process is called (c) _____.

Additional Reading

Levitan, I. B., and Kaczmarek, L. K. (eds.). *The Neuron: Cell and Molecular Biology* (2nd ed.). New York: Oxford University Press, 1997.

Shepherd, G. M. (ed.). *The Synaptic Organization of the Brain* (4th ed.). New York: Oxford University Press, 1998.

Waxman, S. G., Kocsis, J. D., and Stys, P. K. (eds.). *The Axon: Structure, Function, and Pathophysiology.* New York: Oxford University Press, 1995.

TWO

LONGITUDINAL SYSTEMS

The Cerebrospinal Fluid System

Objectives

1. Define or identify the following: dura mater, arachnoid, pia mater, epidural space, subdural space, subarachnoid space, dural sinuses, falx cerebri, tentorium cerebelli, blood–brain barrier, choroid plexuses, lateral ventricles, foramen of Monro, third ventricle, aqueduct of Sylvius, fourth ventricle, and foramina of Luschka and Magendie.
2. Describe and trace the formation, circulation, and absorption of cerebrospinal fluid (CSF).
3. Define communicating hydrocephalus and noncommunicating hydrocephalus. Give an example of each type, describe its location, and state the anatomicopathologic consequences of a lesion in that location.
4. Discuss the relationship between the contents of the cranial cavity and intracranial pressure, and give examples of general pathologic states that may result in increased pressure.
5. Interpret the significance of abnormalities in CSF color, cellular composition, serologic findings, total protein level, gamma globulin concentration, sugar level, and culture, and list the CSF findings in meningitis, encephalitis, subarachnoid hemorrhage, and traumatic puncture.
6. Describe or list the features of the syndrome of meningeal irritation.
7. Describe or list the features that indicate increased intracranial pressure.
8. Describe the neuroanatomical basis for the following neurodiagnostic studies: myelography, computed tomography, magnetic resonance imaging, and radioisotope cisternography.

Introduction

The meninges, ventricular system, subarachnoid spaces, and CSF constitute a functionally unique system that has an important role in maintaining a stable environment within which the nervous system can function. The membranes that constitute the meninges serve as supportive and protective structures for nerve tissue. The CSF itself provides a cushioning effect during rapid movements of the head and a mechanical buoyancy to the brain. The density of brain tissue is only slightly greater than that of CSF, and the average weight of the brain is 1,500 g. However, the CSF exerts a considerable buoyant effect on the brain. In addition, it provides a pathway for the removal of brain metabolites and functions as a chemical reservoir, protecting the local environment of the brain from some of the changes that may occur in the blood, thus ensuring the brain's continued undisturbed performance. The CSF system is found at the supratentorial, posterior fossa, and spinal levels. Because of the extensive anatomical distribution and function of the CSF system, pathologic alterations to it can occur in a wide variety of neurologic disorders.

Overview ■

Structures included in the CSF system are the meninges and meningeal spaces formed between the meningeal linings and the brain, the ventricular system, and the CSF itself.

The *meninges* consist of three mesodermally derived membranes—the dura mater (outermost); the arachnoid; and the thin pia mater (innermost), which adheres closely to the structures of the central nervous system. The epidural space is external to the dura mater, between it and bone. The subdural space is between the dura mater and the arachnoid, and the subarachnoid space is between the arachnoid and the pia mater and contains CSF. CSF is also contained in the cavities in the brain: the two lateral ventricles, the third ventricle, the aqueduct of Sylvius, and fourth ventricle.

The composition of CSF is similar but not identical to that of plasma. CSF is formed by a combination of processes, including passive diffusion, facilitated diffusion, and active transport, and is produced primarily but not exclusively by the choroid plexus of the ventricular system. There is a slow circulation of the CSF through the ventricular system into the subarachnoid space and over the surface of the brain and spinal cord. Most of the CSF passes through the arachnoid villi into the venous sinuses.

Because of the close relationship between the CSF system and the neural tissue, pathologic processes that primarily alter the function of the CSF system may secondarily alter nervous system function. Furthermore, because the central nervous system is bathed and surrounded by CSF, disease processes that primarily affect the nervous system may be secondarily reflected by changes in the anatomy and physiology of this system. Therefore, examination of the composition of the CSF and the structure of this system is

an important and useful neurodiagnostic tool.

Anatomy of the CSF System ■

Dura Mater and Its Major Folds

The *dura mater* is a tough, fibrous membrane. In the cranial cavity, it consists of two almost inseparable layers. The outer (periosteal) layer of the dura mater corresponds to the periosteum of the cranial bones. Therefore, the *epidural space* between the dura mater and bone normally is not present. It is a potential space that becomes of pathologic importance if the dura mater is separated from bone by blood (epidural hematoma) or by pus (epidural abscess). The inner (meningeal) layer of the dura mater remains attached to the outer layer except where they are separated to form venous channels, the *dural venous sinuses.*

The *falx cerebri* is a sickle-shaped reflection of meningeal dura that extends into the interhemispheric fissure to separate the two cerebral hemispheres. It extends from the base of the anterior fossa to the internal occipital protuberance. Its upper margin contains the *superior sagittal sinus,* and its lower free edge, which arches over the corpus callosum, contains the *inferior sagittal sinus* (Fig. 1).

At the level of the internal occipital protuberance, the dura mater forming the falx cerebri extends laterally to form a winglike structure, the *tentorium cerebelli.* The outer border of the tentorium cerebelli is attached to the occipital bone and along the upper edges of the petrous bones. Thus, it separates the ventral surface of the cerebral hemispheres from the dorsal surface of the cerebellum and divides the cranial cavity into the supratentorial compartment (anterior and middle cranial fossae and their contents) and the infratentorial, or posterior fossa, compartment (see Chapter 3, Fig. 3). The cerebellar hemispheres are partially separated by a downward extension of dura mater, the *falx cerebelli.* The wings of the tentorium cerebelli converge and

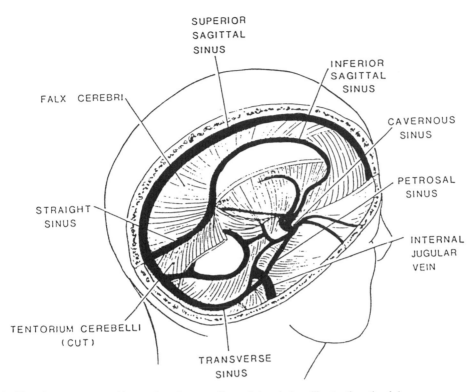

FIG. 1. The dura mater and its major sinuses. Dorsolateral view illustrating the falx cerebri (located at the midline in the interhemispheric fissure), the tentorium cerebelli (separating the supratentorial compartment from the infratentorial, or posterior fossa, compartment), and the dural lining of the base of the skull. The dural venous sinuses are shown in *black.*

attach to the posterior clinoid process of the sella turcica. The free border of the tentorium cerebelli thus forms an opening, the *tentorial notch,* that surrounds the midbrain at the transition between the posterior fossa and the middle fossa.

The two layers of the dura mater remain tightly attached as they pass through the foramen magnum into the spinal canal. At the level of the second or third cervical vertebra, the meningeal dura separates widely from the inner periosteum of bone and forms a narrow sac extending to the level of the second sacral vertebra. The spinal epidural space thus formed between the dura mater and the periosteum contains fat and vascular structures (principally veins). The conus medullaris, the lower end of the spinal cord (Fig. 2), terminates at the level of the second lumbar verte-

bra. A thin remnant of central nervous system tissue, the *filum terminale,* extends caudally from the conus medullaris to the termination of the dural sac at the second sacral level. The filum terminale is composed of glial cells, ependyma, and astrocytes covered by pia mater. The dura mater is pierced by the roots of the spinal and cranial nerves along the length of the brainstem and spinal cord.

Leptomeninges (Arachnoid and Pia Mater)

Embryologically, the leptomeninges (the arachnoid and pia mater) begin as a single membrane that becomes separated by numerous confluent subarachnoid spaces containing CSF. The arachnoid, however, remains attached to the pia mater by numerous weblike trabeculae (Fig. 3). Although the pia mater

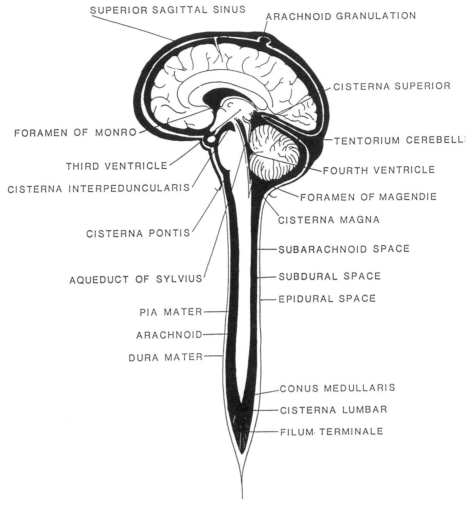

SUPERIOR SAGITTAL SINUS

ARACHNOID GRANULATION

CISTERNA SUPERIOR

FORAMEN OF MONRO

TENTORIUM CEREBELL

THIRD VENTRICLE

FOURTH VENTRICLE

CISTERNA INTERPEDUNCULARIS

FORAMEN OF MAGENDIE

CISTERNA MAGNA

CISTERNA PONTIS

SUBARACHNOID SPACE

SUBDURAL SPACE

EPIDURAL SPACE

AQUEDUCT OF SYLVIUS

PIA MATER

ARACHNOID

DURA MATER

CONUS MEDULLARIS

CISTERNA LUMBAR

FILUM TERMINALE

FIG. 2. The cerebrospinal fluid (CSF) system, illustrating the meningeal layers, ventricles, and subarachnoid cisterns. The CSF is produced primarily in the choroid plexus. It circulates from the lateral ventricles through the foramen of Monro into the third ventricle and then through the aqueduct of Sylvius into the fourth ventricle. The CSF passes from the fourth ventricle into the subarachnoid space through the foramina of Luschka and Magendie. It is reabsorbed through the arachnoid granulations into the superior sagittal sinus. (Modified from Noback, C. R., and Demarest, R. J. *The Nervous System: Introduction and Review* [2nd ed.]. New York: McGraw-Hill, 1977. With permission.)

adheres tightly to the surfaces of the brain and spinal cord, the arachnoid is closely applied to the inner surface of the meningeal dura mater throughout the neuraxis. The potential space between the dura mater and the arachnoid is termed the *subdural space*. It normally contains a thin layer of fluid. In pathologic states,

blood may accumulate in this space and produce a *subdural hematoma.*

As a result of the relationship of the arachnoid to the dura mater and of the pia mater to neural tissue, the *subarachnoid space* varies greatly in size and shape, particularly over the surfaces of the brain and in the lumbar re-

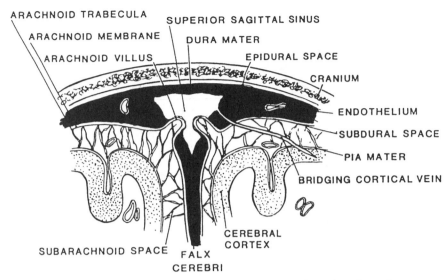

ARACHNOID TRABECULA
ARACHNOID MEMBRANE
ARACHNOID VILLUS
SUPERIOR SAGITTAL SINUS
DURA MATER
EPIDURAL SPACE
CRANIUM
ENDOTHELIUM
SUBDURAL SPACE
PIA MATER
BRIDGING CORTICAL VEIN
CEREBRAL CORTEX
SUBARACHNOID SPACE
FALX CEREBRI

FIG. 3. Meninges and meningeal spaces. Diagrammatic coronal section through the paramedian region of the cerebral hemispheres. Note bridging vein extending from the cerebral cortex to the superior sagittal sinus. Tearing of this type of vein is a common cause of subdural bleeding.

gion of the spinal canal (see Fig. 2). In the cranial cavity, these enlargements of the subarachnoid space are called *cisterns,* which usually are named for their anatomical location (for example, the interpeduncular cistern is located between the cerebral peduncles). The large subarachnoid cistern below the cerebellum is the *cisterna magna.* In the spinal canal, where the spinal cord ends at the level of the second lumbar vertebra and the arachnoid remains closely applied to the dura mater to the level of the second sacral vertebra, a large lumbar subarachnoid space is formed that contains a reservoir of CSF, the filum terminale, and the nerve roots of the cauda equina as they pass to their intervertebral foramina.

The major arterial channels of the brain are located in the subarachnoid space. Bleeding from these vessels results in subarachnoid hemorrhage.

On gross inspection, the pia mater cannot be seen except at intervals in the spinal canal, where it extends laterally to attach to the dura mater as the *denticulate ligaments* (Fig. 4). Throughout the rest of its distribution, the pia

mater closely invests the central nervous system, with its few cell layers being separated from the outermost neural tissue, the *astrocytic glia limitans,* by a thin layer of collagen. In the arachnoid trabeculae, the cells of the pia mater and arachnoid are contiguous and are called pia-arachnoid (Fig. 5). Arterioles, as they dip into the parenchyma of the brain, are invested with a sheath of pia-arachnoid that disappears at the capillary level to leave only the endothelium of the blood vessel and its basement membrane in direct contact with the astrocytic glia limitans (Fig. 5). This forms the so-called blood–brain barrier.

Blood–brain barrier is a descriptive term first used many years ago when it was observed that certain dyes injected intravenously would stain all body organs except the brain; yet, the same dyes injected into the CSF would produce staining of brain tissue. Therefore, it was postulated that a barrier for the passage of the dye was located between the blood and the brain. The tight junctions of the unfenestrated endothelial cells are of major importance in maintaining the integrity of the blood–brain barrier. These junctions are not,

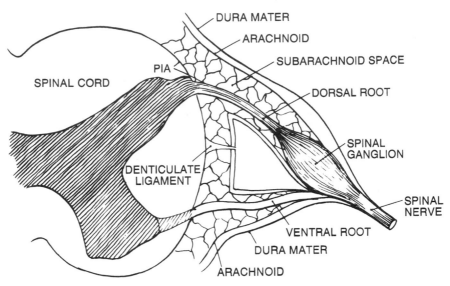

FIG. 4. Meningeal relationships at the spinal level. Note investments of the spinal nerve root by dura mater as it leaves the spinal canal. The denticulate ligaments attach the spinal cord to the dura mater laterally.

however, the only blood–brain barrier but merely part of a system of barriers (some anatomical, others physiologic) that serve to produce differences in the chemical composition of the brain, CSF, and blood.

Arachnoid villi (or granulations) (Fig. 2) are invaginations of the arachnoid into the dural venous sinuses. Fluid circulating through these villi passes into the venous blood and systemic circulation.

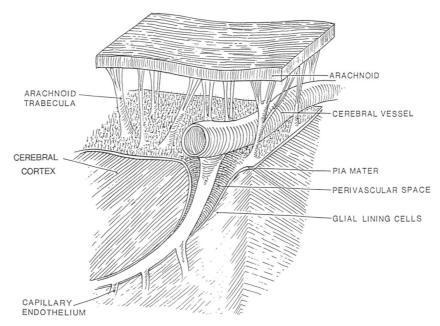

FIG. 5. Detailed relationships of the meninges and structures in the subarachnoid space. An arteriole carries pia mater into the cerebral cortex.

Ventricular System of the Brain

The ventricular system (Fig. 6) is lined with ciliated cuboidal epithelium (derived from ectoderm) called the *ependyma*. *Tanycytes* are specialized ependymal cells that lack cilia and are located in the lining of the floor of the third ventricle. They may be involved in the release of hypophysiotropic hormones from the hypothalamus into the portal circulation. *Choroid plexuses* are found in the lateral, third, and fourth ventricles. They are multitufted vascular organs that arise embryologically when ependyma, leptomeninges, and blood vessels fold into the ventricles. These structures, rich in the enzymes that are found in other secretory organs, are the main (but not the only) source for the production of the CSF. *Pinocytosis* is the movement of substances across the cell membrane in the form of tiny vesicles formed by pinching off a section of the surface membrane. The process of pinocytotic transport has been identified in the choroid plexus.

A *lateral ventricle* (Fig. 7) is located in each of the cerebral hemispheres and is divided into an anterior horn located in the frontal lobe, body and atrium (or trigone) in the parietal lobe, posterior horn in the occipital lobe, and inferior horn in the temporal lobe. The lateral ventricles communicate with each other and the *third ventricle* of the diencephalon via the *interventricular foramina of Monro*. The *aqueduct of Sylvius* traverses the mesencephalon and leads from the third ventricle to the *fourth ventricle,* located dorsal to the pons and medulla. The communication between the ventricular system and the subarachnoid space occurs in the fourth ventricle via two *foramina of Luschka* and the *foramen of Magendie.* A small and discontinuous *central canal* extends for a short distance from the caudal aspect of the fourth ventricle. At the spinal level, this canal is usually obliterated, and in normal adults only a few ependymal cells remain as remnants of the once prominent central canal of the embryo.

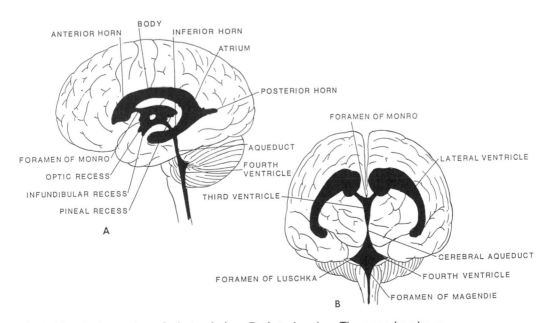

FIG. 6. Ventricular system. **A:** Lateral view. **B:** Anterior view. The pons has been removed from the illustration to display the anatomy of the fourth ventricle. (**A** modified from Noback, C. R., and Demarest, R. J. *The Nervous System: Introduction and Review* [2nd ed.]. New York: McGraw-Hill, 1977. With permission.)

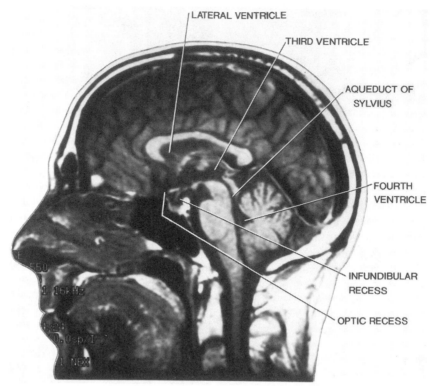

LATERAL VENTRICLE

THIRD VENTRICLE

AQUEDUCT OF SYLVIUS

FOURTH VENTRICLE

INFUNDIBULAR RECESS

OPTIC RECESS

FIG. 7. Sagittal magnetic resonance image of a normal human brain showing the ventricular system and its anatomical relations.

The Cerebrospinal Fluid

Formation and Circulation of CSF

The rate of CSF formation remains relatively constant at approximately 0.35 ml per minute (500 ml/day). Because the total volume of CSF in the adult is 90 to 150 ml, the processes of CSF formation and resorption must remain in delicate balance in order to prevent alteration in structure and function of the brain.

The production of CSF is an active process, mediated partly by the enzyme carbonic anhydrase. CSF production is relatively independent of hydrostatic forces; however, a decrease in choroid plexus perfusion pressure to 50 mm Hg causes a decrease in CSF production. In contrast, the rate of CSF absorption is proportional to the hydrostatic pressure, with greater absorption oc-

curring in the presence of increasing CSF pressure.

Nerve terminals have been identified on plexus arterioles and on the cells of the secretory epithelium. Thus, alterations in CSF production may occur in response to both intrinsic and extrinsic neurotransmitter systems, including norepinephrine and vasopressin.

Most of the CSF is actively secreted into the ventricular system by the choroid plexuses; however, these are not the only source of CSF. Some is derived directly from the interstitial fluid of the brain and crosses the ependyma to enter the ventricles. Additional exchange may take place between the neural tissue and the subarachnoid space across the pia mater.

Circulation of the CSF is pulsatile and promoted by the beating of the cilia of the ependymal cells and the pulsatile changes in the volume of intracranial blood that occurs with cardiac systole and respiratory movements. The to-and-fro movement of CSF results in a directional flow that is from the lateral, third, and fourth ventricles to the subarachnoid space, where it then circulates in two major directions. The more important pathway is rostrally through the tentorial notch and dorsally toward the intracranial venous system, where CSF exits through arachnoid villi that project into the dural venous sinuses, particularly the superior sagittal sinus. Although the exact mechanism of transfer of CSF to venous blood through the arachnoid villi is incompletely understood, transcellular transport via giant vacuoles seems most likely. The villi act as one-way valves, preventing entrance of blood into the CSF. A hydrostatic pressure of 70 mm H_2O or greater forces the CSF into the sinuses. The second pathway, a quantitatively less important and slower route taken by the CSF after its exit from the ventricular system, is downward through the foramen magnum into the spinal subarachnoid space, where it is partially resorbed through the leptomeninges.

CSF Pressure

The craniovertebral cavity and its dural lining are a closed space. Any increase in the volume of one of the three compartments (blood, CSF, brain) in the cavity can occur only in conjunction with an equal reduction in the volume of the others or with a consequent increase in pressure. Normally, however, the contents of the three compartments are relatively constant, producing a CSF pressure of 50 to 200 mm H_2O when recorded in the lumbar subarachnoid sac with the patient in a lateral recumbent position.

Minor oscillations occur in CSF pressure recorded in this manner in response to respiration and arterial pulsation, as varied amounts of blood enter and leave the craniovertebral cavity. Certain additional maneuvers cause wider oscillations in CSF pressure. Compression of the jugular veins, for example, impedes the outflow of blood from the brain, expands the venous vascular bed,

and causes a rapid increase in intracranial pressure. Because the lumbar subarachnoid sac is directly continuous with the intracranial subarachnoid space, this increase in pressure is transmitted throughout the ventricular system and subarachnoid space (as long as there is no obstruction to the flow of CSF). The spinal epidural venous plexuses normally contribute to the CSF pressure by continuous tamponade of the spinal dural sac. Increased intrathoracic or intraabdominal pressure (coughing, sneezing, straining at stool, or abdominal compression) can thereby increase CSF pressure.

In certain pathologic conditions, the increase in the volume of some of the components of the cranial cavity cannot be compensated for by readjustments in the volume of the other constituents. In this situation, intracranial pressure increases to abnormal levels. In addition, *plateau waves,* a pathologic increase in intracranial pressure, are occasionally noted. These acute increases in pressure may be as high as 600 to 1,300 mm H_2O and may be 5 to 20 minutes in duration. The cause of these pressure increases, which are accompanied by a reduction in cerebral blood flow, is not known.

Monitoring of CSF pressure has been used in various clinical situations (most notably in cases of head trauma) to help guide the management of patients with known or suspected increased intracranial pressure. The symptoms and consequences of increased intracranial pressure are discussed later in the chapter.

The Blood–Brain–CSF Barrier System

The central nervous system contains two basic fluid compartments: extracellular (CSF and interstitial fluid) and intracellular (primarily fluid within the cytoplasm of neurons and glial cells). The chemical compositions of these two fluid compartments are dissimilar, and the composition of each fluid differs significantly from that of blood. The chemical composition of the central nervous system fluid compartments is maintained within relatively narrow limits despite large fluctuations in the composition of extracellular fluid elsewhere in the body. Therefore, factors other than simple diffusion must be responsible for the passage of chemicals from one compartment to another.

Historically, reference has been made to a blood–brain barrier, implying an anatomical structure that would explain the variable distribution of substances in each compartment. Although not the sole explanation for the blood–brain barrier, anatomical considerations do have an important role. Morphologically, the choroidal epithelium, arachnoid, and capillary endothelial cells have *tight junctions* that obliterate the intercellular clefts normally between cells. This anatomical feature impedes the diffusion of larger molecules. Some areas of the brain, however, are excluded from this blood–brain barrier system (perhaps as a means of allowing neuronal receptors to sample plasma directly). In these regions, the capillary endothelium contains fenestrations that allow proteins and small molecules to pass from the blood to adjacent tissue. These regions are termed *circumventricular organs.* They include the *area postrema* located in the walls of the fourth ventricle (chemicals acting at this level may produce vomiting), the *subfornical organ* and neighboring structures located in the anterior wall of the third ventricle (chemicals acting here regulate thirst, water balance, and body temperature), the median eminence of the hypothalamus, the neurohypophysis, and the pineal gland. These areas have fenestrated capillaries rather than tight junctions, abundant capillary loops, and large perivascular spaces. Because of their unique structure and connections (neural and humoral sampling), circumventricular organs are important for homeostasis.

There are also other physicochemical factors, such as lipid solubility, protein binding, and state of ionization, that alter the passage of substances from one fluid compartment to another. In addition, certain substances are transported across membranes by carrier-mediated, facilitated diffusion systems, and others are transported by energy-requiring active transport systems. Therefore, although one commonly refers to a blood–brain barrier, one is in effect referring to a wide variety of barrier systems, some anatomical and physicochemical, that act together to maintain homeostasis.

With the breakdown of the blood–brain barrier in various pathologic conditions, several changes occur that are reflected as alterations in the composition of CSF. Four major mechanisms are believed to be involved in the increased vascular permeability noted in disease states: (1) interendothelial passage across tight junctions, (2) transendothelial flow, (3) vesicular transport, and (4) neovascularization.

Composition of CSF

One additional function of the CSF is to provide a pathway for the removal of the products of cerebral metabolism. In this regard, the CSF has been referred to as a large metabolic sink, a reservoir that allows metabolites of the brain to drain into it and then to enter the systemic circulation. Thus, the composition of the CSF is a reflection of the processes described above as well as the metabolic activity of the central nervous system.

Appearance

The CSF is normally clear and colorless; turbidity or discoloration is always abnormal. Turbidity most commonly is due to increased numbers of red or white blood cells. The most important cause of discoloration of the CSF is bleeding in the subarachnoid space. With subarachnoid hemorrhage (usually due to trauma or rupture of an intracranial vessel), the fluid is initially pink to red, depending on the severity of the bleeding. During the 2 to 10 hours after such an event, the red blood cells undergo lysis, and the liberated hemoglobin is broken down to form bilirubin, which imparts a yellow color (xanthochromia) to the CSF. A yellow discoloration also may be due to a markedly elevated level of CSF protein or may be secondary to an increase in the level of plasma bilirubin.

Cellular Elements

Normal CSF contains no more than five lymphocytes per microliter. A cell count of six to ten cells is very suspicious, and a count greater than ten is definitely abnormal and suggests the presence of disease in the central nervous system or in the meninges. The presence of polymorphonuclear leukocytes is always indicative of disease.

Microbiologic Features

CSF is normally sterile. Therefore, results of microbiologic studies (Gram's stain, cultures) should be negative.

Protein

The normal total CSF protein concentration is no greater than 45 mg per deciliter. The capillary endothelial membrane is highly effective in limiting the concentration of protein in the CSF, and increase in the CSF protein concentration is a frequent (but nonspecific) pathologic finding, suggestive of disease involving the central nervous system or meninges.

The amount of protein normally present in CSF is much less than that in plasma, although the relative proportions of the protein fractions are similar. Most of the CSF protein is probably derived from the plasma. One protein of clinical significance is the gamma globulin fraction. Normally, gamma globulin is synthesized outside the central nervous system. The normal concentration of gamma globulin in lumbar fluid is less than 13% of the total CSF protein concentration. In conditions such as multiple sclerosis, neurosyphilis, and some other subacute or chronic infections of the central nervous system, the gamma globulin level increases in association with a normal or slightly increased total protein level. (For this observation to be valid, there must be no change in the level of serum gamma globulin.) Such an increase in the gamma globulin in the CSF suggests an abnormal formation of gamma globulin by chronic inflammatory cells within the nervous system, with diffusion of the protein from brain to CSF.

Measurement of immunoglobulin G (IgG), which accounts for almost all the gamma globulin in normal CSF and in most disease states,

is a more sensitive indicator of central nervous system inflammation and immunoglobulin production than is total gamma globulin in disorders such as multiple sclerosis. Agar gel electrophoresis of concentrated CSF allows identification of qualitative changes in the IgG fraction. In normal CSF and in most noninflammatory neurologic diseases, the IgG fraction forms a diffuse, homogeneous zone of migration. Normal CSF IgG is less than 8.4 mg per deciliter. In multiple sclerosis and some other subacute and chronic inflammatory diseases, two or more discrete subfractions, which represent specific antibody populations called *oligoclonal bands,* are identified within the IgG migration zone. Another protein fraction derived from the central nervous system, myelin basic protein, can be identified by radioimmunoassay. It is not present in normal CSF and is an indicator of active demyelination.

Glucose

The glucose in CSF is normally about 60% to 70% of that in plasma. Therefore, the normal range in patients with blood levels of 80 to 120 mg per deciliter is between 45 and 80 mg per deciliter. Values less than 35 to 40 mg per deciliter are abnormal.

Glucose enters the CSF from plasma by facilitated diffusion via a specific transport system. Similar mechanisms are responsible for its removal. In addition, glucose is metabolized by arachnoidal, ependymal, neuronal, and glial cells, or it may leave the CSF with water (bulk flow).

Changes in levels of CSF glucose reflect similar changes in the blood, but a variable time is required before the CSF glucose equilibrates with the blood glucose. Thus, the CSF concentration does not reach a maximum for about 2 hours after the rapid intravenous injections of hypertonic glucose, and there is a similar delay in the lowering of the CSF glucose level after insulin-induced hypoglycemia. Therefore, when the CSF glucose determination is of diagnostic importance, CSF and blood levels should be obtained simultaneously, with the patient in a fasting state.

An increased CSF glucose level is of little diagnostic importance and likely reflects an increase in the serum glucose level. However, a low CSF glucose level (in the presence of a normal blood concentration) is very important. The CSF glucose level is characteristically low in acute bacterial and chronic fungal infections of the central nervous system. (It is frequently normal in viral infections.) Low CSF glucose values are thought to be primarily due to a breakdown of facilitated diffusion of glucose, which effectively slows the rate of entry of glucose into the central nervous system.

Clinical Correlations I: Disorders of the CSF System   ■

Syndrome of Increased Intracranial Pressure

An uncompensated increase in the volume of any of the constituents of the cranial vault results in an increase in intracranial pressure. Such an increase can occur from an increase in the total volume of brain tissue (as with diffuse cerebral edema), a focal increase in brain volume (as with an intracerebral hemorrhage, neoplasm, or other mass lesion), an increase in CSF volume without an associated loss of brain tissue (as in hydrocephalus), or diffuse vasodilatation or venous obstruction (from any of several causes). Whereas many clinical symptoms may be associated with increased intracranial pressure, none is individually diagnostic of this condition; yet, together they form a characteristic clinical pattern consisting of the following:

1. *Headache* is believed to be due to traction on the pain-sensitive structures within the cranium. Factors that tend to increase this traction, such as coughing, straining, or position change, tend to precipitate or aggravate the headache.
2. *Nausea* and *vomiting* are associated with the vagal motor centers, which are located in the floor of the fourth ventricle and mediate motility of the gastrointestinal tract. Increased ventricular pressure

transmitted to these centers may account for nausea and vomiting.
3. *Increased blood pressure* is related to intracranial pressure; as intracranial pressure increases, arterial blood pressure also must increase if brain blood flow is to continue. This response is mediated by neurons located in the ventrolateral medulla.
4. *Bradycardia* is presumed to be due to pressure on a vagal control mechanism similar to that proposed for nausea and vomiting.
5. *Papilledema* is characterized by elevation and blurring of the optic disk margin, as viewed with an ophthalmoscope (Fig. 8). The subdural and subarachnoid spaces of the brain extend along the course of the optic nerve (Fig. 9). Thus, increased pressure within the skull and subarachnoid space can be transmitted to the nerve, causing impairment of axonal transport. This results in edema of the nerve head.
6. *Alterations in consciousness* occur if the pressure increase is large, and as further pathologic change develops, consciousness may be lost because of diffuse hypoperfusion and secondary brainstem compression (see Chapter 10).
7. *Changes in the skull* occur in children and adults. In children, in whom the bones of the cranial vault have not yet permanently fused, chronic increases in pressure may be partially compensated for by a modest separation of the bones along the suture lines. In infants, in whom a soft spot (fontanelle) is not yet ossified, this membranous structure located at the vertex of the head may become tense and bulge outward. In adults, in whom bony fusion is complete and the skull is incapable of further expansion, some demineralization of bone, especially around the sella turcica, is occasionally seen.

The clinical syndrome of increased intracranial pressure may occur in isolation, but more commonly it is superimposed on the signs and symptoms of the underlying patho-

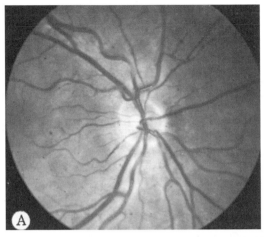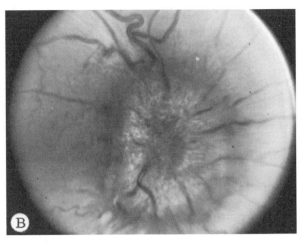

FIG. 8. Optic fundus and optic nerve head. **A:** Normal optic disk. **B:** Papilledema. Disk margins are elevated and blurred; venous congestion and hemorrhages are seen surrounding the disk.

logic lesion. If this syndrome occurs with signs of a focal lesion, whether acute, subacute, or chronic in their evolution, the diagnosis of a mass lesion becomes highly likely.

Intracranial Hypotension

Intracranial hypotension due to leakage of CSF is a common complication following lumbar puncture. It also can occur spontaneously. Usually, it is manifested by postural headache, which occurs or is made worse by assuming an upright position.

Hydrocephalus

In certain pathologic conditions, the pathway for CSF circulation is blocked and absorption is impaired. The rate of CSF formation by the choroid plexus remains relatively constant, and because the relative amount of CSF increases, there is a corresponding increase in ventricular pressure, and progressive dilatation of the ventricles (hydrocephalus) occurs in regions proximal to the blockage (Fig. 10). Signs and symptoms of increased intracranial pressure also may develop.

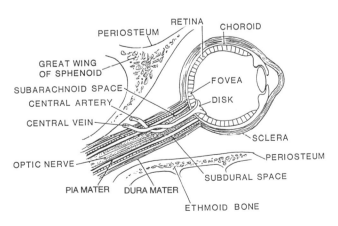

FIG. 9. Relationships of the meninges and meningeal spaces to the optic nerve. Increased intracranial pressure may result in edema of optic nerve head.

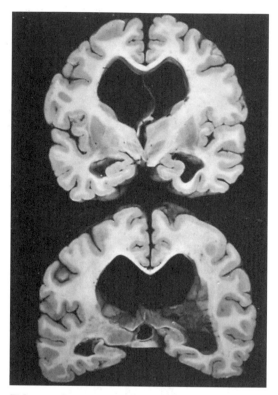

FIG. 10. Coronal sections of the cerebral hemispheres showing hydrocephalus. Note marked dilatation of the lateral ventricles, with thinning of the cerebral walls at the expense of the white matter. In the lower (more posterior) section, the thin septum has been artifically torn.

Before adequate techniques for visualization of the ventricular system were available, clinicians devised a method for determining the site of blockage in hydrocephalus. Histologic studies of the pathology had shown that the obstruction was most commonly either (1) within the ventricular system itself, that is, proximal to the outlets of the fourth ventricle as in, for example, aqueductal stenosis; or (2) outside the ventricular system where inadequate circulation over the convexities of the brain prevents adequate resorption, for example, after meningitis or subarachnoid hemorrhage (Fig. 11). To differentiate these two conditions, a cannula was inserted through the skull into the ventricular system and a second cannula was inserted into the lumbar subarachnoid space. If dye that was injected into the ventricles could be recovered later in the lumbar sac, then a *communicating hydrocephalus* indicating an extraventricular blockage was present; if no dye was recovered, then a *noncommunicating hydrocephalus* indicating a blockage within the ventricular system was present. Although clinicians no longer use this method of diagnosis, the responsible lesions are still often referred to as producing either a communicating or a noncommunicating hydrocephalus.

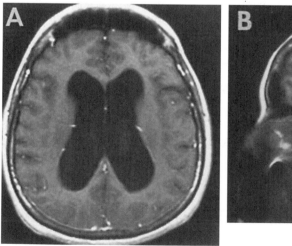
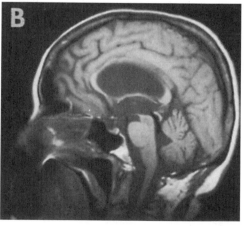

FIG. 11. Communicating hydrocephalus as shown by magnetic resonance imaging. **A:** Horizontal view. **B:** Sagittal view.

The term *hydrocephalus* also describes the situation that occurs in brain atrophy. Coincident with the reduction in volume of brain tissue, there is enlargement of the ventricles and subarachnoid spaces, with an increase in the amount of CSF. The total volume of the intracranial contents remains unchanged, however, and there is no increase in intracranial pressure. This type of process is referred to as *hydrocephalus ex vacuo.*

Cerebral Edema

Brain swelling, or *edema,* is an increase in brain volume due to an increase in the water content of the brain. It is a nonspecific condition that can be associated with a wide variety of cerebral disorders, including hypoxia, meningitis, neoplasm, abscess, and infarction. Three major types of brain edema have been described:

1. *Vasogenic edema* results from an increase in permeability of brain capillary endothelial cells and produces an increase in extracellular fluid volume.
2. *Cytotoxic edema* is an increase in the intracellular fluid volume of the brain. This form of edema is presumably caused by a failure of the ATP-dependent sodium pump mechanism, with the result that sodium efflux is altered and water enters the cell in order to maintain osmotic equilibrium.
3. *Interstitial edema* is a periventricular transudate seen in cases of communicating hydrocephalus with increased CSF pressure and passive movement of CSF from the ventricles to the surrounding periventricular regions.

Although vasogenic edema is most often seen surrounding focal brain lesions and cytotoxic edema is seen in association with hypoxia, either type may be relatively well localized or diffuse and widespread. Both types result in an increase in intracranial volume and pressure, causing symptoms of increased intracranial pressure that may be superimposed on the underlying pathologic process (Fig. 12). Clinical monitoring of intracranial pressure can be accomplished with a transducer surgically placed through the skull. The constant assessment of pressure-related changes provides a physiologic basis for therapeutic intervention.

Syndrome of Acute Meningeal Irritation

Several noxious agents produce meningeal irritation, but regardless of the cause, the clinical manifestations are similar and consist of the following:

1. *Headache* is usually prominent and severe and due to vasodilatation or chemical irritation or inflammation (or both) of the major pain-sensitive structures.
2. *Stiff neck* is caused by irritation of the meninges in the posterior fossa and upper cervical spinal canal, which stimulates spinal nerve roots and results in reflex spasm and contraction of the posterior neck muscles. This increased resistance to neck flexion is termed *nuchal rigidity.*
3. *Alteration in consciousness* results from a pathologic process that is widespread and severe, causing diffuse depression of cortical function and change in the level of consciousness.

The most common causes of the syndrome of acute meningeal irritation are bacterial meningitis, viral encephalitis, and subarachnoid hemorrhage. Each of these superimposes its own characteristic signature on the general pattern of meningeal irritation.

Bacterial Meningitis

An inflammation of the CSF system can be caused by bacterial invasion and can be accompanied by a characteristic leukocytic exudate in the pia mater and arachnoid as well as in structures adjacent to the leptomeninges (Fig. 13). Bacteria may be found in the CSF and within neutrophilic white blood cells. The type of leukocytic exudate reflects the nature of the invading organism. Most commonly, acute infections are caused by meningococ-

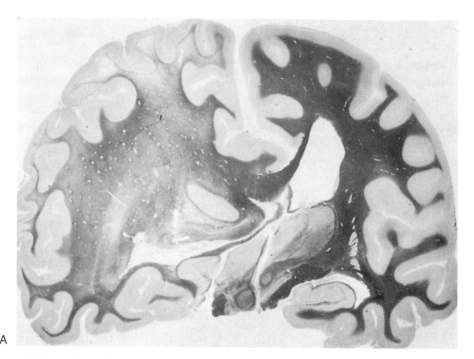

A

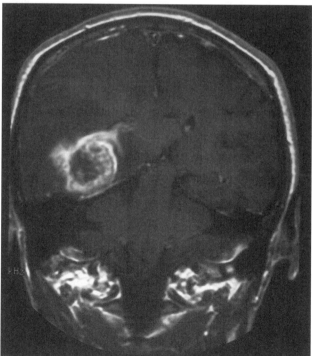

B

FIG. 12. A: Cerebral edema (associated with neighboring meningioma, not shown). Note pallor and swelling of the white matter of the left cerebral hemisphere, with marked shift of the midline structures from left to right. (Luxol-fast blue stain; ×1.) **B:** Magnetic resonance imaging of the brain showing vasogenic edema surrounding a malignant glioma in the right temporal lobe. The increased permeability of the blood–brain barrier is demonstrated by leakage of the contrast material gadolinium (shown as *white*). Note the mass effect, with distortion and shift of the midbrain to the opposite side.

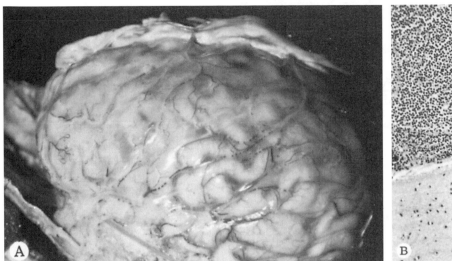
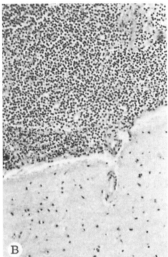

FIG. 13. Acute purulent bacterial meningitis. **A:** Brain *in situ* viewed from the left side showing marked clouding of the subarachnoid space. **B:** Section of cerebral cortex, with the adjacent subarachnoid space filled with acute inflammatory cells. (H&E; ×250.)

cus, *Haemophilus influenzae,* and pneumococcus organisms, and are accompanied by a polymorphonuclear exudate. More indolent infections, such as those caused by the tubercle bacillus or fungi, are associated with a predominance of lymphocytes. Immunosuppressed patients, for example, those with acquired immunodeficiency syndrome (AIDS) or those who take drugs to prevent rejection of a transplanted organ, commonly have meningitis due to opportunistic organisms such as fungi or parasites. In these cases, the cellular response may be poor. The pathologic reaction is distributed widely throughout the leptomeninges, but it may be most extensive in the basal subarachnoid cisterns. The clinical-anatomical-temporal profile of this disorder is that of diffuse, subacute, and progressive involvement of the nervous system, with the superimposed features of fever and systemic reaction and the syndrome of meningeal irritation, and with or without evidence of increased intracranial pressure. After treatment or subsidence of the infection, reactive changes may occur within the CSF system, impairing CSF absorption and producing hydrocephalus.

Viral Encephalitis

Viral infections usually induce remarkably few gross pathologic changes in the brain. Vascular dilatation, congestion, and edema are not uncommon, and occasional petechial hemorrhages may be seen in the cerebral cortex. Histopathologically, there are necrosis of nerve cells and neuronophagia, perivascular cuffing by lymphocytes and mononuclear leukocytes, and meningeal infiltration by similar cells. The clinical-anatomical-temporal profile of this disorder is virtually identical to that noted for bacterial meningitis (diffuse, subacute, and progressive); however, because of the difference in inflammatory response, the findings on examination of the CSF may differ (Table 1).

Subarachnoid Hemorrhage

The acute rupture of an intracranial vessel may produce little pathologic change in the brain itself. As red blood cells intermix with CSF, the signs and symptoms of meningeal irritation are to be expected. Most commonly,

TABLE 1. *CSF findings in syndromes involving meningeal irritation*

CSF	Normal	Subarachnoid hemorrhage	Bacterial meningitis	Viral encephalitis
Appearance	Clear	Bloody	Cloudy	Clear to slightly cloudy
Cell count	<5 lymphocytes	Red blood cells present; white blood cells in proportion to red blood cells in the peripheral blood cell count	Usually >1,000 white blood cells; mostly polymorphonuclear leukocytes	Usually 25–500 white blood cells, mostly lymphocytes
Protein	<45 mg/dl	Normal to slightly increased	Usually increased >100 mg/dl	Minimally increased, usually <100 mg/dl
Glucose	>45 mg/dl	Normal (rarely decreased)	Decreased	Normal
Microbiologic findings	Negative	Negative	Positive Gram's stain; positive cultures	Negative Gram's stain; negative viral cultures usually

CSF, cerebrospinal fluid.

subarachnoid hemorrhage occurs as a result of trauma, rupture of an intracranial aneurysm, or leakage from an arteriovenous malformation. Although the bleeding is often from a single well-localized source, blood rapidly mixes with CSF and is distributed throughout the neuraxis (Fig. 14). A diffuse, acute, and sometimes progressive disorder results. Only rarely does the aneurysm produce focal signs.

Examination of the CSF by lumbar puncture is the usual means of initially differentiating the disorders that produce the syndrome of meningeal irritation (see Table 1).

Intracranial Epidural Hematoma

The epidural hemorrhage lies between the dura mater and the inner table of the skull and most commonly occurs from a skull fracture or traumatic laceration of the *middle meningeal artery*. Blood dissects the dura mater from the bone, forming a localized, rapidly expanding intracranial mass. Typically, the patient receives an injury to the head of sufficient degree to produce a period of unconsciousness. Thereafter, depending on the rate of bleeding, the patient becomes increasingly drowsy and lapses into stupor and finally into deep coma. The cerebral hemisphere is pushed medially by the enlarging mass and compresses the midbrain against the unyielding free edge of the tentorium cerebelli. The

patient will die unless emergency measures are taken to evacuate the blood clot.

The clinical-anatomical-temporal profile of this lesion is that of an acute, focal, and progressive lesion, with evidence of increased intracranial pressure. A history of trauma is often present.

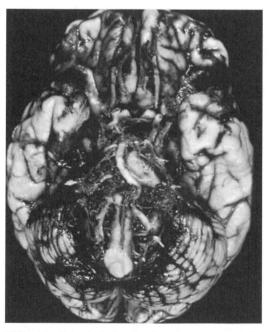

FIG. 14. Base of the brain after acute subarachnoid hemorrhage due to a ruptured aneurysm. Note that blood occurs throughout the subarachnoid space but is concentrated in major cisterns.

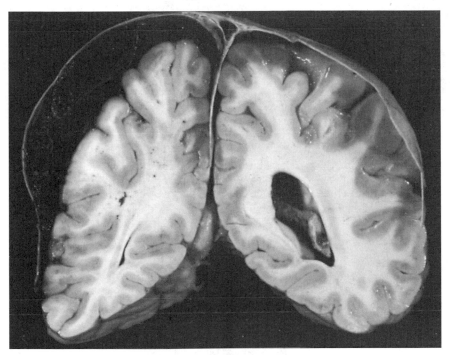

FIG. 15. Left subdural hematoma. Note accumulation of blood between the dura mater and arachnoid, with compression of the left cerebral hemisphere.

Intracranial Subdural Hematoma

Subdural hematomas are seen most commonly in infants and adults of middle age and older, particularly adults who are likely to suffer head injury (for example, alcoholics). The injury that produces the hematoma may be either severe or so mild that it is forgotten.

At the time of injury, a tear usually occurs in a cortical vein at the point where it attaches to the superior sagittal sinus. As a result, a small amount of bleeding occurs in the subdural space. This initial blood often is not enough to cause noticeable symptoms. Fibroblasts and capillaries proliferate and surround this blood with a fibrous membrane derived from the dura mater. Enlargement of the hematoma results from recurrent bleeding of the neomembrane or from increased osmotic activity of disintegrating red blood cells. With further increase in size, the intracranial volume increases, compressing the underlying brain (Fig. 15). The typical clinical-anatomi-cal-temporal profile of this not uncommon and potential treatable disorder is that of a chronic, focal, progressive lesion with symptoms of increased intracranial pressure.

Clinical Correlations II: Diagnostic Studies Utilizing the CSF System ■

The anatomy, physiology, and known pathologic changes that may occur within the CSF system serve as the basis for many neurodiagnostic tests.

Lumbar Puncture

Although lumbar puncture is a procedure with little risk or discomfort to the patient, examination of the CSF via puncture of the lumbar subarachnoid sac is not a routine diagnostic test. Lumbar puncture is indicated only when it is necessary to obtain specific information about the cellular or chemical constituents of the CSF. The procedure usually is contraindicated if there is known or suspected increased intracranial pressure, because in certain instances (especially those of localized mass lesions) sudden alteration in CSF pressure dynamics can lead to herniation of the brain contents through the foramen magnum and clinical decompensation or death. Usually, when increased intracranial pressure is suspected, a brain imaging study (such as computed tomography or magnetic resonance imaging) is performed to help define the nature of the intracranial pathologic process before deciding whether lumbar puncture is needed.

The examination usually is performed in one of the three lower lumbar interspaces (Fig. 16). Puncture above the L2-3 interspace (the region of the conus medullaris) is inadvisable. In infants or children in whom the spinal cord may be situated at a lower level, the puncture should be performed in the L4-5 or L5-S1 interspace.

With the patient in a lateral recumbent position, the use of a simple manometer allows measurement of CSF pressure (normally less than 200 mm H_2O). To ensure that the needle is properly placed in the subarachnoid sac, the pressure response to gentle coughing, straining, or abdominal compression should be observed. Normally, a prompt increase in pressure of at least 40 mm H_2O results from the elevation of central venous pressure that accompanies these maneuvers.

After determination of the initial pressure, the appearance of the fluid is noted, and 5 to 15 ml of CSF is removed for cell count, protein analysis, glucose determination, and microbiologic and other studies. A serologic test for syphilis is generally performed on all spinal fluid specimens because that disease, characterized partly by a chronic inflammatory reaction in the central nervous system, may mimic many other disorders.

Even with the most experienced examiners, occasionally one of the veins lying in the spinal epidural space is nicked by the lumbar puncture needle; a "traumatic tap" results, bloody fluid is obtained, and one must differentiate this from a true subarachnoid hemorrhage. In a traumatic tap, fluid collected in successive test tubes usually shows decreasing amounts of red blood cells, whereas in cases of hemorrhagic disease the blood staining of fluid remains uniform. Furthermore, in a hemorrhagic disorder, several hours often elapse between the onset of symptoms and the performance of a lumbar puncture, and xanthochromic staining of the supernatant fluid is seen in a centrifuged specimen; this staining is not noted in the case of a traumatic puncture.

Myelography

Myelography consists of the introduction of a radiopaque substance, usually via lumbar puncture, into the subarachnoid space. Myelography can be used to study the spinal canal (Fig. 17A) and posterior fossa (Fig. 17B) and is often combined with computed

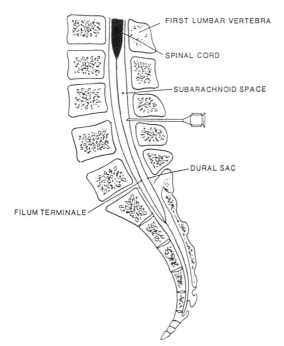

FIRST LUMBAR VERTEBRA

SPINAL CORD

SUBARACHNOID SPACE

DURAL SAC

FILUM TERMINALE

FIG. 16. Site of lumbar puncture. Note that in a normal adult, the caudal border of spinal cord lies at the L-1–L-2 vertebral level.

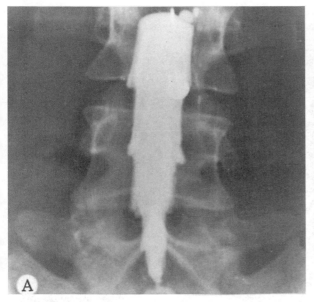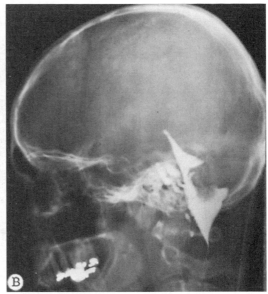

FIG. 17. Myelograms. **A:** Anteroposterior view showing filling of the lumbar subarachnoid space. **B:** By tilting the patient downward, contrast medium can be used to visualize the entire spinal canal and structures contained in the posterior fossa (lateral view).

tomography for better definition of abnormality at the spinal level.

Computed Tomographic Imaging

Computed tomography is another method of studying the anatomy of the intracranial space in patients. This technique, which is rapid, painless, and almost free of risk, permits visualization of the ventricular system, subarachnoid space, and parenchymal structures at the spinal, posterior fossa, and supratentorial levels (Fig. 18).

All computed tomographic imaging techniques are based on four general principles. First, they all look at a physical characteristic of small volumes of tissue (voxels) within a "slice" of the body in a particular plane. Second, they have an array of detectors that allow measurement of that characteristic in each voxel from many different directions. Third, they use a computer to mathematically process the data collected in the detectors in such a way that it localizes each voxel

within the slice and assigns it a relative value. Fourth, they use a display module to create a map of the location and relative value of the characteristic in each voxel addressed. This produces a picture in which each voxel is represented by a dot (pixel) of relative intensity on a black-white (or sometimes color) scale. The shade is proportional to the magnitude or intensity of the tissue characteristic measured. The resolution of anatomical and pathologic detail of the resulting picture depends on the matrix (number of pixels per unit area) and the range of differences in the characteristic under study that can be measured. In x-ray computed tomographic scanning, the tissue characteristic measured is electron density as manifested by attenuation of an x-ray beam. In positron emission tomographic scanning, it is the ability of tissue to take up molecules containing positron-emitting isotopes. In magnetic resonance imaging, it is the density and physical state of mobile hydrogen nuclei (protons) in the tissue.

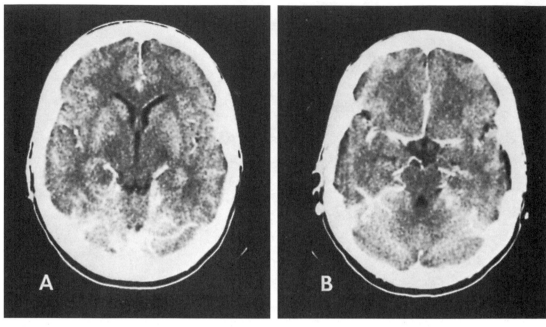

FIG. 18. Computed tomograms (horizontal sections). **A:** Level of the caudate nucleus and thalamus. **B:** The base of the brain at the level of the midbrain.

X-Ray Computed Tomography

Computed tomographic techniques using x-rays to generate the scan were the first to be developed for clinical use. Thin beams of x-ray are passed through the patient's head, and the amount of energy transmitted (not absorbed by structures in its path) is measured by an x-ray detector on the opposite side of the head. This is repeated thousands of times (within a few seconds) from every point around the circumference of the head. The absorption data are processed by a computer, which reconstructs a horizontal section of the head about 1 cm thick. The entire cranial contents can be demonstrated by generating a series of adjacent sections. The ventricular system and any distortions and displacements can be identified. Most hemorrhages, infarcts, and tumors in the substance of the brain can be detected because their density (x-ray absorption) differs from that of normal brain. Intravenously administered contrast media (iodine-containing compounds) aid in visualizing lesions that are

vascular or in which the blood–brain barrier is disturbed.

Magnetic Resonance Imaging

Magnetic resonance imaging is the most recently developed technique for imaging the internal structures of the body, including the central nervous system (Fig. 19). The physics of magnetic resonance imaging are complicated and beyond the scope of this discussion. Briefly, hydrogen nuclei (protons) in tissue, mostly as part of water molecules, normally are aligned randomly. When the body is placed in a strong magnetic field, the protons, which behave as tiny magnets because of their spin, align longitudinally in the direction of the flux lines of the field. When a pulse of energy in the form of radio-frequency waves is delivered to the tissue, the aligned protons absorb energy and tilt away from the longitudinal toward the transverse axis of the magnetic field. When the radio-frequency pulse is turned off, the protons begin to realign in the axis of the main magnetic field. It is during this process

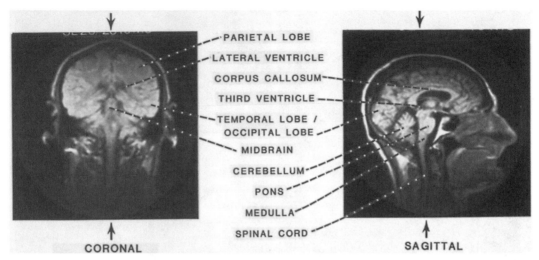

PARIETAL LOBE
LATERAL VENTRICLE
CORPUS CALLOSUM
THIRD VENTRICLE
TEMPORAL LOBE /
OCCIPITAL LOBE
MIDBRAIN
CEREBELLUM
PONS
MEDULLA
SPINAL CORD

CORONAL   SAGITTAL

FIG. 19. Magnetic resonance imaging of the head in computer-reconstructed coronal and sagittal planes. *Arrows* indicate the level of the images of the other plane.

that they emit radio-frequency energy that is picked up by the detectors. Protons spin at a frequency directly proportional to the local magnetic field. The frequency of this spin is the frequency picked up by the detectors. The different frequencies seen by the detector array allow the voxels to be localized in space.

Signals are only sent from the tissue during the return, or relaxation phase, from transverse magnetization back to longitudinal magnetization. Loss of transverse magnetization occurs from reorientation of protons in the main magnetic field and from magnetic interactions of spinning protons in the tissue, causing them to become out of phase with one another. These two phenomena occur at exponential rates that have time constants referred to as T1 and T2, respectively. In addition to local tissue factors, the intensity of the signal in each voxel is determined by the sequence of radio-frequency pulses, the interval between the pulses, the interval between excitation and detection, and the number of times the sequence is repeated. These factors are under operator control and can be manipulated to emphasize signals generated by either T1 or T2 relaxation phenomena. The resulting images are referred to as being T1- or T2-weighted. They display somewhat different tissue characteristics and, therefore, different signal intensities in the same tissue. The T1-weighted images are better for defining normal anatomy (Fig. 19). The T2-weighted images are most sensitive for most pathologic conditions, including those producing edema (for example, infarcts, tumors) or loss of myelin (for example, multiple sclerosis). Magnetic resonance imaging is especially useful in visualizing posterior fossa structures, the craniocervical junction, and the cervical and thoracic spinal cord. Contrast materials such as gadolinium can be used to enhance lesions associated with increased permeability of the blood–brain barrier.

From a practical clinical standpoint, the major advantage of magnetic resonance imaging over computed tomography is the greater sensitivity of the technique and greater anatomical detail of the images generation (Fig. 20). Other advantages are listed in Table 2. Currently, the drawbacks to the use of magnetic resonance imaging are the need for much greater patient cooperation because of the time required to generate images (which are degraded by any motion), the inability to scan patients with pacemakers or other electronic or metallic implants that could be affected by a magnetic field, and the cost.

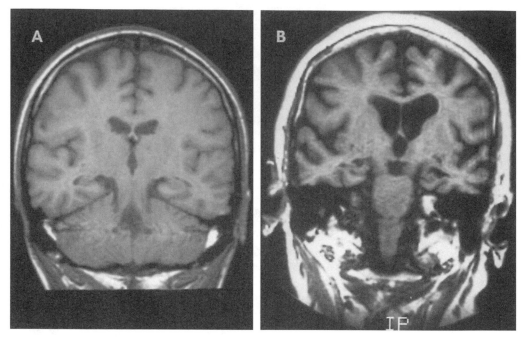

FIG. 20. Magnetic resonance imaging—coronal sections of the brain. **A:** Normal brain. **B:** Brain with atrophy and enlarged ventricles.

Nuclear Medicine Techniques

Radioisotope brain scan is based on detection of focal areas of increased permeability of the blood–brain barrier (for example, tumor, abscess) shown by leakage and accumulation of a normally nondiffusible molecule labeled with a radioisotope and injected intravenously. This technique has been replaced by computed tomography and magnetic resonance imaging.

By injecting a radioisotope into the lumbar subarachnoid space, physiologic observations can be made on the circulation of CSF. Normally, the injected material will rise and accumulate both within the ventricular system and over the convexity of the brain. Localization of the indicator within the ventricles and failure to circulate over the brain surface after 48 hours are suggestive of a blockage in the extraventricular CSF pathways. Both signs are frequently seen in cases of communicating hydrocephalus. This technique is called *radioisotope cisternography.* A similar procedure can be used to evaluate a *CSF leak* in patients with intracranial hypotension. For example, after a skull fracture, CSF may leak through the cribriform plate and produce CSF rhinorrhea. The site of the leak can be identified by detecting where the isotope accumulates.

TABLE 2. *Advantage of magnetic resonance imaging compared with x-ray computed tomography*

No exposure to ionizing radiation
No interference by surrounding bone
Superior resolution of soft tissue
Images can be produced in virtually any plane
Able to image flowing blood
Physiologic imaging

Neurologic Examination of the CSF System

As part of the neurologic examination of patients with suspected disease of the CSF system, it is necessary to search specifically for signs of increased intracranial pressure and meningeal irritation. In addition, assessment of this system occasionally requires lumbar puncture.

An increase in intracranial pressure is suspected on the basis of the clinical-anatomical-temporal profile of the illness and the constellation of signs and symptoms outlined above. Not all patients with increased intracranial pressure have papilledema; however, ophthalmoscopic visualization of the optic nerve head in search of papilledema should be carefully performed on all such patients. One must be cautious; although the presence of edema of the nerve head should always raise the possibility of an increase in intracranial pressure, it may be associated with other conditions.

The presence of meningeal irritation is best determined by examining for *nuchal rigidity.* When there is meningeal irritation, the side-to-side movement of the neck causes little discomfort, and frequently the first 10 to 15 degrees of neck flexion meet with little resistance, but with additional flexion resistance and discomfort increase rapidly. To reduce the effects of traction on the lumbosacral roots when the neck is flexed, a patient with meningeal irritation may automatically flex the hips and knees. (This type of abnormal response seen with meningeal irritation is referred to as *Brudzinski's sign.*) An additional and related test can be performed with the patient recumbent and the legs flexed at the hips and knees. In this position, the lumbosacral nerve roots are relatively slack, and maneuvers designed to stretch these nerve roots (such as extension of the knee) normally produce no discomfort. In the presence of meningeal irritation, there are pain and increased resistance (Kernig's sign). When Kernig's sign is encountered in the absence of nuchal rigidity (and especially if it is unilateral), it is indicative of an irritative process involving the lumbosacral nerve roots rather than of diffuse meningeal irritation.

Clinical Problems

1. A 10-month-old infant presents with an enlarging head and a delay in reaching developmental milestones. The neurologic examination confirms developmental delay and also reveals a tense, bulging, enlarged anterior fontanelle; ophthalmoscopic examination reveals normal fundi; and the head circumference is 50 cm. An opening pressure of 200 mm H_2O is found on lumbar puncture. Based on these findings, answer the following questions:
   a. How do we know the head is abnormally large?
   b. What are the possible causes of a large head?
   c. What tests might be useful in obtaining information about the infant's ventricular system?
   d. Does the lesion found in this patient (see answer to previous question) produce a communicating or noncommunicating type of hydrocephalus?
   e. What changes would you expect to find in the configuration of the ventricular system in a computed tomographic scan or magnetic resonance image of
      i. this patient.
      ii. a patient with chronic obstruction of the foramina of Luschka and Magendie.
      iii. a patient with inflammatory obliteration of the intracranial arachnoid villi.
      iv. a patient with an acute subarachnoid hemorrhage.

2. A 38-year-old man with the same pathologic condition as the infant in problem 1 has a normal head size, papilledema, and an opening pressure of 500 mm H_2O on lumbar puncture. How can you explain the differences in these two cases?

3. A 37-year-old man is evaluated because of a 6-month history of progressive weakness in his legs and loss of pain and thermal sensation to the level of his nipples. Based on your findings on physical examination and normal radiographic findings in the head and in the cervical, thoracic, and lumbar regions of the spinal

column, you perform a lumbar puncture with the following results:

a. Hydrodynamics:
   i. Opening pressure of 80 mm H_2O
   ii. Spontaneous pulsations
      Respiratory: 10 to 20 mm H_2O
      Cardiac: None
   iii. Abdominal compression gives prompt increase of 70 mm H_2O, with rapid decrease to 80 mm H_2O on release of pressure

b. Spinal fluid examination:
   i. Appearance: Slightly yellow, clear fluid
   ii. Cells:
     (a) White blood cells = 4 lymphocytes per microliter
     (b) Red blood cells = 0
   iii. Chemistry:
     (a) Protein = 700 mg/dl
     (b) Glucose = 65 mg/dl
     (c) Blood sugar = 100 mg/dl

Based on these findings, answer the following questions:

a. What is the location of this lesion? (level? lateralization?) Is this a mass lesion? What is the cause?
b. How would you explain each of the hydrodynamic findings on the lumbar puncture?
c. What structures did the lumbar puncture needle penetrate before it reached the subarachnoid space?
d. What radiologic study might help you locate the lesion(s) accurately?

4. You are called to the emergency room to see a semicomatose elderly woman who responds to painful stimuli with movement of all four extremities. She was brought to the hospital by police ambulance after being found in her apartment by neighbors who had not seen her for 3 days. The physical examination reveals blood pressure 120/80 mm Hg, pulse 120 per minute, respiration 124 per minute, and temperature 39.5°C rectally. There is marked resistance to flexion but not to lateral rotation of the neck. Results of the remainder of the examination are normal. Lumbar puncture reveals an opening pressure of 270 mm H_2O. CSF examination reveals the following:

a. Appearance before centrifugation:
   Tube #1: 2+ pink; 2+ turbid
   Tube #3: slightly pink; 2+ turbid
b. Appearance after centrifugation:
   All tubes clear and colorless
c. Cell counts:
   Tube #1: 300 white blood cells (90% polymorphonuclear leukocytes), 2,800 red blood cells
   Tube #3: 320 white blood cells (90% polymorphonuclear leukocytes), 700 red blood cells
d. Protein:
   Tube #1: 180 mg/dl
   Tube #3: 176 mg/dl
e. Glucose:
   10 mg/dl in all tubes

Based on these findings, answer the following questions:

a. What is the location of this lesion? (level? lateralization?) Is this a mass lesion? What is the cause?
b. How do you explain the differences in appearance and cellular count of the CSF between tubes #1 and #3?
c. What would you expect to find on Gram's stain of the CSF? On culture of the CSF?
d. How would you explain the CSF glucose result?

Additional Reading ■

Davson, H., Welch, K., and Segal, M. B. *Physiology and Pathophysiology of the Cerebrospinal Fluid.* Edinburgh: Churchill Livingstone, 1987.

Fishman, R. A. *Cerebrospinal Fluid in Diseases of the Nervous System* (2nd ed.). Philadelphia: W. B. Saunders, 1992.

Lyons, M. K., and Meyer, F. B. Cerebrospinal fluid physiology and the management of increased intracranial pressure. *Mayo Clin. Proc.* 65:684, 1990.

North, B., and Reilly, P. Comparison among three methods of intracranial pressure recording. *Neurosurgery* 18:730, 1986.

The Sensory System

Objectives ■

1. Define receptor, sensory unit, and receptive field.
2. Define receptor potential, frequency and population coding, receptor adaptation, and receptor specificity.
3. Define in physiologic terms the differences between rapidly adapting (phasic) and slowly adapting (tonic) receptors.
4. List the types of somatic receptors.
5. Define hierarchical and parallel organization of somatosensory systems, and list the differences between the direct and indirect somatosensory pathways.
6. Describe the main features of wide dynamic neurons in the dorsal horn.
7. Name the function of the following pathways and trace their paths:
   a. Direct dorsal column–lemniscal tract
   b. Direct spinothalamic (neospinothalamic) tract
   c. Indirect spinothalamic (paleospinothalamic) tract
   d. Dorsal spinocerebellar tract
   e. Ventral spinocerebellar tract
8. Explain the differential effects of lesions involving all large afferents versus lesions restricted to the dorsal columns.
9. Describe the two main types of primary nociceptive units.
10. Explain the concepts of lateral inhibition, gate control, and windup phenomenon.
11. Name the main components of the central pain regulation system. Describe the functions of substance P, opioids, sero-

tonin, and norepinephrine in pain processing.
12. Describe the clinical manifestations of lesions involving the five pathways listed in objective 7, and list the differences that may be encountered when the lesion is located at the peripheral, spinal, posterior fossa, or supratentorial level.
13. Describe sacral sparing, cortical sensory loss, and Brown-Séquard's syndrome, and describe the anatomical basis for these conditions.
14. Describe the mechanisms of sensory dissociation in syringomyelia and selective lesions of large compared with small dorsal root ganglion neurons and fibers.
15. Differentiate between sensory and motor ataxia.
16. Given a patient problem, list the aspects of the history and physical examination that point to a disturbance in the sensory system, localize the area of disturbance to a particular portion of the neuraxis, and state the pathologic nature of the responsible lesion.

Introduction ■

The function of the sensory system is to provide information to the central nervous system about the *external* world, the *internal* environment, and the *position* of the body in space. Impulses traveling toward the central nervous system are called *afferent impulses*. Afferent information may be transmitted (1) as conscious data that are perceived by the organism and then used to modify behavior; (2) as unconscious data that, although used to modify behavior, remain unperceived by the organism; and (3) as both conscious and unconscious data. *Sensory pathways* are afferent pathways involved in conscious perception. Afferent impulses are functionally subdivided into the following:

1. General somatic afferent (GSA)—sensory information from skin, striated muscles, and joints
2. General visceral afferent (GVA)—sensory information, largely unconscious in nature, from serosal and mucosal surfaces and smooth muscle of the viscera
3. Special somatic afferent (SSA)—sensory information relating to vision, audition, and equilibrium
4. Special visceral afferent (SVA)—sensory information relating to taste and smell

Although introductory comments are made in relation to each of these subdivisions, this chapter is concerned primarily with the organization and function of the *general somatic afferent system.*

Overview ◼

The translation of information from the environment is the function of the *receptor organs.* The function of these specialized portions of the peripheral nervous system is to convert mechanical, chemical, photic, and other forms of energy into electrical potentials, one of the forms of information used by the nervous system. Action potentials are then transmitted by specific *sensory pathways* to those regions of the central nervous system where the information is integrated and perception occurs. The peripheral region from which a stimulus affects a central sensory neuron in the *sensory field* of that neuron.

The pathways involved in conscious perception have both a hierarchical and a parallel organization. Hierarchical organization

means that sensory information is transmitted sequentially via several orders of neurons located in *relay nuclei* and processed at each relay station under the control of higher stations in the pathway. Parallel organization implies that different submodalities within tactile, visual, and other sensations are transmitted via separate, parallel channels and that a given sensory modality, such as simple touch, is transmitted by different ascending pathways.

Somatosensory pathways from the trunk and extremities course in the spinal cord, and those transmitting information from the face form the trigeminal system. The trigeminal system is discussed further in Chapter 15.

Somatosensory pathways can be subdivided according to three different functions: (1) transmission of precise information about the type, intensity, and localization of a sensory stimulus; (2) initiation of arousal, affective, and adaptive responses to the stimulus; and (3) continuous unconscious monitoring and control of motor performance.

The first group of pathways is referred to as *direct,* or *discriminative,* pathways. These pathways commonly are tested clinically because they allow localization of lesions in the nervous system. The two most important direct pathways are the *direct dorsal column pathway,* involved in transmission of tactile-discriminative and conscious proprioceptive information, and the *spinothalamic tract,* involved in transmission of pain and temperature sensation (Table 1). These direct pathways consist of three orders of neurons.

The *first-order neurons* are the receptor neurons; they are derivatives of the neural crest. Their cell bodies lie outside the central nervous system in *dorsal root ganglia* of the spinal nerves or in sensory ganglia of cranial nerves, and their axons bifurcate into a peripheral branch and a central branch. The peripheral branch contributes to a *sensory nerve* and innervates receptor organs. The central branch enters the spinal cord or the brainstem via a *dorsal,* or *sensory, root.* The area of the skin innervated by a single dorsal root is called a *dermatome.*

TABLE 1. *Direct pathways commonly tested clinically*

	Direct dorsal column pathway	Spinothalamic tract
Receptors	Proprioceptors	High-threshold mechanoreceptors
	Tactile receptors	Polymodal nociceptors
		Tactile and thermoreceptors
First-order neuron	Dorsal root ganglion	Dorsal root ganglion
Second-order neuron	Medulla (dorsal column nucleus)	Dorsal horn
Third-order neuron	Ventral posterolateral nucleus of thalamus	Ventral posterolateral and posterior nuclei of thalamus
Decussation	Medulla	Spinal cord
Localization	Ipsilateral dorsal column	Contralateral anterolateral quadrant
Function	Spatiotemporal discrimination (e.g., stereognosis)	Discriminative pain and temperature
	Two-point vibration, joint position	Simple touch

The *second-order neurons* have cell bodies located in regions of the embryonic alar plate, that is, in the gray matter of the dorsal horn of the spinal cord or in relay nuclei of the medulla. The axons of these second-order neurons decussate (cross the midline) and continue cephalad. The axons of first- or second-order neurons, as they ascend in the spinal cord, are grouped into tracts (fasciculi) located primarily in the white matter (funiculi) of the spinal cord (Fig. 1). In the brainstem, the axons of second-order neurons continue to ascend in tracts (in this region, some are referred to as *lemnisci*) to reach the *thala-mus*, where they terminate in specific sensory nuclei. Along their ascending course, these sensory pathways maintain a *somatotopic organization,* so that the surface of the body is represented in a topographic manner both in the pathways and in the relay stations.

The *third-order neurons* have cell bodies in the sensory relay nuclei of the thalamus. Somatosensory thalamic neurons are located in the *ventral posterior complex* of the thalamus, which includes the *ventral posterolateral* nucleus for sensory inputs from the trunk and extremities and the *ventral posteromedial* nucleus for sensory inputs from the

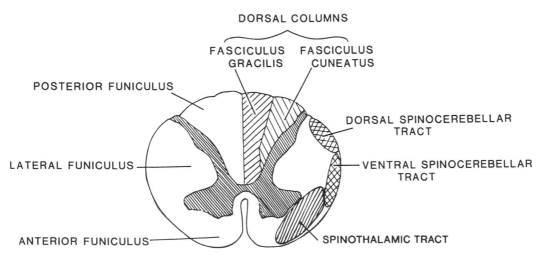

FIG. 1. Cross section of upper cervical spinal cord illustrating the location of the major ascending sensory pathways and their relationship to the posterior, lateral, and anterior funiculi.

face (via the trigeminal system). Like other relay stations, thalamic relay nuclei have a somatotopic and submodality-specific organization. Axons of somatosensory thalamic neurons pass via the thalamocortical radiation to the *primary somatosensory cortex* of the parietal lobe (Fig. 2).

The primary somatosensory cortex is located in the postcentral gyrus of the parietal lobe and is concerned with discriminative aspects of reception and appreciation of somatic sensory impulses. It consists of at least four functionally distinct areas, each containing a complete somatotopic map. Fibers terminate in the postcentral gyrus in an organized fashion, with the lower extremity represented on the medial surface of the hemisphere and the arm and hand represented on the lateral surface. The face, mouth, and tongue are represented in the suprasylvian region (Fig. 3).

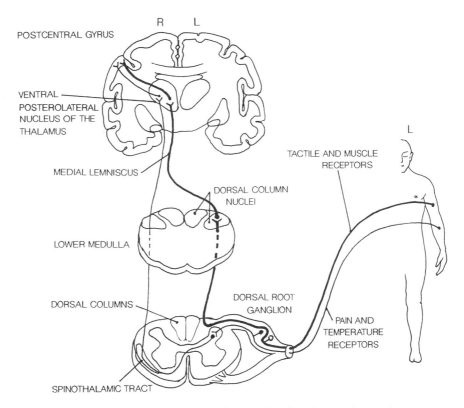

FIG. 2. Diagram of the pathway for discriminative touch, vibration, and proprioception *(thick line)* and for pain and temperature *(thin line)* of the left arm. The first-order neurons are the large and small dorsal root ganglion neurons. Large-diameter afferents for touch and proprioception ascend ipsilaterally in the left dorsal column at the cervical level (fasciculus cuneatus), and synapse on second-order neurons in the lower medulla (nucleus cuneatus). Axons from the second-order neurons decussate and ascend in the right (contralateral) medial lemniscus to synapse in the ventral posterolateral nucleus of the thalamus, which projects to the primary sensory area in the postcentral gyrus. Small-diameter afferents for pain and temperature synapse on second-order neurons in the dorsal horn of the spinal cord. Axons of these second-order neurons decussate in the anterior commissure and ascend, as the spinothalamic tract, in the contralateral ventrolateral quadrant. This tract joins the medial lemniscus and terminates in the ventral posterolateral nucleus and other nuclei in the thalamus.

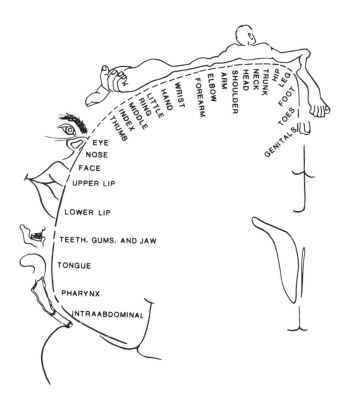

FIG. 3. Coronal section of cerebral hemisphere showing the distribution of third-order sensory fibers in the postcentral gyrus (sensory homunculus). (Modified from Penfield, W., and Rasmussen, T. *The Cerebral Cortex of Man: A Clinical Study of Localization of Function. New York: Macmillan, 1950. With permission.)*

An important feature of the somatosensory and other sensory cortices is that the representation of the body map is dynamic, *use-dependent cortical plasticity*. The shape and size of the representation of a particular body part may be modified in response to peripheral injury or training. Cortical representation of pain occurs not only in the parietal cortex but also in the insular cortex and the *cingulate gyrus*.

A second group of somatosensory pathways, referred to as *indirect pathways*, mediate arousal-affective aspects of somatic sensation (particularly pain) and visceral sensation (Table 2). Unlike direct pathways, indirect pathways are not helpful in the localization of lesions in the central nervous system, because they have poor somatotopy, ascend bilaterally, and terminate diffusely in the reticular formation, intralaminar thalamic nuclei, and other

TABLE 2. *Functional classification of somatosensory pathways*

	Direct (lemniscal)	Indirect (extralemniscal)
Location in the neuraxis	Outer tube	Inner tube (core)
Number of synapses in the central nervous system	2 or 3	Multiple
Receptive fields	Small	Large
Body representation	Contralateral	Bilateral
Somatotopy	Yes	No
Thalamic station	Ventral posterior complex	Midline nuclei
Cortical station	Parietal cortex	Cingulate gyrus
Function	Discriminative	Affective-arousal
Pathways	Dorsal column pathways, spinothalamic pathway, dorsolateral quadrant pathways	Spinoreticulothalamic, spinoreticular, propriospinal pathways

subcortical and cortical regions. Indirect pathways are important for mechanisms of pain and analgesia and for visceral and sexual sensation. They include the *paleospinothalamic*, *spinoreticular*, and *spinomesencephalic tracts* and the *propriospinal multisynaptic system*. Propriospinal neurons interconnect several segments of the spinal cord.

A third group of somatosensory pathways, the *dorsal and ventral spinocerebellar tracts*, transmit information for unconscious control of posture and movement. These are two-neuron pathways that do not relay in the thalamus but terminate in the ipsilateral cerebellum.

The direct somatosensory pathways are of major importance in understanding and interpreting neurologic disease. Lesions at different levels of the neuraxis alter sensory function in different ways; by correlating the patient's signs and symptoms with the anatomical distribution of these pathways, neurologic disorders can be localized. Abnormalities in the peripheral nerves or spinal roots are distributed in a segmental fashion, often involve all sensory modalities, and may be associated with the sensation of pain. Lesions involving the spinal cord may be associated with segmental sensory loss at the level of the lesion and varied sensory loss at all levels below the lesion. Lesions in the posterior fossa produce contralateral sensory loss over the trunk and extremities and may be associated with ipsilateral sensory disturbance in the face. Supratentorial lesions produce entirely contralateral sensory deficits. Because each somatosensory pathway subserves different functions, loss of a particular sensory modality with preservation of others allows anatomical localization of lesions in the nervous system. Lesions of the direct dorsal column pathway affect tactile discrimination, whereas lesions of the spinothalamic system predominantly affect pain and temperature sensation. Because of overlap, or redundancy, of parallel somatosensory pathways, some somatosensory modalities, particularly touch, can still be perceived in cases of interruption of an individual pathway.

Other sensory pathways, such as the visual pathway, are also important for localization in clinical neurology. Similar to the somatosensory pathways, the visual pathway has a topographic organization (called *retinotopy*), a hierarchical organization (with synaptic relays in the thalamus and primary visual cortex), and parallel organization (with submodality-specific channels transmitting information about object movement or shape and color).

Receptors: General Organization and Mechanisms

Sensory receptors are highly specialized structures that respond to environmental changes by producing action potentials for transmission to the central nervous system. This process is called *transduction*. There are many types of receptors subserving different sensory functions.

Receptor Specificity

Each receptor type is generally specialized so that it is more sensitive (that is, has the lowest threshold) to one particular kind of stimulus. Thus, receptors can be classified according to their sensory modality as *mechanoreceptors, chemoreceptors, thermoreceptors*, and *photoreceptors* (Table 3). Receptors also can be classified according to the origin of the stimulus as *exteroceptors* (skin mechanoreceptors for touch and pain, skin thermoreceptors, labyrinthine mechanoreceptors for hearing, retinal photoreceptors, and chemoreceptors for taste and smell), *proprioceptors* (mechanoreceptors in muscles, tendons, and joints and vestibular mechanoreceptors), and *visceral receptors* (mechanoreceptors and chemoreceptors encoding signals related to internal body functions) (Table 3).

Impulse Initiation in Sensory Receptors

Although the mechanism by which receptor potentials are produced varies with the re-

TABLE 3. *Classification and comparison of receptor types*

Receptor type	Receptor	Modality
Mechanoreceptors		
Somatosensory system	Low-threshold mechanoreceptors	Light touch, vibration
	Muscle spindles	Proprioception
	Tendon organs	Proprioception
	Free nerve endings	Pain, temperature
Vestibular system	Hair cells	Head position and motion
Auditory system	Hair cells	Audition
Internal regulation system	Free nerve endings	Visceral distention, pain
Chemoreceptors		
Taste system	Taste buds	Taste
Olfactory system	Olfactory receptor cells	Olfaction
Internal regulation system	Visceral chemoreceptors	Pain
Photoreceptors	Rods and cones	Vision

ceptor organ, certain principles of receptor physiology are common to all. The process starts with the application of a *specific stimulus*, that is, the stimulus for which the receptor has the lowest threshold. *Threshold* is the minimal intensity of stimulus necessary to produce excitation in the appropriate class of first-order neuron.

The major steps in sensory processing are transduction, receptor potential generation, electrotonic spread, and impulse generation. In most cases, transduction of sensory stimuli takes place in a specialized site in the membrane of the receptor cell, leading to gating of an ion current in the membrane channel.

Somatic receptors, including skin and muscle receptors and hair cells of the inner ear, contain *mechanically sensitive cation channels* that open in response to deformations of the cell membrane. Transduction in photoreceptors, odor receptors, and some taste receptors involves *cyclic nucleotide-gated channels* that constitute a large gene family of related proteins that are either nonselective cation or selective potassium channels. Some are particularly permeable to calcium.

In all sensory receptors, the common result of transduction is the production of a change in conductance of a membrane ion channel. This change constitutes the receptor potential, also called the *generator potential*. In most receptors, the receptor potential is depolarizing, either by opening of a sodium or calcium channel or closing of a potassium channel. In

photoreceptors, however, the receptor potential is hyperpolarizing, because light produces closure of a cyclic nucleotide-gated cation channel.

Receptor potentials affect the primary sensory neuron either directly or indirectly, according to the type of receptor. Skin and muscle mechanoreceptors and olfactory receptors consist of the axon of the first neuron of the sensory pathway. In contrast, photoreceptors, hair cells, and taste receptors are specialized cells that tonically release an excitatory transmitter, L-glutamate, which maintains a basal level of activity in the first-order neuron. In response to the specific stimulus, the receptor cell may generate a depolarizing receptor potential, which results in increased release of glutamate and thus increased activity in the primary afferent. The exception is photoreceptors, which are depolarized at rest and undergo transient hyperpolarization in response to light; this produces a transient decrease in the tonic release of glutamate.

Like the synaptic potential, the receptor potential does not give rise directly to an impulse discharge; frequently, the site where receptor potentials are generated is separated from the site where impulses are generated. In somatosensory receptors, receptor potentials and impulses are generated on axons. In other systems, the sites are on different cells, requiring one synaptic relay (for example, vision, hearing, taste). The spread of a receptor potential, like that of a synaptic potential, is accomplished by means of electrotonic potentials.

Encoding of Sensory Information

The final step is the encoding of the electrotonically transmitted receptor impulse into an impulse discharge in the primary afferent that conducts the information to the central nervous system. The receptor potential is graded smoothly and continuously in relation to the intensity of the stimuli. Sensory reception involves the transformation of this graded response into a pattern of all-or-none impulses. The frequency of discharges varies continuously in relationship to the underlying level of depolarization of the receptor potential and its rate of change.

Cell ensembles are needed to encode spatial and temporal information about the stimulus that cannot be encoded in a single cell. Stimulus location is encoded by the firing of a specific population of neurons located at specific points in each relay nucleus. Stimulus intensity is encoded in the somatosensory system through both the frequency of firing of specific neuronal populations (*frequency coding* or *temporal summation*) and the size of the active population (*population coding* or spatial summation).

Receptor Adaptation

Receptor adaptation is a function of the intrinsic properties of the receptor. It is the mechanism by which the amplitude of the generator potential, and thus the firing of action potentials, progressively decreases in response to a continuous stimulus (Fig. 4). Receptors can be subdivided into *rapidly adapting*, or *phasic*, and *slowly adapting*, or *tonic*, receptors. They transmit different types of information to the central nervous system. Rapidly adapting receptors detect transient and rapidly changing stimuli. They fire a few impulses on application of a sustained stimulus but are silent during its steady continuation; they may discharge again when the stimulus is removed. The number of action potentials initiated in their axon is related to the rate of change of the stimulus. Rapidly adapting receptors serve to alert the nervous system to any change in the environment and are particularly suitable for spatiotemporal discrimination. Slowly adapting receptors respond to a sustained stimulus with fairly sus-

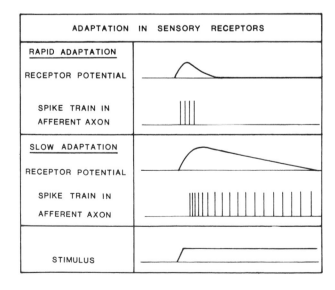

FIG. 4. Rate of adaptation in sensory receptors to prolonged stimulus. Adaptation of receptor potentials and spike trains in primary afferent axons in rapid- and slow-adapting receptors is shown.

tained firing. The time course and peak frequency of discharge of rapidly adapting receptors may reflect the final intensity as well as the rate of application of the stimulus. Slowly adapting receptors keep the nervous system constantly appraised of the status of the body and of its relationships with its surroundings.

Receptor fatigue is the transient abolition of the excitability of a sensory receptor in response to repetitive stimulation. Repetitive stimuli produce successively smaller amplitude generator potentials to the point that the receptor no longer responds either to the stimulus or to change in the stimulus.

Functional Organization of the Sensory Pathways

Serial and Parallel Processing of Sensory Inputs

After the stimulus is transformed into a frequency code, it is transmitted to the central nervous system via a *primary afferent pathway*. In the central nervous system, sensory information is relayed through a series of *relay centers*, and at each center the signal is processed and integrated with other signals. A *sensory pathway* is the series of modality-specific neurons connected by synapses.

The pathways of different sensory systems share some characteristics. A pathway consists of connections in series that determine the temporal sequence of events. In addition, sensory circuits are organized in parallel, so that different forms of information can be transferred and combined at the same time. The axon of a primary afferent neuron divides and synapses on more than one central neuron (this is referred to as *divergence*), and a single central sensory neuron may be contacted synaptically by more than one axon (this is referred to as *convergence*).

Some central pathways transmit inputs from one type of receptor and are referred to as *specific sensory pathways*; they provide for precise transmission of sensory information. Other pathways, through convergence and divergence, become *multimodal* or *nonspecific*; they are involved in sensory integration and behavioral adjustments of the organism.

Sensory Unit and Receptive Field

The *receptive field* of a neuron consists of all the sensory receptors that can influence its activity. The connections with a cell may be excitatory (through a projection relay neuron) or inhibitory (through interneurons). There is a topographic organization of the receptive fields. For example, in the somatosensory system, each point of the body surface is topographically represented at each level of the sensory pathway; this is known as *somatotopy*. In the visual system, there is topographic representation of the visual field of each eye at each relay station, *retinotopy*.

The somatosensory and visual representations of the receptive fields, or maps, are primarily contralateral (contralateral hemibody or visual field). In the auditory system, the representation is mainly contralateral, but bilateral representation is also prominent. The somatotopic and retinotopic maps are distorted in that the size of the population of central neurons with a particular receptive field is proportional to the density of innervation. Areas of high sensory discrimination (fingertips in the somatosensory system, macula in the visual system) have a large number of receptors per unit area and are innervated by a large number of neurons, each with a small receptive field. The size of a receptive field is not fixed. It may vary in response to denervation and other factors.

Receptive fields have a *center-surround organization*. In the somatosensory system, the discharge of a receptor or central sensory neuron is greatest when the stimulus is applied to the center of the receptive field, and the discharge decreases gradually as the stimulus moves toward the periphery of the receptive field. Stimulation of the area immediately surrounding the receptive field may cause inhibition of the central neuron. This is the inhibitory surround.

The organization of a sensory relay station is characterized by a synaptic arrangement that includes three elements: an afferent fiber, a projection neuron, and local inhibitory interneurons. The afferent axon produces excitation of both the projection neuron and the inhibitory interneurons. This excitation is thought to be mediated by L-glutamate. The projection neuron (also called a relay neuron) sends its axon to the next relay station. This neuron also has L-glutamate as a transmitter agent.

Thalamic Station

All sensory modalities, except olfaction, relay in specific relay nuclei of the thalamus. The thalamus is not only the relay station for most sensory channels but it also is important in gating sensory transmission to the cerebral cortex. Each thalamic relay nucleus contains excitatory neurons that project to a specific area of the cerebral cortex. The activity of these thalamocortical neurons is controlled by interneurons in the nucleus.

Primary Sensory Areas of the Cerebral Cortex

Axons from each sensory nucleus in the thalamus terminate in a specific area of cerebral cortex known as a *primary sensory area*. Each of these areas contains neurons that respond selectively to specific characteristics of stimuli; for example, certain neurons in primary somatosensory cortex respond to texture and certain neurons in primary visual cortex respond to color. Each primary sensory area projects to *association areas* of cerebral cortex. Neurons in cortical association areas often respond selectively to a specific combination of features. For example, neurons in one association area respond selectively to faces or images of faces. Mature brains retain the capacity to undergo reorganization, which allows dynamic changes in sensory maps in response to peripheral injury or experience.

This is referred to as *plasticity* of the cortical sensory field.

General Organization of the Somatosensory Systems ▪

Somatosensory Receptors

Somatosensory receptors include cutaneous receptors, joint receptors, and muscle receptors. Cutaneous receptors consist of low-threshold mechanoreceptors, which are innervated by large myelinated fibers and transmit touch sensation, and high-threshold mechanoreceptors, chemoreceptors, and thermoreceptors, which are innervated by small myelinated or unmyelinated fibers and mediate pain and temperature sensation. Joint and muscle receptors are mainly innervated by large, rapidly conducting myelinated fibers. Muscle receptors include muscle spindles, which signal muscle length and rate of change in length, Golgi tendon organs, which respond to changes in muscle tension, and free nerve endings, which respond to muscle pressure and pain (Table 4).

Dorsal Root Ganglion Neurons

Information from somatic receptors is transmitted to the spinal cord by the first-order neurons. The cell bodies of these neurons are located in the dorsal root ganglia (spinal ganglia). Each of these neurons has a single nerve process that divides into two branches. The distal, or peripheral, branch corresponds to the sensory afferent that innervates the receptor, and the proximal, or central, branch enters the spinal cord via the dorsal root. As noted above, the area of the skin innervated by a single dorsal root is called a *dermatome*. The dermatomes are arranged in a highly ordered way on the body surface. The sensory field of each dorsal root is continuous and tends to form a strip perpendicular to the spinal cord. Each spinal nerve receives afferents from several peripheral nerves; therefore,

TABLE 4. *Receptors of the somatosensory system*

Receptor	Innervation	Function
Encapsulated superficial skin receptors (Meissner corpuscles, Merkel disks)	Large myelinated fibers	Detection of edges, texture
Paccinian corpuscle	Large myelinated fibers	Vibration
Free endings in skin, muscles, and joints	Small myelinated or unmyelinated fibers	Pain
Free endings in skin (thermoreceptors)	Small myelinated or unmyelinated fibers	Cold or warmth
Muscle spindles	Large myelinated fibers	Muscle length (proprioception)
Golgi tendon organ	Large myelinated fibers	Muscle tension (proprioception)

the area innervated by an individual dorsal root is less well defined than the area innervated by a single peripheral nerve. Furthermore, the areas innervated by different dorsal roots overlap significantly. Whereas damage of a peripheral cutaneous nerve produces a circumscribed area of sensory loss in the skin, damage to the spinal nerve or dorsal root often results in only a moderate sensory deficit.

The two main types of neurons in a dorsal root ganglion are *large neurons*, with large myelinated axons that innervate low-threshold mechanoreceptors (touch) and proprioceptors, and *small neurons*, with small myelinated or unmyelinated axons that innervate nociceptors, thermoreceptors, and visceral receptors (Table 5). This subdivision is relevant clinically because diseases that selectively affect large sensory fibers or large dorsal root ganglion neurons produce severe loss of all tactile modalities and proprioception but

leave pain and temperature sensation intact. Diseases of small sensory fibers or small dorsal root ganglion neurons affect pain and temperature but spare touch and proprioceptive sensation.

Dorsal Root Entry Zone and Termination in Spinal Cord

Primary afferent fibers from the dorsal root ganglion cells mainly enter the spinal cord in the posterolateral sulcus at the *dorsal root entry zone*. In this zone, the larger and most heavily myelinated proprioceptive and tactile fibers are located medially (medial division), and the finely myelinated and unmyelinated fibers mediating pain and temperature sensation are located laterally (lateral division) (Fig. 5). From this common entry zone, the dorsal root fibers branch to ascend and descend in the white matter and to arborize in

TABLE 5. *Comparison of large neurons and small neurons in dorsal root ganglia*

	Type	
	Large	Small
Sensory function	Touch	Pain
	Vibration	Temperature
	Joint position	Visceral sensation
	Proprioception	
Axon	Large myelinated	Small myelinated
		Unmyelinated
Receptor	Low-threshold mechanoreceptors	High-threshold mechanoreceptors
	Muscle and joint proprioceptors	Polymodal nociceptors
		Chemoreceptors
		Thermoreceptors
Conduction of stimuli	Orthodromic	Orthodromic and antidromic (axon reflex)
Neurotransmitter	L-Glutamate	L-Glutamate and neuropeptides (e.g., substance P)

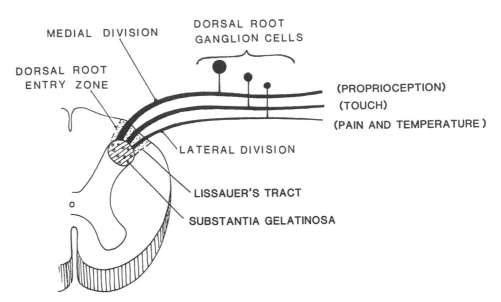

FIG. 5. Dorsal root entry zone. Largest, most heavily myelinated fibers mediating proprioception occupy the medial division. Medium-sized myelinated fibers mediating touch are located centrally, and finely myelinated fibers carrying pain and temperature sensation are located in the lateral division.

the gray matter. The pathways for the different sensory modalities diverge as they ascend in the spinal cord to higher centers.

The medially located large myelinated fibers bifurcate into branches that may (1) ascend directly in the ipsilateral dorsal columns, without synapsing in the spinal cord, as the *direct dorsal column pathway*; (2) synapse on dorsal horn neurons that in turn contribute axons to the dorsal column (the *postsynaptic dorsal column pathway*), dorsolateral funiculus, and spinothalamic tract; (3) synapse in the intermediate gray matter on neurons that give rise to the spinocerebellar tract; (4) synapse on interneurons and motor neurons in the ventral horn for segmental, or myotatic, reflexes; and (5) synapse in the dorsal horn on interneurons that provide segmental modulation of pain transmission.

The laterally located small myelinated and unmyelinated fibers bifurcate into ascending and descending branches that run longitudinally in *Lissauer's tract*, part of the dorsolateral funiculus (see Fig. 4). Within several

segments, these axons leave Lissauer's tract to enter the dorsal horn and the intermediate gray matter of the spinal cord. In the gray matter, they may (1) synapse on different groups of dorsal horn and intermediate gray matter neurons that form the spinothalamic and other tracts ascending in the contralateral ventrolateral quadrant, (2) synapse on dorsal horn interneurons involved in segmental modulation of pain and in intrinsic (propriospinal) intersegmental pathways, and (3) synapse on interneurons and activate somatic and preganglionic autonomic motor neurons to initiate segmental visceral and somatic reflexes.

Spinal Somatosensory Neurons

The second-order spinal somatosensory neurons occupy the dorsal horn and the intermediate gray matter of the spinal cord. These neurons contribute to all somatosensory pathways except the direct dorsal column pathway. Spinal neurons, similar to other central somatosensory neurons, can be subdivided into several types on the basis of their response characteristics: *nociceptive-specific* neurons, *low-threshold mechanoreceptive* neurons, and *wide dynamic range* neurons (Table 6). Wide dynamic range neurons are the most abundant and contribute to all ascending pathways relaying in the spinal cord. One important feature is that an individual type of neuron may change its response characteristics according to segmental and suprasegmental control mechanisms. This is relevant for mechanisms of central pain.

Somatosensory Pathways

From the standpoint of anatomical organization, somatosensory pathways can be subdivided into three groups.

The *direct*, or *lemniscal, pathways* are contralateral, somatotopically organized pathways that synapse in the ventral posterior complex of the thalamus, whose neurons in turn send axons to primary sensory cortex. These pathways are involved in sensory discrimination and are useful clinically for localizing central lesions. They run in the outer tube of the neuraxis and include the following: (1) pathways for tactile discrimination and conscious proprioception—the *direct dorsal column–lemniscal pathway* and parallel pathways in the dorsal column and dorsolateral quadrant; and (2) pathways for dis-

criminative aspects of pain and temperature sensation—the *direct spinothalamic*, or *neospinothalamic, tract*. Note that simple touch and spatial discrimination are transmitted by the dorsal column, the neospinothalamic tract, and other parallel pathways. Therefore, abnormalities of simple touch are less helpful than other sensory modalities in localizing lesions in the central nervous system.

The *indirect pathways* have poor somatotopy, ascend bilaterally, have multiple interconnections with the reticular formation and other subcortical regions, relay in midline thalamic nuclei, and affect limbic and paralimbic cortical areas. The indirect pathways are not helpful for localization, but they are important for transmission of affective-arousal components of pain and visceral sensation and for initiation of reflex somatic, autonomic, and hormonal responses to external stimuli. These pathways are part of the inner tube of the neuraxis and include the following: (1) the *paleospinothalamic, spinoreticular*, and *spinomesencephalic tracts*, which ascend predominantly in the anterolateral quadrant of the spinal cord; and (2) the *propriospinal multisynaptic pathway* (see Table 2).

The *spinocerebellar tracts* are two-neuron pathways that transmit unconscious proprioceptive information to the ipsilateral cerebellum.

TABLE 6. *Functional classification of dorsal horn neurons*

Type of neuron	Primary afferent input	Pathway	Function
Nociceptive-specific	Small myelinated Unmyelinated	Spinothalamic Spinoreticular Spinomesencephalic	Pain
Low-threshold mechanoreceptive	Large myelinated	Postsynaptic dorsal column Spinothalamic Dorsolateral funiculus	Touch Proprioception
Wide dynamic range	Large myelinated Small myelinated Unmyelinated	Spinothalamic Spinoreticular Spinomesencephalic Postsynaptic dorsal column Dorsolateral funiculus	Pain Temperature Touch Visceral sensation
Thermoceptive	Small myelinated Unmyelinated	Spinothalamic	Temperature

Specific Somatosensory Pathways ■

Pathways for Tactile Discrimination and Conscious Proprioception: The Direct Dorsal Column–Lemniscal Pathway

The *direct dorsal column–lemniscal pathway* is important in humans and is critical for highly discriminative tactile sensation, called *stereognosis*, and for fine motor control. The dorsal columns also provide the most important pathway for transmission of conscious proprioception (for example, joint position sense), static tactile discrimination (for example, two-point discrimination), and vibration. These last three modalities are also carried in parallel pathways. All these pathways contribute to the *medial lemniscus* located in the brainstem.

Primary Afferents

Tactile discrimination involves an active process with multiple contacts on the skin and integration of low-threshold mechanoreceptive cutaneous and proprioceptive information (see Table 4). There are four main types of low-threshold mechanoreceptors in the skin. Proprioception involves activity of low-threshold mechanoreceptors in the joints, tendons, and muscles. Muscle spindles have a significant role in position sense of the fingers, which is critical for the ability to recognize the form of objects. In humans, the hand, particularly the fingertips, has the highest innervation density and tactile acuity of any body surface and is the most important tactile organ for object identification. This involves the process of *active exploration*.

Low-threshold tactile and proprioceptive information is carried by large myelinated, high-conduction velocity axons of large dorsal horn neurons. Large primary afferents ascend directly in the ipsilateral dorsal column to synapse on second-order neurons in the medulla (the direct dorsal column pathway). Some of these primary afferents also synapse on second-order neurons in the dorsal horn or intermediate gray matter, which have axons that ascend ipsilaterally in the dorsal columns and the dorsolateral funiculus. All these pathways relay in the lower medulla and then decussate to ascend with the contralateral medial lemniscus.

Dorsal Column–Lemniscal System

The *direct dorsal column pathway* is the most important component of the lemniscal system and consists of large myelinated, primary dorsal root axons that ascend ipsilaterally to reach the dorsal column nuclei in the medulla (Fig. 6). This pathway is critical for spatiotemporal tactile discrimination and fine motor control.

The two major anatomical divisions of the dorsal columns are the *fasciculus gracilis*, which is medial and carries information from the lower extremities and the lower trunk (spinal segment T-7 and lower), and the *fasciculus cuneatus*, which is lateral and carries input from the upper extremities and the upper trunk (spinal segment T-6 and higher).

The cutaneous and muscle afferents from the upper and lower limbs are segregated anatomically in the dorsal columns.

Below spinal segment L-1, the *fasciculus gracilis* contains a mixture of rapidly adapting afferents from skin and muscle receptors in the lower trunk and lower extremities. However, above segment L-1, the input from the majority of muscle receptors in the lower extremities leaves the fasciculus gracilis to terminate in Clarke's nucleus in the thoracic cord, the origin of the dorsal spinocerebellar tract. Thus at cervical levels, the fasciculus gracilis contains almost exclusively rapidly adapting cutaneous afferents, which relay in the *nucleus gracilis* of the medulla.

The *fasciculus cuneatus* is present only at cervical levels and contains a mixture of rapidly adapting afferents from cutaneous and muscle receptors in the upper trunk and upper extremities. Cutaneous and proprioceptive inputs terminate in the *nucleus cuneatus* of the medulla. Muscle receptor afferents traveling in the fasciculus cuneatus leave this tract in the medulla and terminate in the external, or

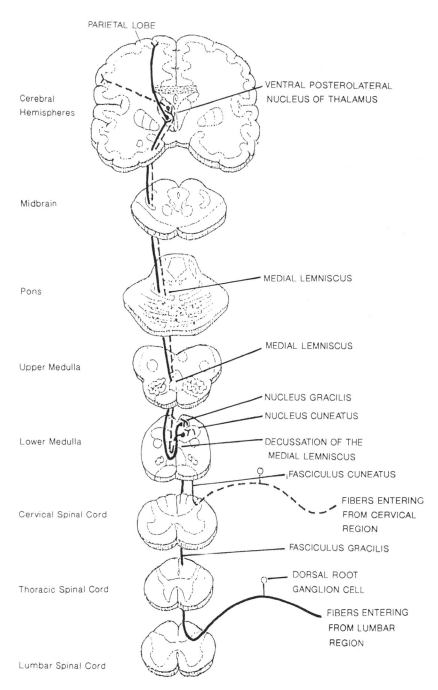

FIG. 6. Dorsal column–lemniscal pathway. Conscious proprioception and discriminative sensation.

accessory, cuneate nucleus (analogous to Clarke's nucleus).

Therefore, the dorsal columns are functionally heterogeneous and carry mostly cutaneous and some proprioceptive inputs to the dorsal column nuclei and proprioceptive input to cerebellar relay nuclei. Lesions in the dorsal columns at any spinal cord level interfere with input from rapidly adapting cutaneous mechanoreceptors, but lesions above the thoracic cord largely spare input from muscle receptors in the lower trunk and lower extremities.

The second-order neurons of the direct dorsal column pathway are located in the dorsal column nuclei of the lower medulla. They are the *nucleus gracilis*, which receives cutaneous inputs from the lower extremity via the fasciculus gracilis, and the *nucleus cuneatus*, which receives cutaneous and some proprioceptive inputs from the upper extremities via the fasciculus cuneatus. The dorsal column nuclei are not simple relay stations but are sites of modulation of sensory transmission critical for sensory discrimination (see below). Second-order axons from the dorsal column nuclei cross to

the opposite side in the lower medulla as the *internal arcuate fibers* (the decussation of the medial lemniscus) and form the medial lemniscus, which ascends to the thalamus.

The medial lemniscus maintains a somatotopic organization, but its position varies at different levels of the brainstem (Fig. 7). In the upper medulla, the medial lemniscus is arranged dorsoventrally on either side of the midline, with the cervical segments represented dorsally and the sacral segments ventrally. In the pons, the medial lemniscus is arranged mediolaterally, with the cervical segments represented medially and the sacral segments laterally.

The medial lemniscus terminates in the *ventral posterolateral nucleus* and other subdivisions of the ventral posterior complex of the thalamus. The ventral posterolateral nucleus receives rapidly adapting cutaneous inputs from the upper and lower extremities and forms a functional unit with the ventral posteromedial nucleus, which receives similar inputs from the face via the trigeminal system. Other subdivisions of the ventral posterior complex receive muscle spindle and slowly

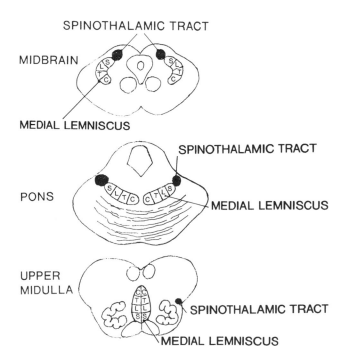

FIG. 7. Localization and somatotopic organization of the medial lemniscus and the spinothalamic pathway in the brainstem. *C,* cervical; *Th,* thoracic; *L,* lumbar; *S,* sacral segments.

adapting mechanoreceptive inputs. Thus, the thalamus contains somatotopically organized, modality-specific maps of the body surface, with the head represented medially, the hand centrally, and the leg laterally in the ventral posterior complex. Somatosensory thalamic neurons project via the posterior limb of the internal capsule to *primary somatosensory cortex* located in the postcentral gyrus of the parietal lobe.

Primary somatosensory cortex consists of at least four functionally distinct areas; each one contains a separate somatotopic representation of body receptors, with specific representation of cutaneous or proprioceptive inputs. In each area, the lower extremity is represented on the medial surface of the hemisphere, and the upper extremity and the head are represented on the lateral surface (see Fig. 3). Neurons in primary somatosensory cortex have a high degree of submodality specificity and are organized into separate submodality-specific columns. Processing of somatosensory information also occurs in the secondary and supplementary sensory cortices and in the somatosensory association cortex in the posterior parietal lobe.

Mechanisms of Sensory Discrimination in the Direct Dorsal Column–Lemniscal System

Features of the dorsal column–lemniscal system crucial for sensory discrimination include small receptive fields, mechanisms of contrast sharpening, and parallel modality-specific channels.

The fingertips have the smallest receptive fields and the largest cortical representation (larger than the trunk and legs together). The density of innervation of the fingertips is four times that of the palm, and the threshold for discrimination of two points in these areas is 1 mm and 10 mm, respectively.

The dorsal column nuclei and the ventral posterolateral nucleus of the thalamus are not simple relay stations but also sites of information processing necessary for spatial and temporal discrimination. This involves a process of *contrast sharpening*, which depends on a mechanism known as *lateral inhibition*. Long ascending dorsal column afferents contain the neurotransmitter L-glutamate and excite not only the relay cells in the nucleus but also local interneurons containing γ-aminobutyric acid (GABA). These inhibitory GABAergic interneurons also receive excitatory input from somatosensory cortex, and they make presynaptic and postsynaptic inhibitory contacts with both afferent terminals and relay projection cells. Thus, input to a given projection neuron produces, via inhibitory interneurons, lateral inhibition of surrounding projection neurons. This prevents the fusion of the excitatory zones when two stimuli are brought close together and thus allows spatial discrimination.

At all relay stations of the dorsal column–lemniscal pathway, there are specific and spatially segregated sensory channels for the various submodalities. In the dorsal column nuclei, thalamus, and primary somatosensory cortex, a single neuron responds only to one sensory submodality (for example, touch or muscle spindles). All cells responding to one submodality are located together and segregated from cells responding to other submodalities. In the cerebral cortex, each neuron in a vertical column is activated by the same sensory submodality; thus, neurons in a vertical column form the elementary topographic and modality-specific unit of function.

Parallel Pathways for Proprioceptive and Tactile Discriminative Function

In addition to the direct dorsal column–lemniscal pathway, other parallel pathways contribute to the lemniscal system and transmit tactile discriminative and proprioceptive information. All these spinal pathways consist of second-order axons from low-threshold mechanoreceptive or wide dynamic range neurons in the dorsal horn. These pathways include (1) the *postsynaptic dorsal column pathway*, which contributes to the ipsilateral gracile and cuneate fasciculi; (2) two pathways that ascend ipsilaterally in the *dorsolat-*

eral funiculus—the *spinocervical tract*, which relays in the lateral cervical nucleus in the upper cervical cord, and the *spinomedullary tract*, which relays in a nucleus of the lower medulla; third-order axons from these two pathways and the postsynaptic dorsal column pathway decussate and join the contralateral medial lemniscus; and (3) the *spinothalamic tract*, which joins the medial lemniscus before reaching the thalamus.

Summary

The lemniscal system consists of several parallel pathways that relay contralateral tactile discriminative and proprioceptive information to the ventral posterior nucleus of the thalamus. Only the direct dorsal column pathway has no spinal station, maintains strict modality specificity, and has mechanisms of contrast sharpening in all its relay stations. Thus, this system is critical for spatiotemporal tactile discrimination and fine motor control. The parallel pathways allow relative sparing of static tactile discrimination and proprioception despite lesions in the dorsal column. Within the dorsal columns, there is a segregation of tactile and proprioceptive inputs arising from the upper and lower extremities. To some degree, the pathways transmitting proprioceptive information to the cerebral cortex (medial lemniscus) and to the cerebellum (spinocerebellar tract) overlap anatomically.

Effects of Lesions in the Dorsal Column–Lemniscal System

The clinical signs of injury to the dorsal column–lemniscal pathway vary according to the site of involvement. Diffuse involvement of large dorsal root ganglion neurons or large myelinated fibers causes loss of tactile discrimination and inability to detect joint position and vibration. These lesions result in the inability to manipulate objects without visual guidance and erratic movements of the fingers in the absence of visual clues (pseudoathetosis). These lesions also cause *sensory ataxia*, which is loss of muscle coordination and severe disturbance of gait because of lack of proprioceptive information.

Unless the patients can watch the movements of their limbs and correct the errors, they stumble, stagger, and fall. Central lesions of the dorsal column system produce similar but less severe or partial abnormalities, because of the redundancy of ascending pathways for transmission of tactile and proprioceptive inputs carried by large afferents.

Lesions of the dorsal columns in humans produce major defects in vibration sense and in the ability for spatiotemporal discrimination, or stereognosis (the deficit is called *astereognosis*). Stereognosis includes graphesthesia (recognition of numbers drawn on the skin), detection of speed and direction of moving cutaneous stimuli, detection of shapes and patterns, and detection of other stimuli requiring object manipulation and active exploration with the digits (*active touch*). These highly discriminative functions are also affected by lesions in primary somatosensory cortex, thalamus, medial lemniscus, and dorsal column nuclei. In addition to astereognosia, lesions of the fasciculus cuneatus may produce deficits similar to those produced by corticospinal lesions, including loss of dexterity of the fingers and disruption of spatiotemporal motor precision.

Spatial discrimination of static stimuli, such as two-point discrimination, stimulus localization, and joint position sense, is relayed not only by the dorsal column–lemniscal pathways but also by several parallel channels. Thus, this ability may not be permanently impaired after lesions restricted to the dorsal columns. Gross touch-pressure may also travel via parallel pathways, particularly the spinothalamic pathway. Only lesions that involve *both* the dorsal column and the dorsolateral funiculus result in severe deficit of conscious proprioception. Sensory ataxia may require associated involvement of the spinocerebellar pathways.

Pathways for Pain and Temperature: Ventrolateral Quadrant System

The mechanisms and pathways for pain sensation have been studied more extensively than those for temperature sensation. On the basis of clinical data, it is likely that these two pathways travel a similar course through the nervous system; therefore, these two modalities are considered together. The sensation of pain has two components: a *sensory-discriminative* component that informs about quality, intensity, and location of the stimulus, and an *arousal-affective* component that is involved in the emotional, behavioral, and autonomic responses to pain. These two components are carried in a direct pathway and several indirect pathways, respectively. These pathways are intermingled and ascend mainly in the *spinothalamic tract* in the anterolateral quadrant of the spinal cord.

Primary Afferents

There are specific low-threshold thermoreceptive fibers that are excited by either warming or cooling but not by tactile stimulation. The peripheral receptors for pain are *free nerve endings*. The two main types of *nociceptive units* are *high-threshold mechanoreceptive units* innervated by small myelinated axons and *polymodal nociceptive units* innervated by unmyelinated axons (Table 7). High-threshold mechanoreceptive units respond to noxious mechanical stimuli (pressure) and mediate the so-called *first*, or *fast, pain*, which is the well-localized, sharp sensation (pricking pain) induced by pinprick or laceration. Polymodal units respond not only to noxious mechanical but also to noxious thermal and chemical (substances released during inflammation) stimuli and mediate the so-called *second*, or *slow, pain*, which is a dif-fuse, dull-aching or burning discomfort that may outlast the stimulus.

The first-order nociceptive neurons include (1) medium-sized dorsal root ganglion neurons with small myelinated fibers that use L-glutamate and correspond to high-threshold mechanoreceptors; and (2) small dorsal root ganglion neurons with unmyelinated axons that contain not only glutamate but also various neuropeptides, including *substance P* and calcitonin gene-related peptide, and correspond to polymodal nociceptors. Axons of small nociceptive dorsal root neurons branch extensively to innervate several sensory fields, and some of their proximal projections enter the spinal cord via the ventral roots instead of the dorsal roots (*ventral root afferents*) to reach the dorsal horn.

Small dorsal root ganglion neurons may release neuropeptides antidromically from their peripheral branches at the site of stimulation. Antidromic release of neurotransmitters by peripheral branches is called *axon reflex*. Nociceptive axon reflexes are the basis for the *neurogenic inflammation*, or *flare, response*. Stimulation of nociceptive endings by mechanical damage or local substances released during inflammation (histamine, prostaglandins, potassium ions) not only produces pain but also causes the antidromic release of substance P and other vasoactive neuropeptides, which produce vasodilatation and increase vascular permeability at the site of injury.

Pain fibers, together with fibers involved in temperature and visceral sensation, enter the spinal cord in the lateral division of the dorsal root entry zone and divide into short ascending

TABLE 7. *Types of nociceptive fibers*

	High-threshold mechanoreceptive type	Polymodal nociceptive type
Axon	Small myelinated	Unmyelinated
Stimulus	Noxious pressure	Noxious pressure, pinch
		Noxious thermal
		Chemicals (potassium ions, histamine)
Neurotransmitter	L-Glutamate	Substance P
		Calcitonin gene-related peptide
Sensation	First, or fast, pain	Second, or slow, pain
	Well-localized	Diffuse
	Sharp	Dull
	Prickling	Aching
		Burning

and descending branches that run longitudinally in the dorsolateral funiculus (Lissauer's tract). Within several segments, they leave the tract to provide excitatory synapses to second-order neurons in the dorsal horn. The excitatory neurotransmitters include L-glutamate and several neuropeptides, particularly substance P.

Dorsal Horn Neurons

The second-order nociceptive neurons include (1) *nociceptive-specific neurons*, which predominantly are located superficially in the dorsal horn and receive input solely from small myelinated and unmyelinated fibers; and (2) *wide dynamic range*, or *multiceptive*, neurons, which predominantly are located deep in the dorsal horn and in the intermediate gray matter and receive input not only from small myelinated and unmyelinated fibers but also from visceral afferents and large myelinated fibers. Wide dynamic range neurons are functionally important because they contribute most of the axons to the spinothalamic system. Also, these neurons transmit both nociceptive and nonnociceptive information, are the site of viscerosomatic convergence for *referred visceral pain*, and can change their functional properties according to local modulatory influences by central pain-modulating mechanisms.

Second-order axons from both nociceptive-specific and wide dynamic range neurons, together with axons from thermoreceptive neurons, cross to the opposite site to continue rostrally in the anterolateral quadrant of the spinal cord, primarily in the spinothalamic pathways.

Spinothalamic Tract

The sensations of pain and temperature are transmitted primarily via the *spinothalamic tract*, which ascends in the ventrolateral quadrant of the spinal cord contralateral to the side of entry of the primary afferents (Fig. 8). The spinothalamic tract is complex and functionally heterogeneous. It mediates the discriminative and arousal-emotional components of pain sensation as well as thermal, visceral, and simple tactile information. The different components of the spinothalamic tract include (1) a direct pathway, the *neospinothalamic pathway*, which mediates the discriminative aspect of pain and temperature and is important for localization; and (2) several indirect pathways—the *paleospinothalamic, spinoreticular*, and *spinomesencephalic tracts*—for the affective-arousal components of pain; they form part of the core, or inner tube, of the neuraxis (Table 8).

The *neospinothalamic tract* consists of second-order axons from both nociceptive-specific and wide dynamic range neurons. The axons cross through the ventral white commissure and ascend strictly contralaterally in the anterolateral quadrant of the spinal cord. The neospinothalamic tract has a somatotopic organization in the spinal cord, with the sacral dermatomes represented dorsolaterally and the cervical dermatomes ventromedially.

The spinothalamic tract ascends in the lateral portion of the brainstem. In the medulla it is dorsal to the lateral aspect of the inferior olivary nucleus, and in the pons and midbrain it is lateral to the medial lemniscus. At the mesodiencephalic junction, the spinothalamic tract and medial lemniscus join (see Fig. 7). Throughout its course, the spinothalamic tract maintains a somatotopic organization, with cervical segments represented medially and sacral segments laterally.

The spinothalamic tract axons synapse on third-order neurons in several thalamic nuclei, particularly the *ventral posterolateral nucleus* that, in turn, projects to the *primary sensory cortex* in the postcentral gyrus. Other spinothalamic tract axons terminate in relay nuclei that project either to the insular cortex or the anterior cingulate gyrus.

The spinothalamic tract is involved in rapid transmission of nociceptive and thermal information for localization and intensity of pain and temperature sensation. Thus, this pathway is important clinically for localization of lesions in the central nervous system. A second important function is to provide a parallel channel for transmission of tactile in-

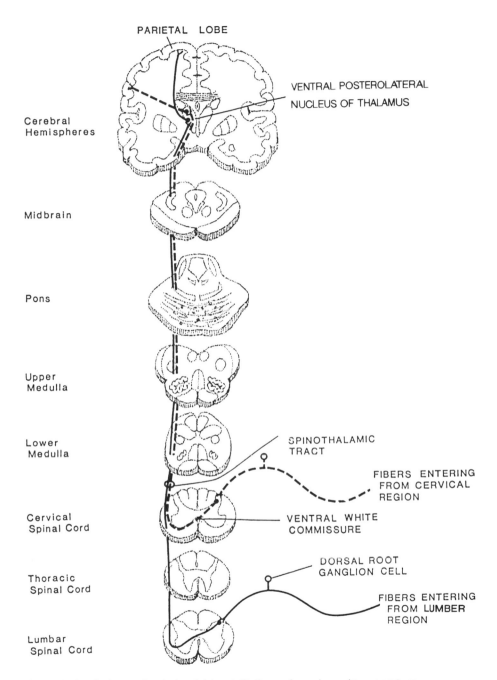

PARIETAL LOBE

VENTRAL POSTEROLATERAL
NUCLEUS OF THALAMUS

Cerebral
Hemispheres

Midbrain

Pons

Upper
Medulla

Lower
Medulla

SPINOTHALAMIC
TRACT

FIBERS ENTERING
FROM CERVICAL
REGION

VENTRAL WHITE
COMMISSURE

Cervical
Spinal Cord

DORSAL ROOT
GANGLION CELL

Thoracic
Spinal Cord

FIBERS ENTERING
FROM LUMBER
REGION

Lumbar
Spinal Cord

FIG. 8. Spinothalamic (neospinothalamic) tract. Pathway for pain and temperature sensation.

formation, including simple touch and static-discriminative touch modalities.

The spinothalamic pathway transmits information about pain and temperature from the contralateral upper and lower extremities and trunk. Transmissions of pain and temperature sensations from the face and cranium are carried by the trigeminal system. Pain fibers from the face are carried primarily in the trigeminal nerve (cranial nerve V). The cell bodies of

TABLE 8. *Pathways for pain transmission*

	Direct or lateral (outer tube)	Indirect or medial (inner tube)
Pathway	Neospinothalamic	Paleospinothalamic Spinoreticular Spinomesencephalic Propriospinal
Somatotopy	Yes	No
Body representation	Contralateral	Bilateral
Synapse in reticular formation	No	Yes
Subcortical targets	None	Hypothalamus Limbic system Autonomic centers
Thalamic nucleus	Ventral posterolateral nucleus	Intralaminar nuclei Other midline nuclei
Cortical region	Parietal lobe	Cingulate gyrus
Role	Discriminative pain	Affective-arousal component of pain
Other function	Temperature Touch	

these primary sensory neurons are located in the *gasserian*, or *semilunar, ganglion* (Fig. 9). On entering the brainstem at the pons, these fibers descend in the ipsilateral *descending*, or *spinal, tract of the trigeminal nerve* to the upper cervical cord. Axons of this tract synapse with second-order neurons in the adjacent *nucleus of the spinal tract of the trigeminal nerve.* The axons of the second-order neurons cross to the opposite side of the brainstem and ascend to the ventral posteromedial nucleus of the thalamus. Third-order neurons in this thalamic nucleus project to the parietal lobe via the posterior limb of the internal capsule.

Pathways for Affective-Arousal Components of Pain

The indirect pathways involved in the affective and arousal aspects of pain sensation originate mainly from wide dynamic range neurons in the deep dorsal horn and intermediate gray matter. Their second-order axons ascend bilaterally in the spinal cord, have poor

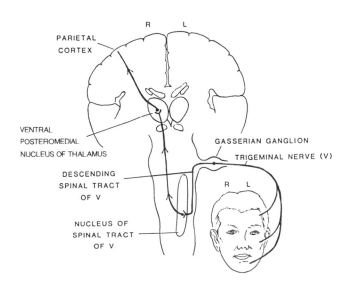

FIG. 9. Pathway of pain fibers of the face.

somatotopy, and make multiple synapses in the reticular formation. These pathways are components of the inner tube systems. Collaterals of these pathways reach the hypothalamus and other areas of the limbic system. Neurons involved in these complex, multisynaptic pathways have large bilateral receptive fields and receive convergent input from not only cutaneous but also visceral and other receptors. These pathways initiate arousal, autonomic, endocrine, and motor responses to pain stimulation. The two main groups of these pathways are (1) ventrolateral quadrant pathways, which include the *paleospinothalamic, spinoreticular,* and *spinomesencephalic* tracts (Fig. 10); and (2) the *propriospinal* multisynaptic ascending system.

In the spinal cord, second-order axons that contribute to these pathways ascend contralaterally and ipsilaterally in the ventrolateral quadrant (they intermingle with those of the neospinothalamic pathway), the dorsolateral quadrant, and the propriospinal system. The paleospinothalamic tract provides multiple input to the reticular formation and terminates in the *midline and intralaminar thalamic nuclei,* which project diffusely to the cerebral cortex, particularly to the cingulate gyrus. The spinoreticular tract terminates in sensory, motor, autonomic, and endocrine-relay areas of the medullary and pontine reticular formation. The spinomesencephalic tract synapses in the *periaqueductal gray matter.*

The *multisynaptic ascending propriospinal system* originates from neurons in the substantia gelatinosa of the dorsal horn and in the intermediate gray matter. This system forms a functional continuum with the reticular formation of the brainstem.

In addition to transmitting affective-arousal components of pain sensation, all these indirect pathways are important for activation of central

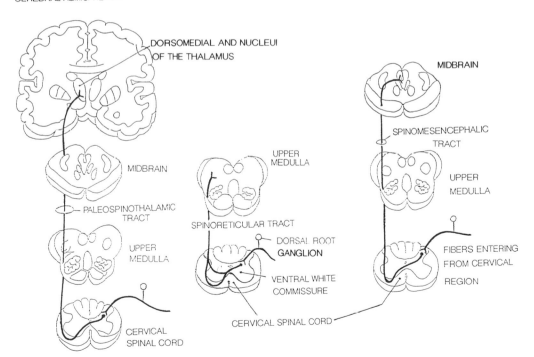

FIG. 10. The three individual pain pathways of the inner tube systems that transmit affective and arousal components of pain. **A:** Paleospinothalamic tract. **B:** Spinoreticular tract. **C:** Spinomesencephalic tract.

antinociceptive (pain inhibition) mechanisms (discussed below).

Summary

Pain and temperature pathways overlap in the spinal cord. The most important pathway for central transmission of pain and temperature is the spinothalamic system. This system originates predominantly from wide dynamic range neurons of the dorsal horn and intermediate gray matter and ascends in the ventrolateral quadrant of the spinal cord. It is a functionally heterogeneous system that includes both a direct spinothalamic, or neospinothalamic, pathway involved in discriminative aspects of pain and temperature (as well as tactile sensation) and a group of indirect pathways involved in arousal-affective aspects of pain sensation. Pain sensation can be transmitted not only via the contralateral ventrolateral quadrant system but also via indirect pathways ascending bilaterally in the spinal cord. This may explain the failure of ventrolateral cord lesions to produce permanent relief from pain.

Effect of Lesions of the Spinothalamic System

Lesions that involve the peripheral level may cause either the sensation of pain or some loss of pain and temperature in the distribution of the affected nerves. Lesions of the central nervous system seldom produce pain unless pain-sensitive structures are involved or central pain-controlling pathways are interrupted. A central lesion that interrupts the spinothalamic tract results in the inability to perceive painful stimuli and to discriminate between hot and cold in the areas below the level of the lesion. A lesion at the spinal level involving the spinothalamic tract results in contralateral loss of pain and temperature sensation. A lesion at the posterior fossa level produces contralateral loss of pain and temperature in trunk and extremities, but if the same lesion also involves the pain fibers in the descending tract of the trigeminal nerve, there is ipsilateral loss of pain and temperature sensation of the face. The separate pathways for body and limb pain

and for facial pain are the neuroanatomical basis for this clinical observation. Thus, lesions at the level of the medulla produce *crossed anesthesia*, whereas those rostral to the medulla produce *complete contralateral hemianesthesia*, which includes the face. Lesions at the supratentorial level produce contralateral loss of pain and temperature. With suprathalamic lesions, crude pain perception may remain intact, but precise localization of painful stimuli is impaired.

Pathways for Transmission of Simple Touch

Tactile sensation is initiated by stimulation of low-threshold mechanoreceptors in the skin. These receptors vary in degree of adaptation and size of receptive field. The axons of primary, large dorsal root ganglion neurons are in the medial division of the dorsal root entry zone. These large myelinated fibers either ascend directly in the dorsal columns or stimulate low-threshold mechanoreceptive and wide dynamic range neurons in the deep dorsal horn. Thus, simple tactile information is carried rostrally by several parallel pathways, including the direct and postsynaptic dorsal column pathways, the spinocervical tract in the dorsolateral funiculus, and the neospinothalamic tract in the anterolateral quadrant.

All these pathways are part of the outer tube systems. They contribute to the lemniscal system, terminate in the contralateral ventral posterolateral nucleus of the thalamus, and activate low-threshold cutaneous mechanoreceptive neurons in the primary somatosensory cortex. These pathways overlap with the ones that mediate discriminative touch and proprioception (dorsal columns) and discriminative pain and temperature (neospinothalamic tract).

The transmission of simple tactile modalities (detection, localization, and, to some extent, two-point discrimination) via several parallel pathways explains the preservation of sensation of touch despite lesions affecting other sensory modalities. Thus, touch is not very useful clinically for localizing lesions in the central nervous system.

Mechanisms of Pain and Analgesia ■

Pain is a frequent manifestation of neurologic as well as nonneurologic disease. Organic pain can be subdivided into *nociceptive pain* and *neurogenic pain*. *Nociceptive pain* is related to activation of normal pain mechanisms in response to tissue injury or inflammation; *neurogenic pain* is due to peripheral or central nervous system lesions that affect processing of information in the pain transmission pathway. Transmission of nociceptive information is regulated by a balance between excitatory and inhibitory influences acting on spinothalamic and other neurons of the pain pathways. Endogenous antinociceptive mechanisms are activated by stress, exercise, sexual activity, and previous nociceptive stimulation of peripheral tissues.

Nociceptive Afferents

As mentioned above, the two types of nociceptive afferents are the small myelinated high-threshold mechanoreceptors and the unmyelinated polymodal nociceptors (see Table 7). Primary nociceptive afferents contain L-glutamate and various neuropeptides. The most abundant are calcitonin gene-related peptide and substance P. Neuropeptides are released in the dorsal horn from the central process and in the periphery from the peripheral process. The release from the peripheral process occurs via an axon reflex. The release from the end of the peripheral process triggers vasomotor and other phenomena referred to as *neurogenic inflammation* or the *flare response*. Neuropeptides are released in response to many different stimuli, including potassium and hydrogen ions, histamine, serotonin, cytokines, and nerve growth factor.

Dorsal Horn

The dorsal horn is not simply a station for pain transmission. It contains many complex, dynamic circuits that support not only transmission of sensory input but also a high degree of sensory processing. One of the important aspects of this sensory processing is the central modulation of pain transmission.

The transmission of pain is modulated by both *segmental mechanisms* and descending *suprasegmental mechanisms* via complex circuits at the spinal or medullary levels. These regulatory circuits involve primary afferents, descending pathways, and local interneurons.

Interneurons in the Dorsal Horn

Interneurons in the dorsal horn are located primarily in the *substantia gelatinosa*, or lamina II. They may be excitatory or inhibitory. Inhibitory interneurons contain GABA, enkephalins, or other neuropeptides and are important for local processing and modulation of pain transmission. They receive input from segmental large and small primary afferent fibers and from descending supraspinal fibers.

Segmental Mechanisms

There are two important segmental mechanisms for modulation of pain transmission. The first involves inhibition of pain transmission by activation of large-diameter afferents; that is, stimulation of low-threshold, large myelinated mechanoreceptive afferents *inhibits* pain transmission in the dorsal horn, probably by the activation of local inhibitory interneurons. This is the basis for the *gate control theory* of pain modulation. A second mechanism involves exaggeration of pain transmission after repetitive activation of small nociceptive fibers; that is, repetitive firing of nociceptive fibers results in increased activity of dorsal horn nociceptive neurons (Fig. 11). This mechanism, known as the *windup phenomenon*, may explain the pain present with nerve injury and during nerve regeneration.

Several reciprocally connected brain regions form a *central pain-controlling network*. The nuclei and pathways of this *endogenous analgesia system* are part of the internal regulation system of the inner tube and are diffusely distributed. They include the cerebral

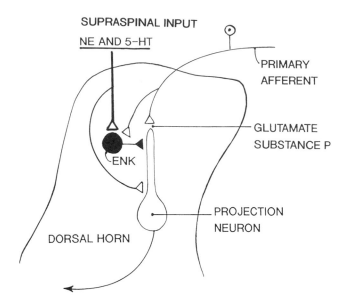

SUPRASPINAL INPUT
NE AND 5-HT

PRIMARY
AFFERENT

GLUTAMATE
SUBSTANCE P

ENK

PROJECTION
NEURON

DORSAL HORN

FIG. 11. Local circuit in the dorsal horn involved in transmission and modulation of pain sensation at the spinal level. Primary afferents release L-glutamate and substance P to excite second-order relay neurons (projection neuron) of the spinothalamic system. This transmission is inhibited by local interneurons containing enkephalin (ENK) or other transmitters and by descending brainstem pathways containing serotonin (5-HT) and norepinephrine (NE).

cortex, thalamus, hypothalamus, brainstem, and dorsal horn. Important components of this system are the *periaqueductal gray matter* of the midbrain; the rostral *ventromedial medulla*, particularly the *raphe nucleus*, which produces serotonin; and the *locus ceruleus* and adjacent medullary neurons that produce norepinephrine (Fig. 12). All these central structures have several properties in common: (1) they contain endogenous opioid neurons and receptors; (2) they are stimulated by opioids and mediate the analgesic effects of morphine-like drugs; (3) they receive input from the indirect ascending nociceptive pathways and thus provide *feedback inhibition* of pain transmission; (4) when stimulated, they produce analgesia, and they *selectively affect pain transmission* and do not affect transmission of nonnociceptive information in the dorsal horn.

Opioids disinhibit antinociceptive neurons of the periaqueductal gray matter. These neurons, in turn, activate the serotoninergic and noradrenergic bulbospinal neurons that project to the dorsal horn via the dorsolateral funiculus of the spinal cord. Noradrenergic and serotoninergic inputs inhibit pain transmission either directly or through inhibitory

GABA-containing or opioid-containing interneurons in the dorsal horn.

Organic pain can be divided into *nociceptive pain* and *neurogenic pain*. *Nociceptive pain* is related to activation of normal pain mechanisms in response to tissue injury. This symptom is most important in calling attention to pathologic processes that occur in many organ systems. Lesions located outside the nervous system frequently stimulate pain-sensitive free nerve endings and produce the subjective sensation of pain. Acute nociceptive pain is initiated by stimulation of nociceptive fibers by several chemical mediators of inflammation (for example, potassium ions, histamine, bradykinin, and prostaglandins) and is potentiated by antidromic release of substance P and other neuropeptides from nociceptive axon terminals (neurogenic inflammation, or flare response). The parenchyma of internal organs, including the brain, is not supplied with pain receptors. However, the wall of arteries, the dura mater, mesothelial surfaces (for example, synovial surfaces, pleura, pericardium, and peritoneum), the wall of hollow viscera, and muscle are subject to inflammation or mechanical traction. Unlike somatic pain, visceral pain is poorly lo-

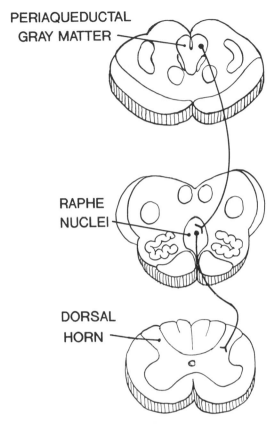

PERIAQUEDUCTAL
GRAY MATTER

RAPHE
NUCLEI

DORSAL
HORN

FIG. 12. Brainstem components of the central pain-controlling network (endogenous analgesic system). The periaqueductal gray matter stimulates serotoninergic neurons in the raphe nuclei and norepinephrine-synthesizing cell groups of the reticular formation in the ventral medulla. Descending serotoninergic and noradrenergic pathways inhibit pain transmission in the dorsal horn. The periaqueductal gray matter and ventral medulla are sites for analgesic action of opioids.

calized and the sensation generally occurs in a surface area of the body remote from the actual source of stimulation. This is the phenomenon known as *referred pain*.

Headache is an important example of nociceptive pain. The pain-sensitive structures in the cranium are the wall of blood vessels, the dura mater, and the periostium. *Migraine* is the typical example of a vascular headache. Headache in migraine is believed to reflect inflammation and antidromic vasodilatation at the *trigeminovascular junctions*. The extracra-

nial blood vessels receive sensory innervation from the trigeminal nerve. Several triggering factors may activate trigeminal afferents that innervate blood vessels; these afferents antidromically release substance P and calcitonin gene-related peptide. These neuropeptides are potent vasodilators and elicit the release of inflammatory mediators. Stretching of the blood vessel wall and inflammation increase impulse conduction in the trigeminal afferents and the antidromic release of vasodilator neuropeptides. This mechanism may contribute to headache that occurs in association with meningeal irritation or mechanical distortion of pain-sensitive structures during increase in intracranial pressure.

Neurogenic pain includes *neuropathic pain, deafferentation pain*, and *sympathetically maintained pain*.

Neuropathic pain occurs in cases of painful nerve compression or after formation of post-traumatic neuroma following a nerve lesion. This may produce abnormal discharges in the areas of demyelination, selective loss of large-fiber–mediated segmental inhibition, and increased activity of small nociceptive fibers.

Deafferentation pain may complicate any type of injury along the course of the somatosensory pathways. This can occur at the peripheral level (for example, phantom pain after limb amputation), along the ascending pathways (for example, demyelinating spinal cord lesions in multiple sclerosis), or at the level of the thalamus (thalamic syndrome). In these conditions, pain occurs in the area of sensory loss. It is due to perturbation in the central processing of pain information that results from interference with normal pain-controlling mechanisms.

Sympathetically maintained pain is characterized by simultaneous occurrence of pain; local autonomic dysregulation (edema, vasomotor disturbances, and sweat abnormalities); and trophic changes in the skin, soft tissues, and bone. It mainly occurs with lesions of peripheral nerves or roots.

Neurogenic pain involves plastic changes (referred to as *sensitization*) at the level of the nociceptors, dorsal root ganglion, and dorsal horn. Normally, polymodal nociceptors have no spontaneous activity. In response to injury, the nociceptors become sensitized by cytokines and other products of inflammation. This sensitization is characterized by increased spontaneous (background) activity, decreased threshold and supernormal discharge in response to noxious stimulation, increased size of receptive fields, increased sensitivity to heat or cold stimuli, increased discharge in response to sympathetic stimulation, and antidromic release of neuropeptides. One mechanism that contributes to the development of neuropathic pain is the activation of so-called *silent nociceptors* by products of inflammation.

Increased activity of nociceptive afferents results in the phenomenon of *central sensitization* at the level of the dorsal horn. The mechanisms are similar to those involved in the *windup phenomenon*; the result is increased discharge, reduced threshold, and enlarged receptive fields of spinothalamic neurons. The mechanisms include increased release of L-glutamate and neuropeptides, and triggering of different calcium-dependent biochemical cascades in spinothalamic neurons (see Chapter 14).

Neurogenic pain has several clinical characteristics: (1) spontaneous pain (burning, aching, shock-like), (2) increased sensitivity to noxious stimulation (referred to as *hyperalgesia*), and (3) and pain sensation following innocuous (for example, tactile) stimulation (referred to as *allodynia*). Spontaneous pain and hyperalgesia involve the small myelinated and unmyelinated nociceptive fibers. Allodynia is mediated by myelinated, nonnociceptive fibers. These fibers normally evoke nonnociceptive responses in spinothalamic neurons and trigger segmental inhibition of nociceptive neurons via local GABAergic mechanisms. In central sensitization, the increased excitability of spinothalamic neurons and impaired local inhibition cause a normally innocuous stimulus to provoke increased firing of spinothalamic neurons, resulting in pain sensation.

Another positive manifestation of nerve injury is *paresthesia* (pins-and-needles sensation), which reflects increased spontaneous activity in large myelinated fibers and can be elicited in normal subjects by nerve compression, hyperventilation, or repetitive nerve stimulation. The mechanism is *ectopic discharge* of the nerve produced by sustained depolarization, which is the result of increased permeability to sodium (for example, with decreased extracellular ionized calcium after hyperventilation) or accumulation of extracellular potassium (for example, after a period of nerve ischemia). The positive sensory symptoms of spontaneous pain and paresthesia typically occur with lesions that affect a peripheral sensory nerve or nerve root. However, these symptoms can occur with lesions that involve any part of the somatosensory pathways, including the spinal cord, thalamus, and parietal cortex.

Lancinating pain in the head or face that occurs spontaneously or in response to minimal stimuli is referred to as *neuralgia*. A typical example is *trigeminal neuralgia*, which consists of paroxysmal, electric shock-like facial pain in the distribution of the trigeminal nerve.

Somatosensory Pathways and Control of Motor Function

Inputs from muscle spindles, Golgi tendon organs, joint proprioceptors, and low-threshold mechanoreceptors are not only processed centrally for conscious sensation but are also crucial for unconscious reflex adjustments of posture and muscle tone and for continuous monitoring of motor performance. Inputs from the muscles, joints, and skin provide continuous information about the position and movement of the limbs and trunk. This information is fed back to all components of the motor system, including the motor cortex, cerebellum, brainstem, and motor neurons in the spinal cord.

The main sources of somatosensory information that acts as feedback to the motor system are the muscle spindles, Golgi tendon organs, and low-threshold mechanoreceptors of the skin and tendons. Joint and muscle receptors are innervated by rapidly conducting, large myelinated peripheral axons of large dorsal root ganglion neurons (first-order neurons). Their proximal axons constitute the primary afferent fibers that enter the spinal cord via the medial division of the dorsal root entry zone. These proprioceptive fibers may (1) course directly through the dorsal gray matter to the ventral gray matter; (2) ascend directly in the dorsal columns or synapse on second-order neurons in the spinal cord to form the lemniscal system; and (3) synapse on second-order neurons in the intermediate gray matter, which contribute to the *spinocerebellar tracts*.

Primary afferent fibers that synapse directly on ventral horn motor neurons initiate a two-neuron muscle stretch reflex that is the anatomical basis for the *muscle-stretch*, or *deep tendon, reflexes* that are commonly tested in clinical neurology. A sudden muscle stretch, as elicited by tapping a tendon with a reflex hammer, stimulates muscle spindle receptors. This in turn produces action potentials in the afferent fibers that enter the spinal cord and synapse on motor neurons in the ventral horn. These ventral horn cells then initiate action potentials that travel back to the muscle of origin and cause it to contract. This is a *local segmental reflex* (see Chapter 14). This reflex is lost whenever disease involves the primary proprioceptive axon or other component of the reflex arc at that segment.

More important is the role of primary afferent input to the *interneuronal pool* in the ventral horn. These interneurons integrate primary afferent, supraspinal, and local circuit information to control motor neuron activity for maintenance of muscle tone (degree of stiffness) and execution of coordinated motor acts.

Motor Function of the Dorsal Column–Lemniscal System

The dorsal column system has extensive interconnections with the corticospinal motor system. Afferent inputs from the dorsal column–lemniscal system affect firing of corticospinal neurons via thalamocortical and corticocortical connections. Fibers from somatosensory cortex travel in the corticospinal tract to modulate sensory processing

in the thalamus and dorsal column nuclei. The lemniscal and corticospinal systems are the afferent and efferent components, respectively, of transcortical *long loop reflexes*, which complement the segmental myotatic reflexes for control of motor neuron activity (see Chapter 8).

Primary afferent fibers that ascend in the dorsal column–lemniscal system constitute the afferent limb; the efferent limb consists of axons in the corticospinal tract.

Spinocerebellar Tracts

The *spinocerebellar tracts* transmit information about the activity of the effector muscles or motor neuron pools to the cerebellum, where it is integrated and processed. The cerebellum is capable of modifying the action of different muscle groups so that movements are performed smoothly and accurately. Because the information carried by these pathways does not reach consciousness directly, it is referred to as *unconscious proprioception*.

The two spinal cord pathways that convey unconscious proprioceptive information to the cerebellum are the *dorsal* and *ventral spinocerebellar tracts*. They are part of the outer tube system and have some features in common, but they also have important anatomical and functional differences. Both tracts (1) originate from neurons in the intermediate gray matter; (2) contain large-diameter, rapidly conducting secondary axons (they are among the fastest conducting pathways in the central nervous system); (3) are located in the periphery of the lateral white matter of the spinal cord; (4) transmit information from the *lower extremities*; and (5) provide input predominantly to the *ipsilateral cerebellum*.

Dorsal Spinocerebellar Tract

The *dorsal spinocerebellar tract* originates in neurons of the *nucleus dorsalis of Clarke (Clarke's column)*. These neurons are potently excited by first-order proprioceptive fibers from muscle spindles of a single muscle or few agonists and from low-threshold cutaneous mechanoreceptors. Second-order axons from

Clarke's column enter the ipsilateral lateral funiculus to form the dorsal spinocerebellar tract. Fibers ascend near the lateral margin of the spinal cord. At the level of the medulla, they enter the cerebellum through the inferior cerebellar peduncle, or restiform body.

Because Clarke's column is found only between spinal cord segments T-1 and L-1, two modifications of the basic organization of this pathway occur above and below these levels:

1. Fibers carrying proprioceptive information from the lower extremities and entering *below* L-1 course in the dorsal column (fasciculus gracilis) until they reach segment L-1. Thus, there is no dorsal spinocerebellar tract in the lumbosacral spinal cord.

2. Proprioceptive fibers entering *above* T-1 (carrying information from the upper extremities to the cervical cord) do not have access to Clarke's column or to the dorsal spinocerebellar tract. Proprioceptive input from the upper extremities ascends in the dorsal column (fasciculus cuneatus) to synapse in the lower medulla in the *lateral*, or *accessory, nucleus cuneatus*, which is analogous to Clarke's column. Second-order neurons in the lateral nucleus cuneatus give rise to axons that form the *cuneocerebellar tract*, which joins the dorsal spinocerebellar tract in the ipsilateral restiform body.

The dorsal spinocerebellar tract and the cuneocerebellar tract are important in the rapid, efficient transmission of proprioceptive and exteroceptive signals from a single muscle or a few muscles to the cerebellum. This allows *feedback control* of motor performance through cerebellar influences on neurons in motor cortex and subcortical motor nuclei.

Ventral Spinocerebellar Tract

The *ventral spinocerebellar tract* originates in *spinal border cells* in the lateral region of the ventral horn of the lumbar spinal cord. These neurons receive information simultaneously from primary proprioceptive and exteroceptive afferents and descending supraspinal pathways affecting ventral horn motor neurons and interneurons. Axons of the spinal border cells cross the midline to form the ventral spinocerebellar tract. This tract is lateral to the ventrolateral quadrant and ascends through the spinal cord, medulla, and pons to enter the cerebellum via a circuitous route through the superior cerebellar peduncle, or brachium conjunctivum. Within the posterior fossa, most of these fibers again cross so that the ventral spinocerebellar tract provides the cerebellum with bilateral but predominantly ipsilateral input about activity in the lower extremities. Input from the upper extremities relays on interneurons at spinal cord level C-7 and C-8. Axons of these interneurons ascend as the *rostral spinocerebellar tract*, reaching predominantly the ipsilateral cerebellum via either the superior or inferior cerebellar peduncle.

The ventral spinocerebellar tract neurons act as comparators between the action of inhibitory and excitatory inputs to spinal motor neurons and interneurons and thus provide the cerebellum with information about the state of excitation of these spinal cord neurons. Therefore, the ventral spinocerebellar tract provides *feed-forward information* to the cerebellum about the activity of motor neuron pools, whereas the dorsal spinocerebellar tract conveys *feedback information* about the resulting movement.

Effect of Lesions

The clinical manifestation of disease involving these pathways is motor incoordination (ataxia) of the extremities. Although these pathways are of great physiologic importance, clinically it is extremely difficult to identify abnormalities from damage of these pathways, which are commonly involved along with the dorsal columns.

The Differential Diagnosis of Ataxia

Definition

Sensory information is vital to the smooth, harmonious production of motor activity. A failure to produce normally smooth motor acts is referred to as *ataxia*. Ataxia may be manifest in the motion of a single limb but is more commonly evident during walking. With ataxia, movements become jerky and uncoordinated. The central nervous system must be constantly apprised of the position, tone, and movement of the limbs and trunk. It accomplishes this task by integrating (primarily in the cerebellum) proprioceptive input and information from the receptors for equilibrium, which are located in the labyrinths of the ear, and by relaying these data back to the appropriate motor effectors. Visual input may be used in part to compensate for a defect in this integrating mechanism.

Types of Ataxia

Sensory ataxias include conditions in which motor performance is faulty when the motor pathways and the cerebellum are intact. This occurs because there is a defect in transmitting proprioceptive or equilibratory information to higher centers. Sensory ataxia frequently can be compensated for by using visual input to guide limb position; hence, the ataxia is often worse in the dark or when the eyes are closed. *Motor ataxias* include conditions in which the sensory pathways are intact but motor performance is faulty and there is a defect in the integration and processing of proprioceptive information. Motor ataxia is usually due to disease in the cerebellum. This type of ataxia is often poorly compensated for by visual input.

Differentiation

The Romberg test is a quick and convenient method of distinguishing between sensory and motor ataxias. A patient who shows no unsteadiness when standing with feet together and eyes open but who displays unsteadiness with the eyes closed has a Romberg sign, indicating that the patient has a sensory ataxia. Patients with a motor (cerebellar) ataxia may or may not be unsteady in the Romberg position but show little or no increase in unsteadiness when they close their eyes and thus do not have the Romberg sign.

Patients who have sensory ataxia generally have difficulty with either vestibular function or proprioception, as a result of peripheral nerve or spinal cord disease. Ataxic patients without a Romberg sign often show abnormalities in cerebellar function.

Other Sensory Systems

The pathways discussed above mediate the major general somatic sensations. Sensation from visceral structures (general visceral sensations), including visceral pain and sexual sensations, are mediated primarily by the spinothalamic and other anterolateral quadrant pathways, as discussed in Chapter 9. The special visceral afferent sensations of taste and smell and the special somatic sensations of hearing and balance are discussed in association with the posterior fossa (see Chapter 15) and the supratentorial (see Chapter 16) levels. Because of the importance of the special somatic sensation of vision in clinical neurologic diagnosis and in localizing lesions, an overview of this pathway is warranted.

Visual Pathway

The visual pathway has many features typical of the lemniscal pathways, including a precise contralateral topographic representation (in this case, of the visual field). Therefore, like the dorsal column and spinothalamic pathways, the visual pathway is commonly tested clinically to localize lesions in the nervous system. In contrast, the central organization of the pathways for audition, taste, and smell is largely bilateral and thus of limited value in the precise localization of a lesion to one side of the neuraxis.

The visual pathways are located entirely at the supratentorial level and are discussed in detail in Chapter 16. Some of its features are considered here to emphasize important differences with the somatosensory pathways (Table 9). The receptor for light stimulus, or *photoreceptor*, is a specialized cell that responds to

TABLE 9. *Comparison of the somatosensory and visual pathways*

	Somatosensory pathways	Visual pathway
Stimulus	Mechanical or thermal	Light
Receptor	Terminal of dorsal root ganglion neuron	Photoreceptor
Ionic mechanism	Opening of a mechanosensitive cation channel	Closing of a cyclic nucleotide-gated cation channel
Response to stimulus	Depolarization of the axon of the first-order neuron	Hyperpolarization and decrease of tonic release of glutamate at the synapse with the first-order neuron
First-order neuron	Dorsal root ganglion cell	Bipolar cell of the retina
Second-order neuron	Dorsal horn or dorsal column nuclei	Ganglion cell of the retina
Third-order neuron (thalamus)	Ventral posterolateral nucleus	Lateral geniculate nucleus
Cortical termination	Postcentral gyrus of the parietal lobe	Calcarine cortex of the occipital lobe

light stimulation with the closing of a cyclic nucleotide-gated channel. Thus, unlike the response of other receptors, the response to a light stimulus is hyperpolarization. This results in a decrease in the tonic release of L-glutamate and its effects on the first-order neurons of the visual pathway, the *bipolar cell.* Bipolar cells synapse on the second-order neurons of the pathway, the *ganglion cells.* The axons of the ganglion cells form the *optic nerve* (Fig. 13). Thus, the receptor, the first-order neurons, and the second-order neurons of the visual pathway

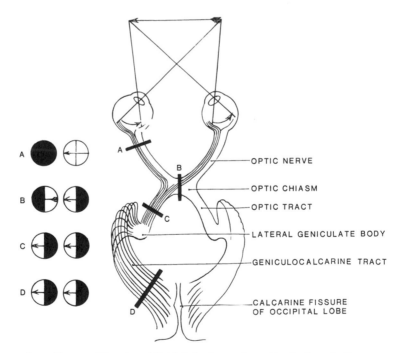

FIG. 13. The optic pathways. The visual field defects produced by lesions in these pathways are shown at the *left.* The visual field of the left eye is shown in the *left circle,* that of the right eye in the *adjacent circle.* Lesions anterior to the optic chiasm **(A)** produce monocular visual loss. Lesions at the optic chiasm **(B)** produce bitemporal hemianopia due to involvement of nasal-retinal crossing fibers. Unilateral lesions behind the optic chiasm affecting the optic tract **(C)**, lateral geniculate body, optic radiations **(D)**, or occipital cortex produce contralateral homonymous hemianopia.

are located in the retina, a derivative of the diencephalon, and the optic nerve is a tract of the central nervous system. There is topographic representation of the visual field in the visual pathway, referred to as *retinotopy*. The nasal portion of the visual field is projected onto the temporal portion of the retina and the temporal portion of the visual field onto the nasal portion of the retina. The axons of ganglion cells in the nasal retina (which relay information from the temporal portion of the visual field) decussate in the *optic chiasm*, and the axons of ganglion cells in the temporal retina (which relay information from the nasal portion of the visual field) remain uncrossed. Crossed (contralateral) nasal and uncrossed (ipsilateral) fibers join at the optic chiasm and form the *optic tracts*. Thus, axons related to the right visual field travel in the left optic tract, and axons related to the left visual field travel in the right optic tract. Like other second-order axons, the right and left optic tracts project to the thalamus and synapse in the ipsilateral *lateral geniculate body*. Neurons of the lateral geniculate body project axons via the *optic radiations* to the primary visual area, located in the *calcarine cortex* of the occipital lobe.

Thus, the visual images of the right half of the visual field project to the left occipital cortex, and the images of the left visual field project to the right occipital cortex.

Lesions located anterior to the optic chiasm in the optic nerves interfere with vision only in the ipsilateral eye (monocular visual loss). Lesions in the center of the optic chiasm interfere only with the nasal crossing fibers, producing a loss of function of the nasal retina and of temporal vision in both eyes (bitemporal hemianopia). Lesions located behind the optic chiasm, that is, in the optic tracts, lateral geniculate body, optic radiations, or occipital cortex, produce a loss of vision in the contralateral visual fields of both eyes (homonymous hemianopia).

Clinical Correlations   ▪

Disease processes involving the sensory system produce various symptoms, including pain, hypesthesia (reduced sensation), anesthesia (a complete loss of cutaneous sensibility), dysesthesia (an altered or perverted interpretation of sensation, such as a burning, tingling, or painful feeling in response to touch), and paresthesia (spontaneous sensation of prickling or tingling). In some instances, sensory stimuli are felt more keenly than normal (hyperesthesia). It is extremely important in every case of pain or sensory loss to determine its exact distribution.

Lesions at the Peripheral Level

The distal axons of the primary sensory neurons mediating all types of afferent input are gathered together, along with motor and autonomic fibers, in peripheral nerves. Thus, a lesion that affects peripheral nerves would be expected to produce a variable sensory loss for all modalities and a loss of muscle-stretch reflexes in the anatomical distribution of that nerve. Some motor or autonomic deficit usually can be found if such fibers are present in the involved nerve. This type of deficit may occur in a focal distribution when only a single peripheral nerve is involved (such as might occur from trauma) and is called *mononeuropathy*. When these symptoms and signs occur in a diffuse distribution, the deficit is called *polyneuropathy*. Pain, paresthesias, or dysesthesias are common accompaniments of peripheral nerve lesions. Figure 14 shows the cutaneous distribution of the major peripheral nerves.

Lesions at the Spinal Level

Disease processes located within the spinal canal typically produce (1) a *segmental* neurologic deficit limited to one level of the body and usually caused by involvement of the nerve roots or spinal nerves, and (2) an *intersegmental* sensory deficit involving all of the body below a particular level and caused by interruption of the major ascending sensory pathways.

Mechanical compression or local inflammation of a dorsal nerve root or spinal nerve

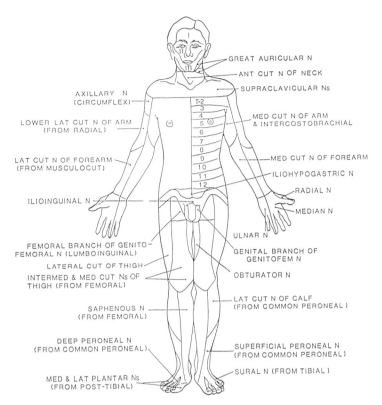

FIG. 14. Cutaneous distribution of the major peripheral nerves. (*ANT,* anterior; *CUT,* cutaneous; *INT,* intermediate; *LAT,* lateral; *MED,* medial; *N,* nerve.) (Modified from Haymaker, W., and Woodhall, B. *Peripheral Nerve Injuries: Principles of Diagnosis* [2nd ed.]. Philadelphia: W. B. Saunders, 1953. With permission.)

produces pain along the anatomical distribution of the affected root. Pain due to nerve root involvement in the distribution of one or more *dermatomes* (Fig. 15) is known as *radicular pain.* This type of pain, which may vary in intensity, is often lancinating (a sharp, darting type of pain). Maneuvers that increase intraspinal pressure (and presumably increase the traction on irritated nerve roots), such as coughing, sneezing, and straining, produce a characteristic increase in this type of pain. In addition to producing radicular pain, lesions of the dorsal root or spinal nerve produce areas of paresthesia, hyperesthesia, or loss of cutaneous sensation in a dermatomal distribution. At appropriate levels, segmental loss of muscle-stretch reflexes, weakness, and autonomic disturbances can be seen.

Commissural Syndrome

A special type of segmental deficit can result from a lesion involving the central regions of the spinal cord, usually over several segments. This deficit is characterized by a loss of pain and temperature sensation from interruption of the second-order axons as they decussate to form the spinothalamic tracts (Fig. 16). The sensory loss is bilateral (because fibers from both sides are interrupted by such a lesion), and it involves the crossing fibers of several adjacent segments. Thus, a lesion involving the central regions of segments T-2 through T-5 produces loss of pain and temperature only in those segments. The commissural syndrome can be produced only by a lesion in the substance of the spinal cord.

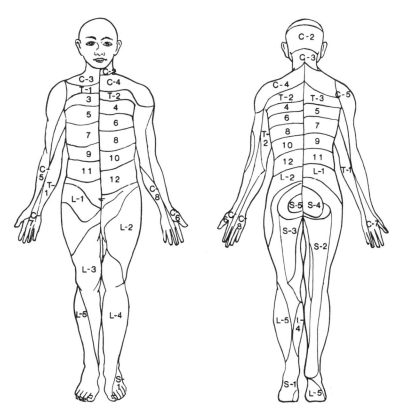

FIG. 15. Cutaneous, or dermatomal, distribution of spinal nerve roots. Note considerable overlap between segments, and note that the distribution differs from that of peripheral nerves.

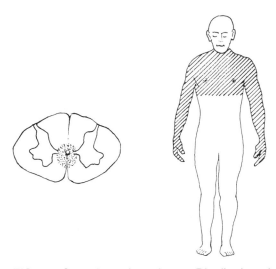

FIG. 16. Commissural syndrome. Distribution of loss of pain and temperature sensations, with a lesion in the location shown on the left.

As the lesion enlarges, other adjacent sensory tracts become involved. This type of lesion may result from trauma (hematomyelia), neoplasm, or other conditions, including syringomyelia.

Syringomyelia is a common cause of the commissural syndrome and consists of cavitation occurring within the central area of the spinal cord (Fig. 17). Whether the cavity develops as a result of dilatation of the primitive central canal (hydromyelia) or as a result of some other destructive process in the central region of the cord, such as an intramedullary neoplasm, is not always clear. Although initially the cavity is centrally located, expansion of the cavity and surrounding gliosis tends to extend the syrinx irregularly throughout the gray matter and at times into the white matter

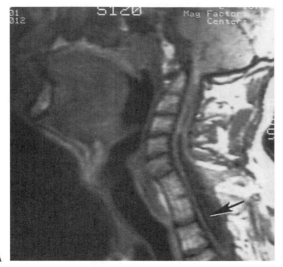

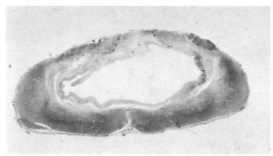

FIG. 17. Syringomyelia. **A:** Magnetic resonance image of syringomyelia at the level of the cervical spinal cord *(arrow).* **B:** Transverse section of cervical spinal cord showing the central cavity lined by a thickened glial membrane and associated with degeneration of the surrounding tissue. (H&E; ×4.)

of the dorsal and lateral columns. The lesion most commonly occurs in the cervical area.

Spinothalamic Tract Syndrome

A lesion involving the spinothalamic tract causes a loss of pain and temperature sensation on the opposite side of the body, involving all segments below the level of the lesion. Pain and temperature fibers enter through the dorsal root branch and extend rostrally in Lissauer's tract for up to two segments above their entry zone before synapsing with the spinothalamic tract neurons of the dorsal horn. Therefore, the sensory level on the side opposite a spinothalamic tract lesion is usually at least two segments below the level of the actual lesion. Within the spinothalamic tract, the fibers are arranged in a laminar fashion, with the sacral fibers near the periphery and fibers from higher levels toward the center. Hence, lesions arising within the substance of the spinal cord (intramedullary lesions) may involve only the central portions of the tract and spare the peripheral fibers, to produce a loss of pain and temperature in all levels below the lesion except the sacral level. This is referred to as *sacral sparing.* When present, sacral sparing is an important clue to an intramedullary spinal cord lesion (Fig. 18).

In certain instances of intractable pain involving the lower extremity, pain may be relieved by placing a lesion in the spinothalamic tract (spinothalamic tractotomy). It is usually done by surgically cutting the ventral portion of the lateral funiculus in the cervical area. Although there is probably some damage to

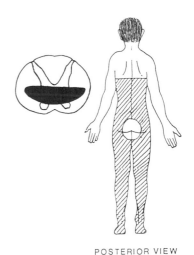

POSTERIOR VIEW

FIG. 18. Sensory loss with sacral sparing due to the intramedullary lesion shown on the *left.* The lesion involves the spinothalamic tracts bilaterally. (Note that the figure in the diagram is viewed from behind.)

the ventral spinocerebellar tract, no permanent symptoms are produced except loss of pain and temperature sensibility on the contralateral side.

Brown-Séquard's Syndrome

This syndrome is seen in pure form with hemisection of the spinal cord. In clinical practice, the syndrome is often partial and incomplete; however, the findings of ipsilateral motor deficit, ipsilateral dorsal column deficit, and contralateral loss of pain and temperature usually are present and are characteristic of a unilateral spinal cord lesion (Fig. 19).

Lesions at the Posterior Fossa Level

Disease processes affecting the posterior fossa level are characterized by a contralateral intersegmental loss of sensory function in the trunk and limbs because of interruption of the major ascending pathways. However, there frequently is also a loss of sensory function (primarily pain and temperature) over the ipsilateral face because of segmental involvement of the trigeminal nerve or its descending tract and nucleus (Fig. 20).

Lesions at the Supratentorial Level

At this level, all major sensory pathways have crossed to the contralateral side; therefore, lesions at this level alter sensory function over the entire contralateral side of the body.

Two important variations of sensory loss may be encountered with lesions at this level.

Thalamic Syndrome

The thalamus is an important integrating and relay station for sensory perception. A lesion affecting the specific sensory nuclei of the thalamus causes a relatively complete loss of all forms of general somatic afferent sensation in the contralateral face, trunk, and limbs (Fig. 21). If the portion of the thalamus related to vision is also involved, a contralateral homonymous hemianopia is produced. After a localized lesion of the thalamus, perhaps due to faulty integration of sensory information, a severe burning (dysesthetic) pain in the area of sensory loss is sometimes produced.

Suprathalamic Syndrome

Lesions that involve sensory pathways from the thalamus to the cerebral cortex or in

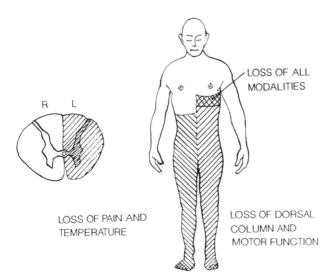

LOSS OF ALL MODALITIES

LOSS OF PAIN AND TEMPERATURE

LOSS OF DORSAL COLUMN AND MOTOR FUNCTION

FIG. 19. Brown-Séquard's syndrome. Sensory loss produced by damage to one-half of the spinal cord by the lesion shown on the left. A motor deficit would also be present (see Chapter 8).

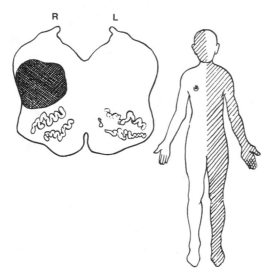

FIG. 20. Distribution of pain and temperature sensation loss characteristic of lesions at the posterior fossa level, as shown on the *left.*

the cortex itself also alter all forms of general somatic afferent sensation on the contralateral side of the body. However, in contrast to the dense loss of sensation found with thalamic lesions, suprathalamic involvement is characterized by only minimal involvement of pain, temperature, touch, and vibratory sensibility

and a severe deficit in the discriminative sensations that require cortical participation (Fig. 22). These sensations are joint position sense, two-point discrimination, touch localization, and the recognition of objects placed in the hand (stereognosis), and suggest that discriminative sensations require intact thalamocortical pathways for their full appreciation, whereas the primary modalities of superficial sensation are perceived and integrated at the thalamic level. This type of discriminative sensory loss is often found with lesions of the parietal lobe and is commonly referred to as a *cortical sensory deficit.* If the optic radiations are also involved, a contralateral visual field defect is produced. In the absence of a visual field defect or other signs of supratentorial involvement, this type of sensory deficit may be confused with the findings of dorsal column disease. A severe deficit in conscious proprioception, bilateral involvement, and associated alteration in vibratory sense all favor a lesion of the dorsal columns. When the deficit is unilateral, the distinction between a suprathalamic and a high-cervical spinal cord lesion can be extremely difficult unless other signs and symptoms are present to aid with localization.

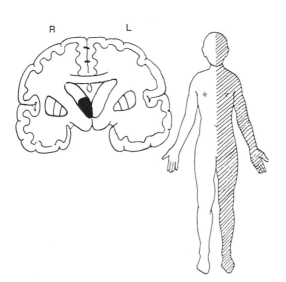

FIG. 21. Thalamic syndrome. Loss of all modalities of sensation contralateral to the lesion.

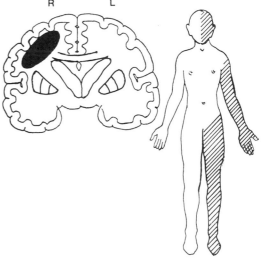

FIG. 22. Suprathalamic syndrome. Loss of cortical sensory functions contralateral to the lesion.

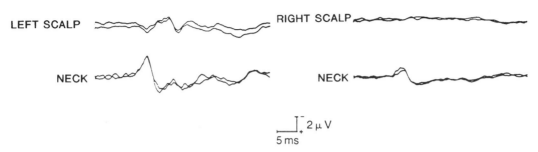

FIG. 23. Somatosensory evoked responses recorded from the neck and scalp in a patient with multiple sclerosis. Note the decrease in the amplitude of the potential recorded from the right neck and scalp compared with those recorded from the left side.

Irritative lesions located in the region of the postcentral gyrus may initiate seizures. The clinical manifestations of seizures in this area consist primarily of a feeling of tingling (paresthesias) on the opposite side of the body. As the localized neuronal discharge spreads from its focus of origin, these sensations may be experienced as moving in an orderly fashion dictated by the topographic organization of the gyrus. Further spread to the adjacent precentral gyrus may produce associated motor activity, and spread to subcortical structures may produce a loss of consciousness.

Somatosensory Evoked Response

The somatosensory evoked response is an electrodiagnostic test that is used to evaluate the sensory system (Fig. 23). Evoked responses are electrical potentials that occur with a fixed latency in response to a stimulus. Because these potentials are very small, a number of successive responses need to be averaged and amplified to be seen. The somatosensory evoked responses are potentials occurring in response to stimulation of a peripheral nerve, which can be recorded from the nerve, the plexus, the sensory pathways within the spinal cord and brainstem, the thalamocortical pathways, and the somatosensory

cortex. Abnormalities of the somatosensory evoked responses occur with lesions or disease processes involving the sensory pathways at any of these levels and are manifested either by an increase in latency or by a reduced amplitude or an absence of response. The somatosensory evoked responses are used to document or to diagnose multiple sclerosis, degenerative processes, traumatic lesions, and other structural lesions affecting the peripheral or central sensory system.

Neurologic Examination: Sensory System

A complete sensory examination includes the evaluation of touch, pain, temperature, joint position, and vibratory senses as well as various discriminatory modalities. Comparison of one side of the body with the other and with the examiner's own sensory abilities is useful for establishing normal and abnormal. Much of the sensory examination is best performed with the patient's eyes closed to eliminate visual cues. Examination of sensation consists of three portions: (1) qualitative, to determine the elements of sensation that are affected; (2) quantitative, to determine the degree of involvement when sensation is impaired; and

(3) anatomical, to map out the areas of sensory impairment.

Sensation is tested in the following ways:

1. *Touch.* Lightly place a piece of cotton on the face, trunk, and extremities, and ask the patient to respond when it is felt.
2. *Pain.* Gently prick the patient with a pin. A more accurate determination can be made by randomly touching the patient with the point or head of a pin and noting whether the patient can appreciate sharp and dull sensations.
3. *Temperature.* Randomly apply warm and cool objects to the skin, and note the patient's ability to distinguish between them.
4. *Vibration sense.* Place a vibrating tuning fork over bony prominences, and note whether the patient can detect the sensation and can determine when the vibration ceases. (In patients older than 50 years, vibratory sense is often reduced in the feet.)
5. *Joint position sense.* Firmly grasp the sides of the great toe or a finger, and ask the patient to detect and respond to movements in an upward or downward direction.
6. *Two-point discrimination.* A two-point caliper is used. This sensation is normally examined only on the fingertips by asking the patient to respond to the tactile stimulus of one or two points. The threshold (minimal recognizable separation) is determined and compared on the two sides of the body.
7. *Tactile localization.* Touch the patient, and request that the point of contact be identified.
8. *Graphesthesia.* Ask the patient to identify numbers or letters traced on the palm of his or her hand with a blunt object.
9. *Stereognosis.* Ask the patient to close his or her eyes and identify objects of different sizes, shapes, and textures (such as a coin, key, clip, or safety pin) placed in the hand.

In the absence of any sensory symptoms or the patient's subjective sensation of pain, a brief screening examination consisting of a test of touch, pain, joint position, and vibratory sense in both hands and both feet and of a test of pain and touch perception on the face is all that is required. When a sensory deficit is suspected or identified, the examiner must determine the modality of sensation involved and map its distribution to see if it conforms to that found with lesions of the peripheral nerve, spinal nerve or dorsal root, spinal cord, posterior fossa, or supratentorial region.

Clinical Problems

Each of the following clinical problems illustrates some aspect of dysfunction in the sensory system. For each problem, determine the anatomicopathologic diagnosis (as outlined in the objectives in Chapter 4), and answer the related questions.

1. A 48-year-old woman experienced the abrupt onset of pain followed by paresthesia and loss of feeling in a rather circumscribed area along the lateral aspect of her right thigh. Examination revealed a localized area of decreased perception of pinprick, temperature, and touch in this region only. Results of the rest of the examination were normal.
   a. What is the anatomicopathologic diagnosis?
   b. What specific anatomical structure is involved?
   c. How would the distribution of symptoms differ if the lesion involved the median nerve at the wrist?
2. A 40-year-old man had onset of neck pain and paresthesias over the occipital region of the head 6 months ago. These symptoms were aggravated by coughing and sneezing. Three months ago, his symptoms became worse and he noted a tingling sensation up and down his spinal column whenever he bent his neck. One month ago, he noted progressive difficulty in walking in the dark. On examina-

tion, he was found to have decreased perception to touch and pinprick over the posterior scalp region, reduced position sense in his arms and legs bilaterally, decreased vibratory sensation in both upper and lower extremities, and decreased ability to perceive discriminative tactile sensation bilaterally.

a. What is the anatomicopathologic diagnosis?

b. What segmental structures provide sensory innervation to the posterior scalp region?

c. What sensory structures are involved by the lesion?

d. What is the precise level of the responsible lesion?

e. What most likely are the precise pathologic lesions responsible for this clinical syndrome?

f. How would the symptoms and signs differ if the lesion were located at the T-6 spinal level?

3. A 41-year-old woman noted a painless, slowly progressive loss of sensation in an area involving the back of her head, neck, shoulders, and both upper extremities. Neurologic examination revealed a sensory loss involving only pain and temperature in this area. Specific testing of all other modalities of sensation in the affected areas and elsewhere revealed no abnormalities, and there were no changes in motor performance, strength, or deep tendon reflexes.

a. What is the anatomicopathologic diagnosis?

b. What sensory structure(s) is (are) involved by the lesion?

c. What is the most likely pathologic lesion responsible for this clinical syndrome?

4. A 21-year-old soldier returned from battle after sustaining a gunshot wound in his spinal column. On examination, you note that he has weakness of the left lower extremity. In addition, he has loss of pain and temperature perception on the right side from about the level of his navel downward. Vibration, joint position sense, and discriminatory function are reduced in the left leg. Touch is normal.

a. What is the anatomicopathologic diagnosis?

b. What is the precise level of the lesion?

c. What is the name given to this type of syndrome?

d. Why was the sensation of touch preserved in this patient?

e. Where in the nervous system would you expect to find evidence of wallerian degeneration?

5. A 68-year-old hypertensive woman awoke one morning noting that she was unable to feel anything over the entire left side of her body. On examination, motor strength and reflexes were normal, as were the visual fields; however, she did not respond to pinprick, temperature, or touch over the left side of her face, trunk, and extremities, and she could not perceive joint motion or vibration in her left arm and leg.

a. What is the anatomicopathologic diagnosis?

b. What specific sensory system structure(s) is (are) most likely involved?

c. Where in the nervous system would you expect to find evidence of wallerian degeneration?

6. A 31-year-old man noticed the gradual onset of headaches. On several occasions during the last month, he experienced spells consisting of a curious tingling, burning sensation that began in the left thumb and the left corner of his mouth. This gradually became more intense and spread to involve his left hand and the left side of his face and then extended up his arm, trunk, and leg. In 5 minutes, the spell would cease, and he would feel tired and sleepy. Examination reveals a striking inability to perceive joint position, motion, and other discriminative testing over the left side. Touch, pain, temperature, and vibratory sense are preserved.

a. What is the anatomicopathologic diagnosis?

b. What is the nature of the spell experienced by the patient?

c. Why were some forms of sensation involved and others not?

Additional Reading ▪

Bonica, J.-J. Anatomic and physiologic basis of nociception and pain. In Bonica, J.-J. (ed.), *The Management of Pain,* vol 1. (2nd ed.). Philadelphia: Lea & Febiger, 1990, pp. 28–94.

Davidoff, R. A. The dorsal columns. *Neurology* 39:1377, 1989.

Fields, H. L., Heinricher, M. M., and Mason, P. Neurotransmitters in nociceptive modulatory circuits. *Annu. Rev. Neurosci.* 14:219, 1991.

Kaas, J. H. Somatosensory systems. In Paxinos, G. (ed.), *The Human Nervous System.* San Diego: Academic Press, 1990, pp. 813–844.

Kandel, E. R., and Jessell, T. M. Touch. In Kandel, E. R., Schwartz, J. H., and Jessell, T. M. (eds.), *Principles of Neural Science* (3rd ed.). New York: Elsevier, 1991, pp. 367–384.

Talbot, J. D., Marrett, S., Evans, A. C., Meyer, E., Bushnell, M. C., and Duncan, G. H. Multiple representations of pain in human cerebral cortex. *Science* 251:1355, 1991.

Willis, W. D., Jr., and Coggeshall, R. E. *Sensory Mechanisms of the Spinal Cord* (2nd ed.). New York: Plenum Press, 1991.

The Motor System

■

Introduction ■

The entire range of human activity—from walking and talking to gymnastics to control of the space shuttle—depends on the motor system coordinating the actions of muscles, bones, and joints with external sensory information and centrally determined goals. These unique capacities of the motor system cannot be duplicated by even the most sophisticated robots, especially the ability to learn new patterns and to adapt to unexpected changes. The inability to duplicate the capabilities of the motor system is a reflection of its complexity and our incomplete understanding of how it works.

All bodily movements, including those of internal organs, are the result of muscle contraction, which is under neural control. The muscles of the limbs, trunk, neck, and head are *general somatic efferent* in embryologic origin and are under control of the somatic motor pathways. The internal organs are part of the internal regulation system. The *general visceral efferent* structures that control smooth muscle are described in Chapter 9. *Special visceral efferent* structures, such as the neurons for phonation and swallowing, are embryologically derived from the branchial arches and receive both limbic and somatic motor input.

The motor system, like the sensory system, includes a complex network of structures and pathways at all levels of the nervous system. This network is organized to mediate many types of motor activity. An understanding of this organization and of the integration of the motor system with the sensory system is necessary for the accurate localization and diagnosis of neurologic disease. Weakness, paralysis, twitching, jerking, staggering, wasting, shaking, stiffness, spasticity, and incoordination involving the arms, legs, eyes, or muscles of speech are all due to impairment of the motor system. This chapter introduces an organization of the motor system that can help in the identification of disorders of the motor system.

Overview

The functions of the motor system are control of posture and movement. Its general organization is depicted in Fig. 1.

The final output from the central nervous system to the effector muscles arises from *alpha motor neurons* (also called *lower motor neurons*) located in the ventral horn of the spinal cord (and motor nuclei of the brainstem). This output is referred to as the *final common pathway*. The alpha motor neurons receive segmental inputs from the limbs via primary afferents and descending inputs from

supraspinal structures. Segmental and supraspinal inputs affect motor neuron activity either directly or, more commonly, via interneurons. The descending pathways originate from motor areas of the cerebral cortex and the brainstem. Cortical motor neurons give rise to the *corticospinal tract*, or *direct activation pathway*, which controls fine movements of the distal portions of the limbs, particularly the fingers. The descending pathways from the brainstem, referred to as *indirect activation pathways*, primarily control postural and reflex movements. The activity of these pathways is regulated by *two control circuits* centered on the *basal ganglia* and the *cerebellum*. The basal ganglia are important in the selection and initiation of specific motor programs. The cerebellum controls the execution of the motor acts and motor learning (Fig. 1). The cortical motor areas project to both the basal ganglia and the cerebellum. Both of these structures project back to the cortex via a relay in the motor nuclei of the thalamus.

Final Common Pathway

The somatic, or skeletal, muscles that perform the work of moving parts of the body are all under direct control of *lower motor neurons (alpha motor neurons)* and contract only in response to activation by these neurons. Each muscle performs a particular movement, but each muscle may be involved in several different motor activities organized by the lower motor neurons and their pools of interneurons. These neurons are located in the ventral horn of the spinal cord and brainstem. A lower motor neuron and the muscle fibers under its control constitute a *motor unit*.

Each motor unit includes an *alpha motor neuron*, with a cell body in the brainstem or spinal cord and an axon that travels peripherally in a nerve to a specific muscle and divides into a number of terminal axons, and all the muscle fibers on which the terminals synapse.

Acetylcholine is the only neurotransmitter in the final common pathway. Alpha motor

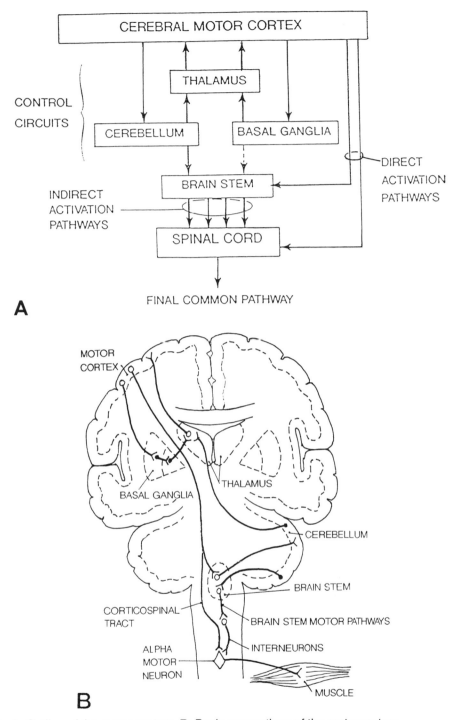

FIG. 1. A: Outline of the motor system. **B:** Basic connections of the motor system. The motor neurons of the ventral horn of the spinal cord and of the motor nuclei in the brainstem are the final common pathway for muscle control. They receive input from the contralateral motor cortex via the corticospinal tract and the corticobulbar tract (direct activation pathway) and from several brainstem nuclei (indirect activation pathways). The cerebellum controls the ipsilateral limbs via connections with the spinal cord, brainstem, and contralateral motor cortex through the thalamus. The basal ganglia participate in motor planning via reciprocal connections with ipsilateral motor cortex (that is, contralateral to the limb).

neurons and their surrounding interneuronal pool integrate activity from central and peripheral sources and transmit action potentials to the muscles to produce the appropriate level of contraction. Disease processes that impair the function of a motor unit prevent the normal activation of muscle fibers in that motor unit. This is manifested as an inability of the muscle to contract fully (weakness or paralysis).

The final common pathway responds to local input from the sensory system and from descending direct and indirect activation pathways. Local sensory input produces simple reflex responses, such as the knee jerk. This type of activity is involuntary, specific, and localized to limited areas of the body. This input is lost if there is damage to the sensory pathways. Thus, loss of a particular reflex could result from damage to either the final common pathway or the sensory input pathway.

Direct Activation Pathway

The largest, best-defined motor pathway is the direct activation (single-neuron) pathway that extends from the cerebral cortex to the spinal cord, called the *corticospinal tract*.

This pathway provides a direct route by which information can travel from the cerebral cortex to the brainstem and spinal cord without an intervening synapse. Its major function is to effect voluntary activity, in particular skilled movements under conscious control. The direct activation pathway carries signals from three somatotopically organized cortical areas—the primary motor cortex, premotor cortex, and supplementary motor cortex (see Chapter 16)—to the lower motor neurons and interneuron motor pools in the brainstem and ventral horn of the spinal cord.

The direct activation pathway descends from the cerebral cortex through the white matter of the cerebral hemispheres, the brainstem, and the spinal cord to end on ventral horn cells. The axons cross the midline at the junction of the brainstem and spinal cord to end on the opposite side. The effectiveness of this pathway depends on an intact final common pathway to carry information to the muscles. The neurotransmitter in the direct activation pathway is glutamate (excitatory). Damage to the direct activation pathway results in weakness, with loss of voluntary movements, especially fine, skilled movements, but preservation of other forms of movements, including segmental reflexes.

Indirect Activation Pathways

The older, more diffuse, indirect motor pathways are sometimes called e*xtrapyramidal pathways*. These pathways mediate the enormous number of automatic activities involved in normal motor function. For example, the maintenance of erect posture when sitting or standing requires the coordinated contraction of many muscles. This coordination is under subconscious control and is mediated by the indirect activation pathways, which include the reticulospinal, vestibulospinal, and rubrospinal tracts. Disease affecting these pathways is manifested in many ways, depending on the location and structures involved, but the abnormalities are particularly those of abnormal muscle tone and reflexes.

Control Circuits

Two parallel pathways, the cerebellar and the basal ganglia pathways, control and modify motor activity. The *cerebellum* and *basal ganglia* both receive input from several motor and sensory cortical areas and project back to the cerebral cortex via the thalamus. They integrate and modulate motor activity primarily through the cerebral cortex and direct activation pathways. However, the cerebellum and basal ganglia also send information to the brainstem and the indirect activation pathways. The basal ganglia are concerned primarily with learned, automatic behavior and with preparing and maintaining the background support, or posture, needed for voluntary motor activity. The major neurotransmitters in the basal ganglia are dopamine and γ-aminobutyric acid (GABA). The cerebellum accomplishes the coordination and correction of movement errors of muscles during active movements. Glutamate and GABA are the major neurotransmitters in the cerebellar circuits. Abnormalities of the control circuits result in disorders of posture and coordination, at times accompanied by *tremor* or other abnormal involuntary movements. Control circuit damage does not produce weakness.

Sensory-Motor Integration

The integration of sensory pathway and motor pathway activity to provide an appropriate response to a particular sensory stimulus is best demonstrated by reflexes. *A reflex is a stereotyped response to a specific sensory stimulus*. In reflexes, action potentials from sensory pathways activate cells in the motor system, which then initiate a specific motor response. One of the most familiar examples of a reflex is the knee jerk, in which the lower leg moves involuntarily in response to tapping of the quadriceps tendon. This is a simple reflex that involves only a primary sensory neuron, a localized portion of the spinal cord, and the final common pathway. Other reflexes are more complex and involve structures at many levels.

Final Common Pathway

The final common pathway is the effector mechanism by which all motor activity is mediated. It includes the motor neurons in the ventral horn of the spinal cord and brainstem and their axons that extend peripherally via nerves to innervate muscles. These motor neurons are called *alpha motor neurons or alpha efferents*. The alpha efferents innervate the muscle fibers that are responsible for skeletal muscle contraction.

Anatomy

The basic functional component of the final common pathway is the *motor unit*. The concept of the *motor unit*, that is, an alpha motor neuron in the ventral horn and the muscle fibers innervated by it, is a physiologic one, developed largely as a result of the work of Sir Charles Sherrington and his colleagues on the reflex activity of the spinal cord. By definition, each unit consists of the cell body of a motor neuron, its single axon (which leaves the spinal cord in the ventral root and extends through the peripheral nervous system before ramifying to innervate the muscle fibers in a particular muscle), and all the muscle fibers innervated by the terminal axons (Fig. 2).

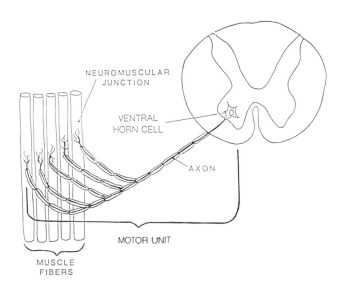

NEUROMUSCULAR JUNCTION

VENTRAL HORN CELL

AXON

MOTOR UNIT

MUSCLE FIBERS

FIG. 2. A single motor unit and its components: the lower motor neuron and muscle fibers innervated by it. The final common pathway contains hundreds of thousands of such units innervating skeletal muscle.

Ventral Horn Cells

The ventral horn (also called the anterior horn) of the spinal cord is derived from the basal plate and contains the output neurons and interneurons involved in motor control of the neck, trunk, and limbs. Similar neurons located in the motor nuclei of the brainstem control the craniofacial muscles. *Alpha motor neurons* are relatively large (50 to 80 µm in diameter) and are arranged in well-defined columns. They innervate contractile skeletal muscle fibers. A second type of motor neuron, *gamma motor neurons*, innervates muscle spindles. In addition to the output motor neurons, the ventral horn contains several types of *interneurons*. The interneurons integrate the activity from the direct and indirect pathways and peripheral sensory input.

A motor neuron not only excites but also exerts a trophic effect on the muscle fiber that it innervates. Destruction of the ventral horn cell of a motor unit results in degeneration of the axon and the loss of innervation of the muscle fibers of that motor unit. The muscle becomes weak or paralyzed, and the muscle fibers atrophy.

Motor Axons

The motor axons are large myelinated fibers (6 to 20 µm in diameter) located in the peripheral nerves. Nearly half of the fibers are the large alpha motor neuron fibers (extrafusal fibers); the others are the gamma motor fibers to the muscle spindles (intrafusal fibers).

Branching of motor nerve fibers occurs along the course of nerves at the nodes of Ranvier and is greatest distally in the muscle. Each terminal ramification of a nerve fiber ends at a *neuromuscular junction*, a motor end plate on a single muscle fiber. The nerves that go to muscle also contain many sensory fibers arising mainly from the muscle spindles. Mild damage to the motor axons in a peripheral nerve can block the conduction of action potentials to the muscle; severe damage can produce wallerian degeneration of the axon distal to the site of the lesion. In either instance, muscle function is lost.

The Neuromuscular Junction

The points of contact between the terminal ramifications of motor axons and muscle fibers innervated by them are known as *motor end plates*, or *neuromuscular junctions*. Each motor end plate is a composite structure belonging partly to the motor axon and partly to the muscle fiber. The terminal axon lies in a hollow indentation of the surface of the muscle fiber, the *synaptic gutter*. The membrane of the nerve terminal and that of the muscle fiber are separated by a narrow space, the *synaptic cleft*. The nerve terminal holds many vesicles that contain the neurotransmitter acetylcholine.

Organization of Muscle Fibers in a Motor Unit

The nerve terminals of a single motor axon innervate muscle fibers that may be distributed widely throughout the muscle, intermingling with muscle fibers innervated by other neurons. A muscle may contain from 50 to 2,000 motor units.

The size of a motor unit is determined by the number of extrafusal fibers innervated by a single motor neuron. This is expressed as the *innervation ratio*, the number of muscle fibers per axon. Muscles concerned with fine movements have smaller innervation ratios than those that perform cruder movements. The motor units of the powerful limb muscles, for example, each contain from 500 to 2,000 muscle fibers. In contrast, motor units in intrinsic hand muscles have innervation ratios of only 50 to 400 and eye muscles have ratios of 3 to 10.

After destruction of isolated ventral horn cells, for example, in poliomyelitis, reinnervation of some of the denervated fibers may occur by branching of the remaining motor nerve fibers. These new collateral sprouts of intact axons form new motor end plates on the denervated muscle fibers, resulting in an increase in the number of muscle fibers in the remaining motor units and, thus, an increase in the innervation ratio.

Muscle

Muscle fibers of skeletal muscles are long cylindrical structures, each of which is a syncytium containing hundreds of nuclei. The cytoplasm of the muscle fiber contains mitochondria, sarcoplasmic reticulum, and *myofibrils*, the contractile elements of the muscle. The myofibrils have a banded structure that subdivides them into units called *sarcomeres*. The fine structure of muscle is described in more detail in Chapter 13.

Individual muscle fibers may be several centimeters long. They may run from one end of the muscle to the other or they may be attached to tendinous insertions within the muscle. The fibers are arranged in groups, or *fasciculi*, each of which is a bundle of parallel fibers bound together and surrounded by connective tissue containing blood vessels and nerves. Adult muscle fibers range from 30 to 90 μm in diameter. Differences in fiber diameter between different muscles and between the muscles of different people occur because of differences in build and muscular development. The size of muscle fiber also depends on the activity of the muscle and on *trophic factors* released from the nerve terminals. Lack of use causes muscle fibers to shrink, but they do so more severely and rapidly with immobilization or with loss of innervation. In cases of loss of innervation, this loss of size, or *atrophy*, of the fiber is limited to the muscle fibers that are innervated by the damaged neuron. In abnormalities of the muscle itself, atrophy involves all fibers in the muscle.

Physiology

The motor unit is the physiologic unit of reflex and voluntary contraction. Under normal conditions, the motor unit behaves in an all-or-none manner, which means that an impulse in the motor nerve fiber produces an action potential in and synchronous contraction of all the muscle fibers it supplies. Thus, the resulting contraction of the motor unit is the sum of the mechanical responses of the component muscle fibers.

Neuromuscular Transmission

Activation of a lower motor neuron in the spinal cord or brainstem produces an action potential that spreads to each of the terminal branches of the motor axon in the muscle. Each of these axons releases the neurotransmitter *acetylcholine*, which diffuses rapidly across the synaptic cleft and acts on the postsynaptic membrane of the muscle fiber.

Acetylcholine produces fast excitation of the muscle fiber via activation of *nicotinic receptors*, which are cation channels. This results in opening of the channel and depolarization of the muscle. This is referred to as the *end-plate potential*. The end-plate potential initiates an action potential in the muscle fiber, which then spreads along the entire length of the muscle fiber. The electrical currents generated by the muscle action potential invade the depths of the muscle fiber via a tubular system to turn on the contractile mechanism that produces the actual twitch of the muscle. This sequence of steps converts the activation of motor neurons to muscle contraction.

The motor nerve terminal releases several other substances in addition to acetylcholine; these substances exert a trophic action on the muscle by modifying its biochemical properties. An important example of these trophic interactions is the clustering of muscle acetylcholine receptors exactly opposite to the sites of release of acetylcholine from the motor nerve terminal. Interruption of innervation of the muscle produces muscle atrophy and redistribution of the nicotinic receptors along the membrane.

Motor Units

Normal movements involve the coordinated activity of hundreds to thousands of motor units in many muscles. The speed and strength of a movement are controlled by the number of motor units active, their rate of firing, and the characteristics of the motor units activated.

The size of the motor unit depends on the number of muscle fibers innervated by a single motoneuron, that is, the innervation ratio.

Units with low innervation ratios are needed for some tasks. For example, extrinsic ocular muscles, which must fixate accurately, need very fine control and therefore have low innervation ratios. The number of muscle fibers in a motor unit is also related to the load that it must move. For example, to move the mass of the lower limb even slightly requires the simultaneous action of many muscle fibers; consequently, in the muscles responsible for such movements, high innervation ratios are found. Because activation of a normal ventral horn cell results in contraction of all the muscle fibers in the motor unit, gradation of contraction is accomplished by varying the frequency of firing of single motor units and the number of motor units activated. When effort is increased, more motor units are brought into action.

In general, the motor units in limb muscles may be divided into two groups according to their speed of contraction: *fast twitch and slow twitch*. The distinction is based on the differences in time from the start of the contraction to the time at which the motor unit develops its peak tension in response to a single stimulus. In a typical fast-twitch motor unit, this contraction time is approximately 25 milliseconds, and in a slow-twitch unit it is approximately 75 milliseconds. The motor nerve innervating the muscle fibers of the motor unit determines the twitch time by some trophic (chemical) substance liberated at the nerve endings independently of acetylcholine, by the pattern of nerve impulses reaching the motor end plate, or by a combination of these.

Slow-twitch motor units tend to be found in certain muscles, for example, the soleus muscle. This has led to the use of the term *slow muscle*. Other muscles containing predominantly fast-twitch motor units are designated *fast muscles*. The segregation of more motor units of a particular speed into certain muscles is of functional significance. It is generally agreed that slow limb muscles, such as the soleus muscle, subserve a predominantly postural role, whereas the fast limb muscles are concerned more with phasic, voluntary movements. However, fast- and slow-twitch motor units are intermingled in most muscles.

The biochemical and physiologic properties of the muscle fibers of a motor unit depend on the type of alpha motor neuron that innervates them. In general, smaller alpha motor neurons innervate slow muscle fibers that are able to generate small but sustained tension, are resistant to fatigue, and are rich in oxidative enzymes. Larger alpha motor neurons innervate fast muscle fibers that generate large but short-lasting tension, fatigue rapidly, and are rich in glycolytic enzymes (see Chapter 13).

The mechanisms by which an alpha motor neuron determines the twitch time and other properties of the muscle fibers it innervates are not completely known but include trophic influences and the pattern of impulses reaching the motor end plate.

The trophic interactions between the motor axon and the muscle fibers are reciprocal. After injury of a motor axon, the denervated muscle fibers produce signals that attract collaterals of the surviving axons. This process, referred to as *collateral sprouting*, incorporates the denervated muscle fibers into the motor unit of the neuron supplying the axon collaterals. Thus, although the number of motor units decreases because of the loss of motor axons, the size of the surviving motor units increases, and this helps maintain strength.

Increasing force of muscle contraction is attained by two mechanisms, increasing rates of firing of individual motor units (temporal summation) and recruitment of other motor units (spatial summation). In the normal activation of lower motor neurons, the neurons discharge repetitively at rates of 5 to 20 per second. At these rates, the twitch of slow muscles is not completed before the next action potential arrives, so that smooth movements or steady contractions can be obtained from repetitive action potentials.

During muscle contractions of increasing force, alpha motor neurons are recruited according to the *size principle*: small, slow twitch units are recruited earlier and large, fast twitch units are recruited later.

Control of Lower Motor Neuron Activity

The activity of an alpha motor neuron, and thus the motor unit, depends on the integration of many different excitatory and inhibitory synaptic inputs that act on cell body and dendrites of the neuron. These inputs originate *segmentally* and *suprasegmentally*.

Segmental inputs include afferents from muscle and other receptors and generate various local reflexes. Suprasegmental inputs arise from the motor cortex (direct activation pathway) and brainstem (indirect activation pathways). With few exceptions, most segmental and suprasegmental inputs affect motor neurons indirectly through excitatory and inhibitory interneurons (Fig. 3).

Segmental Reflexes

The segmental control of the final common pathway is through reflexes triggered by primary afferents from peripheral receptors.

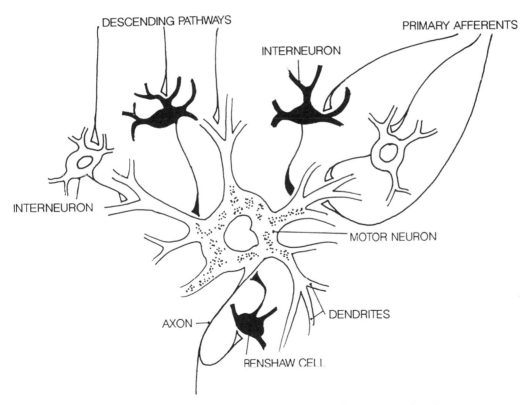

FIG. 3. Influences on motor neurons. Alpha motor neurons receive segmental and suprasegmental input. The segmental input arises from primary afferents of muscle and skin receptors that initiate segmental reflexes. Suprasegmental input arises from descending pathways from the motor cortex (direct activation pathway) and brainstem (indirect activation pathway). With few exceptions, segmental and suprasegmental inputs affect motor neurons through local neurons. The principal neurotransmitter of the primary afferents and descending pathways is glutamate, an excitatory neurotransmitter. Excitation of motor neurons may be direct or via excitatory *(light)* interneurons. Inhibition occurs via inhibitory *(dark)* interneurons.

These afferents include large and small myelinated fibers from muscle and skin receptors. The cell bodies of these afferents are in dorsal root ganglia. Striated muscles are rich in sensory receptors, including *muscle spindles*, *Golgi tendon organs*, and bare endings. In general, segmental afferent inputs are integrated with suprasegmental influences by interneurons that in turn control the excitability of the alpha motor neurons. The exception is the monosynaptic stretch reflex discussed below. All these afferents also contribute to the ascending sensory pathways.

Segmental reflexes involving the final common pathway include the *stretch*, or *muscle spindle reflex*, the *Golgi tendon organ reflex*, and the *flexion reflex*. Of these, the stretch reflex is the most important clinically because it is the basis for neurologic testing of tendon reflexes.

The Stretch Reflex

The classic stretch reflex is a simple two-neuron reflex elicited by stimulation of a muscle spindle and producing activation of the motor unit (Fig. 4).

The stretch reflex provides a mechanism for controlling motor neuron activity in response to a change in length of the muscle. The receptors for a stretch reflex are the *muscle spindles*. Lengthening of a muscle activates its muscle spindles, and their afferents directly activate the motor neuron that innervates the muscle. Motor neuron activity elicits contraction and thus shortening of the muscle, as follows:

Increased muscle length
↓
Activation of muscle spindle
↓
Activation of alpha motor neuron
↓
Muscle contraction
↓
Decreased muscle length

The *muscle spindle* is a group of specialized muscle fibers with two types of sensory receptors, the *primary* and *secondary endings*, which measure the length and velocity of stretch in a muscle. The muscle spindle fibers are referred to as intrafusal fibers (inside the muscle spindle) in contrast to the ex-

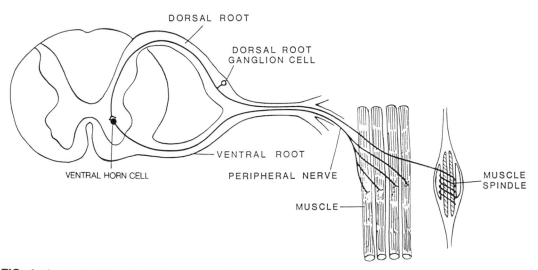

FIG. 4. Anatomical basis of the stretch reflex. This reflex is a two-neuron reflex mediated by stretch receptors in the muscle spindle, sensory axons with their cell bodies in the dorsal root ganglion, a synapse in the spinal cord, and an anterior horn cell innervating the striated muscle.

trafusal fibers, which make up the bulk of the muscle.

The muscle spindles are arranged in parallel with the extrafusal muscle fibers. Each spindle is surrounded by a connective tissue capsule that connects the spindle to the origin and insertion of the muscle. Within the connective tissue capsule are two types of intrafusal muscle fibers, the large-diameter, longer *nuclear bag* fibers and the smaller *nuclear chain* fibers. The former have a number of nuclei close together in the middle, whereas in the latter the nuclei are distributed evenly throughout the length of the intrafusal fiber (Fig. 5).

The *primary sensory ending,* or *annulospiral ending,* of the muscle spindle forms a spiral around both the nuclear bag fibers and the nuclear chain fibers. This sensory ending gives rise to a large-diameter fast-conducting afferent nerve fiber (type Ia), which ends monosynaptically in the spinal cord on the motor neurons of the muscle of origin and synergistic muscles. Collateral branches from the primary afferent fibers ascend in the dorsal columns to other levels and also connect via interneurons to the motor neurons of antagonistic muscles. The spindle *secondary sensory endings,* or *flower-spray endings,* are almost exclusively on nuclear chain fibers. They give rise to smaller diameter and therefore slower conducting (type II) afferent axons, which connect with motor neurons only via interneurons.

Both primary and secondary sensory endings are sensitive to stretch in the intrafusal fibers. They may be activated by stretch of the skeletal muscle containing the spindle or by contraction of the intrafusal muscle fibers in the spindle. Because of differences in viscos-

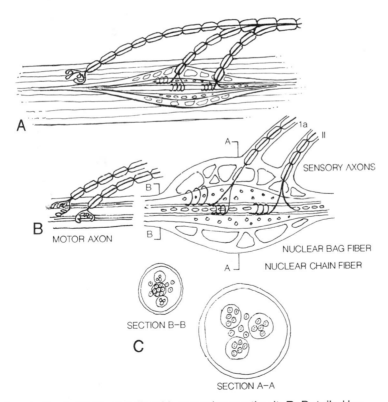

FIG. 5. Muscle spindle. **A:** Entire spindle with axons innervating it. **B:** Detailed longitudinal view of a muscle spindle at its center and at one end. **C:** Cross-sectional view of a muscle spindle at the middle *(A-A)* and the end *(B-B)*.

ity, the two types of intrafusal fibers differ in their response to stretch, and their discharges are divided into dynamic (phasic) and static (tonic) phases. The dynamic phase occurs during the period of stretching, and the static phase occurs while the sensory endings are held stretched (Fig. 6).

The prototypic stretch reflex is initiated by stimulation of Ia muscle spindle afferents. Rapid lengthening of the spindle increases the discharge of the Ia afferents, which monosynaptically stimulate the alpha motor neurons that innervate the agonist and synergistic muscles. Collaterals of Ia afferents also synapse on inhibitory interneurons (referred to as *Ia inhibitory interneurons*) that inhibit the alpha motor neurons that innervate the antagonistic muscles (Fig. 7). The neurotransmitter of these inhibitory interneurons is GABA.

Thus, sudden activation of the spindles in a muscle results in a brisk muscle contraction. The response of the primary endings in the muscle spindle to a quick stretch is the basis of stretch reflexes, called *myotatic reflexes*, in which the physician taps a tendon with a reflex hammer and produces a stretch of the muscle. The resulting discharge of a large number of type Ia afferents is sufficient to activate the anterior horn cells on which these afferents end and to cause a muscle twitch. Therefore, loss of either the afferent fibers or the lower motor neuron results in a loss of myotatic reflexes.

The central connections of the type II axons from the secondary spindle endings are more complex than those of the primary endings. Like the type Ia endings, they have excitatory connections with synergistic muscles and have inhibitory connections with antagonistic muscles so that they may participate in the myotatic reflexes. However, they also have more widespread, polysynaptic connections that have a longer duration of action, which may be part of flexion reflexes in which a limb is withdrawn from noxious stimuli.

The excitability of the myotatic reflex arc is controlled by several types of inhibitory interneurons. For example, on the afferent side of the reflex, release of the excitatory neurotransmitter (glutamate) from the Ia afferent is inhibited by a *presynaptic inhibitory neuron* that has GABA as a neurotransmitter. Lack of presynaptic inhibition of Ia afferents may lead to exaggeration of the myotatic reflexes, called *hyperreflexia*.

For a muscle spindle to respond appropriately to a stretch or change in muscle length, the spindle length must be adjusted as the length of the muscle changes. This is accomplished through a separate motor innervation of the spindle fibers. The motor innervation of the intrafusal muscle fibers is known as the *fusimotor system* (and comes from gamma motor neurons) (Fig. 8). Different classes of gamma motor neurons can preferentially increase either the phasic (changing) discharge

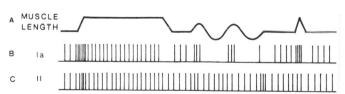

FIG. 6. Responses of afferent fibers from a muscle spindle. **A:** Length of muscle containing muscle spindle. Muscle length is changed with various waveforms of stretch. **B:** Response of type Ia afferent fibers from a primary ending of the muscle spindle. **C:** Response of type II afferent fibers from a secondary ending of the muscle spindle. Type Ia afferents respond to rapid stretch; type II afferents respond to length.

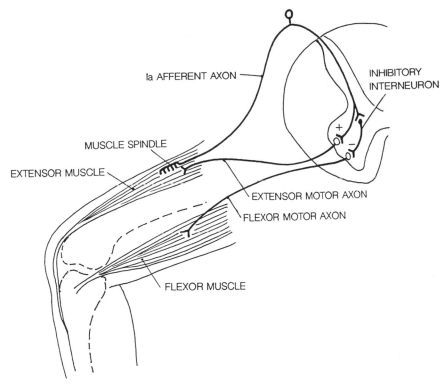

FIG. 7. Central connections of a type Ia afferent fiber from a muscle spindle. Spindle activity activates the muscle in which the spindle is located and inhibits the antagonist.

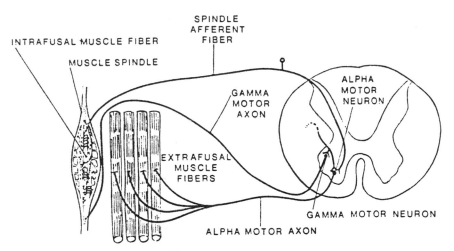

FIG. 8. Gamma motor system. Contraction of intrafusal fibers by gamma motor neurons can maintain a muscle spindle at the proper length to respond to muscle stretch even though the muscle changes length.

from the muscle spindle or the tonic (maintained) discharge. The independent motor control of the spindle's phasic and tonic discharges is of considerable importance in maintaining stability of the stretch reflex during movements.

During muscle contraction, the type Ia fiber discharge would be completely suppressed by unloading if the gamma motor neuron were not simultaneously active. Therefore, gamma motor neurons are coactivated with the alpha motor neurons to a muscle in order to maintain the spindle receptor sensitivity to unexpected movements (Fig. 9).

Muscle spindles are not distributed equally throughout the muscles. More are present in slow muscles, such as the soleus, than in fast muscles, such as the gastrocnemius. Within the spinal cord, there is a concentration of monosynaptic spindle afferents on the synergistic slow motor neurons. Thus, the spindle mechanism is of greater importance in control of the tonic activity of slow muscles.

The Golgi Tendon Reflex

Another important sensory structure in the muscle is the *Golgi tendon organ*. The Golgi tendon organ increases its discharge rate in response to increased tension; it is exquisitely sensitive to tension generated by muscle contraction (Fig. 10). The Golgi tendon organ is innervated by Ib afferents and provides a tension feedback mechanism. Increased tension due to active muscle contraction or to passive muscle stretch activates Ib afferents. Inputs carried by Ib afferents lead to disynaptic inhibition of the alpha motor neurons that innervate the muscle, resulting in muscle relaxation. This is mediated by Ib inhibitory interneurons. Together, the muscle spindles (the length servo) and the Golgi tendon organ (the tension servo) provide the nervous system with the information necessary to control muscle stiffness (Figs. 11 and 12).

The Flexion Reflexes

The flexion reflexes are polysynaptic reflexes that involve several spinal cord segments and mediate withdrawal responses to nociceptive (painful) stimuli. *Flexion reflex afferents* include type II axons from secondary spindle endings, small-diameter muscle afferents, and skin and joint afferents. In general, flexion reflex afferents produce activation of ipsilateral flexor motor neurons and inhibition of extensor motor neurons via polysynaptic connections. Opposite effects occur in the contralateral muscles through interneurons mediating *reciprocal inhibition*. The flexion reflex is under powerful inhibitory control by interneurons and descending supraspinal pathways.

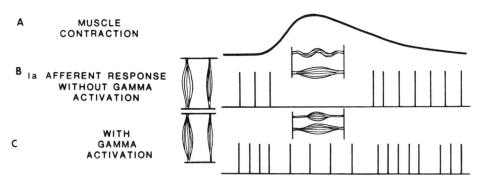

FIG. 9. Effect of gamma motor neuron activation. **A:** Length of muscle (muscle contraction) as it actively contracts. **B:** Action potential discharges in type Ia afferent fibers during muscle contraction without gamma motor neuron activation. **C:** Type Ia afferent firing during muscle contraction with gamma motor neuron activation.

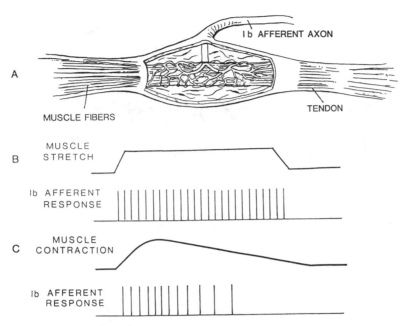

FIG. 10. Golgi tendon organ. **A:** Diagram of a Golgi tendon organ. **B:** Action potentials in afferents from a Golgi tendon organ are shown as the muscle is passively stretched. **C:** Afferent activity with active muscle contraction.

Local Circuit Neurons

Activity of motor neurons in response to reflex and descending inputs is regulated through local circuit neurons, including interneurons and propriospinal neurons. These neurons may be excitatory (with glutamate as the neurotransmitter) or inhibitory (with GABA or glycine as the neurotransmitter). Interneurons are interposed between the afferent and the efferent components of the reflex pathway and include the Ia and Ib inhibitory interneurons described above in relation to muscle spindle and Golgi tendon organ activity. Presynaptic inhibitory neurons inhibit neurotransmitter release from primary afferents via a GABAergic axoaxonic synapse.

Renshaw cells are excited by collaterals of motor axons and inhibit alpha motor neurons, a mechanism referred to as *recurrent inhibition*. The function of the Renshaw loop is to stabilize the discharge frequency of motor neuron pools and generally to prevent the neurons from discharging at excessive rates.

The Renshaw loops originate mainly from the motor neurons innervating fast-twitch motor units, but they act primarily on the smaller alpha motor neurons that innervate slow-twitch skeletal muscle fibers. The primary function of slow motor units is to subserve static postural functions, and the primary function of the fast motor units is to produce phasic movements. Thus, the asymmetric Renshaw inhibitory distribution also acts to subdue the postural stretch reflexes in slow muscle during the activity of phasic motor neurons.

Integration in the Final Common Pathway

We have just discussed some of the input that impinges on a motor neuron: afferent activity from the muscle spindles, the Golgi tendon organs, and the Renshaw cells. In addition to sensory input, the ventral horn cells receive input from three other major sources: the direct activation pathway, the indirect activation pathways, and other segments of the spinal cord. Each of these sources may transmit exci-

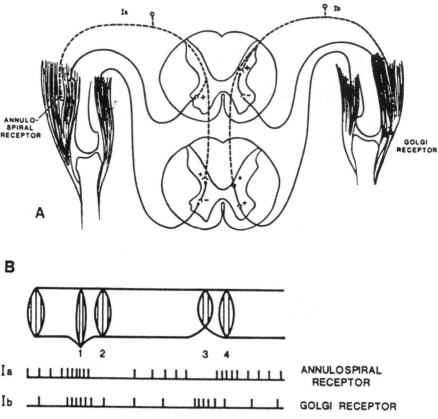

FIG. 11. Muscle spindle and Golgi tendon organ. **A:** Central connections of types Ia and Ib afferents. On the left, the type Ia connections produce excitation (+) of synergistic muscles (myotatic reflex) and inhibition (–) of antagonistic muscles through inhibitory interneurons. On the right, the type Ib connections produce inhibition of synergistic muscles through an inhibitory interneuron (–). **B:** Effects of passive muscle stretch *(1)* and active muscle contraction *(3)* on action potential firing in type Ia axons from muscle spindle and type Ib axons from tendon organ (*2* and *4* indicate resting muscle state).

tatory or inhibitory impulses to the final common pathway, and all this input is integrated by the ventral horn cells before they respond. Table 1 summarizes the major spinal reflexes.

Muscle Tone

A common clinical test is to gauge the resistance of a muscle to passive movement. Normally, when the examiner moves a limb and a muscle is stretched, there is mild resistance to the passive movement, referred to as *muscle tone*. Muscle tone depends on the intrinsic elasticity of the tissue and activation of motor units based on the state of excitability of their corresponding motor neurons. One component of muscle tone arises from activation of motor units by stretching the muscle spindles. Other components include the Golgi tendon afferents, flexor reflex afferents, long loop reflexes, and descending pathways. Muscle tone, like segmental reflexes, is determined by the central state of excitability of the motor unit. An increase in the excitability of the alpha or gamma motor neurons due to increased central excitation or to lack of segmental inhibition re-

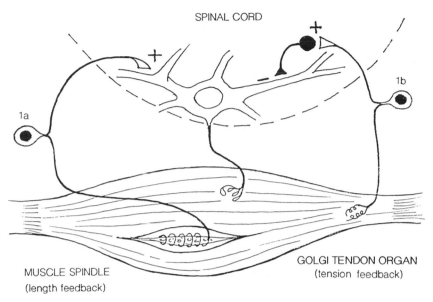

SPINAL CORD

1a

1b

MUSCLE SPINDLE
(length feedback)

GOLGI TENDON ORGAN
(tension feedback)

FIG. 12. Control of muscle stiffness by interaction of the length feedback (muscle spindle) producing Ia afferent-mediated monosynaptic excitation and a tension feedback (Golgi tendon organ) producing a Ib afferent-mediated disynaptic inhibition of the alpha motor neuron innervating the muscle.

sults in increased muscle tone, called hypertonia. A decrease in either the afferent input from the muscle spindles or the efferent activity of the lower motor neurons results in a reduction of muscle tone, called hypotonia.

Pattern Generation in the Spinal Cord

Propriospinal neurons, unlike interneurons, project to other segments of the spinal cord and thus participate in intersegmental coordination of motor output. Motor neurons, interneurons, and propriospinal neurons form a neuronal network in the spinal cord. The term *neuronal network* refers to groups of neurons that are anatomically interconnected by synapses. Networks that produce specific patterns of movement are referred to as *central pattern generators*. Spinal pattern generators initiate rhythmic patterns of activity involved

TABLE 1. *Spinal cord reflexes*

	Reflex type		
	Stretch	Golgi tendon	Flexor
Receptor	Muscle spindle	Golgi tendon organ	Touch, pressure, and pain receptors
Stimulus	Change in muscle length	Tension generated by active contraction	Various (noxious, tactile)
Afferent	Ia	Ib	II,III,IV
Interneuron	Ia inhibitory	Ib inhibitory	Interneuronal pool
Effects			
On agonist	Mono- (and poly-) synaptic excitation	Disynaptic inhibition	Excitation of ipsilateral flexors
On antagonist	Disynaptic inhibition	Di/trisynaptic excitation	Inhibition of ipsilateral extensors
Result	Muscle contraction	Muscle relaxation	Withdrawal

in alternative activation of flexor and extensor muscles involved in automatic activities, including *locomotion*. A pattern generator has a self-maintained oscillatory activity that depends on the intrinsic properties of its neurons and their reciprocal synaptic interactions via interneurons. However, the function of the pattern generator is modulated by supraspinal influences and segmental afferents.

Effects of Damage to the Final Common Pathway

Diseases may affect the final common pathway at the level of the ventral horn cell, the axon, or the muscle fiber. However, damage to any of these sites has common clinical features that permit the clinician to identify disease of the motor unit. These include weakness, atrophy, loss of reflexes, and loss of tone. Other features that may indicate abnormal function of the motor unit include fasciculations, cramps, and excessive contraction.

In the weakness or paralysis due to final common pathway disease, there is a loss of voluntary contraction, a loss of involuntary movements, and a loss of reflex contraction of the muscle. The weakness occurs either because the action potentials cannot be transmitted to the muscle owing to disease of the lower motor neuron or because diseased muscle fibers cannot respond to the action potentials of the lower motor neurons.

The strength of a muscle is generally proportional to its size: an elderly lady has less strength than a young weight lifter, although both have normal muscle function. A physician must evaluate strength in proportion to size. The loss of muscle bulk in disease is referred to as *atrophy* and is often found with weakness due to disease of the final common pathway. Two types of atrophy must be differentiated. The first, *neurogenic atrophy*, occurs with loss of innervation, when a muscle undergoes atrophy and is weak (out of proportion to its size). The second, *disuse atrophy*, occurs with lack of use of the muscle. In disuse atrophy, strength is appropriate to the size of the muscle. Disuse atrophy is not a sign of

disease of the neuromuscular system, whereas neurogenic atrophy is. Atrophy may also occur in muscle disease.

In general, if the lower motor neurons are lost, reflexes—particularly the stretch reflexes—are also lost. They are most consistently lost if the disease process damages the afferent fibers of the reflex arc. Disruption of the reflex arc also results in the loss of normal tone or response to passive movement. This state is called *flaccidity*, and the weakness with disease of the final common pathway is *flaccid paralysis*.

Weakness, flaccidity, and atrophy also occur in the face, tongue, and pharyngeal muscles with disease of the lower motor neurons in the brainstem. This results in a characteristic breathy, imprecise, nasal speech called *flaccid dysarthria* (*dysarthria* means abnormal utterances).

Diseases of the motor unit also may be associated with excessive activity or spontaneous firing with a low threshold for discharge. This may take the form of a single spontaneous discharge of a motor unit, a *fasciculation*. A fasciculation can be seen on the surface of the skin as a brief localized twitch. A continuous high-frequency discharge of fascicles of muscle fibers is a *cramp*. Fasciculations and cramps may be manifestations of disease or may be due simply to physiologic irritability, as can occur after excessive exertion. After destruction of the lower motor neuron, the muscle fibers that have lost their innervation generate slow repetitive action potentials and contract regularly, a process called *fibrillation*. Fibrillations are not visible through the skin.

Direct Activation Pathway: The Corticospinal Tract

Anatomy

The direct activation pathway is the route by which the motor areas of the cerebral cortex in each hemisphere control motor neurons in the ventral horn on the opposite side of the spinal cord and in the motor nuclei of the brainstem. The fibers in the direct activation pathway are corticospinal and corticobulbar. Those traveling to the spinal cord are called the *corticospinal*, or *pyramidal, tract*. Those ending on brainstem nuclei are *corticobulbar fibers*. The neurons from which these tracts arise are known as *upper motor neurons* (Fig. 13). The major function of the direct activation pathway is to initiate and control skilled voluntary activity.

Each corticospinal tract arises primarily from cells in the cortex of the frontal lobe of

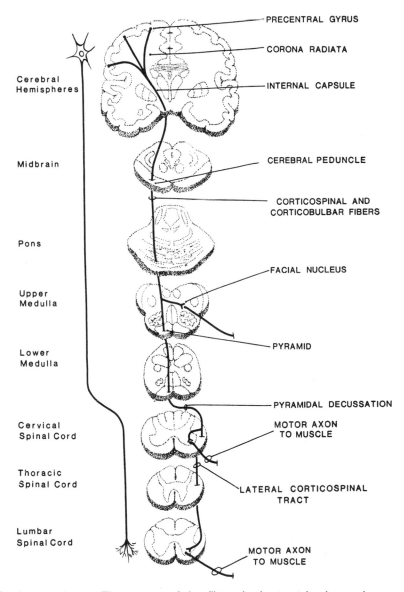

FIG. 13. Corticospinal tract. The course of the fibers in the tract is shown descending through the cerebral hemispheres, brainstem, and spinal cord. Some of the axons in the tract extend the entire length of the spinal cord as shown schematically for a single neuron on the *left*.

one hemisphere and descends through the corona radiata into the internal capsule. The tract passes from the internal capsule via the cerebral peduncles to the base of the brainstem, where it forms the medullary pyramids. At the junction between the medulla and spinal cord, most of the fibers in each pyramid cross the midline (the corticospinal decussation) to lie in the lateral funiculus of the opposite half of the spinal cord. These crossed fibers form the *lateral corticospinal tract* of the cord.

The term *corticospinal tract* is based on its origin and termination. The *pyramidal tract* is so named because of its association with the *medullary pyramids*, the large paired fiber tracts on the ventral surface of the medulla. Properly speaking, only the corticospinal fibers, in contradistinction to corticobulbar fibers, pass through the pyramids, but it is common to include in the pyramidal tract the upper motor neurons to the spinal cord (corticospinal) and similar (so-called supranuclear) fibers to the brainstem motor nuclei (corticobulbar).

Motor Cortex

The corticospinal tract is formed by axons of neurons located in several areas of the cerebral cortex. These include the *primary motor cortex (area 4)* and several nonprimary cortical motor areas, namely the *lateral premotor cortex (area 6a)*, the *supplementary motor area* (or *medial premotor cortex, area 6b*), and the *anterior cingulate motor area* (on the medial surface of the hemisphere) (Fig. 14). All these areas are closely interconnected and project to the ventral horn. In addition, the corticospinal tract contains axons of neurons in the primary sensory cortex (areas 3, 1, 2) and posterior parietal cortex (area 5); these axons project mainly to the dorsal horn for control of sensory processing. Each corticospinal tract contains more than one million fibers. Only 3% to 4% of all the fibers originate from *giant pyramidal cells of Betz* in the primary motor cortex.

The primary motor cortex occupies the anterior lip of the central sulcus of Rolando and the adjacent precentral gyrus (area 4) (Fig.

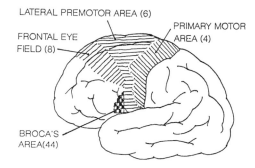

A

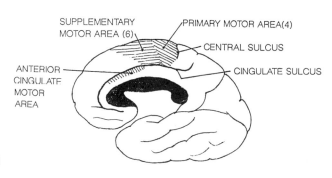

B

FIG. 14. Motor areas of the cerebral cortex. **A:** Lateral view of the cerebral hemisphere showing the primary motor area (area 4), lateral premotor area (lateral area 6), frontal eye fields (area 8), and Broca's area (area 44). **B:** Medial view of the cerebral hemisphere showing the supplementary motor area (medial area 6) and the anterior cingulate motor area. The numerals in parentheses refer to Brodmann's areas.

14). The primary motor cortex integrates input from multiple sources and has a somatotopic organization, with the contralateral body represented upside down just as in the sensory cortex (see Chapter 7, Fig. 3): the head area is located above the fissure of Sylvius, the upper extremity next (with the thumb and index finger in proximity to the face), the trunk interposed between the shoulder and hip areas high on the convexity, and the lower limb representation extending onto the paracentral lobule in the longitudinal fissure. The size of the cortical representation varies with the functional importance of the part represented. Thus, the lips, jaw, thumb, and index finger each have a large representation; the forehead, trunk, and proximal portions of the limbs have a small one. As in other areas of the central nervous system, there are more neurons in the areas subserving delicate and complex functions.

Three important features regarding the somatotopic organization of the primary motor cortex are (1) the convergence of inputs from wide territories of the primary motor cortex to individual motor units, (2) the divergence of output from a single cortical neuron to alpha motor neurons innervating different muscles, and (3) the *plasticity* of cortical representation—the area representing a given muscle can be modified in response to injury or acquisition of specific motor skills.

The cortical areas in the frontal lobe anterior to the precentral gyrus are involved in the programming and planning of motor acts. These acts may be initiated automatically in response to visual or other sensory clues or they may be a component of an emotional response. The *lateral premotor area* is implicated in motor programming of visually guided movements of the limbs. The medial premotor area corresponds to the *supplementary motor area* and is immediately anterior to the foot and leg representations in the primary motor cortex. The supplementary motor cortex is important in the planning of voluntary movements. The *anterior cingulate motor area*, located in the superior margin of the anterior cingulate sulcus, is involved in motor responses initiated by emotional and motivational cues (Fig. 14B). The primary motor, premotor, supplementary motor, and anterior cingulate motor cortices all contribute axons to the corticospinal tract. Immediately rostral to the lateral premotor area is the *frontal eye fields (area 8)*, which contain neurons involved in the generation of spontaneous and visually guided rapid eye movements. This cortical area does not contribute to the corticospinal tract. Broca's area is immediately ventral to the lateral premotor area, in the frontal operculum of the *left* cerebral hemisphere near where the face is represented. Neurons in Broca's area participate in the motor programming necessary for speech.

Internal Capsule

Axons from the motor cortex converge in the corona radiata toward the internal capsule, where they are compactly gathered. Here, too, there is a topographic localization. The corticobulbar fibers occupy a more anterior location in the posterior limb of the internal capsule than the corticospinal fibers. Thus, the projection fibers are located from anterior to posterior in the following order: face, arm, leg, bladder, and rectum. Anterior to the pyramidal tract fibers are frontopontine fibers and fibers reciprocally connecting the frontal lobe and the thalamus; posterior to the pyramidal fibers are the ascending sensory tracts from the thalamus to the parietal lobe (Fig. 15).

Brainstem

The pyramidal fibers remain grouped together as they pass from the internal capsule to the cerebral peduncle in the midbrain. In the midbrain, the corticospinal and corticobulbar fibers occupy the middle two-thirds of the cerebral peduncle, with the corticobulbar fibers being more medial. During their course in the brainstem, the corticobulbar fibers leave the pyramidal pathway at several levels, some crossing the midline and some remaining uncrossed. These fibers synapse in the motor centers and nuclei of the cranial nerves—trigeminal, facial, vagus, spinal accessory, and hypoglossal.

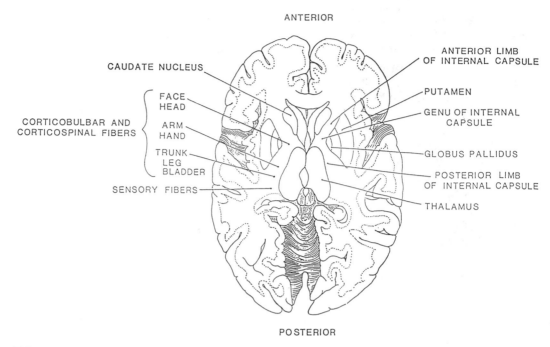

FIG. 15. Horizontal section through the cerebral hemispheres showing the somatotopic representations of motor function in the internal capsule.

In the pons, the pyramidal fibers are split into small bundles by the interspersed pontine nuclei. The topographic localization persists, with the face medially, the leg laterally, and the upper limb in the intermediate position. The fibers reunite in the medulla to form the medullary pyramids. At the lower border of the medulla, the main pyramidal decussation occurs, and about 80% of the fibers cross to the opposite side of the spinal cord.

Spinal Cord

In the spinal cord, the crossed pyramidal fibers occupy the lateral column (the *lateral corticospinal tract*) (Fig. 16), and the much smaller number of uncrossed pyramidal fibers descend in the ventral column (the *ventral corticospinal tract*) to the cervical and thoracic levels. There is doubt whether the ventral corticospinal fibers ultimately cross or remain uncrossed; it is likely that some of them remain uncrossed and are responsible for the ipsilateral innervation of certain muscle groups.

Crossed Innervation

Because of the decussation of most of the fibers of the pyramidal tracts, the voluntary

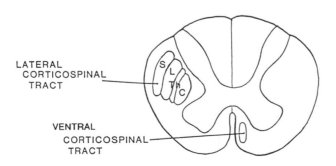

FIG. 16. Somatotopic representation of motor function in the lateral corticospinal tract. (*C,* cervical; *Th,* thoracic; *L,* lumbar; *S,* sacral.)

movements of one side of the body are under the control of the opposite cerebral hemisphere. However, there are some exceptions to this rule that are of importance in clinical diagnosis. In general, muscle groups of the two sides of the body that habitually act in unison tend to have a bilateral cortical innervation, whereas muscle groups that act alone in isolated, delicate, and especially in learned movements tend to have a unilateral innervation from the opposite hemisphere. Thus, paraspinal muscles are innervated by both hemispheres, as are the muscles in the upper half of the face (Fig. 17). Because of this arrangement, a massive lesion of one hemisphere causes severe weakness of the opposite side of the body but not of upper facial or paraspinal muscles. These principles do not apply in all cases. Even in muscles such as those of the tongue and the palate, which

might be expected to work in unison, there is a greater innervation from the contralateral hemisphere.

Physiology

The corticospinal tract is needed for skilled movements of the fingers and feet and recruitment of motor neurons during increasing force.

Cortical Motor Control

Unlike the primary sensory cortex, the motor cortex is the site of convergence from a large number of cortical and subcortical areas. The discharge pattern of motor cortical neurons results from this convergence. Movement generation and control involve populations of cortical neurons, and a given cell participates in movements in many directions.

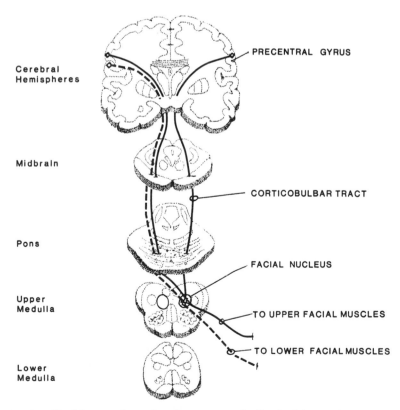

FIG. 17. Crossed cortical innervation of motor neurons to the facial muscles on one side. The upper facial muscles have bilateral control; lower facial muscles have unilateral control from the contralateral hemisphere.

Except for the direct corticomotoneuronal termination in motor nuclei innervating distal muscles of the limbs, most neural signals from the motor cortex activate motor neurons indirectly through influences on interneurons of the spinal cord. This results in a converging and diverging pattern of influences on motor neuron pools via interneurons. Axons that send collaterals to several motor neuron pools mediate activity of functionally related muscle groups, and this allows the direct motor pathway to control the limb as a whole.

The primary motor, premotor, and supplementary motor areas are interconnected and project axons through the corticospinal tract. These regions are activated during natural movements and are involved in the generation of motor commands. They all provide collaterals to motor nuclei of the brainstem—but not to the oculomotor (cranial nerve [CN] III), trochlear (CN IV), and abducens (CN VI) nuclei—and send axons to the basal ganglia and cerebellar control circuits.

An important feature of motor cortex is its functional flexibility. Plasticity of the motor cortex has been demonstrated following cortical lesions, motor training, and disconnection between the primary motor cortex and its peripheral targets. For example, after the arm area of the primary motor cortex has been ablated, neurons in the face area are activated during finger movements. In patients who have recovered from lesions that involved the motor cortex or internal capsule, the activity in the premotor and supplementary motor areas is increased in comparison with that in normal control subjects during performance of motor tasks.

Effect on the Final Common Pathway

The neurotransmitter of the corticospinal and corticobulbar pathways is glutamate. Thus, direct cortical inputs produce depolarization of motor neurons, and this allows both an increase in the frequency of firing and the recruitment of additional motor units. Therefore, the corticospinal system is important in increasing the force of muscle contraction.

Motor neurons that receive direct input from motor cortex (direct corticomotor neuronal connections) innervate the small intrinsic muscles of the hand and are involved in finger movement. The effects on agonist and antagonist motor neuron groups depend on the pattern of movement. For example, during the precision grip, many arm and forearm muscles are activated simultaneously for precise control of their force.

Effects of Lesions of the Direct Activation Pathway

Knowledge of the clinical manifestations of disease of the direct activation pathway comes equally from experimental studies and from observation of clinical disorders.

Disturbances of the corticospinal system may be irritative (positive) or paralytic (negative). These two types of disturbance are exemplified clinically by seizures and paralysis and experimentally exemplified by the results of stimulation and ablation. John Hughlings Jackson, from his study of the attacks that now bear his name (jacksonian seizures), surmised that there must be somatotopic representation of motor function in the brain. Focal motor seizures are likely to start in the cortical areas governing the thumb and index finger, the corner of the mouth, or the great toe, because of the relatively large extent of those areas. The spread (march) of the attack is determined by the pattern of cortical localization. Thus, a seizure starting in the thumb and index finger may spread to involve the wrist, elbow, shoulder, trunk, and lower limb, spreading from hip to foot. Seizures arising from premotor cortex or supplementary motor cortex can cause complex motor actions, such as raising the contralateral hand and turning the head and eyes toward the hand.

Although the terminations of the corticospinal pathways act on all the cells of the ventral horn, they seem to have their major influence on the motor neurons in the lateral portions of the ventral horns, that is, on those controlling the distal movements of the extremities. Therefore, lesions limited to the corticospinal pathways result in a characteristic clinical pattern. There is weakness or paralysis of muscles, especially the distal muscles of the extremities. The impairment is greatest for fine movements, skilled movements, and movements under voluntary control. The paralysis is not associated with atrophy, and reflexes may be preserved, although they are often mildly decreased.

The corticospinal pathway provides background excitation to motor neurons. After interruption of the corticospinal input, alpha and gamma motor neurons become unresponsive to segmental stimuli for a period of time. Therefore, acute interruption of the corticospinal input produces not only immediate weakness but also decreased reflexes and muscle tone. With recovery of excitability, alpha motor neurons regain their ability to respond to afferent stimuli from the muscle. Reflexes may then become exaggerated because of the loss of inhibition through the concomitant involvement of the indirect activation pathways (see below).

The distribution of the weakness is a function of the site of the lesion. If the lesion is localized in a limited area of cortex, then a single limb or one side of the face only may be involved. If the lesion involves only the pyramidal tract fibers in the pyramids of the medulla, one side of the body below the level of the lesion is affected. The distribution also depends on whether innervation is unilateral or bilateral. For example, the upper part of the face is spared when corticobulbar lesions involve facial fibers. If the lesion involves the frontal eye fields, there is paralysis of conjugate eye movements to the opposite side.

In addition to the weakness, hypotonia, and reduction in reflexes, certain specific signs occur with lesions of the corticospinal pathway. The abdominal and cremasteric reflexes are segmental reflexes that depend on an intact pyramidal tract. With a corticospinal tract lesion, these reflexes are lost on one side. Some abnormal reflexes become manifest after a corticospinal tract lesion.

The plantar response to noxious stimulation of the sole of the foot is part of a reflex that in-

volves all muscles that shorten the leg. In the newborn, this response, referred to as the *triple flexion reflex*, is brisk and includes the toe extensors, which also shorten the leg on contraction and thus are flexors from the physiologic standpoint. As the corticospinal tract myelinates and gains control over alpha motor neurons, this response becomes less brisk, and in normal subjects after age 2 the toe extensors are no longer part of it. The toes curl down in response to noxious stimulation of the sole that elicits segmental reflex involving the small foot muscles under the skin, comparable to the abdominal or cremasteric reflexes. When the corticospinal tract is damaged, noxious stimulation of the sole of the foot elicits extension (dorsiflexion) of the great toe and spreading of the other toes. This is the *extensor plantar response*, or *Babinski's sign*. In a similar fashion, gentle stroking of the palm elicits an abnormal grasping response, the *grasp reflex*, when the motor cortex is damaged.

The occurrence of distal flaccid paralysis with Babinski's sign is unusual and occurs *only* with small lesions in the medullary pyramids or in the primary motor cortex. Such lesions selectively involving the direct corticospinal system in isolation are rarely seen clinically.

The corticospinal pathway provides numerous collaterals that innervate motor nuclei of the brainstem that give rise to the indirect pathways. The corticospinal and descending brainstem indirect pathways are intermingled at the level of the internal capsule, cerebral peduncles, basis pontis, and spinal cord. Thus, a lesion at any of these levels produces a combined effect that accounts for the typical clinical manifestations of the *upper motor neuron syndrome*. This includes not only distal weakness, loss of cutaneous reflexes, and Babinski's sign (all due to damage of the corticospinal pathway) but also increased muscle tone and reflexes due to interruption of cortical input to brainstem inhibitory areas or their projections to the spinal cord (see below).

Lesions involving the anterior portions of the frontal lobe may spare the primary motor cortex and produce no weakness. However, such lesions can result in impairment of the voluntary activation of the motor system. The loss of the ability to perform skilled motor acts by will when they can still be elicited automatically or reflexly is called *apraxia*. Apraxia may be considered the highest-level abnormality of motor function in which the initiation of complex movements is lost. Apraxia may involve any of the motor activities, including speech and movements of the arms, legs, or eyes. Apraxia of *speech* is characterized by an inability to say a word at will, although still being able to think of it and to utter it correctly automatically or reflexly. Motor apraxia of speech is sometimes referred to as a type of aphasia (loss of speech).

The localization of lesions along the pyramidal pathways is relatively straightforward. Widespread cortical lesions may involve all of one side of the body, but a facial, arm, or leg monoplegia is more likely with a lesion of the cerebral cortex. Occasionally, the arm and face are involved together because of their proximity (often with apraxia of speech if the lesion is in the dominant hemisphere). More anterior lesions of the frontal cortex may result in impaired voluntary eye movements or apraxia of motor activity. Lesions in the internal capsule or cerebral peduncles typically produce weakness of the opposite arm and leg and opposite side of the face.

Cortical lesions also may have positive manifestations such as focal seizures. However, seizures do not occur with a lesion of the direct activation pathway at lower levels, for example in the internal capsule or below, where the findings are those of a loss of function such as weakness.

The level of lesions along the pathway sometimes can be identified by the associated segmental involvement of other structures, such as one of the cranial nerves in the case of a brainstem lesion or one of the spinal nerves in the case of a spinal cord lesion.

Motor Neuron Disease

Some diseases seem to selectively affect the motor system. One of these is *amy-*

otrophic lateral sclerosis, or *motor neuron disease*. It is a progressive, degenerative disease of unknown cause. Pathologically, this condition is characterized by degeneration of the motor cells in the spinal cord, brainstem, and cerebral cortex, associated with secondary axonal degeneration in the peripheral nerves and in the lateral funiculus of the spinal cord (corticospinal tract).

Motor neuron disease expresses itself with varying degrees of involvement in the final common pathway and the direct and indirect activation pathways. Damage to the final common pathway results in diseased lower motor neurons, which are initially irritable, producing frequent, widespread fasciculations. After death and degeneration of the lower motor neurons, there is a combination of flaccid weakness and atrophy of muscle. The denervated muscle fibrillates, although this is not seen clinically. Involvement of the descending pathways may produce Babinski's sign and hyperactive reflexes as well.

Brainstem Motor Pathways

Anatomy

In addition to direct input to the ventral horn, motor cortex sends projections to several regions of the brainstem that contain neurons whose axons contribute to pathways that are in parallel with the corticospinal system and synapse on lower motor neurons and interneurons. These indirect pathways originate in the *red nucleus, superior colliculus, vestibular nuclei*, and *reticular formation*. All these areas also receive input from the cerebellum and are involved in the maintenance of equilibrium, posture, muscle tone, and coordination (Fig. 18).

The *red nucleus*, located in the midbrain, receives direct input from the motor cortex and cerebellum. Large neurons of the red nucleus give rise to axons that cross in the midbrain and form the *rubrospinal tract*. This

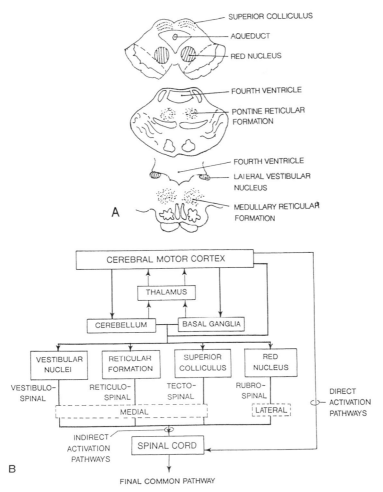

FIG. 18. A: Brainstem nuclei that project to the ventral horn and contribute to the indirect activation pathways. These nuclei (except the vestibular nucleus) receive input from motor areas of the cortex and the cerebellum. The red nucleus primarily controls flexor muscles of the contralateral upper limb. The superior colliculus controls neck muscles in coordination with eye movements. The lateral vestibular nucleus and nuclei in the paramedian pontine and medullary reticular formation control postural reflexes and balance between extensor and flexor tone in the limbs. **B:** Basic circuitry of the direct and indirect activation pathways.

crossed pathway descends in the lateral funiculus of the spinal cord. The importance of the rubrospinal tract in humans has not been determined. It reaches at least as far as the cervical spinal cord, where it innervates predominantly alpha motor neurons that innervate flexors of the upper limb (Fig. 19).

The *vestibular nuclei* are located at the level of the medulla and lower pons. They re-

ceive input from the vestibular organs in the inner ear (signaling changes in position and angular and linear acceleration of the head), spinal cord, and cerebellum. Connections to the spinal cord via the *vestibulospinal tracts* are critical for postural adjustments of the trunk, neck, and limbs. The lateral vestibular nucleus gives rise to the *lateral vestibulospinal tract*, which descends uncrossed in

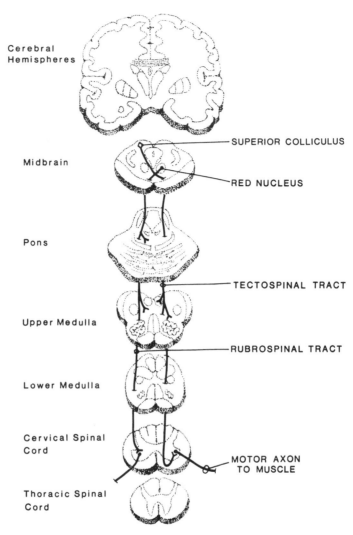

Cerebral
Hemispheres

Midbrain

SUPERIOR COLLICULUS

RED NUCLEUS

Pons

TECTOSPINAL TRACT

Upper Medulla

RUBROSPINAL TRACT

Lower Medulla

Cervical Spinal
Cord

MOTOR AXON
TO MUSCLE

Thoracic Spinal
Cord

FIG. 19. Rubrospinal and tectospinal pathways, though both bilateral, are shown unilaterally. The rubrospinal tract is shown descending on the left. It arises in the red nucleus on the opposite side. The tectospinal tract is shown descending on the right after arising in the colliculus on the left.

the ventral and ventrolateral funiculi to control extensor motor neurons at all levels of the spinal cord (Fig. 20).

The *reticular formation* consists of diffuse groups of neurons located throughout the brainstem. These neurons are intimately interconnected, receive input from most motor and sensory pathways, and are critical for sensorimotor integration. Reticular formation neurons in the midbrain and rostral pons give rise to ascending projections and are a major component of the consciousness system (Chapter 10). Reticular formation neurons in the lower pons and medulla project to the spinal cord via the *reticulospinal tracts*. These tracts descend bilaterally in the ventral and ventrolateral funiculi to all segments of the spinal cord (Fig. 21). Similar to the lateral vestibulospinal tract, the reticulospinal tracts innervate predominantly motor neurons controlling axial

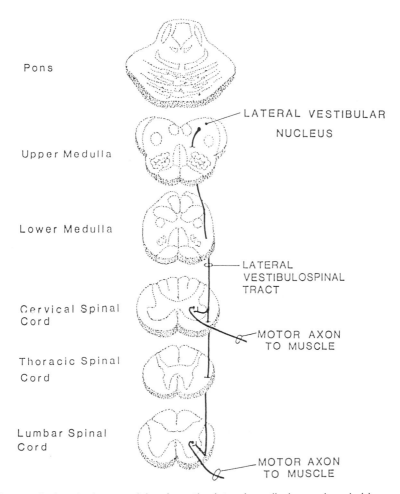

Pons

LATERAL VESTIBULAR
NUCLEUS

Upper Medulla

Lower Medulla

LATERAL
VESTIBULOSPINAL
TRACT

Cervical Spinal
Cord

MOTOR AXON
TO MUSCLE

Thoracic Spinal
Cord

Lumbar Spinal
Cord

MOTOR AXON
TO MUSCLE

FIG. 20. The vestibulospinal tract arising from the lateral vestibular nucleus is bilateral but is shown on only one side.

and proximal limb muscles. Many inputs from the reticulospinal pathways are relayed via spinal neurons that give rise to *propriospinal pathways*. The position of the vestibulospinal, reticulospinal, and propriospinal pathways in the ventral and ventrolateral quadrant vary at different levels of the spinal cord.

The *tectospinal tract* and the *medial vestibulospinal tract* are descending motor pathways that reach only the cervical cord level and participate in the control of neck muscles and the coordination of movements of the head and eyes in response to various stimuli. The tectospinal tract originates in the

superior colliculus, located in the tectum of the midbrain. The superior colliculus is a critical reflex center for oculomotor and head control in response to visual, auditory, and somatosensory stimuli. The medial vestibulospinal and tectospinal tracts constitute the descending component of the *medial longitudinal fasciculus*.

Physiology

The indirect activation pathways are subdivided into two main groups, medial and lateral, that reflect their course, termination in the spinal cord, and function.

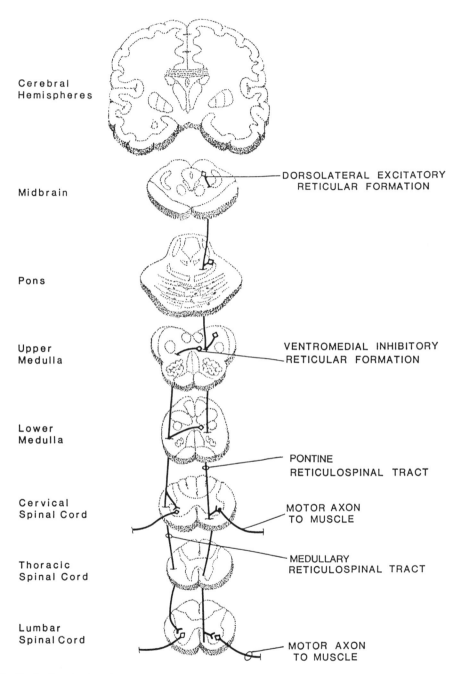

FIG. 21. Reticulospinal pathways. Both tracts are present bilaterally but are shown only on one side. The pontine reticulospinal tract arising from the excitatory dorsolateral reticular formation in the pons is shown on the *right*. The medullary reticulospinal tract arising from the inhibitory ventromedial reticular formation is shown on the *left*.

Medial Pathways

The *medial pathways* control posture, synergistic (particularly extensor) whole limb movements, and orienting movements of the head and body. They include the vestibulospinal, reticulospinal, and tectospinal pathways. All these pathways synapse either directly with motor neurons or, more commonly, with interneurons and propriospinal neurons. An important group of propriospinal neurons is located in the ventral horn of the upper cervical cord. The *propriospinal pathways* interconnect different levels of the spinal cord and are important for automatic patterns of movement involving all the limbs and trunk, as in locomotion.

The *reticulospinal tract* is functionally heterogeneous, reflecting its multiple origins in the reticular formation of the lower pons and medulla. Neurons of the medullary and pontine reticular formation receive input from the motor cortex, the *corticoreticular* pathway. Corticoreticular axons are distributed bilaterally, but they are predominantly crossed.

The *medullary* reticulospinal tract exerts a predominantly *inhibitory* effect on segmental reflexes, primarily via inhibitory interneurons. The corticoreticulospinal pathway is important in making the adjustments needed to execute cortically directed movements by inhibiting potentially interfering segmental reflexes. Cortical input activates the medullary reticulospinal pathway, which in turn, inhibits the myotatic and flexion reflexes via interneurons. Interruption of the corticoreticular or reticulospinal components of the indirect activation pathways impairs local inhibitory mechanisms and results in an exaggeration of segmental (and suprasegmental) reflexes.

The *pontine reticulospinal tract*, like the lateral vestibulospinal tract, facilitates extensor and inhibits flexor motor neurons.

The *lateral vestibulospinal tract* terminates predominantly on interneurons that activate motor neurons innervating extensor muscles in the trunk and ipsilateral limb. Activity in this tract is important for postural adjustments in response to gravity and to changes in the position and acceleration of the head. The lateral vestibulospinal tract is also important in mediating cerebellar control of posture. The ascending component of the medial longitudinal fasciculus coordinates activity of the vestibular and oculomotor nuclei.

Lateral Pathways

The *lateral pathways*, like the corticospinal tract, provide the capability for independent flexor movements, especially of the upper limb. These pathways are represented by the *rubrospinal tract*. This tract crosses in the midbrain and descends ventral to the corticospinal tract in the lateral funiculus of the spinal cord. Motor cortex innervates the red nucleus, and the corticorubrospinal system provides a mechanism parallel to the corticospinal pathway for control of the upper limb. In humans, the importance of the rubrospinal tract for normal motor control is undetermined.

Effects on the Final Common Pathway

The brainstem motor pathways contain L-glutamate and other neurotransmitters. They affect motor neuron activity primarily via interneurons and propriospinal neurons. Propriospinal neurons are located in the dorsal portion of the ventral horn and project to various segments via propriospinal fibers that course in close to the gray matter. Interneurons include the various inhibitory interneurons that have GABA or glycine as a neurotransmitter. These include the presynaptic axoaxonic interneurons, Ia and Ib interneurons, and Renshaw cells. The indirect pathways control the excitability of alpha and gamma motor neurons through this interneuronal pool.

The most important brainstem motor pathways are summarized in Table 2.

Effects of Lesions of the Brainstem Motor Pathways

Lesions that interrupt either the cortical input to brainstem motor nuclei or the projec-

TABLE 2. *Brainstem motor pathways*

Feature	Medial pathways	Lateral pathway
Origin	Vestibular nuclei Reticular formation Superior colliculus	Red nucleus
Projection	Ipsilateral or bilateral (tectospinal tract is contralateral)	Contralateral
Course	Ventromedial or ventrolateral spinal cord	Dorsolateral spinal cord
Target	Medial pool of motor neurons and interneurons that control axial and proximal muscles, predominantly extensors	Lateral pool of motor neurons and interneurons that control predominantly distal muscles, mainly flexors
Primary actions	Lateral vestibulospinal and pontine reticulospinal tracts—increase extensor tone Medullary reticulospinal tract—inhibit extensor and nociceptive reflexes Tectospinal and medial vestibulospinal tracts—coordinate movements of head and neck with those of the eyes	Facilitate flexors of the arms
Cerebellar control	Vermis	Intermediate zone
Cortical control	Excitatory	Inhibitory via interneurons (likely)
Function	Control of posture, balance, and whole limb movements	Control of independent flexor muscles in the arm

tions of these nuclei to the spinal cord produce physiologic changes in the spinal cord, including impaired activation of local inhibitory interneurons. The effects of the interruption of these pathways evolve over time as a manifestation of the functional plasticity of local spinal cord circuits. The characteristic manifestation is spasticity, generally in association with hyperreflexia.

Spasticity

Spasticity is a velocity-dependent increase in tonic stretch reflexes (hypertonia) usually associated with exaggeration of the stretch reflexes (*hyperreflexia*). A common manifestation of hyperreflexia is *clonus* (repeated jerking of a muscle), which occurs when stretch reflexes occur in series and relaxation in one muscle initiates contraction in another one. Spasticity is commonly associated with other phenomena such as flexor or extensor spasms and the *clasp-knife phenomenon*. In the clasp-knife response, increased resistance to passive movement with initial stretch subsides with continuous stretch. All these phenomena re-

flect a state of increased excitability of segmental and intersegmental reflex arcs, including myotatic stretch reflexes and flexion reflexes.

Spasticity and hyperreflexia are the result of the loss of activity of inhibitory interneurons, including the presynaptic axoaxonic and Ia and Ib inhibitory interneurons. The activity of inhibitory interneurons in the spinal cord depends on descending indirect activation pathways, particularly the medullary reticulospinal tract. Hyperexcitability of alpha motor neurons may also result from primary changes in their membrane properties (for example, decreased membrane resistance) or alteration of their synaptic input (for example, sprouting of terminals from surviving presynaptic fibers). Without medullary reticulospinal inhibition, the lateral vestibulospinal (and pontine reticulospinal) tract contributes to increased motor neuron excitability. When the tonic stretch reflexes are exaggerated, the limbs adopt abnormal postures caused by exaggerated activity of the postural reflexes in *antigravity muscles*. The mechanism of the clasp-knife response is poorly understood, but it may represent an exaggerated flexor reflex triggered by activation of group II muscle afferents.

Postural Responses in Comatose Patients

Large bilateral lesions of the brainstem affect descending cortical control of the reticular formation and other brainstem motor pathways, and produce coma and specific abnormal postural responses to external stimuli (see Chapter 10). Loss of forebrain control over the inhibitory medullary reticular formation results in overactivity of extensor motor neurons activated by the lateral vestibular nucleus and pontine reticular formation. The posturing of comatose patients in response to passive movement or pain has localizing value and helps physicians to determine the level of the brainstem involved.

If the damage occurs rostral to the red nucleus, interrupting both the cortical inhibitory input to the red nucleus and the cortical excitatory input to the inhibitory medullary reticular formation, the excitatory effect of the red nucleus on the flexor muscles of the arms results in flexor posturing of the arms. The legs show extensor posturing because the lack of activity of the inhibitory medullary reticular formation unmasks the excitation of leg extensor motor neurons via input from the vestibulospinal pathway. Flexion of the arms with extension of the legs is called *decorticate posture*.

If the lesion is in the midbrain or upper pons caudal to the red nucleus but rostral to the vestibular nuclei, the vestibulospinal tract stimulates the hyperexcitable extensor motor neurons and produces extensor posturing in all the extremities. This condition is called *decerebrate posture*.

Lesions caudal to the level of the vestibular nuclei result in flaccidity, the total loss of muscle tone. Lesions in the lower brainstem that are severe enough to damage the vestibular nuclei and the reticular formation are not compatible with life.

Upper Motor Neuron Syndrome

The term *upper motor neuron* refers to cortical motor neurons and their projection to the spinal cord, either directly or via the brainstem motor pathways. Lesions of the motor pathways in the cerebral hemispheres, brainstem, or spinal cord typically interrupt the corticospinal tract (direct activation pathways) and the cortical projections to the inhibitory medullary reticular formation (corticoreticulospinal tracts) as well as to the red nucleus and excitatory reticular formation. Because of the intermingling of the direct and indirect pathways, only rarely are they damaged selectively. The clinical findings constitute the *upper motor neuron syndrome* and usually include a combination of the effects already described for pure lesions of the corticospinal (direct activation pathway) and the cortico-brainstem-spinal pathways (indirect activation pathways).

The distribution of neurologic findings of the upper motor neuron syndrome varies with the localization of the lesion. The combined paralytic and release phenomena are exemplified by a lesion in the internal capsule. Such a lesion produces a characteristic pattern of impaired motor activity on one side of the body. If paralysis is severe, the pattern is called a *hemiplegia*. If mild, it is called a *hemiparesis*. The typical findings of hemiparesis are as follows:

Movement. Motor activity is slowed, and weakness is present in a characteristic distribution: the upper portion of the face is spared and the lower portion is weak contralateral to the lesion. Volitional facial movements are weak, but emotional and associated movements such as smiling are spared or exaggerated. There may be slight weakness of the palate contralateral to the lesion and a tendency for the tongue to deviate on protrusion to the side of the hemiplegia. In the upper extremity, the weakness affects the extensor muscles more than the flexors, whereas in the lower extremity the flexors are weaker than the extensors. Chiefly affected are skilled, delicate, precision movements. Thus, the fin-

TABLE 3. *Origin of signs with an upper motor neuron lesion*

Component	Corticospinal tract (direct activation pathway)	Corticoreticulospinal and other indirect pathways
Deficit	Distal motor weakness Loss of dexterity Fatigability Absence of cutaneous reflexes	
"Release" phenomenon	Babinski's sign	Increased muscle tone—decorticate or decerebrate posture Hyperreflexia—clonus Clasp-knife phenomenon—flexor or extensor spasms

gers are particularly involved. There also is greater weakness of extension of the wrist and elbow and of abduction and elevation of the shoulder. In the lower limb, the weakness involves chiefly the dorsiflexors of the toes and ankle and the flexors of the knee and hip.

Movements tend to be massive and crude. The patient may not be able to carry out selective movements; for instance, he or she may be able to flex and extend all the fingers together but not individually, and on attempting to dorsiflex the ankle, may also flex the knee. The patient walks with a characteristic circumduction of the affected leg. Movements that the patient is unable to carry out voluntarily may occur reflexly; when the patient yawns or is tickled, the paretic upper limb may elevate and the fingers extend and abduct. Involuntary associated movements also occur in the paralyzed limb when powerful movements are carried out on the nonparalyzed side.

Muscle Tone and Posture. With an upper motor neuron lesion, there is increased resistance to passive movement (spasticity) and overactivity of the spinal reflexes that maintain upright posture, and a corresponding increase of tone in the antigravity muscles. In humans, the *antigravity muscles* are the flexors in the upper limb and the extensors in the lower limb. Lesions of the upper motor neuron result in a characteristic posture: the upper limb is adducted and flexed at the elbow, wrist, and fingers; the lower limb is adducted and extended at the hip and knee. The response to passive movement includes the clasp-knife response, in which the increased resistance to passive movement present with

initial stretch subsides with continued stretch. Large, acute, supratentorial lesions may produce a transient flaccid paralysis.

Impaired speech also occurs with upper motor neuron lesions. Because of bilateral innervation of bulbar muscles, these findings are most common with bilateral disease. They are referred to as *spastic dysarthria*, characterized by a harsh, labored, slow, monotonous, and weak speech with poor articulation.

Reflexes. The stretch reflexes in upper motor neuron disease differ from normal in that the threshold is lowered and the response is exaggerated and more protracted (hyperreflexia) and they are associated with clonus. (Clonus must be distinguished from the clonic, jerking movements in a seizure.) The abdominal and cremasteric reflexes are impaired or lost, but Babinski's sign appears.

The sources of these phenomena are listed in Table 3.

Control Circuits

The basal ganglia and cerebellum control different aspects of motor activity and are considered together as *control circuits.* The basal ganglia and cerebellum both receive extensive input from widespread areas of the cerebral cortex and send information back to the cortex through different nuclei of the thalamus. These systems are organized into several parallel loops: cerebral cortex–basal ganglia–thalamus–cerebral cortex and cerebral cortex–cerebellum–thalamus–cerebral cortex. The basal ganglia and cerebellum control motor activity through nonoverlapping thalamic projections to similar cortical motor areas, including primary motor cortex and premotor cortex (lateral premotor and supplementary motor areas). In addition to their role in motor control, the basal ganglia and cerebellum are involved in cognitive functions via projections to association areas of the cerebral cortex, particularly the prefrontal cortex and cingulate cortex. Only the motor functions of these structures are considered in this chapter.

The functions and connections of the basal ganglia and cerebellar control circuits are different despite the general features they have in common. The basal ganglia are concerned with selective activation and inhibition of specific *motor programs* necessary for automatic performance of learned movements and postural adaptations. The cerebellum is involved in the control of the *execution of motor acts*, including maintenance of balance and posture, planning and execution of coordinated limb movements, adjustments of motor performance, and learning of new motor tasks. The general anatomical organization and differences between the basal ganglia and the cerebellar control circuits are summarized in Table 4.

Basal Ganglia Control Circuit

The precise function of the basal ganglia is still undetermined. They are thought to enable the automatic performance of learned motor acts and postural adjustments. When movement is generated by cerebral cortical or cerebellar mechanisms, the basal ganglia act by selectively reinforcing the desired motor act and by broadly inhibiting competing motor mechanisms that would interfere with the desired movement.

Anatomy

Components and Neurochemistry

The basal ganglia include the striatum, globus pallidus, subthalamic nucleus, and substantia nigra (Fig. 22). The *striatum* is the receptive component of the basal ganglia and receives input from the cerebral cortex. It includes the *putamen, caudate nucleus*, and *nucleus accumbens*. The putamen is the primary striatal component of the circuit involved with controlling motor function. GABAergic neurons in the striatum project to the globus pallidus.

TABLE 4. *Comparison of the basal ganglia and cerebellar control circuits*

Feature	Basal ganglia	Cerebellum
Cortical input	Widespread (predominantly frontal lobe)	Widespread
Receptive component	Striatum (caudate and putamen) Subthalamic nucleus	Cerebellar cortex, Purkinje cells
Effector component	Globus pallidus, internal segment	Cerebellar nuclei
Regulatory component	Substantia nigra pars compacta	Inferior olivary nucleus
Thalamic nucleus	Ventral anterior (and others)	Ventral lateral
Motor cortex target	Supplementary and premotor cortices (primary motor cortex)	Primary motor cortex (supplementary and premotor cortex)
Brainstem target	Pedunculopontine nucleus Superior colliculus	Red nucleus Vestibular nuclei Reticular formation
Direct spinal input	No	Yes
Function	Selection of motor programs	Initiation and execution of motor acts
Clinical correlation	Hypokinesia Rigidity Tremor at rest Abnormal movements (hyperkinesia)	Disequilibrium Incoordination Ataxia Action tremor
Localization of clinical findings	Contralateral to lesion	Ipsilateral to lesion

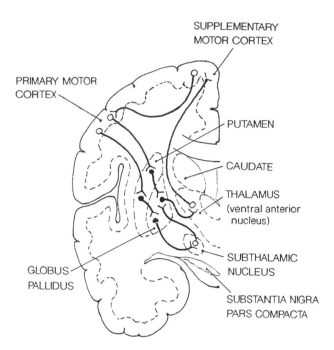

SUPPLEMENTARY
MOTOR CORTEX

PRIMARY MOTOR
CORTEX

PUTAMEN

CAUDATE

THALAMUS
(ventral anterior
nucleus)

SUBTHALAMIC
NUCLEUS

GLOBUS
PALLIDUS

SUBSTANTIA NIGRA
PARS COMPACTA

FIG. 22. The main nuclei and connections of the basal ganglia circuit. The basal ganglia include the striatum (putamen, caudate nucleus, and the accumbens nucleus [not shown]), globus pallidus (including external and internal segments), subthalamic nucleus, and substantia nigra. The striatum (especially the putamen) is the receptive component of the basal ganglia control circuit and it receives excitatory (glutamate-mediated) input from the motor cortex. Neurons of the striatum contain GABA and project to both segments of the globus pallidus and the substantia nigra (projection not shown). The internal segment of the globus pallidus contains GABAergic neurons that constitute the output of the basal ganglia. The main target is the ventral anterior and other thalamic nuclei that project to the supplementary motor cortex and other areas of the frontal lobe. The external segment also contains GABAergic neurons that project to the internal segment and the subthalamic nucleus. The subthalamic nucleus sends an excitatory (glutamatergic) projection to the internal segment of the globus pallidus. The substantia nigra pars compacta contains dopaminergic neurons that project to the striatum. The basal ganglia circuits consist of extrinsic and intrinsic connections. The extrinsic connections include input from the cerebral cortex and substantia nigra pars compacta to the striatum (and subthalamic nucleus) and output from the internal segment of the globus pallidus to the thalamus and brainstem motor nuclei. The intrinsic connections include projections from the striatum to both segments of the globus pallidus, reciprocal connections between the substantia nigra and the striatum, and reciprocal connections between the subthalamic nucleus and the globus pallidus.

The *globus pallidus* includes an internal segment and an external segment. The internal segment is the output structure of the basal ganglia. The external segment is part of the intrinsic basal ganglia circuit. Neurons of the globus pallidus also have GABA as their neurotransmitter.

The *subthalamic nucleus* receives input from the cerebral cortex and has reciprocal connections with the globus pallidus. Unlike other basal ganglia structures, its neurons have glutamate as a neurotransmitter.

The *substantia nigra* is reciprocally connected with the striatum. It has two subdivisions, the *pars compacta* and the *pars reticulata*. Neurons in the pars compacta contain dopamine. The pars reticulata is anatomically and functionally a continuation of the internal segment of the globus pallidus. The pars reticulata controls face and eye movements and is not discussed further in this chapter.

Connections

The striatum receives three main inputs: excitatory (glutamatergic) input from the cerebral cortex, excitatory (glutamatergic) input from the intralaminar thalamic nuclei (not discussed further), and modulatory (dopaminergic) input from the substantia nigra pars compacta. The intrinsic circuitry of the striatum includes local neurons that contain acetylcholine. Dopamine (from the substantia nigra pars compacta) and acetylcholine (from local neurons) exert opposite modulatory effects on the output neurons of the striatum, the medium spiny neuron. These neurons are inhibitory GABAergic cells that project to the globus pallidus and substantia nigra.

The internal segment of the globus pallidus, the output component of the basal ganglia, contains GABAergic neurons that project to three main targets: the thalamus, superior colliculus (involved in generation of fast eye movements), and pedunculopontine nucleus of the reticular formation (involved in locomotion). The most important of these projections is to the thalamus, including the ventral anterior and other nuclei that relay information to the premotor and supplementary motor areas and to other regions of the frontal lobe. The output of the basal ganglia affects both the corticospinal and the brainstem motor pathways.

The output of the basal ganglia through the internal segment of the globus pallidus is activated by excitatory (glutamatergic) input from the subthalamic nucleus and is inhibited by GABAergic input from the striatum and external segment of the globus pallidus. The balance between these influences is modulated by the dopaminergic input from the sub-

stantia nigra pars compacta and by other components of the circuit.

Physiology

Through the projection from the internal segment of the globus pallidus to the thalamus, the basal ganglia exert a continuous (tonic) inhibitory effect on the motor thalamocortical circuits and act as a continuous "brake" on motor programs. This tonic inhibition is transiently interrupted (that is, the brake is lifted) to allow selective activation of a specific motor program. Simultaneously, the inhibition is reinforced (that is, the brake is applied) to prevent the execution of other interfering motor acts (Fig. 23).

The tonic inhibitory outflow from the internal segment of the globus pallidus is controlled by two opposite influences: (1) it is tonically activated by the subthalamic nucleus, and (2) it is transiently inhibited by the striatum. Thus, the subthalamic nucleus acts to continuously apply the brake, and the striatum acts to transiently lift the brake. In addition, the external segment of the globus pallidus continuously inhibits the brake through GABAergic input to both the internal segment and the subthalamic nucleus.

Unlike the neurons in the globus pallidus, striatal output neurons are essentially silent and fire only when sufficiently activated by cortical input. The ability of striatal output neurons to respond to excitatory input from the cerebral cortex depends on the modulatory effects of dopamine and acetylcholine. When the striatal neurons discharge, they produce a transient inhibition of the neurons in the globus pallidus. There are two types of striatal GABAergic output neurons. One type projects to the internal segment of the globus pallidus and forms the direct striatopallidal pathway. It directly influences the output of the basal ganglia. This pathway phasically inhibits neurons in the internal segment, allowing the initiation of a motor program. The other type of striatal output neuron projects to external segment of the globus pallidus and forms the indirect stri-

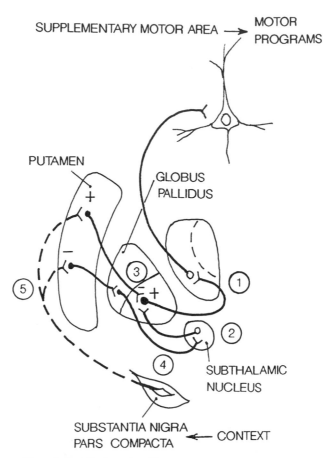

FIG. 23. Mechanism of basal ganglia function. The internal segment of the globus pallidus (GPi) exerts a tonic GABAergic inhibition on neurons of the thalamus that project to motor areas of the cerebral cortex (1). This tonic inhibitory activity depends mainly on two things: continuous activation by glutamatergic input from the subthalamic nucleus (2), and transient inhibition by GABAergic input from the striatum (3). This direct striatopallidal pathway transiently disinhibits the thalamus and allows execution of a specific motor plan. A parallel inhibitory output from the striatum acts indirectly on GPi to facilitate the tonic inhibition of other movements. This output is directed to the external segment of the globus pallidus (GPe), which tonically inhibits both the GPi and the subthalamic nucleus (4). By inhibiting the GPe, this indirect striatopallidal pathway activates both the subthalamic nucleus and the GPi, increasing the tonic inhibitory influence on the thalamus. Dopaminergic input from the substantia nigra pars compacta to the striatum critically modulates the balance between the direct and indirect striatopallidal pathway. Through different receptor subtypes, dopamine exerts a global excitatory effect on the direct striatopallidal pathway (favoring disinhibition of the thalamus) and an inhibitory effect on the indirect striatopallidal pathway (preventing an increase in tonic inhibition of the thalamus) (5). Thus, the dopaminergic input to the striatum is thought to be critical for context-dependent activation of selected motor programs.

atopallidal pathway. It modifies the activity of the internal segment indirectly through the external segment and subthalamic nucleus. This pathway, by inhibiting the external segment, the indirect striatopallidal pathway, allows increased activity of neurons in the internal segment, thus blocking motor programs.

The balance between the ability of the striatum to initiate and to block the initiation of individual motor programs is critically dependent on the dopaminergic input from the substantia nigra. Dopamine has a global excitatory effect on the striatal neurons that project to the internal segment of the globus pallidus (brake lifters) and an inhibitory effect on the striatal neurons that project to the external segment (brake pressers). These opposing effects are mediated by different subtypes of dopamine receptors. Because dopaminergic neurons discharge in response to behaviorally significant stimuli, they provide a contextual framework for activity in the basal ganglia circuit. Local cholinergic neurons also innervate striatal output neurons and exert effects opposite to those of dopamine. Thus, a balance between dopamine and acetylcholine affects the activity of striatal neurons (Fig. 23).

Manifestations of Disorders of the Basal Ganglia Control Circuit

An emerging concept in basal ganglia function is that it is the pattern, rather than the amount, of activity in the internal segment of the globus pallidus that is the critical factor in motor control. When this pattern is affected by disease, symptoms develop that improve after the internal segment has been surgically ablated. The pattern of activity in the internal segment depends on the balance between the direct and indirect striatopallidal connections and the activity of the subthalamic nucleus. This balance is critically affected by the levels of dopamine in the striatum. The lack of dopamine in the striatum impairs the initiation of motor programs, whereas the relative excess of dopamine impairs the suppression

of unwanted movement. Thus, disorders of the basal ganglia may be classified into two main types: hypokinetic disorders (when dopaminergic mechanisms are impaired), and hyperkinetic disorders (when dopaminergic mechanisms are exaggerated). Because these disorders initially were thought to involve direct projections from the basal ganglia to the brainstem, without involvement of the pyramidal system, they were (erroneously) referred to as *extrapyramidal disorders,* a term that is still used.

Hypokinetic-Rigid Syndrome (Parkinsonism)

Hypokinesia refers to the global paucity of spontaneous or associated movements (for example, eye blinking and arm swing). It is associated with slowness in the initiation and performance of voluntary or automatic acts (*bradykinesia*). Hypokinesia commonly occurs in conjunction with an increase in muscle tone, referred to as *rigidity*. Rigidity is increased resistance to passive limb movement that, unlike spasticity, is velocity-independent and occurs throughout the range of motion of the limb. The patient has a stooped, flexed posture of the trunk and limbs, and movement is slow, stiff, and initiated or stopped with great difficulty. The combination of hypokinesia and rigidity in association with postural instability is commonly referred to as *parkinsonism,* because its most common cause is *Parkinson's disease,* a degenerative disorder characterized by hypokinesia, rigidity, postural instability, and *tremor*. Tremor is a regular, alternating movement that occurs in the hands and, less commonly, the lower extremity or head. In parkinsonism, the tremor occurs *at rest* and diminishes with voluntary activity. Parkinson's disease is a degenerative disorder characterized by loss of dopaminergic neurons in the substantia nigra; the diseased neurons usually contain cytoplasmatic hyaline inclusion bodies (Lewy bodies). The mechanism of neuronal degeneration is undetermined but is thought to involve oxidative damage and mitochondrial dysfunction in these cells. The illicit "designer drug" MPTP (1-methyl-4-phenyl-1,2,3,6-tetrahydropyridine) destroys substantia nigra neurons by this mechanism and causes parkinsonism. Parkinsonism may also result from pharmacologic blockade of dopamine receptors, for example, by psychoactive drugs. In Parkinson's disease, depletion of dopamine in the striatum produces an exaggerated activity in the subthalamic nucleus and internal segment of the globus pallidus. Replacement of L-dopa (the substrate for dopamine synthesis) or dopamine antagonists can relieve the symptoms in most patients. Lesions restricted to the internal segment relieve symptoms unresponsive to pharmacologic treatment.

Hyperkinetic Movement Disorders

Disorders of the basal ganglia can produce various involuntary movements. Among the most common are dyskinesias. An example is *hemiballismus*, gross rapid flinging movements of one arm caused by a lesion of the contralateral subthalamic nucleus. *Chorea* refers to brief, rapid, writhing movements of the limbs. These movements are typical of Huntington's disease, a neurodegenerative disorder that is a dominantly inherited disorder characterized by chorea, changes in muscle tone, and progressive dementia and behavioral manifestations. The characteristic pathologic change is a profound cell loss in the caudate nucleus and cerebral cortex. The caudate nucleus shrinks and this produces a characteristic dilatation of the lateral ventricle. The cell loss in the caudate nucleus is selective, affecting predominantly the output GABAergic neurons and sparing certain interneurons. *Dystonia* refers to abnormal sustained posturing of the trunk or an extremity. It may be focal (for example, *torticollis* in the neck) or generalized. Although dystonia is a typical manifestation of basal ganglia disease, the pathophysiologic mechanism is likely heterogeneous. *Athetosis* refers to slow writhing movements of the fingers and is commonly associated with chorea.

Other movement disorders include *tremor, myoclonus* (a fast muscle jerk), and *tics*. These abnormal movements may occur in disorders that affect regions other than the basal ganglia; for example, tremor occurs with lesions of the cerebellar control circuit, and myoclonus occurs with lesions affecting the motor cortex or brainstem reticular formation. Tics may occur with lesions in the circuits of nucleus accumbens.

Cerebellar Control Circuit

The cerebellum and its connections compose the second major control circuit. This control is concerned with the planning and execution of movements, adaptation of motor performance, and motor learning. Its functions include control of posture, balance, and eye movements necessary for maintaining equilibrium; adjustment of ongoing execution of movement; initiation, timing, and planning of coordinated limb movements; and learning new motor tasks.

The cerebellum controls the output of the motor system by acting as a comparator between the motor commands and their actual execution. Thus, it is an error detection system. When an error is detected, the cerebellum corrects it by sending signals to motor areas of the brainstem and cerebral cortex. Cerebellar inputs and outputs are side loops of pathways from the motor cortex, subcortical nuclei, and spinal cord. Information about motor plans is provided to the cerebellum by collateral projections from premotor cortex and motor cortex (relayed to the cerebellum via the *pontine nuclei*) and from brainstem motor regions (red nucleus, vestibular nuclei, and reticular formation). Information about motor performance, or external feedback, is provided by inputs from peripheral receptors (dorsal spinocerebellar tract). The cerebellum corrects motor performance through its output to brainstem nuclei (red nucleus, vestibular nuclei, reticular formation) and to premotor cortex and motor cortex. The cerebellar output to the motor cortex is relayed through the ventral lateral nucleus of the thalamus. Adaptation of motor performance or motor learning involves operation of an error signal relayed to the cerebellum by the *inferior olivary nucleus* (Fig. 24).

Anatomy

The cerebellum is subdivided into a *flocculonodular lobe* and the *body* of the cerebellum, which includes the *anterior lobe* and the *posterior lobe*. The midline portion of the anterior and posterior lobe is called the *vermis*, and the lateral portions are the *cerebellar hemispheres* (Fig. 25).

Gross Anatomy

Each of the lobes is divided into several lobules; each lobule consists of several leaf-like *folia*. Nerve fibers enter or leave the cerebellum in the three *cerebellar peduncles*. The inferior cerebellar peduncle (or *restiform*

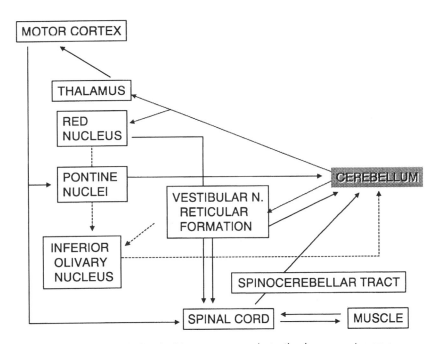

FIG. 24. The cerebellar control circuit. Motor commands to the lower motor neurons from the cerebral cortex (direct activation pathway) and brainstem (indirect activation pathways) are relayed to the cerebellum, which acts as a comparator between these commands and their execution, based on information from feedback pathways from the spinal cord (spinocerebellar tract). Cortical motor commands are relayed to the cerebellum via the pontine nuclei, located in the basis pontis; brainstem motor commands are relayed to the cerebellum directly. The cerebellum modulates the motor output of the indirect activation pathways (rubrospinal, vestibulospinal, and reticulospinal) via direct projections to the brainstem and modulates the motor commands from the cerebral cortex (corticospinal tract) via a relay in the ventrolateral nucleus of the thalamus. The cerebellocortical connections are crossed (for example, the upper limb is controlled by the contralateral motor cortex and the ipsilateral cerebellum).

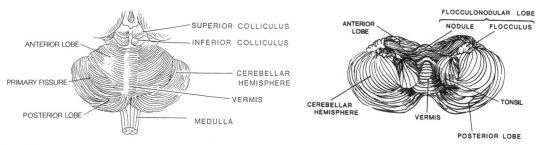

FIG. 25. Gross anatomy of the cerebellum. **A:** Superior (dorsal) view. The body of the cerebellum includes a medially located vermis and the expanded lateral hemispheres. The primary fissure divides the dorsal portion of the cerebellum into an anterior lobe and a posterior lobe. **B:** Inferior (ventral) view. The cerebellum consists of a flocculonodular lobe and a body, which consists of the anterior and posterior lobe. Most of the body of the cerebellum corresponds to the posterior lobe.

body) connects the cerebellum with the medulla and spinal cord; the middle cerebellar peduncle (or *brachium pontis*) connects the cerebellum with the pons; and the superior cerebellar peduncle (or *brachium conjunctivum*) connects the cerebellum with the midbrain and cerebral hemispheres.

The cerebellum controls the ipsilateral limbs. Therefore, it processes input from the ipsilateral spinal cord and vestibular nuclei and the contralateral cerebral hemisphere and red nucleus. The cerebellar projections to the motor cortex and red nucleus travel in the superior cerebellar peduncles, which decussate in the midbrain. Descending input from the cerebral hemispheres provides information to the contralateral cerebellum via the pontine nuclei; the crossed pontocerebellar axons form the entire middle cerebellar peduncle. Reciprocal connections with the spinal cord (dorsal spinocerebellar tract), vestibular nuclei, and reticular formation are primarily ipsilateral and travel in the inferior cerebellar peduncle.

Basic Circuitry

Histologically, the cerebellum consists of three-layered cortex and deep cerebellar nuclei. The large *Purkinje cells* provide the output of the cerebellar cortex to the deep nuclei and vestibular nuclei. Purkinje cells are in-hibitory GABAergic neurons. The cerebellar nuclei transmit the output of the body of the cerebellum. The flocculonodular lobe projects directly to the vestibular nuclei. The body of the cerebellum can be divided into three sagittal regions, with each one containing an output nucleus: (1) the vermis, with output via the *fastigial nucleus*; (2) the paravermis, with output via the *globose* and *emboliform nuclei*; and the large lateral zone (hemisphere), with output via the *dentate nucleus* (Fig. 26).

Information about motor commands and their execution is continuously transmitted to intrinsic cerebellar circuits via the *mossy fiber system* (Fig. 27). Mossy fibers arise from neurons in the spinal cord, vestibular nuclei, reticular formation, and pontine nuclei. These fibers synapse on the *granule cells* of the cerebellar cortex. The granule cells provide a highly divergent excitatory input to a large population of Purkinje cells aligned along a folium via the *parallel fiber* system. The mossy fiber–granule cell–parallel fiber system is a glutamatergic system that excites Purkinje cells and local interneurons. The *inferior olivary nucleus* receives collaterals from all pathways projecting to the cerebellum and from projections leaving the cerebellar nuclei. In response to any unexpected change in motor performance, the inferior olivary nucleus sends an error signal to the cere-

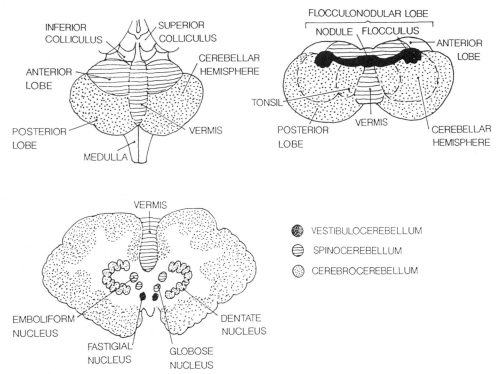

FIG. 26. Horizontal section showing the deep cerebellar nuclei and their relationships with the three main sagittal functional subdivisions of the cerebellum. The flocculonodular lobe *(black)* corresponds to the vestibulocerebellum (also referred to as archicerebellum). The anterior lobe *(horizontal lines)* (and the fastigial and globose/emboliform nuclei) corresponds to the spinocerebellum (or paleocerebellum). The posterior lobe, comprising the bulk of the cerebellar hemispheres, and the dentate nucleus correspond to the cerebrocerebellum *(stippled)* (neocerebellum). The fastigial nucleus is located in the vermis, the globose and emboliform nuclei in the paravermis, and the dentate nucleus in the lateral hemispheres.

bellum through the *climbing fiber* system, another afferent system of the cerebellar cortex. Unlike mossy fibers, each climbing fiber provides a very powerful synapse to only one or a few Purkinje cells. The inferior olive–climbing fiber input is also excitatory to Purkinje cells.

In addition to Purkinje cells, the climbing and mossy fibers provide collateral input to the deep cerebellar nuclei. Therefore, the cerebellar output nuclei receive two main sets of input: an early direct excitation by the mossy and climbing fibers and delayed inhibition via the Purkinje cells.

The cerebellar control system is organized into sagittally oriented *microzones,* the func-

tional unit of the cerebellum. A microzone includes a longitudinal cortical strip of Purkinje cells, a localized area in the inferior olivary nucleus, and a subdivision of the cerebellar nuclei. All these are reciprocally interconnected by sagittally organized olivocerebellar, olivonuclear, and corticonuclear pathways.

Physiology

The cerebellum and its connecting pathways are organized into three functional subdivisions, each with distinct anatomical connections and specific functions. These three functional divisions are the *vestibulocerebellum, spinocerebellum,* and *cerebrocerebel-*

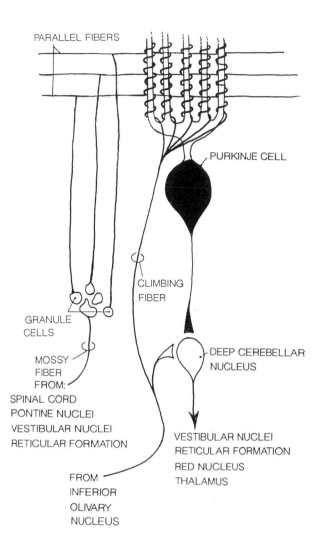

PARALLEL FIBERS

PURKINJE CELL

CLIMBING FIBER

GRANULE CELLS

MOSSY FIBER FROM:
SPINAL CORD
PONTINE NUCLEI
VESTIBULAR NUCLEI
RETICULAR FORMATION

DEEP CEREBELLAR NUCLEUS

VESTIBULAR NUCLEI
RETICULAR FORMATION
RED NUCLEUS
THALAMUS

FROM INFERIOR OLIVARY NUCLEUS

FIG. 27. Basic circuit of the cerebellum. The input to the cerebellum terminates primarily in the cerebellar cortex, including the granule cells, Purkinje cells, and several interneurons. Input from the cerebral cortex (via the pontine nuclei), spinocerebellar tract, vestibular system, and reticular formation reach the cerebellum via the mossy fiber system. The mossy fibers synapse on the granule cells, which in turn provide input to a large number of Purkinje cells via the parallel fiber system. The inferior olivary nucleus is the only source of the climbing fiber system. Each climbing fiber innervates only one or a few Purkinje cells. Both mossy fiber–parallel fiber and climbing fibers are excitatory to Purkinje cells. The Purkinje cell is the output cell of the cerebellar cortex. It is a GABAergic neuron that inhibits neurons in the vestibular nuclei and deep cerebellar nuclei. The deep cerebellar nuclei form the output of the cerebellum. Their neurons project to nuclei in the thalamus and brainstem, including the inferior olivary nucleus.

lum. The terms indicate the major connections of the segments (Table 5 and Figs. 28–30).

Vestibulocerebellum and Control of Equilibrium

The *vestibulocerebellum* (or archicerebellum) corresponds to the flocculonodular node and is reciprocally connected with the vestibular nuclei. Through the vestibular system, the flocculonodular lobe receives information about head position and acceleration; it also receives visual information through the reticular formation. The flocculonodular lobe projects directly to the vestibular nuclei and inhibits them. The vestibular nuclei control the axial musculature (via the vestibulospinal tracts) and compensatory movements of the eyes in response to head motion (vestibuloocular reflex). Thus, the vestibulocerebellum controls equilibrium of the trunk and coordinated movements of the head and eyes (Fig. 28). Disorders of this area produce trunk ataxia, dysequilibrium, and nystagmus.

Spinocerebellum and Control of Posture and Gait

The *spinocerebellum* (or paleocerebellum) corresponds to the anterior lobe and includes

TABLE 5. *Functional subdivisions of the cerebellum*

Division (lobe)	Main input	Output nucleus	Target	Effector	Function	Syndrome
Vestibulocerebellum (flocculonodular)	Vestibulocerebellar tract	Vestibular	Spinal cord Oculomotor nuclei	Vestibulospinal tract Vestibulo-ocular projection	Equilibrium of trunk, head, and eyes	Dysequilibrium Nystagmus
Spinocerebellum (anterior)	Spinocerebellar tracts	Fastigial	Lateral vestibular Reticular formation	Medial motor pathways (vestibulospinal, reticulospinal)	Posture and gait	Imbalance Gait ataxia
		Globose and emboliform	Red nucleus (magnicellular) Thalamus (ventral lateral)	Lateral motor pathways (rubospinal, corticospinal)	Control of proximal movement	Lower limb ataxia
Cerebrocerebellum (posterior)	Corticopontocerebellar tract	Dentate	Thalamus (ventral lateral)	Corticospinal tract	Motor coordination and learning	Upper limb ataxia
			Red nucleus (parvicellular)	Rubro-olivary system		Palatal myoclonus

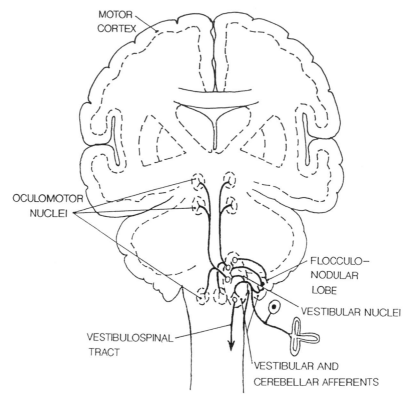

FIG. 28. The vestibulocerebellum. The vestibulocerebellum consists of the flocculonodular lobe. Purkinje cells of the flocculonodular lobe receive vestibular input directly from first-order sensory neurons and from vestibular nuclei and send inhibitory projections to the vestibular nuclei, which control oculomotor neurons (vestibulo-ocular reflex) and spinal motor neurons (vestibulospinal tract). Thus, the vestibulocerebellum is critical for the control of equilibrium and eye movements.

the vermis and paravermis regions. Its main input is from the spinocerebellar tracts. The dorsal spinocerebellar tract ascends ipsilaterally and provides feedback information about motor performance. The ventral spinocerebellar tract crosses in the spinal cord and then crosses again in the superior cerebellar peduncle and provides feed-forward information about the degree of excitability of motor neurons ipsilateral to the spinocerebellum (see Chapter 7). The main output of the spinocerebellum is to the spinal cord through the fastigial nucleus (vermis) and the globose and emboliform nuclei (paravermis) (Fig. 29). The fastigial nucleus receives vestibular, visual, and auditory inputs and projects to the vestibular nuclei and reticular formation. Thus, it controls the medial motor pathways

(the vestibulospinal and reticulospinal tracts). This output regulates postural adjustments of the legs during gait.

The globose and emboliform nuclei receive input from the motor cortex and red nucleus and control the lateral motor pathways. The axons from these deep cerebellar nuclei decussate in the midbrain (decussation of the brachium conjunctivum) and synapse in the contralateral red nucleus (origin of the rubrospinal tract) and ventral lateral nucleus of the thalamus (which contains neurons that project motor cortex). These connections provide continuous feedback correction during the execution of movements of the limbs (primarily the upper limbs). Disorders of the spinocerebellum are manifested predominantly as gait ataxia.

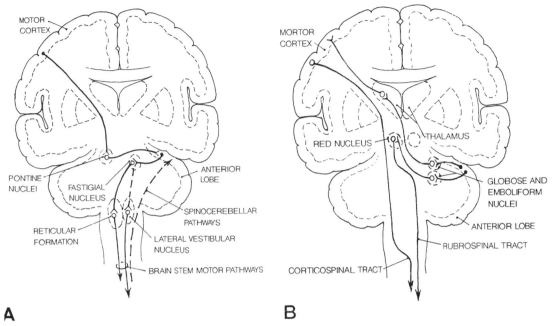

FIG. 29. Connections of the spinocerebellum. **A:** The spinocerebellum (anterior lobe) receives input primarily from the spinal cord (spinocerebellar pathways) and collateral input from the descending corticospinal tract (via the pontine nuclei) and brainstem nuclei of the indirect activation pathways. The spinocerebellum controls the performance of these pathways through two main output systems: the vermis and paravermis. The cerebellar vermis, via the fastigial nuclei, projects to the vestibular nuclei and reticular formation, the origins of the medial motor pathways. **B:** The paravermis, via the globose and emboliform nuclei, controls the lateral motor pathways through projections to the red nucleus (rubrospinal tract) and thalamus, which in turn projects to motor cortex (corticospinal tract).

Cerebrocerebellum and Control of Voluntary Movement

The *cerebrocerebellum* (or neocerebellum) corresponds to the large posterior lobe and projects through the large dentate nucleus to the thalamus (Fig. 30). The evolutionary increase in the size of the cerebellar hemispheres corresponds to a similar increase in the size of the cerebral cortex. The functions of the cerebrocerebellum may not be restricted to motor control but may also include cognitive functions. It projects not only to the motor and premotor regions of the cerebral cortex but also to the prefrontal cortex and other association areas involved in processing of language, learning, and other high cortical functions. The cerebrocerebellum receives input from essentially all areas of the cerebral cortex via the large corticopontocerebellar pathway. The dentate nucleus sends axons through the superior cerebellar peduncle to the ventral lateral nucleus of the thalamus, which projects to the premotor and motor cortices, and to the red nucleus (parvicellular portion), which projects to the inferior olivary nucleus (origin of the error signal relayed via the climbing fiber system).

The projection from the dentate nucleus to the thalamus closes an important feedback loop between the cerebral cortex and the cerebellum: the corticocerebellar-dentothalamocortical loop. This loop is thought to be critical for the initiation, planning, and timing of motor acts, including specification of the di-

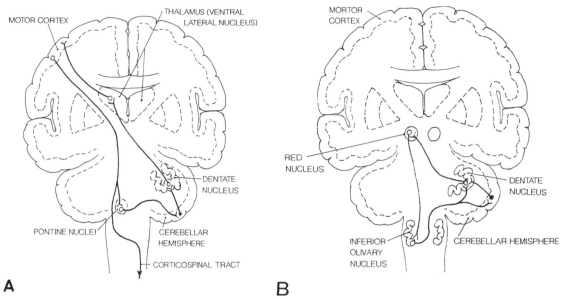

FIG. 30. Connections of the cerebrocerebellum. **A:** The large cerebellar hemispheres receive massive input from several areas of the cerebral cortex via the corticopontocerebellar pathway. Its outflow is via the dentate nucleus. The dentate nucleus projects to the ventral lateral thalamic nucleus for initiation and control of motor performance. The massive dentatothalamic outflow is thought to provide a signal for the initiation and successful completion of a learned movement, independently of sensory feedback. **B:** The dentate nucleus also projects to the parvicellular portion of the red nucleus. This portion of the red nucleus does not give rise to the rubrospinal tract but provides input to the ipsilateral inferior olivary nucleus. The inferior olivary nucleus, in turn, projects to the cerebellum via the climbing fiber system, thus closing a cerebellodentatorubro-olivocerebellar loop. Because the inferior olivary nucleus provides an error signal in response to unexpected changes in motor performance, this system is critical for motor adaptation and motor learning.

rection, pattern, and intensity of movements of the upper extremity.

The projection from the dentate nucleus to the red nucleus (parvicellular part) closes an important feedback loop between the cerebellum and the inferior olivary nucleus, the cerebellodentatorubro-olivocerebellar pathway. Because neurons in the inferior olivary nucleus discharge rhythmically, this pathway is thought to provide a timing sequence for the entire motor system.

Cerebellum and Motor Learning

The cerebellar circuits are modified by experience (motor practice). The functional adaptation of cerebellar circuits following learning of a novel motor task is critically dependent on climbing fiber modulation of mossy fiber inputs to the Purkinje cells. The discharge of the inferior olive–climbing fiber increases markedly as an error signal after an unexpected disturbance in motor execution. Transient activation of a large number of synaptic inputs via the climbing fibers produces a decrease in the response to the mossy fiber input on the same Purkinje cell; this persists after the learning of a motor task and resets the pattern of Purkinje cell firing to a new level. This phenomenon, called *long-term depression*, involves complex postsynaptic interactions between the parallel and climbing fibers, including excitatory amino acid receptors, neuronal depolarization, increased calcium influx, synthesis of nitric oxide, and changes in protein phosphorylation affecting the dendrites and soma of Purkinje cells.

Cerebellar Hemisphere Syndrome

The posterior lobe, particularly the large lateral hemispheres, form a servomechanism for coordination of skilled action. Lesions of the posterior lobe produce irregular movements of the limbs (*limb ataxia*), loss of muscle coordination (*dyssynergia*), loss of ability to measure range of motion (*dysmetria*), irregularity in alternate motion rate (*dysdiadochokinesia*), tremor with voluntary activity (*intention tremor*), delay in movement initiation, and, in some cases, hypotonia. All these manifestations are ipsilateral to the side of the lesion. The mechanism of cerebellar tremors is undetermined. It appears to involve abnormal rhythmic activity in the circuits involving the inferior olivary, dentate, and ventral lateral thalamic nuclei. Neurons in all these regions can generate spontaneous oscillatory activity.

Disorders of oculomotor control and speech also occur in cerebellar disease, particularly if it involves the vermis. Cerebellar speech disorders are manifested as irregularities of speech, loudness, and rhythm and are known as *ataxic dysarthria*. Speech is slowed, with excess stress on some words or syllables and random breakdown of articulation.

Motor System Examination   ■

Movement in a normal person involves the simultaneous, coordinated activities of all the major divisions of the motor system. Therefore, these are tested together in the neurologic examination. The examination is best organized into separate evaluation of strength, reflexes, coordination, gait, tone, and muscle bulk and observation for abnormal movements. The typical findings in disorders of the motor system are summarized in Table 6.

Strength

Strength testing evaluates the power of muscle groups in performing specific actions.

Strength depends on age, occupation, physical activity, and muscular development. It may be apparently reduced in patients with bone deformity, pain, or a lack of understanding of the test. Because the object of strength testing is to detect disease of the neuromuscular system, these extraneous factors must be excluded. Strength cannot be graded as abnormal on the basis of an absolute measure of force. It must be judged for each person on the basis of age and all the other variables noted.

Strength is tested by having the patient resist pressure initiated by the examiner. The position of the extremity during testing is of great importance in isolating the action of specific muscle groups and in providing optimal leverage. Each muscle group should be tested in the position that best isolates its function and puts it at a relative mechanical disadvantage (partially contracted position). Force should not be applied suddenly but should be applied gradually to a maximum.

There are several systems for grading strength (or weakness). A simple and universally understood one uses a verbal description:

Normal. Level of strength expected for that person.
Mild weakness. Level of strength less than expected but not sufficient to impair any daily function.
Severe weakness. Strength sufficient to activate the muscle and move it against gravity but not against any added resistance.
Complete paralysis. No detectable movement.

The following muscle groups are tested as part of a general neurologic examination. The individual muscles participating in these functions are discussed in Chapter 13.

Facial muscles. Upper and lower facial muscles are tested separately by having the patient wrinkle the forehead, squeeze the eyes shut, and show the teeth.
Neck muscles. The patient resists attempts by the examiner to flex and extend the neck by exerting pressure on the occiput and forehead, respectively.

TABLE 6. *Findings on neurologic examination of motor function related to the divisions of the motor system at the four levels of the nervous system*

	Level of damage			
	Peripheral	Spinal	Posterior fossa	Supratentorial
Final common pathway	Weakness, atrophy, hyporeflexia, hypotonia, absent abdominal reflexes, cramp, and fasciculation	Weakness, atrophy, hyporeflexia, hypotonia, absent abdominal reflexes, cramp, and fasciculation	Weakness, atrophy, and fasciculation	
Corticospinal tract		Weakness, loss of abdominal reflex, and Babinski's sign	Weakness, loss of abdominal reflex, Babinski's sign, hyporeflexia, and hypotonia	Weakness, loss of abdominal reflex, Babinski's sign, seizure, apraxia, hyporeflexia, and hypotonia
Brainstem motor pathway		Hyperreflexia, clonus, spasticity, and clasp-knife reflex	Hyperreflexia, clonus, spasticity, clasp-knife reflex, and decerebrate posture	Hyperreflexia, clonus, spasticity, clasp-knife reflex, apraxia, decorticate posture
Cerebellar control circuit			Ataxia, dysmetria, dyssynergia, intention tremor, past pointing, rebound, hyporeflexia, and hypotonia	Ataxia
Basal ganglia control circuit				Rigidity, athetosis, dystonia, chorea, hemiballismus, hyperkinesia, and resting tremor

Arm abductors. The patient holds the arms laterally at right angles to the body, while the examiner pushes down on the elbows.

Elbow flexors and extensors. With the elbow bent at a right angle, the patient resists attempts to straighten it out (flexing to prevent extension) and to bend it (extending to prevent flexion).

Wrist extensors. The patient holds the wrist straight with knuckles up, while the examiner attempts to depress it.

Finger flexors. The patient resists attempts to straighten the fingers of a clenched fist (or squeezes two of the examiner's fingers in his or her hand).

Trunk flexors. The patient attempts to do a sit-up from a supine position, with the legs extended.

Hip flexors. In a sitting position, the patient holds the knee up off the chair against resistance; supine, the patient keeps the knee pulled up to the chest.

Hip extensors. Prone, the patient holds the bent knee off the examining table; supine, the patient resists attempts to lift the leg straight off the examining table; these are the major muscles used in arising from a squatting position (with knee extensors).

Knee flexors. The patient resists attempts to straighten the knee from a 90-degree angle position.

Knee extensors. The patient resists attempts to bend the knee from a 90-degree angle position; these are major muscles used in arising from squatting.

Ankle plantar flexors. The patient's ability to rise onto the toes of one foot or to walk on toes is assessed. This ability is too powerful to test by hand unless it has been severely weakened.

Ankle dorsiflexors. The patient holds the ankle in a resting 90-degree angle position against attempts to depress it.

Reflexes

Two major types of reflexes are tested in the neurologic examination: stretch reflexes and superficial (cutaneous) reflexes. The former depend on a rapid, brisk stretch of the muscle, whereas the latter depend on an uncomfortable stimulus to the skin. Correct positioning and application of the stimulus are extremely important in eliciting reflexes. There are also significant variations among patients and even of a reflex in a single patient on repeated testing. Therefore, much experience with normal reflexes is required before the presence of abnormality can be assessed.

The jaw, biceps, triceps, knee, and ankle reflexes are the most important stretch reflexes. The patient must be completely relaxed in the testing of all these reflexes.

Jaw jerk. The examiner's index finger is placed lightly on the patient's mandible below the lower lip. It is then tapped briskly with the reflex hammer. The reflex is a brisk jaw closure.

Biceps jerk. The patient's elbow is bent to 90-degree angle position, with the forearm resting on the lap or on the examiner's arm. The examiner's thumb is placed on the patient's biceps tendon with slight pressure. The thumb is then tapped firmly and briskly with the reflex hammer. The reflex is a quick biceps muscle contraction with tendon (and forearm) movement.

Triceps jerk. The patient's elbow is bent to 90-degree angle position, with the forearm hanging limply and supported at the elbow by the examiner's hand. A firm, brisk tap is applied directly to the tendon of the triceps 1 to 3 cm above the olecranon. The elbow extends in this reflex.

Knee jerk. The patient's knee is bent to 90 degrees in the sitting position. A firm, brisk tap is applied to the quadriceps tendon 0.5 to 1.0 cm below the patella. The knee extends in this reflex.

Ankle jerk. The patient's ankle is passively bent to 90 degrees and held by the examiner in that position. The examiner gives a firm, brisk tap to the Achilles tendon 2 to 3 cm above the heel. The foot plantar flexes in the reflex.

Abdominal reflex. The patient lies supine, with the abdomen relaxed. By means of a sharp object, the skin of the patient's abdomen is scraped quickly and lightly in each quadrant along a line toward the umbilicus. The umbilicus moves toward the stimulus.

Plantar responses. The sole of the patient's foot is scratched firmly with a blunt instrument such as a key. The stimulus is begun at the heel and smoothly carried forward along the lateral border of the sole to the base of the toes and then medially to the base of the great toe. A normal response is curling of the toes. Babinski's sign is extension of the great toe and fanning of the other toes.

Coordination

The ability to coordinate the movements of multiple muscle groups can be observed during ordinary activity, such as shaking hands, talking, dressing, and writing. Specific tests allow assessment of coordination in localized areas. All may be done with the patient sitting or supine, and each should be done individually for all four extremities.

Finger-to-nose testing. The patient is asked to touch alternately his or her own nose and the examiner's finger with the tip of his or her own index finger. The examiner's finger should be far enough away so that the patient must fully extend the arm. Test this with the patient's eyes open and then closed.

Heel-to-shin testing. The patient places the heel carefully on the opposite knee and slides it slowly along the edge of the tibia to the ankle and back up to the knee again.

Rapid alternating testing. The patient pats each hand or foot as rapidly and regularly as possible against a firm surface. A more difficult variation requires alternately patting the front and back of the hand on the knee as rapidly and regularly as possible.

Gait and Station

Tests of gait and station involve all areas of the motor system. Various patterns of gait abnormality occur with different disorders. The test of gait and station is perhaps the single most useful motor system test and should be observed in all patients.

Gait. The patient walks normally back and forth in a moderate rate; he or she then walks on the heels and toes and tandem along a straight line, touching heel to toe; the patient then hops on each leg.

Station. The patient is asked to stand with the feet together, first with the eyes open and then with the eyes closed. There should be little or no sway.

Muscle Tone

The elbows, wrists, and knees are passively flexed and extended with the patient completely relaxed. There should be only a minimal smooth resistance to the movement.

Muscle Bulk

All major muscle groups should be examined for signs of focal atrophy. The diameters of the extremities may be measured and compared with each other.

Abnormal Movements

Because many motor disorders are manifest as abnormal involuntary movements, the patient should be examined undressed, both sitting and supine and fully relaxed for such movements. Fasciculations in particular require careful observation of each area under good lighting.

Clinical Problems

1. A 26-year-old housewife began having infrequent, brief episodes of twitching of her left hand 10 months ago. These ceased 4 months ago, but she then noted clumsiness when using her left hand. This progressed to moderate weakness and a peculiar feeling in her hand. In the past month, she began having headaches.

On examination, she was lethargic but otherwise mentally intact. There was mild swelling of the optic disks bilaterally. She had a mild droop of the lower part of her face on the left, moderate weakness and slowing of rapid alternating movements of the left hand, and a circumduction gait on the left. Reflexes were hyperactive in the left arm and leg, with Babinski's sign on the left. Muscle tone was increased on the left. Sensation was normal except for inability to recognize some objects in her left hand.

a. Identify the level, side, and type of lesion.
b. Which spinal cord tracts would show wallerian degeneration?
c. How does the firing rate of the gamma motor neurons to left-side extremity muscles compare with normal?
d. What were the transient episodes?
e. Would the jugular compression test be useful?

2. A 23-year-old woman has a slowly progressive disorder that first began in high school when she was noted to be "fidgety." She did well in school and worked as a secretary for 3 years. During this time, she experienced gradually increasing jerking movements of her arms and face, and her speech became slurred, to the point that she was no longer able to work. During the past 2 years, her gait has become unsteady and her movements have slowed. She also has had occasional, uncontrollable, flailing movements of her arms. During the past year, her memory has been poor and her intellectual capabilities have deteriorated.

On neurologic examination, she had occasional, coarse, asymmetric jerks of the upper extremities and neck, with some grimacing. Sensation, strength, and reflexes were unremarkable. Her tone was increased, with rigidity in all extremities. She had a coarse intention tremor of both arms.

a. Identify the level, side, and type of disease.

b. What major divisions of the motor system are involved?
c. What two general types of cause must be considered in this disorder?
d. Name the structures in the diseased pathways.
e. What are the signs of basal ganglia disease?

3. A 21-year-old single woman was found lying unresponsive in bed by her girlfriend, who had stopped off in the morning to drive her to work. She called for an ambulance and brought the patient to the hospital. The following facts were obtained from the friend on questioning. The patient had been in good health. She was well the evening before. She was apparently taking no medications, and no empty or partially filled bottles were in evidence. There were no signs of a struggle or violence and no suicide note. She was in bed as though she had been asleep. There were no unusual findings about the patient: no blood, urine, feces, or injuries. But her skin had a peculiar pink appearance.

On examination she was unresponsive to all but painful stimuli, to which she responded with decerebrate posturing, with her arms, legs, and neck stiffly extended. Her eyes apparently did not respond to threatening stimuli but appeared to close randomly. Her jaw was tightly clenched. There were bilateral extensor plantar responses. Her respirations were irregular. Tone was generally increased with some lengthening reaction. Reflexes were generally hyperactive. All other aspects of the examination were within normal limits.

a. Identify the level, side, and most likely type of disease.
b. What other types of disorders can have this temporal profile?
c. There is evidence of involvement of which components of the motor system?
d. How is decerebrate rigidity produced?
e. Which sensory receptors are responsible for a clasp-knife reflex?

4. A 9-year-old boy had a mild cold, which a day later was associated with fever and severe aching muscle pains, especially in his back. He was generally weak, but by the fourth day, he noted an inability to move his right leg and the fingers on his left hand. Lumbar puncture revealed that the cerebrospinal fluid was clear and colorless, with a blood glucose level of 68 mg per deciliter, a protein level of 86 mg per deciliter, and 46 lymphocytes per microliter. His generalized symptoms cleared over the next week.

On examination at 3 weeks, there was almost complete paralysis of his right leg, moderate weakness of his left arm, and mild weakness of other muscles, including the facial muscles. Results of sensation and coordination tests were normal—where he was able to perform them. Reflexes were hypoactive in the right leg, which was flaccid. There was atrophy of all muscles, most strikingly in the right leg and left arm.

a. Identify the level, side, and type of disease.
b. Are the cerebrospinal fluid findings of any help in identifying the disease?
c. Which component of the motor system is involved?
d. What are the signs of disease in this component?
e. List the major inputs to the final common pathway.

5. A 58-year-old banker suddenly lost the ability to speak, and within a few minutes he was unable to move his right arm. On examination later in the day, there had been no progression in symptoms. He appeared to understand what he was told, but he could not answer questions. In attempting to speak, he uttered nonsense words or garbled words. A very few words came out correctly, such as "hello." His right arm was paralyzed, and the right cheek and right side of his mouth drooped. Forehead movements were normal. Leg strength was normal. Deep tendon reflexes were hypoactive in his right arm but normal elsewhere. He seemed to recognize sensations everywhere. Results of coordination tests were normal, except in the right arm. His gait was normal. Optic fundi were normal.

a. Identify the level, side, and type of lesion.
b. Specifically, what component and what site in the motor system are involved?
c. How do plantar responses and abdominal reflexes change with lesions in this division?
d. What term is used to describe this speech disorder?
e. Why was forehead movement on the right normal?

6. A 7-year-old boy with a history of chronic recurrent otitis media awoke one morning complaining of headache. At school, he was noted to be awkward and to have trouble using his right hand. By the next day, he was unable to hold a glass of milk in his right hand without spilling it, and he veered to the right when walking.

On examination, his neck was slightly stiff, although his fundi were normal. He had an intention tremor of his right arm and leg, with marked dysmetria of these extremities on finger-to-nose and heel-to-shin testing. Reflexes on the right were slightly hypoactive. Sensation was normal.

a. Identify the level, side, and type of lesion.
b. Why should you hesitate to do a lumbar puncture?
c. Which component of the motor system is involved?
d. Which fiber pathways in this component decussate?
e. What are the functional subdivisions of this component of the motor system?

Additional Reading ∎

Burke, R. E. Spinal cord: ventral horn. In Shepherd, G. M. (ed.), *The Synaptic Organization of the Brain* (4th ed.). New York: Oxford University Press, 1998, pp. 77–120.

De Zeeuw, C. I., Strata, P., and Voogd, J. (eds.). The cerebellum: From structure to control. *Prog. Brain Res.* 114:1, 1997.

Llinás, R. R., and Walton, K. D. Cerebellum. In Shepherd, G. M. (ed.), *The Synaptic Organization of the Brain* (4th ed.). New York: Oxford University Press, 1998, pp. 255–288.

Narabayashi, H., Yanagisawa, N., Nagatsu, T., and Mizuno, Y. (eds.). Parkinson's disease: From basic research to treatment. *Adv. Neurol.* 60:1, 1997.

Wilson, C. J. Basal ganglia. In Shepherd, G. M. (ed.), *The Synaptic Organization of the Brain* (4th ed.). New York: Oxford University Press, 1998, pp. 329–375.

The Internal Regulation System

Objectives

1. Describe the main functions and the general organization of the internal regulation system.
2. List the main components of the central circuits of the internal regulation system at the supratentorial, posterior fossa, and spinal levels.
3. List the main functions of the paralimbic cortex, amygdala, hypothalamus, nucleus of the tractus solitarius, ventrolateral medulla, cranial parasympathetic nuclei, intermediolateral cell column, and sympathetic ganglia.
4. Describe the organization and function of spinal and brainstem visceral afferents. List the location and function of the circumventricular organs.
5. Differentiate sympathetic pathways from parasympathetic pathways by their location, function, and pharmacology.
6. List the main differences between the somatic and visceral motor systems with regard to organization of output, neurotransmission, characteristic of the effectors, and consequences of denervation.
7. List the main humoral and somatic motor output mechanisms of the internal regulation system.
8. Describe the clinical effects of lesions of the hypothalamus, medullary reticular formation, oculomotor nerve, superior cervical and stellate ganglia, and conus medullaris.
9. List sites at which lesions can produce abnormalities of the pupil, and describe the types of abnormalities seen with each lesion.
10. List the sites at which lesions can produce bladder disorders and the type of neurogenic disorder produced by a lesion at each site.

Introduction

The internal regulation system is a critical component of the central core of neurons and pathways that control automatic functions necessary for *life and survival of the species.* The internal regulation system controls visceral, endocrine, and behavioral functions that maintain the internal environment of the body in response to internal and external changes. The neural components are located at supratentorial, posterior fossa, spinal, and peripheral levels. The most important functions of the internal regulation system are (1) maintenance of *homeostasis,* or the internal environment, for cell function; (2) integration of adaptative responses to external and internal stimuli, including reactions to fear and stress; (3) drinking, feeding, and sexual behaviors; (4) modulation of pain sensation; and (5) regulation of immune function.

The internal regulation system performs all these important functions through three components: (1) the *autonomic nervous system,* including pathways innervating the heart, smooth muscle, visceral organs, blood ves-

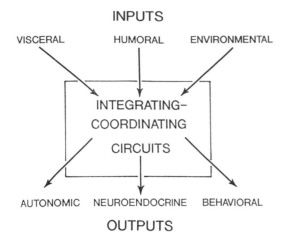

INPUTS

VISCERAL   HUMORAL   ENVIRONMENTAL

INTEGRATING–
COORDINATING

CIRCUITS

AUTONOMIC   NEUROENDOCRINE   BEHAVIORAL

OUTPUTS

FIG. 1. Organization of input, integrating-coordinating, and output components of the internal regulation system.

sels, skin, and eye; (2) the *neuroendocrine system,* including circulating hormones from the pituitary gland and the peripheral endocrine organs; and (3) connections with the *somatic motor system* for expression of com-

plex behaviors such as feeding and drinking and of automatic motor functions such as respiration and swallowing.

Overview ■

The internal regulation system consists of (1) integrating-coordinating circuits; (2) visceral, humoral, and external environmental inputs; and (3) autonomic (visceral motor), neuroendocrine, and somatic motor behavioral outputs (Fig. 1).

The *integrating-coordinating circuits* form a functional unit located at the supratentorial, posterior fossa, spinal, and peripheral levels (Table 1 and Fig. 2). At the *supratentorial level,* the internal regulation system includes the *prefrontal* and *insular cortices,* the *basal forebrain,* and the *preoptic-hypothalamic area.* The prefrontal cortex and insula are involved in high-order visceral sensory and motor functions. The amygdala is critical for ini-

TABLE 1. *Functional anatomy of the internal regulation system*

Level	Area	Function
Supratentorial		
Telencephalon	Insular cortex	Visual sensation
	Anterior cingulate cortex	Visceromotor coordination
	Amygdala	Emotional response (fear)
Diencephalon	Preoptic-hypothalamic area	Homeostasis
		Neuroendocrine control
		Arousal
		Circadian rhythms
		Reproduction
		Feeding and drinking behavior
		Integrated response to stress
		Immunomodulation
Posterior fossa		
Midbrain	Periaqueductal gray matter	Central control of pain
		Response to stress
Pons	Parabrachial complex	Visceral sensory relay
		Micturition
		Respiration
Medulla	Nucleus of the tractus solitarius	First visceral sensory relay
		Integration of brainstem reflexes
		Respiration
	Ventrolateral reticular formation	Vasomotor tone
		Sympathetic activation
		Respiration
		Control of hypothalamic function
	Vagal nuclei	Preganglionic parasympathetic
Spinal		
Spinal cord	Intermediolateral column	Preganglionic sympathetic and parasympathetic

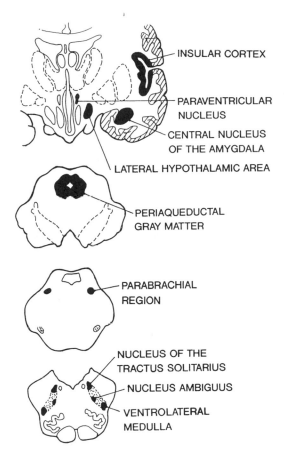

INSULAR CORTEX

PARAVENTRICULAR
NUCLEUS

CENTRAL NUCLEUS
OF THE AMYGDALA

LATERAL HYPOTHALAMIC AREA

PERIAQUEDUCTAL
GRAY MATTER

PARABRACHIAL
REGION

NUCLEUS OF THE
TRACTUS SOLITARIUS

NUCLEUS AMBIGUUS

VENTROLATERAL
MEDULLA

FIG. 2. Principal components of the central integrating-coordinating circuits of the internal regulation system. All these areas are reciprocally connected and contain various neurotransmitters.

tiation of responses associated with emotion. The preoptic-hypothalamic area has a central role in homeostasis.

At the *posterior fossa level,* the internal regulation system includes the periaqueductal gray matter of the midbrain, visceral sensory relay nuclei (particularly the nucleus of the tractus solitarius), autonomic centers of the reticular formation, and cranial parasympathetic nuclei. The periaqueductal gray matter is important for integration of autonomic, motor, and pain-controlling mechanisms associated with response to external stressors, reproduction, and defense behavior. The nucleus of the tractus solitarius is the first relay station for cardiovascular, respiratory, and other visceral afferents. Its main functions are

initiation of cardiovascular and respiratory reflexes and transference of visceral sensory information to other components of the internal regulation system. Neurons of the medullary reticular formation, particularly ventrolateral medulla, maintain such vital functions as vasomotor tone and respiration. The cranial parasympathetic nuclei contain efferent neurons important for control of the pupil, lacrimation, salivation, and visceral organs. The most important output originates from the medullary nuclei that project through the vagus nerve.

At the *spinal level,* the internal regulation system includes the *intermediolateral cell column* (containing thoracolumbar sympathetic and sacral parasympathetic neurons), *phrenic* and other *respiratory motor neurons,* and *sphincter motor neurons* in the sacral cord.

The *autonomic ganglia, peripheral endocrine organs,* and *local circuits* form the internal regulation system at the *peripheral level.*

The integrating-coordinating circuits receive three types of input: visceral, humoral, and exteroceptive (Table 2). Visceral receptive inputs are carried by *general visceral afferent pathways,* which transmit information from visceral receptors via spinal or medullary afferents. Brainstem afferents are carried by the glossopharyngeal nerve (cranial nerve IX) and the vagus nerve (cranial nerve X) and synapse in the nucleus of the tractus solitarius.

TABLE 2. *Input to the internal regulation system*

Input	Source
Visceral	Visceral mechanoreceptors and chemoreceptors
Humoral	Blood temperature, osmolarity, glucose level
	Steroid hormones
	Circulating peptides and monoamines
	Cerebrospinal fluid pH
Exteroceptive	Olfaction
	Taste
	Visual
	Vestibular/auditory
	Somatic sensory (pain)

TABLE 3. *Output mechanisms of the internal regulation system*

Output	Central relay	Effector mechanism
Visceral motor	General visceral efferent column of brain stem and spinal cord	Sympathetic and parasympathetic visceral motor pathways
Neuroendocrine	Hypothalamic-pituitary area	
	Magnocellular system	Vasopressin/oxytocin
	Parvicellular system	Anterior pituitary hormones
	Peripheral endocrine organs	Endocrine cells of adrenal gland, pancreas, kidney, and gut
Somatic motor	Pattern generators of medulla and pons	Automatic motor patterns
	Circuits of limbic system	Complex motivated behavior

Humoral inputs include changes in the composition of the blood and cerebrospinal fluid detected by *central chemosensitive zones* and *circumventricular organs.*

Exteroceptive sensory input is relayed to the paralimbic areas of the brain.

The *three effector mechanisms* of the internal regulation system are the *visceral motor, neuroendocrine,* and *somatic motor* systems (Table 3).

The *visceral motor,* or *autonomic, output* includes the *sympathetic* and the *parasympathetic* outflows. These are two-neuron pathways that synapse in the *autonomic ganglia.* Preganglionic sympathetic neurons form functional units at segments T-1 to L-3 of the spinal cord, the *thoracolumbar outflow.* Preganglionic parasympathetic neurons are located in the brainstem and in segments S-2 to S-4 of the sacral cord, the *craniosacral outflow.* The neurotransmitter of the preganglionic fibers is *acetylcholine,* which acts primarily on nicotinic receptors in the autonomic ganglia (Fig. 3). Postganglionic sympathetic neurons use the neurotransmitter norepinephrine, which acts on adrenergic receptors. Postganglionic parasympathetic neurons use acetylcholine, which acts on muscarinic receptors in target organs. Sympathetic and parasympathetic outputs are continuously active and exert complementary effects in control of the heart and other viscera, blood vessels, and pupillary muscles.

The *humoral,* or *endocrine, output* is mediated by circulating hormones, including peptides secreted by the hypothalamic-pituitary area and hormones secreted by peripheral endocrine cells.

The *somatic motor output* is mediated via connections with the motor system, *central pattern generators* of the medullary reticular formation (which control respiration and swallowing), and the *sphincter motor neurons.*

Circuits of the internal regulation system integrate neural and humoral inputs with neural and humoral outputs. This is critical

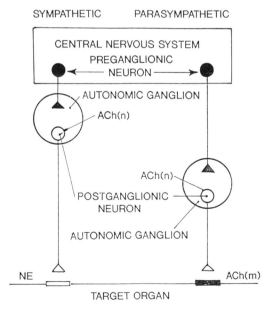

FIG. 3. General organization of the sympathetic and parasympathetic outputs of the internal regulation system. *ACh,* acetylcholine; *NE,* norepinephrine; *(n),* nicotinic receptors; *(m),* muscarinic receptors.

for *tonic maintenance* of vital functions, *reflex adjustments* for homeostasis, and complex *adaptive responses* to change in the internal and external environments.

Abnormal function in the internal regulation system produces several different clinical manifestations. Hypothalamic lesions disrupt control of temperature regulation, water balance, appetite, and endocrine and reproductive functions. With medullary lesions, respiration or vasomotor tone may not be sustained. Central or peripheral autonomic failure produces orthostatic hypotension, inability to sweat, impotence, bladder dysfunction, and abnormal gastrointestinal motility.

Integrating-Coordinating Circuits ■

The *integrating-coordinating circuits* of the internal regulation system are represented at all levels of the nervous system (Table 1). The integrating-coordinating circuits are characterized by reciprocal interactions mediated by several neurotransmitters. Amino acids transmit fast, point-to-point excitatory or inhibitory signals. Monoamines, including catecholamines, and neuropeptides modulate neuronal excitability in central autonomic circuits. Monoamines and neuropeptides may also act by volume transmission, that is, diffusion through the brain extracellular fluid to act on neuronal targets at a distance.

The main interconnecting pathways of the internal regulation system include the afferent and efferent connections of the amygdala, the *medial forebrain bundle,* which interconnects the basal forebrain, preoptic-hypothalamic area, and midbrain, and the *periventricular system,* also called the *dorsal longitudinal fasciculus,* which carries descending inputs to brainstem and spinal cord autonomic nuclei. The medial forebrain bundle and the periventricular system are bidirectional, multisynaptic pathways of the inner tube consisting of unmyelinated or small myelinated axons. Through the medial forebrain bundle, the internal regulation system is interconnected with the diffusely projecting cholinergic and monoaminergic nuclei of the brainstem and forebrain involved in behavioral state control.

Supratentorial Level

At the supratentorial level, the internal regulation system includes visceral areas of the cerebral cortex, the amygdala and associated areas of the basal forebrain, and effector nuclei of the preoptic-hypothalamic area.

Cerebral Cortex

Cortical areas involved in high-order autonomic control include the *insular, orbitofrontal, anterior cingulate,* and *medial temporal cortices* (Fig. 4). These are known as *paralimbic areas* and have connections with the amygdala, hippocampus, and neocortical association areas. The paralimbic areas channel exteroceptive information to the amygdala, hypothalamus, and other components of the internal regulation system. The insula is a primary visceral sensory area and receives general visceral and taste information. The orbitofrontal and anterior cingulate cortices initiate various autonomic responses. These cortical regions are connected with the amygdala and hypothalamus directly or through limbic relay nuclei in the thalamus.

Amygdala

The *amygdala* is critical for initiation and expression of *emotional responses.* It provides emotional significance to internal and external stimuli and initiates the appropriate autonomic and motor responses. These functions depend on the connections of the amygdala with the *cholinergic neurons of the basal forebrain,* the *ventral striatum,* involved in motivated behavior, and the *hypothalamus, periaqueductal gray matter,* and *brainstem autonomic nuclei,* including those in the ventrolateral medulla (Fig. 5).

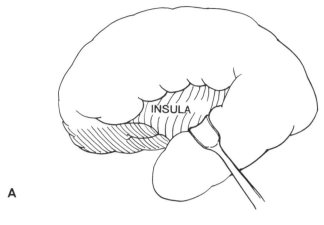

A

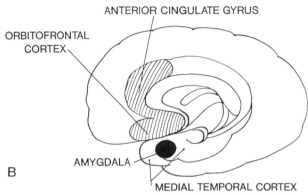

ANTERIOR CINGULATE GYRUS

ORBITOFRONTAL CORTEX

AMYGDALA

B

MEDIAL TEMPORAL CORTEX

FIG. 4. Telencephalic components of the internal regulation system. **A:** The insular cortex is the primary visceral sensory area. **B:** The amygdala is involved in emotions. The orbitofrontal and anterior cingulate cortices integrate autonomic reactions with other behavioral responses.

Preoptic-Hypothalamic Area

The preoptic area and the hypothalamus form a functional unit critical for homeostasis. They receive humoral, visceral, and exteroceptive information and compare this information with a predetermined *set point.* They then initiate compensatory autonomic, humoral, and behavioral responses to regulate the internal milieu around this set point.

The preoptic-hypothalamic area is subdivided into three longitudinally arranged functional zones: the periventricular, medial, and lateral zones (Table 4 and Fig. 6). The *periventricular zone* contains nuclei involved in neuroendocrine control, biologic rhythms such as circadian rhythms, and complex autonomic responses. The *medial zone* contains nuclei that are critical for homeostasis, energy metabolism, and reproduction. The *lateral*

zone participates in arousal, motivated behavior, and autonomic control.

Important hypothalamic nuclei in the periventricular zone include the *suprachiasmatic nucleus* involved in circadian rhythms, the *paraventricular nucleus* involved in integrated hormonal and autonomic responses to stress, and the *arcuate,* or *infundibular, nucleus,* which together with the paraventricular nucleus controls anterior pituitary function.

The medial zone contains several nuclear groups, including the *medial preoptic–anterior hypothalamic region,* which contains sensor neurons for blood temperature, osmolarity, and glucose. Other nuclei in the medial zone are the dorsomedial (autonomic responses to stress) and ventromedial (reproductive behavior) nuclei of the hypothalamus. The *lateral zone,* or *lateral hypothalamic area,* contains the *tuberomamillary nuclei,*

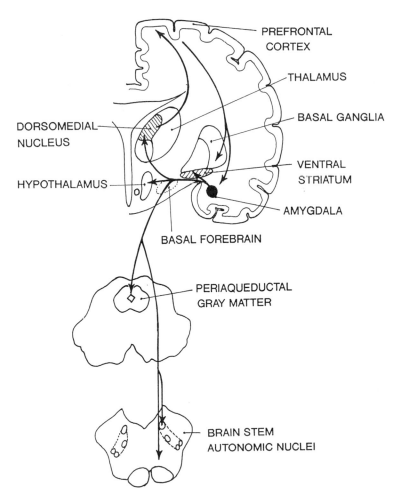

FIG. 5. Main connections of the amygdala. The amygdala coordinates autonomic, motor, and cognitive aspects of the emotional responses.

TABLE 4. *Functional anatomy of the preoptic-hypothalamic area*

Zone	Function
Periventricular	Autonomic responses
	Circadian rhythms
	Neuroendocrine
Medial	Homeostasis
	Energy metabolism
	Reproduction
Lateral	Arousal
	Motivated behavior
	Autonomic control

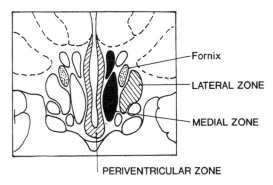

FIG. 6. The three longitudinal functional zones of the preoptic-hypothalamic area (this section is through the hypothalamus).

which project diffusely to the cerebral cortex and are involved in arousal. The lateral hypothalamic area contains the medial forebrain bundle, which includes dopaminergic pathways of the reward system of the brain involved in motivated behavior.

The *autonomic output* of the hypothalamus originates from several regions, particularly the *paraventricular nucleus,* the *lateral hypothalamic area,* and the *dorsomedial nucleus.* These regions contain intermixed populations of neurons that project directly to lower autonomic centers, including the nucleus of the tractus solitarius, medullary reticular formation, and preganglionic sympathetic and parasympathetic neurons (Fig. 7).

The *neuroendocrine output* is mediated via two systems. The *magnicellular system* includes neurons of the *supraoptic* and *paraventricular nuclei* that secrete *vasopressin* (*antidiuretic hormone*) and *oxytocin* (Fig. 8A). The *parvicellular,* or *tuberoinfundibular, system* includes neurons in the *preoptic, paraventricular,* and *arcuate nuclei* that secrete *releasing* or *inhibiting factors* to control anterior pituitary function (Fig. 8B). The interactions of the hypothalamus with the endocrine system are mediated via several feedback mechanisms (Fig. 9).

The *hypothalamic outputs* important in behavior are mainly the connections of the lateral hypothalamic area with the cerebral cortex, basal forebrain, and somatic motor circuits. These outputs are involved with control of arousal and complex motor behavior (Fig. 10).

Posterior Fossa Level

The brainstem components of the internal regulation system include the *periaqueductal gray matter* of the midbrain, the *parabrachial region* of the pons, the *nucleus of the tractus solitarius,* autonomic centers of the reticular formation of the *ventrolateral medulla* and pons, and *preganglionic parasympathetic cranial nerve nuclei* of the midbrain, pons, and medulla (Table 5).

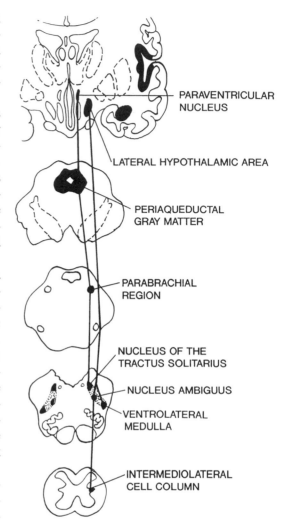

FIG. 7. Important sources of autonomic outputs of the hypothalamus. The hypothalamic area contains mixed populations of neurons controlling sympathetic and parasympathetic outputs.

PARAVENTRICULAR NUCLEUS

LATERAL HYPOTHALAMIC AREA

PERIAQUEDUCTAL GRAY MATTER

PARABRACHIAL REGION

NUCLEUS OF THE TRACTUS SOLITARIUS

NUCLEUS AMBIGUUS

VENTROLATERAL MEDULLA

INTERMEDIOLATERAL CELL COLUMN

The *periaqueductal gray matter* coordinates motor and autonomic responses to stressful external stimuli and plays a critical role in central inhibitory control of pain transmission. The *parabrachial region,* located in the dorsal pons close to the superior cerebellar peduncle (brachium conjunctivum), relays input from the nucleus of the tractus solitarius to rostral visceral sensory areas and contains important "premotor" autonomic neurons. *The nucleus of*

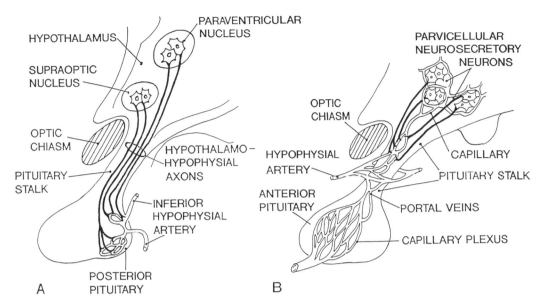

FIG. 8. A: Magnicellular hypothalamic neurosecretory system. Supraoptic and paraventricular nuclei contain separate groups of neurons that produce vasopressin or oxytocin and transport them to the posterior pituitary for release into the general circulation. **B:** Parvicellular hypothalamic neurosecretory system. The nuclei produce releasing or inhibiting factors that control secretory cells in the anterior pituitary.

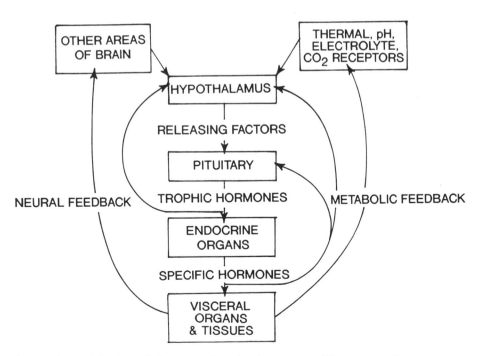

FIG. 9. Interactions of the hypothalamus and endocrine system. Direct *arrows* indicate control, and *loops* show feedback pathways.

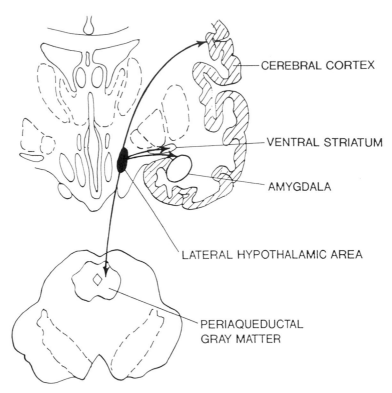

FIG. 10. Hypothalamic outputs important in behavior. Lateral hypothalamic areas project to the cerebral cortex for behavioral arousal and to the ventral striatum, amygdala, and midbrain locomotor region to mediate behavioral responses.

the tractus solitarius is the first brainstem station for the termination of visceral afferents. It has two important functions: it is the site of initiation and integration of many autonomic reflexes, and it provides input to all areas of the autonomic core, particularly the hypothalamus.

Complex networks of neurons in the brainstem reticular formation control preganglionic visceral motor neurons and respiratory and sphincter motor neurons. These neurons are concentrated in the parabrachial region, the nucleus of the tractus solitarius,

TABLE 5. *Autonomic regions of the brainstem*

Level	Region	Function
Midbrain	Periaqueductal gray matter	Pain control
		Defense reaction
Pons	Parabrachial region	Micturition center
		Pneumotaxic center
Medulla	Nucleus of the tractus solitarius	Relay of visceral afferents
		Cardiovascular reflex center
		Dorsal respiratory group
	Ventrolateral reticular formation	Premotor sympathetic neurons
		Ventral respiratory group
		Visceral sensory relay
	Dorsal nucleus of the vagus	Preganglionic vagal
	Nucleus ambiguus	Preganglionic vagal

and the ventrolateral medulla. The ventrolateral medulla contains several groups of neurons that have spontaneous activity and provide continuous excitation to motor neurons that sustain vasomotor tone and respiration.

The *micturition centers* in the pons contain neurons that control bladder and sphincter function. The *respiratory groups* contain inspiratory and expiratory neurons that project to spinal phrenic and intercostal respiratory motor neurons, respectively. Brainstem respiratory neurons located in the parabrachial region, nucleus of the tractus solitarius, and ventrolateral medulla are called *pontine (pneumotaxic center), dorsal,* and *ventral respiratory groups,* respectively. A group of interneurons close to the ventral respiratory group is critical for generation of respiratory rhythm.

An important group of *vasomotor neurons* in the *rostral ventrolateral medulla* projects directly to sympathetic preganglionic neurons and maintains basal arterial blood pressure, mediates sympathetic reflexes, and serves as the relay station for many pathways affecting the sympathetic system. The ventrolateral medulla, in the region of the *nucleus ambiguus,* also contains *cardiovagal neurons* that control heart rate.

The portion of medullary reticular formation that extends from the nucleus of the tractus solitarius to the ventrolateral medulla is called the *intermediate reticular zone.* It contains interneurons that coordinate various respiratory and cardiovascular reflexes. Medullary vasomotor, cardiomotor, and respiratory neurons and control networks are intermingled, functionally related, and have reciprocal connections. The descending brainstem pathways for control of breathing, blood pressure, sweating, and micturition run in the ventral half of the white matter of the lateral columns of the spinal cord.

Autonomic Output Neurons in the Brainstem

The autonomic output neurons of the brainstem occupy the *general visceral efferent column* in the midbrain, pons, and medulla. These neurons are preganglionic parasympathetic neurons located in the nuclei of cranial nerves III (oculomotor nerve), VII (facial nerve), IX (glossopharyngeal nerve), and X (vagus nerve). The most important autonomic output from the brainstem is carried by the vagus nerve and originates from the *dorsal nucleus of the vagus* and the *nucleus ambiguus* (Fig. 11). Vagal output controls respiratory, cardiovascular, and gastrointestinal functions.

Spinal Level

Spinal components of the internal regulation system include *preganglionic visceral motor neurons* and *somatic motor neurons* that innervate respiratory and external sphincter muscles. Preganglionic autonomic neurons occupy the *intermediolateral cell column* of the gray matter and include the *thoracolumbar (sympathetic) cell group* and the *sacral (parasympathetic) cell group.* These neurons are the final common pathway for central control of visceral function. Preganglionic sympathetic neurons are organized in separate functional units (sudomotor, vasomotor, visceral motor), which generate integrated responses throughout the body for control of blood pressure, heart rate, body temperature, and other functions. Sacral parasympathetic neurons control rectal, bladder, and sexual function via *sacral parasympathetic reflexes.*

Respiratory motor neurons include inspiratory neurons at spinal levels C-3 and C-4, which innervate the diaphragm via the phrenic nerve, and intercostal motor neurons at spinal levels T-1 to T-10, which innervate intercostal and abdominal muscles. *Sacral motor neurons* located at the level of S-2 to S-4 innervate the pelvic floor muscles and the external sphincters and are an integral part of reflexes controlling bladder, rectal, and sexual function.

Peripheral Level

Visceral sensory and humoral inputs may initiate visceral motor or endocrine responses via reflex mechanisms that are integrated peripherally. These reflexes may be integrated

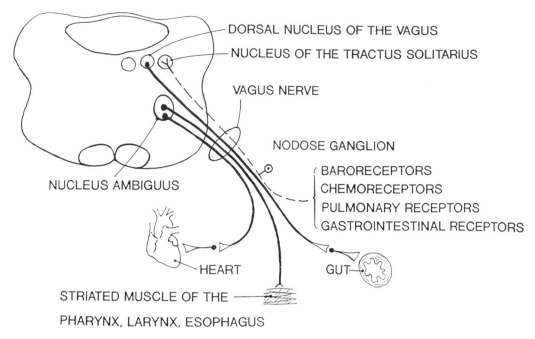

FIG. 11. Components of the vagus nerve. Most of the fibers of the vagus nerve are afferent.

locally at the level of the target organs, at the level of the autonomic ganglia (ganglion reflexes), and at the level of the peripheral endocrine organs. Local reflexes are typical of the *enteric nervous system,* which is located in the wall of the gut. It contains afferent neurons, interneurons, and efferent neurons that respond to local mechanical and chemical influences and control peristalsis and secretions in the gastrointestinal tract. Ganglion reflexes generate topographically restricted visceral motor responses. Inputs integrated at the level of the *peripheral endocrine organs* produce widespread humoral influences.

Input to the Internal Regulation System

Afferents from Visceral Organs

General Characteristics

Visceral receptors are mechanoreceptors or chemoreceptors located in the muscular wall

and the mucosal and serosal surfaces of internal organs, blood vessels, and pleural and peritoneal cavities. Most visceral receptors are innervated by small myelinated and unmyelinated fibers. Visceral afferents, similar to somatic afferents, have cell bodies in the dorsal root ganglia or cranial nerve ganglia. The density of innervation of the viscera is low compared with that of skin and deep somatic tissues. This explains the vague spatial resolution of visceral sensation.

Unmyelinated visceral afferents contain several combinations of neuropeptides and, as nociceptive afferents do, may release neuropeptides centrally (to transmit visceral sensory information) and locally (via axon reflexes to produce vascular and secretory changes at the level of the site of stimulation).

Visceral afferents have two functions. They provide input to central structures for conscious sensation of visceral stimuli, and they initiate visceral reflexes. Most visceral afferent information is concerned with unconscious monitoring of the internal milieu and is used to produce reflex adjustments of visceral function through visceral efferents. General visceral afferent signals follow three main routes. Some remain in the peripheral organ to mediate local reflexes, some provide collateral input to autonomic ganglion cells to mediate ganglion reflexes, and some enter the central nervous system at the level of the spinal cord or brainstem.

In the central nervous system, visceral afferents either synapse on second-order neurons that project to higher levels to initiate integrated arousal, autonomic, and humoral responses or synapse (directly or through interneurons) on visceral or somatic motor neurons to initiate visceral-visceral or visceral-somatic reflexes. General visceral afferents may be subdivided into two groups: afferents that enter the central nervous system at the spinal level (Fig. 12) and those that enter at the brainstem, or posterior fossa, level (Table 6).

Spinal Visceral Afferents

Spinal visceral afferents have an important role in nociceptive (visceral pain) and non-nociceptive visceral sensation and in spinal visceral-somatic and visceral-visceral reflexes (Fig. 13). Spinal afferents have cell bodies in dorsal root ganglia. They pass through the paravertebral ganglia via the sympathetic and sacral parasympathetic nerve trunks and join the spinal roots to enter the spinal cord. The afferents of an organ terminate mainly in one or two segments of the spinal cord, although there is some overlap between afferents from different organs. Some primary afferents may branch peripherally to supply both visceral and somatic structures, and some may enter the spinal cord through the ventral roots.

In the spinal cord, visceral afferents branch extensively to provide divergent input to many

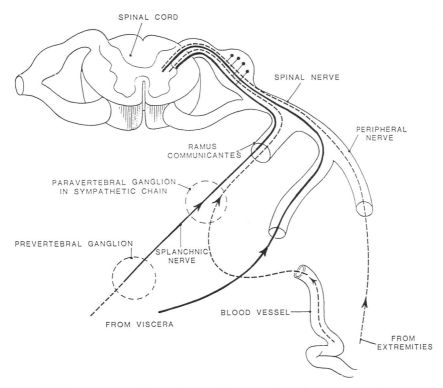

FIG. 12. Visceral afferents reach the spinal cord by several pathways. Afferents travel directly via peripheral nerves or indirectly through sympathetic paravertebral or prevertebral ganglia, whether coming from the extremities or the viscera.

TABLE 6. *Spinal and brainstem visceral afferents*

	Spinal afferents	Brainstem afferents
Peripheral nerve trunk	Sympathetic Sacral parasympathetic	Cranial parasympathetic (CN IX and X)
First-order neuron	Dorsal root ganglion	Nodose ganglion (CN X) Petrosal ganglion (CN IX)
First central relay	Dorsal horn	Nucleus of the tractus solitarius
Mediation of visceral pain	Yes	No
Reflex function	Generally excitatory	Generally inhibitory

CN, cranial nerve.

dorsal horn neurons and interneurons. They synapse on the so-called *viscerosomatic neurons* in the dorsal horn and intermediate gray matter. These special second-order neurons receive convergent inputs from visceral and somatic afferents.

Visceral sensation is carried mainly via ventrolateral pathways in the spinal cord, including the spinothalamic and spinoreticular pathways, which transmit *visceral pain,* and the spinosolitary and spinomesencephalic pathways, which may activate descending input that inhibits pain transmission in the dorsal horn. Some information may be carried by the dorsal columns, including sensations related to micturition, defecation, and gastric distention. Visceral sensory input is relayed in the *midline* and *ventral posteromedial thalamic nuclei* and terminates in the *insular cortex.*

Visceral sensory pathways send numerous collaterals to the ventral medullary reticular formation, which initiates visceral-visceral and visceral-somatic reflexes and gives rise to descending reticulospinal pathways controlling pain transmission in the dorsal horn, and to brainstem, hypothalamic, and limbic regions to initiate adaptive, affective, autonomic, and neuroendocrine responses.

Spinal visceral afferents have an exclusive role in transmission of *visceral pain.* Visceral

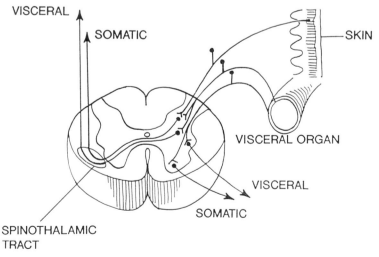

FIG. 13. Visceral afferents make many connections in the spinal cord. Local reflexes are mediated via visceral and somatic motor neurons. Synapses with second-order neurons carry information to the brain through the spinothalamic tract. Some of the visceral afferents may end on second-order neurons in the somatic sensory system as well, resulting in referred pain.

pain may be initiated from mechanoreceptors (signaling visceral distention), chemoreceptors, or thermoreceptors; it is relayed centrally, but there is no clear topographic representation of the viscera. Unlike somatic pain, visceral pain is generally vague and poorly localized—being described as abdominal, thoracic, or pelvic rather than being localized to a specific organ. It commonly activates autonomic and somatic reflex responses. Visceral pain is often referred to overlying or nearby somatic structures; this is called *referred pain* (Fig. 14). Referred pain may be due to convergence of visceral and somatic afferents onto a common viscerosomatic neuron pool in the spinal cord.

Brainstem Visceral Afferents

Brainstem visceral afferents are carried by the vagus and glossopharyngeal nerves. *Vagal afferents,* with cell bodies in the nodose ganglion, carry information from gastrointestinal, tracheobronchial, and cardiopulmonary mechanoreceptors and chemoreceptors and from aortic baroreceptors and chemoreceptors. *Glossopharyngeal afferents,* with cell bodies in the petrosal ganglion, carry input from baroreceptors and chemoreceptors in the carotid sinus and carotid body, respectively. Vagal and glossopharyngeal afferents relay in the *nucleus of the tractus solitarius.* This nucleus transmits visceral information to other brainstem autonomic nuclei and to the hypothalamus, amygdala, medial thalamus, and insular cortex.

Vagal and glossopharyngeal afferents initiate several important medullary cardiovascular and respiratory reflexes. Brainstem visceral afferents have a minor role in visceral sensation and do not mediate visceral pain, although they may trigger central pain-controlling mechanisms. Together with taste and trigeminal afferents, brainstem visceral afferents are also important in initiating such automatic motor acts as swallowing, vomiting, and coughing. These complex motor acts involve *central pattern generators* in the lateral reticular formation of the medulla.

Humoral Input

Humoral input to the internal regulation system may arise from the *blood,* the *cerebrospinal fluid,* or the *circumventricular organs.*

Direct Effects of Blood Composition

Changes in blood glucose, blood gases, electrolytes, temperature, osmolarity, and steroid hormones exert influence at all levels of the internal regulation system. For example, the hypothalamus, medulla, and pancreas contain glucoreceptors, and the skin, viscera, spinal cord, brainstem, and hypothalamus contain thermoreceptors. Some chemical stimuli may act only on specific receptors. For example, a decrease in arterial oxygenation activates mainly chemoreceptors in the carotid body. Steroids exert a widespread influence because steroid hormone receptors are widely distributed in the central nervous system.

Composition of the Cerebrospinal Fluid

Changes in pH and partial pressure of carbon dioxide in the cerebrospinal fluid are detected by *central chemosensitive areas* of the

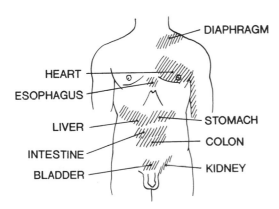

FIG. 14. *Shading* shows dermatomal areas in which pain is felt with disease in visceral organs (referred pain).

ventral surface of the medulla. The cerebrospinal fluid also contains neuropeptides that are released from the hypothalamic-pituitary area and that can exert marked effects throughout the neuraxis.

Circumventricular Organs

Circumventricular organs are specialized structures located in the walls of the ventricles. They characteristically contain fenestrated capillaries and lack a blood–brain barrier (see Chapter 6). Circumventricular organs detect chemical changes in the blood and cerebrospinal fluid and relay this information to the rest of the internal regulation system. For example, the *area postrema* in the walls of the fourth ventricle mediates the emetic effects of dopamine and other substances. Another circumventricular organ, the *subfornical organ,* located in the anterior wall of the third ventricle immediately below the fornix, mediates the important effects of circulating angiotensin II and natriuretic peptides on blood pressure, thirst, and sodium balance.

Exteroceptive Input

The internal regulation system receives input from sensory pathways and association areas of the cerebral cortex.

Pain and Temperature

Spinoreticular and trigeminoreticular pathways relay nociceptive and thermal information to central autonomic circuits in the ventral medulla, dorsal pons, periaqueductal gray matter, hypothalamus, and amygdala and initiate suprasegmental somatic-visceral reflexes. Connections with the medial thalamus and limbic cortex are important for the affective component of visceral pain.

Special Somatic Afferents

Visual input reaches the suprachiasmatic nucleus of the hypothalamus and is important in circadian rhythms. Vestibular input, through connections of the vestibular nuclei and the fastigial nucleus of the cerebellum with the area postrema and the nucleus of the tractus solitarius, mediates vomiting and other manifestations of acute vestibular dysfunction.

Taste and Olfaction

Input from the *taste buds* is transmitted via the facial, glossopharyngeal, and, to a lesser extent, vagus nerves to the rostral portion of the nucleus of the tractus solitarius and relayed to the ventromedial nucleus of the thalamus and then to insular cortex. Olfactory input reaches the anterior medial temporal cortex.

Cortical Input

Information relayed to the cerebral cortex by different sensory pathways is integrated in cortical association areas. This highly integrated exteroceptive and interoceptive information is sent by these cortical areas to the *paralimbic areas* of the cerebral cortex, including the *orbitofrontal, anterior cingulate, insular,* and *medial temporal* regions. These regions project to the amygdala and the hypothalamus, which are involved in elaborating the emotional aspects of sensation.

Output of the Internal Regulation System

General Visceral Efferents

General Organization

General visceral efferents are contained in the sympathetic and parasympathetic divisions of the autonomic nervous system. Autonomic influences are more continuous and generalized and have a longer latency and duration than the effects of the somatic efferent system. The differences between the functional organization of the efferent systems are summarized in Table 7.

TABLE 7. *Comparison between the general visceral efferent system and the general somatic efferent system*

	Visceral	Somatic
Activity	Tonic, slow, diffuse	Phasic, fast, local
Output	Two neurons (preganglionic and postganglionic)	One neuron (alpha motor neuron)
Efferent axon	Small myelinated	Large myelinated
Effector neurotransmitter (receptor)	Acetylcholine (muscarinic) Norepinephrine (adrenergic)	Acetylcholine (nicotinic)
Effectors		
Type	Heart, smooth muscle, glands	Striated muscle
Spontaneous activity	Yes	No
Effect of denervation	Supersensitivity	Paralysis, atrophy

The tonic activity of visceral efferents is due to spontaneous discharge of reticular pacemaker neurons in the brainstem. The visceral output involves a *two-neuron pathway,* with at least one synapse in the *autonomic ganglia.*

Preganglionic Component

The preganglionic neurons occupy the general visceral efferent column of the brainstem and spinal cord. The preganglionic sympathetic neurons are located in the intermediolateral cell column of spinal segments T-1 to L-3 (*thoracolumbar outflow*). The preganglionic parasympathetic neurons are located in the brainstem and in spinal segments S-2 to S-4 (*craniosacral outflow*).

Preganglionic autonomic neurons, similar to somatic motor and branchial motor neurons, originate from the basal plate and use *acetylcholine* as their primary neurotransmitter. Their axons emerge from the brainstem or spinal cord as small myelinated fibers and pass through peripheral nerves to the autonomic ganglia.

Autonomic Ganglia

The peripheral autonomic ganglia are not only synaptic relay stations but also sites of complex interactions affecting the transmission of preganglionic input to postganglionic neurons. Acetylcholine, the neurotransmitter of preganglionic sympathetic and parasympathetic fibers, primarily produces a fast excitation of ganglion neurons via *nicotinic receptors.*

Autonomic ganglion neurons, like dorsal root ganglion neurons, originate from the neural crest. Their axons, called *postganglionic fibers,* are *unmyelinated* and contain varicosities from which acetylcholine or norepinephrine is released together with neuropeptides and other cotransmitter agents.

Visceral Plexuses

Visceral plexuses are complex networks of neurons and axons and consist of four main elements: preganglionic parasympathetic efferents, postganglionic sympathetic efferents, primary visceral afferents, and clusters of peripheral sympathetic or parasympathetic ganglion cells.

Autonomic Neurotransmission

The autonomic terminals are varicosities that release neurotransmitter to interact with receptors at specific postjunctional sites and at extrajunctional sites in the membrane.

The primary postganglionic sympathetic neurotransmitter is *norepinephrine,* which acts via different subtypes of *adrenergic receptors.* As an exception, the sympathetic input to sweat glands is mediated by acetylcholine.

Norepinephrine is inactivated mainly through reuptake by presynaptic terminals. It is metabolized by the enzymes monoamine oxidase and catechol-*O*-methyltransferase.

The primary postganglionic parasympathetic neurotransmitter is *acetylcholine,* which acts via different subtypes of *muscarinic* receptors. Acetylcholine is rapidly hydrolyzed by *acetylcholinesterase.* Adrenergic and muscarinic receptors are G-protein–linked receptors that initiate slow onset and relatively persistent electrical and biochemical effects in their targets. In addition to acetylcholine or norepinephrine, postganglionic autonomic terminals release other cotransmitter substances, including adenosine triphosphate (ATP) and neuropeptides.

Modulation of Autonomic Neurotransmission

Autonomic neurotransmission is modulated by inhibitory feedback effects of norepinephrine or acetylcholine acting via presynaptic autoreceptors, effects of neuropeptide cotransmitters, local factors (for example, histamine, serotonin, prostaglandins, and kinins), and circulating hormones.

Sympathetic Outflow

Descending Pathways

Descending inputs to preganglionic sympathetic neurons originate from several sources, particularly the hypothalamus and ventral medulla. These inputs are neurochemically complex—they contain excitatory amino acids, monoamines, and several neuropeptides—and innervate functionally different subsets of preganglionic sympathetic neurons.

The rostral ventrolateral medulla provides the critical input for tonic maintenance of sympathetic vasomotor activity. Descending sympathetic pathways occupy a narrow band in the lateral column of the spinal cord. This input has three main functions: (1) to provide tonic excitation of preganglionic sympathetic neurons, (2) to mediate reflex and adaptive influences on sympathetic activity, and (3) to allow a functionally selective, rather than a massive, sympathetic discharge.

Preganglionic Sympathetic Neurons

Preganglionic sympathetic neurons are located in the intermediolateral cell column of spinal segments T-1 to L-3 (Fig. 15). They are organized into different *preganglionic sympathetic functional units* that control specific targets and are under specific control of hypothalamic and brainstem areas.

Preganglionic sympathetic fibers have a segmental organization, but their distribution does not follow the dermatomal pattern of somatic nerves. Thus, preganglionic neurons in spinal segments T-1 to T-2 innervate the head and neck; T-3 to T-6, the upper extremities and thoracic viscera; T-7 to T-11, the abdominal viscera; and T-12 to L-3, the lower extremities and pelvic and perineal organs.

Preganglionic sympathetic axons are myelinated, exit through the ventral roots, and pass via the *white rami communicantes* of the corresponding spinal nerve to reach the *paravertebral sympathetic chain.* At this level, preganglionic fibers may (1) synapse on a postganglionic neuron at the same level, (2) branch and run rostrally and caudally in the sympathetic chain to synapse on a large number of postganglionic neurons, (3) pass through the paravertebral chain without synapsing and form the *splanchnic nerves* that innervate *prevertebral ganglia,* or (4) pass through the chain as splanchnic nerves to innervate the *adrenal medulla* (Fig. 16). The adrenal medulla, a homologue of a sympathetic ganglion, releases its neurotransmitters, mainly epinephrine, into the blood stream.

Sympathetic Ganglia

Sympathetic ganglia can be subdivided functionally into two classes: *paravertebral* (or sympathetic trunk) *ganglia* and *prevertebral* (or autonomic plexus) *ganglia* (Table 8 and Fig. 16).

Paravertebral ganglia provide long postganglionic unmyelinated axons to all sympathetically innervated tissues and organs except those in the abdomen, pelvis, and perineum. These fibers follow three main courses: perivascular, spinal, and visceral.

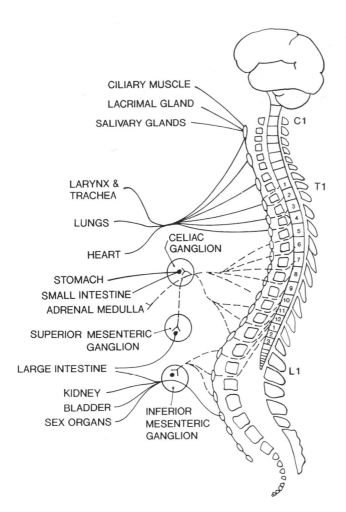

CILIARY MUSCLE
LACRIMAL GLAND
SALIVARY GLANDS

C1

LARYNX &
TRACHEA

T1

LUNGS

CELIAC
GANGLION

HEART

STOMACH
SMALL INTESTINE
ADRENAL MEDULLA

SUPERIOR MESENTERIC
GANGLION

LARGE INTESTINE

L1

KIDNEY
BLADDER
SEX ORGANS

INFERIOR
MESENTERIC
GANGLION

FIG. 15. General organization of the sympathetic outflow system.

Perivascular fibers course along arterial trunks and branches. For example, the axons from the superior cervical ganglion (spinal segments T-1 and T-2) provide pupillodilator and sudomotor innervation to the face and follow the course of branches of the internal and external carotid arteries, respectively. Spinal fibers join the peripheral spinal (somatic) nerves via the gray rami communicantes. Thus, the distribution of postganglionic sympathetic fibers is similar to that of the corresponding somatic nerve. For example, axons from the stellate ganglion innervate the upper extremity via branches of the brachial plexus. Sympathetic fibers traveling in somatic nerve trunks provide *vasomotor, sudomotor,* and *pilomotor* innervation to the extremities and trunk. Visceral fibers from the lower cervical and upper thoracic ganglia innervate the heart via the cardiac plexus to produce cardiac stimulation or reach the tracheobronchial tree via the pulmonary plexus to produce bronchodilatation.

Prevertebral ganglia are anterior to the abdominal aorta, close to the origin of the celiac and mesenteric arteries, and innervate all abdominal, pelvic, and perineal organs. Their preganglionic inputs are carried by the *splanchnic nerves.* Preganglionic input from spinal segments T-5 to L-2 are carried by the splanchnic nerves to the *celiac* and *superior mesenteric ganglia.* These ganglia contribute postganglionic sympathetic fibers to the *celiac plexus,* which innervates all abdominal viscera except the descending colon. The celiac plexus also carries the preganglionic input to the adrenal medulla. Sympathetic input produces

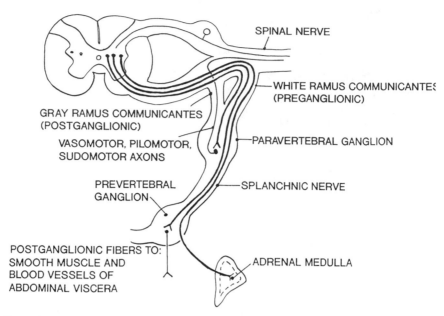

FIG. 16. Organization of the paravertebral and prevertebral sympathetic outflow.

splanchnic vasoconstriction, inhibition of secretion and motility of the gut, and *secretion of epinephrine, renin,* and *glucagon.*

Preganglionic axons from spinal segments L-1 to L-3 travel in the *lumbar splanchnic nerves,* which synapse in the *inferior mesenteric ganglion.* This provides postganglionic axons to the *hypogastric plexus,* which innervates the descending colon and pelvic and perineal organs (rectum, bladder, and genitalia). This input inhibits muscle contractility, allowing storage of urine and feces, and produces *contraction of the vas deferens.* Thus, this sympathetic input is necessary for *ejaculation.*

TABLE 8. *Functional organization of the sympathetic outflow*

Spinal segment	Ganglion	Pathway	Organ	Effect
Paravertebral ganglion				
T-1	Superior cervical	Perivascular (internal carotid)	Pupil	Dilatation (mydriasis)
T-2	Superior cervical	Perivascular (external carotid)	Facial sweat glands	Sweating
T-2 to T-6	Stellate	Gray rami (brachial plexus)	Upper extremity	Vasoconstriction Vasoconstriction in skin Piloerection Sweating
T-9 to L-1	Lumbosacral	Gray rami (lumbo-sacral plexus) Perivascular	Lower extremity	Vasodilatation in muscle
T-2 to T-8	Upper thoracic	Cardiac plexus Pulmonary plexus	Heart Tracheobronchial tree	Stimulation Bronchodilatation
Prevertebral ganglion				
T-6 to T-10	Celiac	Celiac plexus	Gastrointestinal tract	Inhibition of peristalsis and secretion
T-11 to L-1	Superior mesenteric	Celiac plexus	Gastrointestinal tract	
T-12 to L-1	Celiac	Celiac plexus	Kidney	Vasoconstriction Renin secretion
T-10 to L-1	Celiac	Celiac plexus	Adrenal gland	Epinephrine secretion
T-12 to L-3	Inferior mesenteric, hypogastric	Hypogastric plexus	Rectum Bladder Sex organs	Retention of feces Retention of urine Ejaculation

Sympathetic Neurotransmission

Norepinephrine is the primary postganglionic sympathetic neurotransmitter in all organs except sweat glands, which receive sympathetic cholinergic innervation. Epinephrine released by the adrenal medulla acts as a neurohormone that amplifies sympathetic responses. The effects of norepinephrine and epinephrine are mediated by *alpha-* and *beta-adrenergic receptors*. Alpha receptors mediate constriction of smooth muscle in blood vessels and visceral sphincters. Beta receptors mediate cardiac stimulation, relaxation of visceral smooth muscle and some vascular smooth muscle, and metabolic and endocrine effects (Table 9).

Postganglionic sympathetic fibers also release *ATP* and *neuropeptide Y* in addition to *norepinephrine*. Neuropeptide Y is a potent vasoconstrictor; it also modulates noradrenergic transmission by inhibiting presynaptic release and by potentiating postsynaptic effects of norepinephrine.

Parasympathetic Outflow

Cranial Parasympathetic Outflow

Input to cranial parasympathetic nuclei originates in the hypothalamus and the amygdala and descends close to sympathetic pathways in the lateral tegmentum.

The *cranial parasympathetic neurons* are located in the general visceral efferent column of the midbrain, pons, and medulla. Their preganglionic axons are components of cranial nerves III, VII, IX, and X (Fig. 17). The effects of parasympathetic outputs are summarized in Table 10. Parasympathetic output carried in cranial nerve III produces *constriction of the pupil* and *accommodation of the lens*. The output carried in cranial

TABLE 9. *Peripheral autonomic effects*

	Sympathetic		Parasympathetic
	Alpha receptor	Beta receptor	Muscarinic receptor
Heart			
Heart rate		Increases	Decreases
Atrioventricular conduction		Increases	Decreases
Contractility		Increases	Antagonizes
Smooth muscle			
Pupil	Dilatation		Constriction
Lens			Accommodation
Bronchial		Dilatation	Constriction
Gastrointestinal			
Motility		Decreases	Increases
Sphincter		Increases	Decreases
Bladder			
Detrusor		Relaxation	Contraction
Sphincter	Constriction		Relaxation
Sex organs	Ejaculation		Erection
Blood vessels			
Arteries	Constriction (skin, gut, kidney)	Dilatation (muscle, heart)	Dilatation (gut, genital)
Veins	Constriction		
Pilomotor	Contraction		
Glands			
Salivary/lacrimal	Inhibits		Stimulates
Bronchial	Inhibits		Stimulates
Gastrointestinal	Inhibits		Stimulates
Sweat	Stimulates[a]		
Metabolism		Glycogenolysis Lipolysis Renin secretion	Insulin secretion

[a]Postganglionic *sympathetic fibers* that innervate sweat glands are *cholinergic* axons and they act on *muscarinic* receptors.

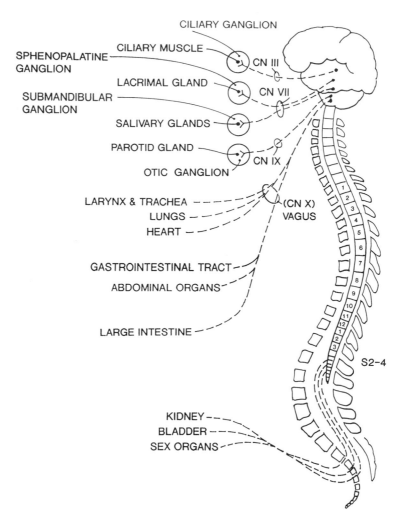

FIG. 17. General organization of the parasympathetic outflow system. *CN,* cranial nerve.

nerves VII and IX stimulates *secretion of lacrimal* and *salivary glands.*

Cranial nerve X, or the *vagus nerve,* provides the most widespread brainstem parasympathetic output. Vagal preganglionic neurons are located in the *dorsal nucleus* of the vagus, which controls respiratory and abdominal viscera, and in the region of the *nucleus ambiguus,* which innervates the heart. The vagus nerve provides input to terminal parasympathetic ganglia located in or near the target organs. Its main effects are *cardioinhibitory, visceral motor,* and *secretomotor.* The cardiac vagus exerts a beat-to-beat control of heart rate. The abdominal vagus facilitates the processes of digestion, absorption, and utilization of nutrients. The vagus nerve innervates neuronal plexuses of the enteric nervous system and stimulates (1) esophageal motility, gastric evacuation, and coordinated peristalsis along the gut; (2) secretion of electrolytes and digestive enzymes by the stomach, liver, pancreas, and intestine; and (3) secretion of insulin and other gastrointestinal peptides.

Sacral Parasympathetic Outflow

The preganglionic neurons are located in the lateral gray matter of spinal segments S-2 to S-4. Their axons pass via the ventral roots

TABLE 10. *Functional organization of the parasympathetic outflow*

	Nucleus	Nerve	Ganglion	Effect
Cranial division				
Midbrain	Edinger-Westphal	CN III	Ciliary	Pupilloconstriction Accommodation
Pons	Superior salivary	CN VII	Sphenopalatine Submandibular	Lacrimation Salivation (submaxillary and sublingual glands)
Medulla	Inferior salivary	CN IX	Otic	Salivation (parotid gland)
	Dorsal nucleus of the vagus	CN X	Near end organs	Bronchoconstriction Bronchosecretory Gastrointestinal peristalsis and secretion
	Ambiguus	CN X	Near end organs	Decreases heart rate and conduction
Sacral division				
Segments S-2 to S-4	Intermediolateral column	Pelvic Splanchnic	Near end organs	Emptying of bladder and rectum Erection

CN, cranial nerve.

to the pelvic splanchnic nerves (nervi erigentes), which join the inferior hypogastric (pelvic) plexus. The sacral parasympathetic system is critical for *defecation, micturition,* and *erection.*

Parasympathetic Neurotransmission

Acetylcholine is the primary postganglionic parasympathetic neurotransmitter at all parasympathetic neuroeffector junctions. It acts via different subtypes of muscarinic receptors (Table 9). These receptors mediate cardiac inhibition, increased contractility of visceral smooth muscle, relaxation of sphincters and visceral blood vessels, and increased secretion of exocrine glands. Postganglionic cholinergic fibers that innervate the exocrine glands also contain *vasoactive intestinal polypeptide,* a potent vasodilator that potentiates the secretomotor effect of acetylcholine. Postganglionic parasympathetic neurons that innervate smooth muscle may also produce *nitric oxide,* which has a potent vasodilator effect and appears to be critical for erection. Nitric oxide is abundant in intrinsic neurons of the gut.

Functional Aspects of Autonomic Control of Visceral Function

The sympathetic outflow responds to stress and facilitates the expenditure of energy. It is particularly active during emotion, fear, cold, exercise, and pain. In contrast, the parasympathetic outflow promotes restoration and conservation of energy stores and is most active during rest and sleep (Table 11).

The sympathetic system may be widely activated; it has widespread influence and relatively long-lasting effects, especially during *fight or flight reactions.* The parasympathetic system has more discrete, localized, and shorter lasting effects. The widespread effects of the sympathetic system may be explained by the considerable divergent output of the preganglionic neurons and by the amplification effects of circulating epinephrine. Also, the longer duration of sympathetic responses may be due to the slower inactivation of norepinephrine by reuptake and metabolism, as compared with the rapid inactivation of acetylcholine by acetylcholinesterase.

Most visceral organs have a dual sympathetic and parasympathetic control. However, peripheral blood vessels, pilomotor muscles, sweat glands, and the spleen receive only sympathetic innervation. Parasympathetic control predominates in the salivary glands, sinoatrial node, and gastrointestinal tract. Sympathetic-parasympathetic interactions are not simply antagonistic but functionally complementary. For example, parasympathetically mediated erection is complemented by sympathetically

TABLE 11. *Comparison between sympathetic and parasympathetic systems*

	Sympathetic	Parasympathetic
Function	Energy expenditure, emergency	Protective, restorative
Effect	Generalized, long lasting	Local, short lasting
Preganglionic neuron	Thoracolumbar cord, T-1 to L-3	Cranial nerves III, VII, IX, X
		Sacral cord, S-2 to S-4
Ganglion	Paravertebral	Near end organ
	Prevertebral	
Preganglionic myelinated fiber	Short	Long
Preganglionic neurotransmitter	Acetylcholine	Acetylcholine
Postganglionic unmyelinated fiber	Long	Short
Distribution	Throughout body	Specific organs
Innervation of limbs	Yes	No
Postganglionic neurotransmitter	Norepinephrine	Acetylcholine
	(except in sweat glands)	
Receptors	Alpha- and beta-adrenergic	Muscarinic
Neurotransmitter inactivation	Slow	Fast
Cotransmitter	Neuropeptide Y	Vasoactive intestinal polypeptide
	ATP	ATP

ATP, adenosine triphosphate.

mediated ejaculation. The interactions between the sympathetic and parasympathetic systems may occur at the level of the central nervous system, autonomic ganglia, neuroeffector junction, or target organ.

Visceral Effectors

The autonomic effectors include the specialized and contractile tissue of the heart, the smooth muscle, and the glandular epithelia. Smooth muscle and cardiac muscles, unlike striated muscle, exhibit the properties of *automatism, adaptation,* and *intramural conduction.* Automatism is the ability to sustain rhythmic contractions in the absence of innervation and is due to generation of impulses by a pacemaker area. This activity tends to spread to other cells, may shift from one region to another, and is affected by autonomic neurotransmitters, local conditions, local neurochemicals, and circulating hormones. Adaptation is the ability of smooth muscle to modify its rhythmicity and contractility in response to mechanical factors, such as stretch or distention of an organ. Intramural conduction involves transmission of electrical input between syncytial fibers through gap junctions (as in the heart and blood vessels) or through local intramural connections (as in the gut).

Whereas the main consequences of denervation in striated muscle are paralysis and atrophy, most autonomic effectors develop *denervation supersensitivity* in response to postganglionic denervation. Denervation supersensitivity is the exaggerated response to the specific neurotransmitter. This phenomenon is clinically important because it indicates a postganglionic lesion.

Humoral Output of the Internal Regulation System

In addition to the fast, short-lasting influences mediated through the autonomic output, the internal regulation system produces longer latency and more prolonged responses via humoral output. This output arises from two main sources: the *hypothalamic-pituitary axis* and the *peripheral endocrine organs.*

Hypothalamic-Pituitary Axis

The neuroendocrine, or humoral, output of the hypothalamus is mediated through two neurosecretory systems: the *magnicellular hypothalamohypophysial system,* which produces *vasopressin* and *oxytocin,* and the *parvicellular tuberoinfundibular system,* which produces *releasing factors* and *inhibiting factors* (regulatory hormones) that regulate anterior pituitary function.

Peripheral Endocrine Organs

Autonomic and pituitary outputs affect the function of peripheral endocrine organs, including the thyroid gland, endocrine pancreas, juxtaglomerular apparatus of the kidney (renin secretion), steroid-producing endocrine glands (adrenal cortex and gonads), and peptide-producing endocrine cells of the gastrointestinal tract. All these peripheral humoral mediators may exert direct effects on target organs, produce local modulation of target responses to autonomic inputs, and influence central neural structures.

Somatic Motor Output

The internal regulation system has important connections with the motor system at all levels of the neuraxis. At the supratentorial level, connections of the lateral hypothalamus and the amygdala with the ventral striatum are important for complex motor behavior. At the posterior fossa level, connections between the nucleus of the tractus solitarius and the central pattern generators of the medullary reticular formation coordinate cranial nerve motor neurons involved in vomiting and respiration. At the spinal level, hypothalamic and brainstem inputs may affect somatic motor respiratory and sphincter motor neurons.

Input-Output Integration in the Internal Regulation System ■

The most characteristic feature of the internal regulation system is the interactions between visceral sensory, humoral, and somatic sensory inputs and visceral motor (autonomic), endocrine, and somatic motor (behavioral) outputs. This interaction occurs at all levels, particularly in the hypothalamus, brainstem, and spinal cord.

Hypothalamic Level

The *paraventricular nucleus* of the hypothalamus is an important output region and is critical for homeostasis and integrated responses to stress. It receives visceral sensory input from the nucleus of the tractus solitarius and the ventrolateral medulla, humoral input from the subfornical organ, and somatic sensory input via spinothalamic pathways or connections with the limbic lobe. The paraventricular nucleus initiates integrated responses to stress. It contains (1) magnocellular neurons that secrete vasopressin and thus regulate water balance; (2) parvicellular neurons that secrete corticotropin-releasing hormone, which stimulates the pituitary-adrenal axis and thus controls glucose metabolism and immune function; (3) central autonomic neurons that project to visceral motor nuclei of the brainstem and spinal cord; and (4) neurons that project to the dorsal horn of the spinal cord to inhibit pain transmission.

Brainstem Level

The medulla is the site of reflex mechanisms critical for control of respiration and circulation. Medullary reflex circuits have several general features. The afferent limb of cardiovascular and respiratory reflexes mediated by the medulla involves input from cardiovascular and pulmonary mechanoreceptors and chemoreceptors carried by the vagus and glossopharyngeal nerves and integrated in the nucleus of the tractus solitarius. The efferent limb is mediated by vasomotor, cardiovagal, or respiratory neurons in ventrolateral medulla and the corresponding spinal outputs. Interneurons in the intermediate medullary reticular formation coordinate the interactions between the nucleus tractus solitarius and neurons in ventrolateral medulla. Vasomotor, cardiovagal, and respiratory medullary neurons form an integrated *cardiorespiratory network,* which is coordinated by local interneurons. Medullary cardiovascular and respiratory neurons are affected by humoral influences, including blood-borne chemicals that act on chemoreceptors in the *area postrema,* a circumventricular organ in the floor of the fourth ventricle. Also, changes in the pH of the cerebrospinal fluid are detected by neurons in the *central chemosensitive zone* of the ventral surface of the medulla. Finally, medullary reflexes may be affected by influences from the hypothalamus and amygdala, which may inhibit or facilitate these reflexes during complex adaptive responses such as exercise and emotion.

Spinal Level

Preganglionic sympathetic neurons are organized into different sympathetic functional units. These include skin vasomotor, muscle vasomotor, visceral motor, pilomotor, and sudomotor units. Therefore, preganglionic neurons do not discharge massively but control specific targets. Thus, instead of there being a generalized sympathetic tone, there is coordinated activity of specific subsets of sympathetic neurons. For example, the sympathetic response to life-threatening conditions includes vasoconstriction in the skin and splanchnic vessels, vasodilatation in skeletal muscle, piloerection, sweating, and release of epinephrine. This is different from the response to a change in posture from supine to standing, which includes predominantly vasoconstriction in skeletal muscle and to a lesser extent in skin but no release of epinephrine, pupillary dilatation, or piloerection. In humans, sympathetic nerve activity in skeletal muscle is finely regulated by baroreflex activity, whereas sympathetic activity in the skin is regulated mainly by environmental temperature and emotional state.

Activity of preganglionic sympathetic neurons depends on supraspinal and segmental inputs. Several parallel pathways descending from the hypothalamus and brainstem exert specific modulatory influences on selective populations of preganglionic neurons. This is critical for their coordinated action. Preganglionic neurons are the efferent limb of various sympathetic reflexes. These reflexes are triggered by skin, muscle, or visceral afferents that are in dorsal roots and generally stimulate preganglionic neurons through local interneu-

rons. The segmental reflexes are controlled by suprasegmental input. For example, innocuous stimulation of the skin or distention of the bladder in normal subjects produces minimal change in preganglionic activity. However, in patients with lesions at a high level in the spinal cord in which descending pathways are interrupted, innocuous stimuli trigger massive sympathetic excitation, including intense sweating, muscle and skin vasoconstriction, tachycardia, and hypertension.

Preganglionic parasympathetic neurons are restricted to spinal segments S-2 to S-4. They innervate the colon, bladder, and sexual organs. Their function involves reciprocal interactions with sacral somatic motor neurons that innervate the sphincters and pelvic floor muscles. Parasympathetic neurons are *excited,* whereas sphincter somatic motor neurons are *inhibited,* during micturition and defecation. The opposite occurs during times of storage of urine and feces.

Specific Circuits ■

Control of the Pupil

The diameter of the pupil is controlled by the balanced activity of two sets of muscles: the *constrictor muscle,* a circular band of muscle fibers; and the *dilator muscle,* a radial band of muscle fibers. The constrictor muscle is innervated by the parasympathetic system, and the dilator muscle is innervated by the sympathetic system. Pupillary constriction is called *miosis,* and pupillary dilatation is *mydriasis.*

Parasympathetic Pathway

The parasympathetic pathway for pupillary constriction is a two-neuron system. Preganglionic axons from the *Edinger-Westphal nucleus* of the midbrain are carried in the *oculomotor nerve* and relay in the *ciliary ganglion* in the orbit. Postganglionic neurons innervate the constrictor (and the ciliary muscle) via the *short ciliary nerves.*

Sympathetic Pathway

The sympathetic pathway for pupillary dilatation is a three-neuron system. The first neuron is located in the hypothalamus. The second neuron is a preganglionic sympathetic neuron in the *ciliospinal center* in the intermediolateral cell column at spinal levels T-1 and T-2. Preganglionic axons enter the sympathetic chain and ascend in the sympathetic trunk to synapse on a third (or postganglionic) neuron, which is in the *superior cervical ganglion*. Postganglionic fibers follow the course of the internal carotid artery and ophthalmic artery to innervate the dilator muscle through the *long ciliary nerves*.

Pupillary Reflexes

Unlike other smooth muscles, pupillary constrictors and dilators do not demonstrate automatic activity in the absence of innervation. The size of the pupil is a function of the relative activity of parasympathetic and sympathetic influences (Fig. 18).

The pathway for pupillary constriction is activated by either stimulation with light (*light reflex*) or near vision (*accommodation*). The pathway for the light reflex is discussed further in Chapter 15. Briefly, it involves afferents in the optic pathway, a synapse in the pretectal area of the midbrain, excitatory input to the Edinger-Westphal nucleus, and efferent axons to the constrictor muscle via the oculomotor nerve and ciliary ganglion. Decussation of the pathway allows stimulation of either eye to produce both an *ipsilateral,* or *direct, response* and a *contralateral,* or *consensual, response*. The *accommodation reflex* is integrated at the level of the oculomotor nucleus and consists of *miosis, gaze convergence,* and *increased curvature of the lens*. Pretectal lesions may result in lack of pupillary response to light but spare pupillary constriction with accommodation.

The pathway for pupillary dilatation is activated mainly by the hypothalamus. The *ciliospinal reflex* consists of pupillary dilatation evoked by noxious cutaneous stimulation, such as pinching the face or neck.

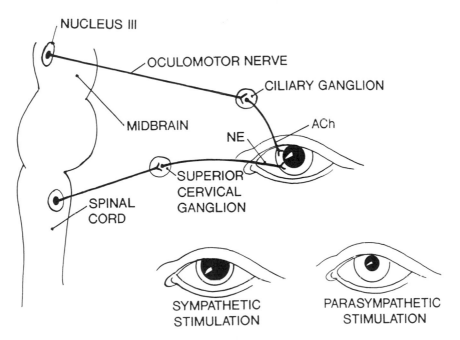

FIG. 18. Effects of sympathetic and parasympathetic activity on pupil size. *ACh,* acetylcholine; *NE,* norepinephrine.

Cardiovascular Control

The autonomic nervous system controls cardiac output and peripheral resistance through its effects on the heart, peripheral vessels, and circulating hormones such as vasopressin and angiotensin II.

Parasympathetic Control

Parasympathetic control of the heart is exerted primarily by neurons in the region of the *nucleus ambiguus* of the medulla and is carried by the vagus nerve. The vagal innervation of the heart decreases heart rate, delays atrioventricular conduction, and antagonizes the stimulating sympathetic effects of myocardial contractility. Vagal influence on the sinus node predominates over that of the sympathetic innervation and allows control of heart rate on a beat-to-beat basis. Vagal effects on heart rate vary during the respiratory cycle and are less marked during inspiration than expiration. This results in inspiratory tachycardia and expiratory bradycardia, known as *respiratory sinus arrhythmia.* This is an important indicator of normal cardiovagal function.

Sympathetic Control

Sympathetic output controls the heart and the blood vessels. Basal sympathetic vasomotor activity originates primarily from *rostral ventrolateral medulla.* Sympathetic output produces (1) an increase in heart rate, atrioventricular conduction, and cardiac contractility via beta receptors; (2) constriction of blood vessels in the skin, kidney, and abdomen via alpha receptors; and (3) dilatation of cardiac and skeletal muscle blood vessels via beta receptors. Constriction of abdominal blood vessels is very important in preventing a decrease in arterial pressure while changing from a supine to a standing position (orthostatic hypotension). Humoral mechanisms, including vasopressin and the renin-angiotensin-aldosterone system, allow longer lasting control of arterial pressure.

Cardiovascular Reflexes

Cardiovascular control centers in the medulla are regulated primarily by two types of influences: by hypothalamic and other descending inputs and by various cardiovascular reflexes integrated at the medullary level. Cardiovascular reflexes include the *arterial baroreflex, arterial chemoreflex,* and *cardiopulmonary reflexes.* They originate from mechanoreceptors or chemoreceptors in the carotid sinus, aortic arch, and cardiac atria and ventricles. Baroreceptor and chemoreceptor inputs from the carotid sinus or the aortic arch are carried to their first central relay station (second-order neuron), the *nucleus of the tractus solitarius,* by afferent branches of the glossopharyngeal and vagus nerves. The cell bodies of these afferents are in the petrosal and nodose ganglia. Inputs from cardiac receptors are carried by either vagal or spinal (sympathetic trunk) afferents. All cardiovascular medullary reflexes are mediated directly or indirectly through the connections of the nucleus of the tractus solitarius with the cardiovagal and sympathoexcitatory neurons in ventrolateral medulla. The arterial baroreflex is a critical buffering mechanism for preventing fluctuations of arterial pressure. This reflex is responsible for rapid adjustments of arterial pressure when adopting erect posture. The carotid sinus and aortic baroreceptors are stimulated by an increase in arterial pressure. Baroreceptor stimulation excites the nucleus of the tractus solitarius, which in turn stimulates cardiovagal neurons and inhibits vasomotor neurons. This produces reflex bradycardia and vasodilatation and a decrease of arterial pressure to basal level. In contrast, a decrease in arterial pressure decreases baroreceptor activity, which results in compensatory tachycardia and vasoconstriction.

Thermoregulation

Changes in body temperature are detected by thermoreceptors in the skin, viscera, spinal cord, brainstem, and, most important, in the hypothalamus. Two regions of the hypothalamus have a major role in thermoregulation: the *preoptic-anterior hypothalamic area* and the *posterior hypothalamic area.* The preoptic-anterior hypothalamic area contains sensor neurons that detect changes in blood temperature and initiate responses leading to heat loss, for example, skin vasodilatation and sweating. The posterior hypothalamic region may integrate the thermoregulatory set point and be involved in responses leading to heat gain, such as vasoconstriction and shivering. There are several effector mechanisms for thermoregulatory control: (1) somatic motor (shivering and behavior in response to thermal discomfort), (2) humoral-metabolic (increased basal metabolism and lipolysis), and (3) autonomic (mainly via effectors in the skin).

Sympathetic innervation of the skin is important in thermoregulation. It includes adrenergic vasoconstrictor, cholinergic sudomotor, adrenergic pilomotor, and vasodilator efferents. The most important effects are regulation of blood flow in the skin and sweating. Exposure to cold temperatures produces skin vasoconstriction (pallor) and pilo-erection, whereas warm temperatures elicit sweating and vasodilatation. Thermoregulatory sweating is mediated by sympathetic cholinergic muscarinic innervation of the eccrine sweat glands. Emotional stimuli (fear, anxiety) and severe decrease in arterial pressure (as in shock) activate vasoconstrictor and sudomotor fibers, resulting in cold, clammy skin.

Control of the Bladder

The control of bladder function is integrated at spinal, posterior fossa, and supratentorial levels.

Spinal Level

At the spinal level, the control of the bladder is exerted via sacral parasympathetic, lumbar sympathetic, and sacral somatic outputs (Table 12 and Fig. 19). The *sacral parasympathetic output* (spinal segments S-2 to S-4), carried via the *pelvic nerve,* is mediated by *muscarinic cholinergic receptors* in the bladder and promotes *bladder emptying,* or *micturition,* by activating the bladder detrusor muscle and relaxing the bladder neck. Sacral parasympathetic mechanisms are critical for bladder function. Lesions of the sacral cord or the cauda equina abolish the micturition reflex. Muscarinic blockade produces urinary retention.

The *lumbar sympathetic output* (spinal segments T-11 to L-3), carried by the hypogastric nerves, produces both relaxation of the detrusor muscle (beta receptors) and contraction of the bladder neck, or internal sphincter (alpha receptors). These actions favor storage of urine. Sympathectomy, unlike parasympathetic denervation, does not significantly affect bladder function.

The *sacral somatic motor output* (motor neurons in spinal segments S-2 to S-4), carried by the pudendal nerve, stimulates the external sphincter via *nicotinic cholinergic receptors* and also promotes urine storage.

TABLE 12. *Innervation of the bladder*

Division	Spinal level	Nerve	Neurotransmitter	Receptor	Mechanism	Effect
Parasympathetic	S-2 to S-4	Pelvic	Acetylcholine	Muscarinic	Contraction of detrusor	Bladder emptying
					Relaxation of sphincter	Bladder emptying
Sympathetic	T-11 to L-3	Hypogastric	Norepinephrine	Beta	Relaxation of detrusor	Retention of urine
				Alpha	Contraction of bladder neck	Retention of urine
Somatic	S-2 to S-4	Pudendal	Acetylcholine	Nicotinic	Contraction of external sphincter	Retention of urine

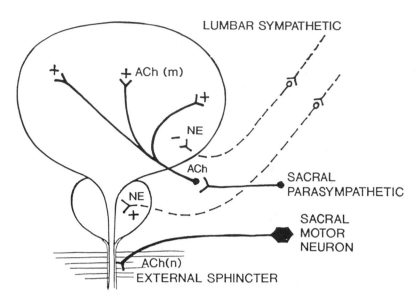

FIG. 19. Innervation of the bladder. *ACh,* acetylcholine; *NE,* norepinephrine; *(n),* nicotinic receptors; *(m),* muscarinic receptors.

Posterior Fossa Level

The *micturition centers* are located in the pons (Fig. 20). They include at least two different regions: a medial region that gives rise to excitatory input to sacral parasympathetic (micturition) neurons, and a lateral region that sends excitatory input to sacral somatic motor neurons (sphincter motor neurons). During micturition, the medial region is activated and inhibits the lateral region. Thus, sacral preganglionic neurons are activated, and sphincter motor neurons are inhibited. This activity produces coordinated bladder contraction and sphincter relaxation, resulting in bladder emptying. Interruption of descending pathways from the pontine micturition centers to the sacral cord, as in cases of spinal cord lesions, may produce incoordinated activity of these effectors, or *detrusor-sphincter dyssynergia.*

Supratentorial Level

Activity of the micturition centers is controlled by input from the hypothalamus and the medial frontal cortex. Cortical input is responsible for voluntary control of the initia-

tion and the cessation of micturition. This control may be interrupted by lesions involving the medial frontal lobes, for example, hydrocephalus and tumors. The result is involuntary micturition that is referred to as *uninhibited bladder.*

Reflex Control of the Bladder

Reflex control of the bladder is initiated by input from volume and tension receptors in the muscular wall that is carried by the pelvic nerve (spinal segments S-2 to S-4), from pain receptors in the submucosa of the base of the bladder that is carried by the hypogastric nerve (spinal segments L-1 to L-3), and from muscle proprioceptors in the external sphincter and pelvic floor that is carried by the pudendal nerve (spinal segments S-2 to S-4) (Fig. 20).

If the neuraxis is intact, micturition primarily involves a supraspinal spinopontospinal reflex that is triggered by stimulation of tension receptors and that is responsible for the coordinated activity of the detrusor and sphincter muscles. If the suprasegmental pathways are interrupted, micturition occurs

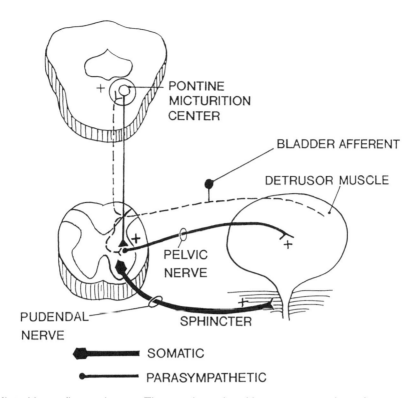

FIG. 20. Micturition reflex pathways. The pontine micturition center consists of a group of neurons that stimulate sacral parasympathetic neurons to activate bladder contraction. In addition, these neurons in the pontine micturition center inhibit other more laterally located neurons that project to and excite the motor neurons that innervate the external sphincter (not shown). Thus, bladder afferents to the pontine micturition center elicit coordinated contractions of the detrusor and relaxation of the sphincter.

via segmental spinospinal sacral reflexes that are triggered by perineal or nociceptive stimulation, but bladder and sphincter contractions are not well coordinated (detrusor-sphincter dyssynergia).

Lumbar sympathetic neurons mediate visceral sympathetic reflexes that are inhibitory. Afferent fibers that are activated by low increases in bladder pressure enter the sacral cord, ascend to the lumbar cord, and stimulate sympathetic efferents that inhibit the detrusor muscle and activate the bladder neck. This promotes *continence.*

In summary, during storage of urine, bladder distention triggers low-level firing of bladder afferents. This stimulates sympathetic outflow, causing contraction of the bladder outlet and inhibition of the detrusor, and pudendal (somatic motor) outflow to the external sphincter. These *spinal guarding reflexes* preserve *continence.* At the onset of micturition, intense activity in bladder afferents activates the pontine micturition center, which simultaneously activates the detrusor and inhibits the spinal guarding reflexes, thus favoring *bladder emptying.*

Reproductive Function

The control of reproductive function includes behavioral, hormonal, and autonomic mechanisms. Sexual and reproductive functions involve interactions among paralimbic, limbic, preoptic-hypothalamic, brainstem, and spinal autonomic centers. The preoptic-anterior hypothalamic region is *sexually dimorphic* (larger in men) and controls sex behavior and release of gonadotropins. In contrast, the arcuate nucleus exerts a tonic, dopamine-mediated inhibition of prolactin release. Both regions are targets of feedback regulation by sex hormones. The autonomic control of sex organs is mediated by the pelvic plexus. In men, sacral parasympathetic output is critical for erection. This involves relaxation of erectile tissue and vasodilatation; these effects may be mediated by nitric oxide or vasoactive intestinal polypeptide (or both) released from parasympathetic neurons. Lumbar sympathetic input produces an alpha-adrenergic–mediated contraction of the vas deferens, which is necessary for ejaculation. In women, parasympathetic input produces increased vaginal secretion and engorgement of the clitoris, whereas sympathetic input facilitates contraction of the cervix and vagina.

Enteric Nervous System

The *enteric nervous system* is a separate division of the autonomic nervous system. It contains a large number of neurons located in the submucosal plexus and the myenteric plexus in the wall of the gut. These plexuses include afferent (sensory) neurons that are stimulated by intestinal distention, excitatory and inhibitory interneurons, and motor neurons. Excitatory and inhibitory motor neurons coordinate peristalsis along the gut. Secretory motor neurons control gastrointestinal exocrine secretions. These neurons contain several neuropeptides in various combinations in addition to acetylcholine, γ-aminobutyric acid (GABA), ATP, and nitric oxide. Enteric neurons are controlled by the vagus and the prevertebral sympathetic ganglia.

Prevertebral ganglia are the site of integration of preganglionic, primary visceral, and enteric sensory inputs. Prevertebral reflexes are stimulated by intestinal distention. Input from enteric cholinergic and primary afferent (peptidergic) axons stimulates noradrenergic ganglion cells, which in turn inhibit myenteric motor neurons, thus providing feedback to reduce the mechanosensitivity of the gut.

Clinical Correlations

Diseases involving the internal regulation system may produce (1) level-specific syndromes, (2) isolated disorders of a particular autonomic effector, or (3) diffuse autonomic failure.

Level-Specific Syndromes

Supratentorial Level

Seizures originating in temporal or frontal limbic and paralimbic areas may produce vegetative auras (olfactory or gastric sensations), autonomic phenomena (tachycardia, pallor or flushing, pupillary dilatation), emotions (anxiety or fear), or complex motor automatisms. Hypothalamic disorders produce complex autonomic and neuroendocrine disturbances that are associated with abnormal thermoregulation, osmolarity, and food intake. The hypothalamus exerts a tonic inhibitory control on the secretion of prolactin. Thus, lesions that interrupt hypothalamic-pituitary connections produce *hyperprolactinemia,* with galactorrhea, amenorrhea, and infertility. Secreting pituitary tumors may produce hyperprolactinemia, gigantism, and hypercorticalism. Pituitary or hypothalamic lesions may also produce *pituitary insufficiency.* Insufficient secretion of vasopressin (antidiuretic hormone) produces *diabetes insipidus.* Excessive secretion of this hormone produces the *syndrome of inappropriate release of antidiuretic hormone.*

Brainstem Level

Brainstem lesions may produce life-threatening disorders affecting respiration (sleep apnea) or cardiovascular disorders (paroxysmal hypertension, intractable hypotension, or cardiac arrhythmias).

Spinal Level

Lesions of the upper spinal cord may interrupt bulbospinal pathways for tonic autonomic control, thus producing respiratory arrest, hypotension, absence of sweating, and urinary retention. Chronic spinal lesions may result in *dysreflexia,* because of lack of modulation of preganglionic neurons by structures above the spinal level.

Peripheral Level

Interruption of either preganglionic or postganglionic output may produce localized or generalized failure of autonomic effectors. An important aspect of peripheral lesions is the development of denervation supersensitivity, which may be useful in localizing the lesion.

Output-Specific Syndromes

Pupil

A *unilateral, large pupil* commonly results from underactivity of ipsilateral parasympathetic outflow. The lesion may occur at the level of the preganglionic neuron (oculomotor nerve), the postganglionic nerve (ciliary ganglion), or receptor (muscarinic blockade) (Table 13).

A *unilateral small pupil* is commonly due to underactivity of the ipsilateral sympathetic outflow. Miosis is commonly associated with ptosis (lid droop due to sympathetic denervation of the tarsal muscle) and facial anhydrosis (loss of sweating), a combination known

as *Horner's syndrome* (Table 14). This syndrome can be caused by (1) central lesions that involve the hypothalamospinal pathway, (2) preganglionic lesions (for example, compression of the sympathetic chain by a tumor in the apex of the lung), or (3) postganglionic lesions at the level of the internal carotid plexus (for example, a tumor in the cavernous sinus).

Cardiovascular Circuits

Baroreceptor dysfunction may produce severe hypertension, arterial pressure fluctuations, or syncope. Lesions involving cardiovascular regulatory centers, descending vasomotor pathways to the spinal cord, or peripheral sympathetic fibers cause *orthostatic hypotension,* a severely disabling symptom of autonomic failure.

Thermoregulation

Sympathetic denervation may produce warm, dry skin, whereas sympathetic hyperactivity produces coldness and sweating. Diffuse sudomotor failure may result in intolerance to heat.

Bladder

Disturbances at different levels of the system for bladder control result in the development of *neurogenic bladder* (Fig. 21). Two types of neurogenic bladder occur: *reflex, or upper motor neuron type,* and *nonreflex, or*

TABLE 13. *Large dilated pupil*

	Preganglionic	Postganglionic	Pharmacologic blockade
Cause	Lesion of oculomotor nerve	Lesion of ciliary ganglion	Muscarinic blockade
Direct light reflex	No	No	No
Consensual reflex	No	No	No
Contralateral eye reflexes	Yes	Yes	Yes
Response to muscarinic agonists (pilocarpine)			
Low dose	No	Yes	No
High dose	Yes	Yes	No

TABLE 14. *Horner's syndrome*

	Central or preganglionic	Postganglionic
Facial sweating	Abnormal	Normal (except above eyebrow)
Response to drugs releasing norepinephrine (methamphetamine)	Yes	No
Response to direct alpha agonist (e.g., norepinephrine)	Normal	Exaggerated (denervation supersensitivity)
Localization of lesion	Hypothalamus Dorsolateral medulla Spinal cord	Superior cervical ganglion Cavernous sinus

lower motor neuron type, depending on the presence and absence, respectively, of bulbocavernous and anal reflexes (Table 15). The two types of reflex bladders include *uninhibited bladder* and *automatic* (or *spastic*) *bladder. Uninhibited bladder* occurs with lesions of the medial frontal cortex and is associated with urinary incontinence but not retention, because of preservation of detrusor-sphincter synergy. *Spastic* (or *automatic*) bladder occurs with lesions of the spinal cord that interrupt the pathway from the pontine micturition centers. Spastic bladder is associated with urgency, frequency, and incontinence and may result in urinary retention, due to detrusor-sphincter dyssynergia. *Flaccid* (or lower motor neuron) bladder is a nonreflex type of neurogenic bladder, such as occurs with lesions

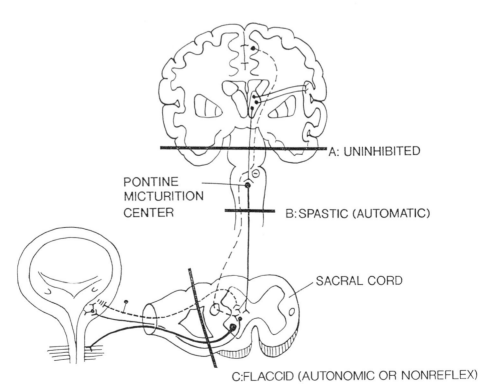

FIG. 21. Sites of lesions producing neurogenic bladder. **A:** Uninhibited reflex bladder. **B:** Spastic (automatic) reflex bladder. **C:** Flaccid (autonomic or nonreflex) bladder.

TABLE 15. *Neurogenic bladder*

	Uninhibited	Spastic (automatic)	Flaccid (autonomic)
Incontinence	Yes	Yes	Yes
Retention	No	No or late (detrusor-sphincter dyssynergia)	Yes
Perianal sensation	Yes	Yes or decreased	No
Anal and bulbocavernous reflexes	Yes	Yes	No
Bladder volume	Normal	Decreased	Increased
Intravesical pressure	Normal	Increased	Decreased
Localization of lesion	Medial frontal lobes	Lower brainstem or spinal cord above level of conus medullaris	Conus medullaris or cauda equina
Example	Hydrocephalus Meningioma	Trauma Multiple sclerosis	Neoplasm Extruded disk Diabetes mellitus Motor radiculopathy

of the cauda equina. It is characterized by urinary retention and overflow incontinence.

Sexual Function

Hypothalamic-pituitary dysfunction may produce amenorrhea, impotence, or infertility. Impotence is also a common manifestation of generalized autonomic failure, lower spinal cord lesions, and peripheral autonomic nerve disease.

Gastrointestinal Function

Dysfunction of the enteric nervous system may result in protracted vomiting, impairment of gastric evacuation, diarrhea, or severe constipation.

Generalized Autonomic Failure

Generalized autonomic failure affects pupillary, cardiovascular, sweating, bladder, sexual, and gastrointestinal functions in several combinations and may occur as a manifestation of central or peripheral lesions. Central lesions occur in neurodegenerative disorders that affect preganglionic autonomic neurons and occasionally sphincter motor neurons and respiratory circuits. Peripheral lesions involve autonomic ganglia or, more

commonly, small unmyelinated postganglionic fibers, as in diabetes mellitus.

Examination of Visceral Function ■

The internal regulation system affects all major organ systems through visceral motor and humoral outputs. The function of each effector system is described above. Several visceral functions are mediated by cranial nerves and are considered in detail in Chapter 15. A limited but important number of specific functions should be tested as part of the neurologic history and examination of visceral function.

Clinical Evaluation

The clinical evaluation of the internal regulation system should include appropriate inquiry into a history of autonomic symptoms and examination of autonomic function in each of the areas listed below.

Pupil

Because the size and symmetry of the pupils and their reactions to light depend on the balance of sympathetic and parasympathetic inputs, these features should be carefully noted. Normal pupils are equal in size (2 to 4 mm in diameter) and react briskly to light in either eye.

Cardiovascular Function

Pulse and blood pressure in supine and standing positions can reflect alterations in neural input and must be part of each examination. A pronounced decrease in arterial pressure when the patient is standing, called *orthostatic hypotension,* particularly when not associated with compensatory increase in heart rate, indicates a dysfunction in the afferent, central, or efferent components of the baroreceptor reflex. Lack of heart rate variability with deep respiration (respiratory sinus arrhythmia) indicates failure of the vagal control of the heart.

Thermoregulation

Skin temperature and sweating are controlled by the sympathetic fibers. A search should be made for the localized absence of sweating, asymmetrical skin temperature or color, and absence of normal oral and conjunctival moisture.

Bladder

The clinical evaluation of neurogenic bladder includes (1) assessment of the ability to voluntarily control initiation or interruption of micturition and bladder sensation; (2) examination of reflexes integrated at the level of the conus medullaris and mediated by sensory and motor roots in the cauda equina (the *bulbocavernous* and *anal reflexes,* which are somatic reflexes integrated at spinal levels S-2 to S-4, and the *scrotal* and *internal anal reflexes,* which are autonomic reflexes integrated at spinal levels S-2 to S-4 and T-12 to L-2, respectively); (3) evaluation of perianal sensation; and (4) quantitation of residual volume, either by palpation and percussion of the bladder for evidence of abnormal bladder dis-

tention or by the postvoid residual after catheterization.

Laboratory Evaluation

Pharmacologic testing with adrenergic and cholinergic agonists is useful for detecting lack of response or denervation supersensitivity of effector organs. These tests are used commonly to assess pupillary control, sweating, and cardiovascular function. *Denervation supersensitivity* is a manifestation of postganglionic, as opposed to preganglionic, autonomic failure.

Pupil

Pharmacologic testing with local instillation of drugs that affect sympathetic neurotransmission in the pupil helps to localize lesions responsible for Horner's syndrome (Table 14).

Cardiovascular Function

Cardiovascular reflex tests used to study patients with autonomic failure include (1) blood pressure and heart rate responses to *head-up tilt;* (2) heart rate fluctuations during deep breathing, or *respiratory sinus arrhythmia;* and (3) the *Valsalva maneuver* (Table 16). During head-up tilt, hypotension with no compensatory tachycardia indicates failure of the afferent, central, or efferent components of the baroreflex arc. Lack of heart rate fluctuations during deep breathing indicates cardiovagal failure. The Valsalva maneuver, a voluntary expiration against resistance, is a complex test that evaluates reflex cardiovagal and sympathetic vasomotor and cardiomotor responses to a transient decrease in cardiac output.

Sweating

The sympathetic innervation of the skin is tested by determining the patient's ability to sweat. The distinction between central and peripheral causes of sudomotor failure can be

TABLE 16. *Findings with clinical testing for autonomic failure*

	Sympathetic dysfunction		Cardiovagal dysfunction
	Central	Peripheral	
Response to head-up tilt			
Blood pressure	Orthostatic hypotension	Orthostatic hypotension	Variable
Heart rate	No increase	No increase	No increase
Respiratory sinus arrhythmia	Normal	Normal	Abnormal
Valsalva maneuver	Abnormal	Abnormal	Abnormal
Thermoregulatory sweat test	Abnormal	Abnormal	Normal
Acetylcholine sudomotor axon reflex	Normal	Abnormal	Normal

made by combining the *thermoregulatory sweat test* and the *acetylcholine sudomotor axon reflex test*. The thermoregulatory sweat test is a test of central and peripheral pathways that measures the sudomotor response to an increase in body temperature. The quantitative sudomotor axon reflex test stimulates receptors in sympathetic sudomotor terminals through local application of acetylcholine. Abnormal results on the thermoregulatory sweat test but normal findings with the quantitative sudomotor axon reflex test indicate central sudomotor failure. Abnormal findings with both tests indicate a peripheral lesion (Table 16).

Bladder

Clinical evaluation of neurogenic bladder is complemented by urodynamic evaluation, including cystometrography, measurement of bladder pressure and urinary flow, and electromyography of the external sphincter.

Sex Organs

Evaluation of impotence includes measuring levels of such hormones as prolactin and testosterone and performing the penile tumescence test during sleep.

Gastrointestinal Tract

Motor function of the gut is tested by measuring the magnitude, frequency, rhythm, and distribution of peristaltic waves with pressure transducers.

Clinical Problems

1. A 52-year-old man was referred for evaluation because of blackouts. The spells began a year before admission and were becoming more frequent. They occurred only when he arose from a supine or sitting position to a standing one and were most severe in the morning. This change in position precipitated a giddy feeling in his head and dimness of vision and often was followed by complete loss of consciousness. No convulsive movements were observed, and shortly after hitting the floor he regained consciousness, only to pass out again if he got up too quickly.

   In addition to this primary symptom, the patient complained that during the last 3 years, he had gradually become sexually impotent. He also noted that he felt very uncomfortable in hot weather and did not perspire as he had before. Occasionally, fever would develop during hot weather, with no evidence of infection.

   On examination, blood pressure was recorded at 130/70 mm Hg when the patient was supine. When he sat up, it decreased to 110/50 mm Hg. When he stood, it was 70/30 mm Hg, and he began to complain of faintness. Pulse rate was 82 to 90 per minute during the entire episode. The skin was warm and dry and remained so after many minutes in a hot examining room. Results of the rest of the physical examination were normal.

a. What is the site of the lesion?
b. What is the type of lesion?
c. Which of the patient's symptoms could be due to a disorder of sympathetic efferents?
d. What effect would pilocarpine (which directly stimulates sweat glands) have on this patient?
e. Which of the following may result in hypotension?
   i. Spinal cord lesion at T-2
   ii. Fear
   iii. Peripheral nerve disease
   iv. Micturition

2. A 51-year-old tree trimmer had gradually experienced difficulty with urination during a 6- to 9-month period. He felt less urge to urinate, had difficulty in starting, and voided only small amounts. Recently, incontinence and a urinary tract infection had developed.

   On examination, he had decreased anal sensation with absent anal and bulbocavernous reflexes. His bladder was distended, but he was unable to empty it.
   a. What is the location of the lesion?
   b. What is the type of lesion?
   c. What type of bladder disturbance is this?
   d. What abnormalities of sexual function might be expected?

3. A 37-year-old man who had had a thyroid carcinoma completely resected had a 2-month progressive history of left shoulder pain, with no motor or sensory symptoms.

   Examination revealed drooping of the left eyelid, the left pupil smaller than the right (though both reacted normally to light), and dry skin on the left side of his face.
   a. What is the location of the lesion?
   b. What is the type of lesion?
   c. What structure is most likely involved?
   d. Does the lesion involve sympathetic or parasympathetic fibers?
   e. List the structures where these pathways could be damaged to produce a similar syndrome.

f. In this patient, a drug that releases norepinephrine from nerve terminals has no effect. What does this indicate?
g. If a drug that causes the release of norepinephrine from nerve terminals evokes pupillary dilatation, where is the lesion most likely located?

4. An elderly retired oil tycoon was brought to the emergency room complaining of severe cramping abdominal pain, vomiting, diarrhea, and shortness of breath. He was able to relate that he became ill about half an hour after ingestion of a hearty meal served to him by his young bride of only a month. The meal consisted of steak smothered in mushrooms, mashed potatoes, and home-canned green beans. His spouse had complained of not feeling well before dinner and had not eaten at all.

   Examination revealed marked tearing. The pupils were pinpoint in size. The patient was salivating profusely. Pulse rate was 50 per minute. Examination of the chest revealed diffuse rales in inspiration and wheezing in expiration. Auscultation of the abdomen revealed markedly active bowel sounds, and the examination was frequently interrupted by the patient's urgent need for a bedpan.
   a. What is the location of the lesion?
   b. What is the type of lesion?
   c. Is the disorder due to an abnormality in the sympathetic or parasympathetic pathway?
   d. What is the most likely cause of the disorder?
   e. What would be the effect of a cholinergic blocking agent on the pupils?
   f. Give examples of situations in which emotional activity in the limbic system alters function in the following organs:
      i. Heart
      ii. Gastrointestinal tract
      iii. Urinary tract
      iv. Skin
      v. Lacrimal glands

5. A 14-year-old boy was examined because of a discharge from his nipples that began 4 months ago. Additional questioning

elicited a 2-year history of headaches when supine, a 20-lb weight gain, and, recently, lethargy and irritability.

Examination revealed mild obesity and sallow skin. He moved slowly, had a hoarse voice, and no secondary sexual characteristics. There was a clear discharge from both nipples. Examination of the cranial nerves showed only partial loss of vision in the temporal fields bilaterally.

a. What are the level and site of the lesion?

b. What is the type of lesion?

c. Which neural structures are involved?

d. What receptors are found in this area?

e. What mechanism produces most of the symptoms?

Additional Reading ■

Bannister, R., and Mathias, C. J. (eds.). *Autonomic Failure: A Textbook of Clinical Disorders of the Autonomic Nervous System* (3rd ed.). Oxford: Oxford University Press, 1992.

Benarroch, E. E. *Central Autonomic Network: Functional Organization and Clinical Correlations.* New York: Futura, 1997.

Dinner, D. S. (ed.). The autonomic nervous system. *J. Clin. Neurophysiol.* 10:1, 1993.

Loewy, A. D., and Spyer, K. M. (eds.). *Central Regulation of Autonomic Functions.* New York: Oxford University Press, 1990.

Low, P. A. (ed.). *Clinical Autonomic Disorders: Evaluation and Management* (2nd ed.). Philadelphia: Lippincott-Raven, 1997.

Swanson, L. W. The hypothalamus. In Björklund, A., and Hökfelt, T. (eds.), *Handbook of Chemical Neuroanatomy,* vol 15. Amsterdam: Elsevier, 1987, pp. 1–124.

Törk, I., et al. Autonomic regulatory centers in the medulla oblongata. In G. Paxinos (ed.), *The Human Nervous System.* San Diego, CA: Academic Press, 1990, pp. 221–259.

ten

The Consciousness System

Objectives

1. Describe the anatomy of the consciousness system, with special reference to the reticular formation, the thalamic nuclei, the ascending projectional system, the basal forebrain, the cerebral cortex, and the neurochemically defined nuclear groups.
2. List the major connections (input and output) of the reticular formation.
3. Describe the projection pathways of the consciousness system to the cerebral cortex.
4. Describe and differentiate the electrical activity of single neurons and neuronal aggregates.
5. Describe the two main types of sleep patterns, the differences between them, and the anatomical regions involved with sleep states.
6. Define and list the characteristics of each of the following: narcolepsy, delirium, confusion, somnolence, stupor, coma, concussion, seizure, and syncope.
7. State the anatomical locations of lesions that result in loss of consciousness, and give examples of specific disease processes that affect each area.
8. Describe the neurophysiologic basis of the EEG and the fundamental waking and sleeping patterns, and describe how the EEG is useful in evaluating patients with disorders of consciousness.

Introduction

The major afferent pathways that provide the central nervous system with direct access to information about the external environment arc described in Chapter 7. These pathways are located in the outer tube portion of the central nervous system. In parallel with these pathways at the posterior fossa and supratentorial levels is another ascending system, the consciousness system, that is located primarily in the inner tube portion of the central nervous system. This system extends from the medulla to the cerebral cortex.

The consciousness system is a diffuse system that regulates consciousness, attention, and the sleep-wake states and modulates cortical reactivity to stimuli. Although the sensory pathways and the consciousness system both transmit sensory information to the cerebral cortex, the primary afferent pathways do so by means of direct pathways that are located in the outer tube and specific thalamic nuclei that project primarily to the sensory cortex. In contrast, the pathways of the consciousness system modulate activity via diffuse multineuronal pathways located in the inner tube that project either directly to the cerebral cortex or indirectly by way of thalamic nuclei.

In this chapter, the anatomy and physiology of the consciousness system, its role in the regulation of wakefulness and sleep, and pathologic states of altered consciousness, which are a reflection of deranged activity within the system, are described.

Overview ■

The consciousness system is a diffuse yet organized neuronal system located in the brainstem, diencephalon, and cerebral hemispheres. Structures in the system are (1) portions of the brainstem reticular formation, (2) neurochemically defined nuclear groups of the brainstem, (3) thalamic nuclei, (4) basal forebrain, (5) ascending projections to the thalamus and cerebral cortex, and (6) widespread areas of the cerebral cortex. Control of the behavioral states of consciousness, attention, and wakefulness and sleep is related to specific changes in neural activity in the brainstem and basal forebrain that result in functional changes in thalamic and cortical circuits.

The reticular formation consists of multiple aggregates of neurons that receive and integrate information from many areas of the neuraxis, including the sensory system, cerebral cortex, basal forebrain, hypothalamus, and cerebellum. The reticular formation also sends projections to widespread areas of the cerebral cortex, either directly or indirectly through the thalamic nuclei, as well as to the motor and internal regulation systems. The neurochemically defined nuclear groups of the reticular formation consist of the cholinergic and monoaminergic nuclei. The latter includes the norepinephrine, serotonin, and histamine cell groups. The reticular formation can modify cortical function directly or indirectly through connections with the thalamus and can selectively modulate the activity of the cerebral cortex and its reactivity to stimuli.

Proper functioning of the consciousness system and hence the regulation of consciousness and attention are predicated on a continuous interaction between the cerebral cortex, basal forebrain, thalamus, and brainstem reticular formation.

The electrical activity of a neuronal aggregate such as the cerebral cortex is a reflection of its own intrinsic activity and of ascending influences, primarily from the thalamus and reticular activating system.

The *electroencephalogram* (EEG) is a means of recording cortical activity. The waveforms that are seen represent summations of the postsynaptic, dendritic potentials generated near the surface in response to the intrinsic, neuronal electrical activity of the cerebral cortex as modified by input from subcortical structures. Thus, the EEG can provide information not only about cortical functioning but also about activity throughout the consciousness system.

Consciousness is an awareness of environment and self and is achieved through the action of the projections of the reticular activating system and basal forebrain on the cerebral cortex. The process of attention by which normal persons can focus their thoughts on specific information is achieved by the modulation of neuronal input to the cerebral cortex through the reticular activating system and basal forebrain. This permits persons to direct their attention to specific aspects of the environment without being continually distracted by multiple simultaneous stimuli.

Sleep is a normal cyclic physiologic alteration of consciousness and is readily reversed by appropriate stimuli. It has been divided into two stages: rapid eye movement and non-rapid eye movement sleep. *Rapid eye movement* (REM) *sleep* is characterized by rapid eye movements, muscle twitches, decreased muscle tone, dreaming, and an EEG pattern resembling that of a recording made during wakefulness. *Non–rapid eye movement* (non-REM) *sleep* is characterized by the absence of rapid eye movements, reduced body movements, and an EEG pattern showing the characteristic waveforms of the sleep state.

Pathologic processes that destroy or depress the function of the reticular formation, of the ascending projection pathways, or of both cerebral hemispheres produce alterations in consciousness. Examples of states of altered consciousness include *coma,* a state of extended unconsciousness from which the patient cannot be aroused; *confusional states,* in which the patient is disoriented, inattentive, and cannot think clearly; *concussion,* a brief loss of consciousness after a blow to the head from which the patient recovers without neurologic sequelae; *seizure,* a transient alteration in brain function due to excessive neuronal discharge, which, when generalized and involves the consciousness system, causes loss of consciousness; and *syncope,* a transient loss of consciousness due to widespread neuronal ischemia.

Evaluation of a patient with a disorder of consciousness requires analysis of associated neurologic signs to determine whether the responsible lesion is (1) located at the supratentorial level, (2) located at the posterior fossa level, or (3) diffusely distributed at both levels.

Anatomy of the Consciousness System

Structures of the consciousness system include portions of the brainstem reticular formation, the basal forebrain, the neurochemically defined nuclear groups of the brainstem and basal forebrain, the thalamus, the ascending projection pathways, and widespread areas of the cerebral cortex (Fig. 1).

Reticular Formation

The reticular formation is a complex aggregate of neurons whose cell bodies form neuronal clusters in the tegmental portion of the brainstem, that is, from the level of the decussation of the pyramids in caudal medulla to the basal forebrain area and thalamus. The

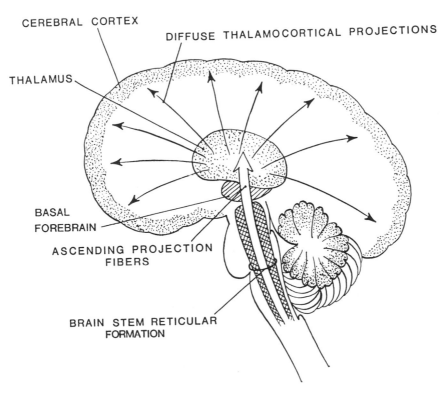

FIG. 1. Lateral view of the brain showing the components of the consciousness system.

neurons are characterized by long radiating dendrites that have few branches and axons that have numerous collaterals and project for long distances along the neuraxis. The diffuse arrangement of the multipolar neurons and their many interconnections allow a single reticular neuron to receive afferents from many sources and to make synaptic contact with numerous neurons. This arrangement gives rise to the term *reticular* ("forming a network"). With phylogenic advancement, this centrally located network becomes surrounded by structures serving specific functions in the motor and sensory systems.

The reticular formation has been subdivided functionally into a *midline region* (the *raphe*), a *medial region* containing large neurons that project to the spinal cord and to oculomotor nuclei, and a *lateral region* that receives axon collaterals from many ascending sensory pathways. At the level of the medulla, the lateral reticular formation participates in the coordination of complex motor patterns such as respiration, swallowing, and vomiting. Neurons in the ventrolateral medulla control the respiratory and circulatory systems via projections to the spinal cord. The reticular formation at the level of the pons and midbrain contains neurochemically defined groups of neurons that project to the cerebral cortex either directly or via the thalamus.

Afferent pathways to the reticular formation (Fig. 2) consist of (1) collateral branches from the primary ascending tracts of the sensory system (spinothalamic and spinoreticular pathways), which synapse with cells in the reticular formation; (2) fibers from the cerebral cortex, consisting of corticoreticular fibers from widespread cortical areas as well as collaterals from the corticospinal and corticobulbar tracts of the motor system; (3) fibers from other structures, including the cerebel-

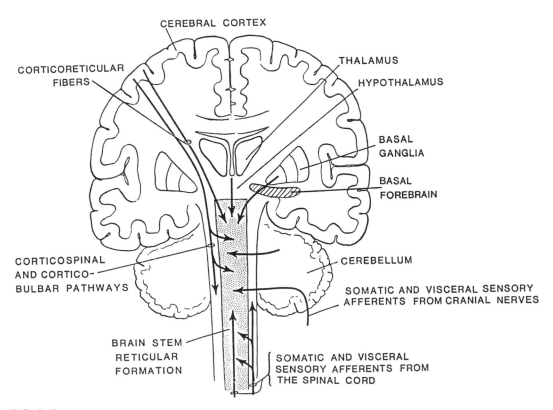

FIG. 2. Input to the brainstem reticular formation.

lum, basal ganglia, hypothalamus, cranial nerve nuclei, and the colliculi; and (4) visceral afferents from the spinal cord and cranial nerves.

The efferent pathways project rostrally to the forebrain and caudally to the spinal cord. In addition to the ascending projections of the reticular formation in the consciousness system, other projections convey information to the motor and internal regulation systems (Fig. 3). By means of these numerous connections and pathways, the reticular formation can integrate information from various levels of the neuraxis and thereby regulate and modify the activity of the nervous system. The concept of the reticular formation as a diffuse interconnected system that receives numerous converging inputs and gives rise to multiple divergent outputs is being revised as different groups of anatomically and func-

tionally defined neurons (each with specific neuronal connections) become characterized.

Neurochemically Defined Nuclear Groups of the Brainstem and Basal Forebrain

The important groups of cells in the reticular formation that are involved with the control of the different behavioral states of wakefulness and sleep are characterized by their neurotransmitters and consist of cholinergic groups and monoaminergic groups (Table 1 and Fig. 4).

The *cholinergic nuclear groups* of neurons are located in the *basal forebrain* and in the dorsal tegmentum of the upper pons and midbrain (referred to as the *mesopontine tegmentum*) and form an anatomically functional unit that has projections to the cerebral cortex and thalamus. The cholinergic structures of the

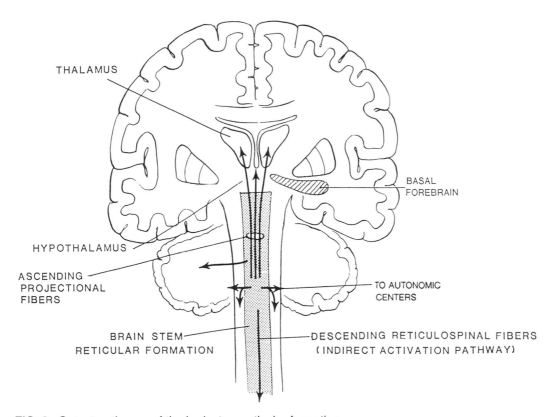

FIG. 3. Output pathways of the brainstem reticular formation.

TABLE 1. *Neurochemically defined nuclear groups*

Neurotransmitter	Location of nuclear group	Modulates
Acetylcholine	Basal forebrain	Attention
	Dorsal tegmentum of pons and midbrain	Wakefulness
		REM sleep
Monoamines		
Norepinephrine	Locus ceruleus	Wakefulness and attention
Serotonin	Raphe nuclei	Wakefulness
Histamine	Hypothalamus	Wakefulness

REM, rapid eye movement.

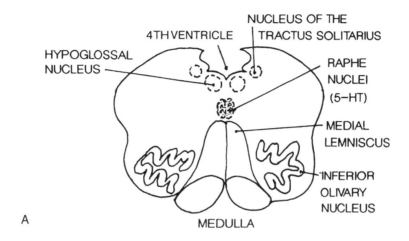

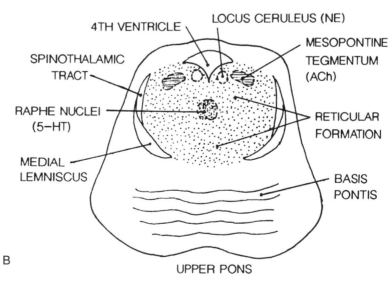

FIG. 4. Location of diffusely projecting neurons of the consciousness system at the level of the medulla **(A)** and upper pons **(B)**. NE, norepinephrine; 5-HT, serotonin; ACh, acetylcholine.

basal forebrain, including the nucleus basalis (of Meynert) and the medial septal nuclei, send diffuse projections to the cerebral cortex. These projections are critical for regulation of behavioral functions, including cortical arousal, wakefulness, sensory processing, learning, and memory. In addition to direct action on the cerebral cortex, some basal forebrain neurons project to the reticular nucleus of the thalamus and to other thalamic nuclei. Cholinergic input to the thalamic reticular nucleus modulates the activity of the thalamus and the thalamocortical projections to the cerebral cortex. Thus, cholinergic neurons of the basal forebrain project directly to the cerebral cortex or to the reticular thalamic nucleus. Cholinergic neurons located in the mesopontine tegmentum project to the thalamus and basal forebrain. Thus, the ascending cholinergic pathways from the brainstem project to the cerebral cortex via the basal forebrain or thalamus, which in turn can affect cortical activity.

The *monoaminergic groups* important in regulating behavioral states and state-dependent cortical activity are the *norepinephrine, serotonin,* and *histamine nuclear groups.* These neurochemically defined nuclear groups are located in the brainstem and hypothalamus and send projections to the basal forebrain and cerebral cortex via the medial forebrain bundle.

The *norepinephrine cells* are located in the *locus ceruleus,* which is in the lateral part of the upper pons (Fig. 4). The locus ceruleus is a group of melanin-pigmented cells rich in norepinephrine; it has a slightly bluish appearance in fresh specimens, hence, the name. It sends projections to areas that mediate responses to sensory stimuli, including the thalamus, hypothalamus, basal forebrain, cerebral cortex, cerebellum, and spinal cord. Neurons in the locus ceruleus increase their activity in response to new and challenging stimuli and thus have an important role in the mechanism of arousal and attention.

The *serotoninergic neurons* form the *raphe nuclei,* which are located in the median area of the brainstem (Fig. 4). The rostral group (upper pons and midbrain) gives rise to as-

cending projections to the thalamus, hypothalamus, basal forebrain, and cerebral hemispheres. The caudal group (lower pons and medulla) gives rise to descending projections to the spinal cord and other areas of the brainstem. Serotoninergic neurons exert a widespread influence on various areas of the central nervous system.

The *histamine neurons* are located in the *posterior lateral hypothalamus.* They enhance arousal mechanisms and wakefulness.

Thalamus

The thalamus is the gateway to the cerebral cortex and subserves two important roles. It acts as a relay station (relaying information to and from the cerebral cortex), and it filters and modulates the flow of information to the cerebral cortex from other areas.

The thalamus is subdivided into two main components: the relay nuclei and the reticular nucleus (Fig. 5). The larger component, or dorsal thalamus, contains the relay nuclei for sensory, motor, and association pathways and has reciprocal connections with the cerebral cortex. These thalamic relay nuclei contain (1) *relay,* or *projection,* neurons that contain glutamate and send excitatory input to the cerebral cortex; and (2) local *interneurons* that contain γ-aminobutyric acid (GABA) and participate in thalamic local inhibitory circuits. The dorsal thalamus in turn is subdivided into (1) specific thalamic relay nuclei that are associated with the sensory and motor pathways and have reciprocal connections with localized areas of the cerebral cortex, (2) association nuclei that have reciprocal connections with association areas of the cerebral cortex (for example, prefrontal cortex and parietotemporal cortex), and (3) nonspecific thalamic nuclei that receive input from the reticular formation and basal forebrain and project axons diffusely to the cerebral cortex (Fig. 6). The nonspecific thalamic nuclei include the *midline nuclei,* which are particularly interconnected with the internal regulation system, and the *intralaminar nuclei*

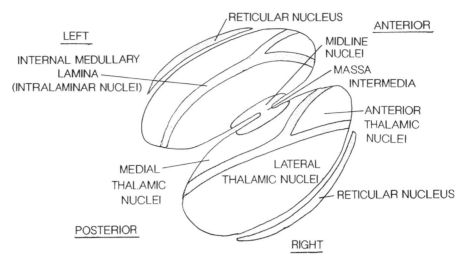

FIG. 5. Thalamic nuclei involved in the consciousness system. The intralaminar, midline, and reticular nuclei of the thalamus receive input from the reticular formation and cerebral cortex. The intralaminar and midline nuclei project diffusely to the cerebral cortex and exert a facilitatory effect on cortical neuronal excitability. The reticular nucleus does not project to the cortex but controls the activity of other thalamic nuclei.

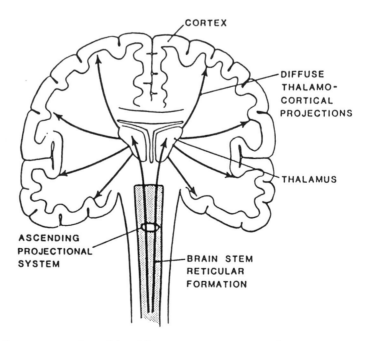

FIG. 6. Schematic representation of the diffuse thalamocortical projections of the thalamus, part of the consciousness system. They arise from the midline and intralaminar nuclei and produce diffuse activation of separate areas of the cortex. These projections are important not only for alertness but also for coordination of activity in numerous cortical areas activated by specific thalamocortical projections and involved in specific sensory or cognitive function.

(located in the internal medullary lamina, a band of myelinated fibers that separates the anterior, medial, and lateral groups of relay and association nuclei).

The second component of the thalamus is the *reticular nucleus,* which contains GABAergic neurons that project to other thalamic nuclei but not to the cerebral cortex. Neurons in the reticular nucleus send inhibitory input to all thalamic nuclei and synchronize thalamic neurons so that rhythmic activity occurs in the nuclei during certain stages of sleep (see below).

Relay nuclei and the reticular nucleus receive abundant input from the cerebral cortex. For thalamic relay nuclei, the cortical input originates from the cortical area to which the nucleus projects. These *cortico-thalamo-cortical loops* are important in coordinating, via the nonspecific thalamic nuclei, activity initiated in different parts of the cerebral cortex. This temporal synchronization of separate cortical areas is critical for processing of sensory information.

Basal Forebrain

The *basal forebrain* consists of a group of structures located at the ventral and medial aspects of the cerebral hemispheres. It includes the *nucleus basalis* (of Meynert) and the *septal nuclei* (Fig. 7). The nucleus basalis consists mainly of cholinergic neurons and sends extensive projections to widespread areas of the cerebral cortex. It serves as the major source of extrathalamic input to cortical areas. The medial forebrain bundle is a large tract that extends from the midbrain tegmentum through the lateral hypothalamus into the septum, preoptic area, hypothalamus, basal olfactory region, and cingulate gyrus. This bundle represents the most rostral extent of the reticular system and contains ascending and descending fibers that interconnect the brainstem and telencephalon. Many of the cholinergic and monoaminergic fibers that originate in the brainstem send projections to cortical regions through the medial forebrain bundle.

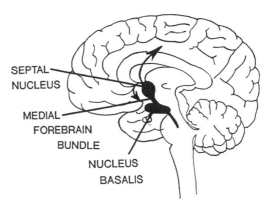

FIG. 7. Lateral view of the brain showing the basal forebrain area. The cholinergic nuclei of the basal forebrain receive input from the cholinergic nuclei of the mesopontine tegmentum as well as from the monoaminergic groups. The nucleus basalis projects to the neocortex, whereas the septal nucleus projects to the hippocampal formation. These projections are important in attention, motivation, and memory.

Ascending Pathways to the Cerebral Cortex

The activating influences of the reticular formation and other subcortical structures are transmitted to the cerebral cortex by two main types of projection pathways: thalamocortical pathways, and extrathalamic pathways that involve the basal forebrain and medial forebrain bundle (Table 2 and Fig. 8).

The thalamic relay nuclei receive information from specific afferent pathways (e.g., medial lemniscus, optic track). The thalamic relay nuclei in turn send projections to specific topographic areas of the cerebral cortex. The specific thalamocortical inputs are phasic and dependent on the arrival of input from the specific afferent pathways. The thalamus not only acts as a relay station but also controls and coordinates neuronal activity in the cerebral cortex. It does so in part via diffuse thalamocortical projections from the intralaminar nuclei.

The extrathalamic pathways originate from cholinergic and monoaminergic neuronal groups located primarily in the brainstem and basal forebrain. These include norepinephrine neurons in the locus ceruleus, serotoninergic neurons in the raphe nuclei, histamine neurons in lateral hypothalamus, and cholinergic

TABLE 2. *Ascending pathways of the consciousness system*

	Thalamocortical pathways	Extrathalamic pathways
Input from	Sensory relay nuclei in spinal cord and brainstem	Cholinergic and monoaminergic neuron groups in brainstem and basal forebrain
Projection pathway	Thalamic radiations	Medial forebrain bundle
Projects to	Specific topographic areas of cerebral cortex	Widespread areas of cerebral cortex and thalamus
Function	Relay information to cerebral cortex Filter flow of information to cerebral cortex	Modulate activity of cerebral cortex and thalamus
Activity	Phasic/excitatory	Tonic-continuous Modulatory
Dependent on	Specific afferent stimulation	Behavior state (wake-sleep)

neurons in the mesopontine tegmentum and basal forebrain. These structures send projections to widespread areas of the cerebral cortex by way of the medial forebrain bundle. In addition, they send projections to the thalamus, which in turn sends projections to the cerebral cortex. Thus, cholinergic and monoaminergic neurons exert a continuous, tonic modulatory influence on cortical and thalamic neurons dependent on the behavioral

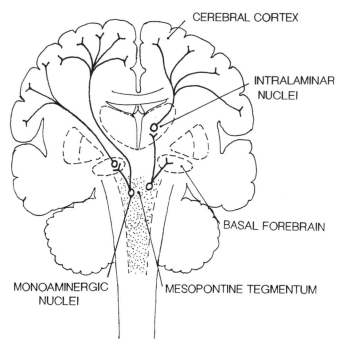

FIG. 8. Schematic representation of the thalamic and extrathalamic pathways of the consciousness system. Thalamic pathways arise not only from specific relay nuclei but also from intralaminar and midline nuclei, whose diffuse excitatory projections have glutamate as a neurotransmitter. These nuclei receive input from the brainstem reticular formation and basal forebrain. The cholinergic neurons of the basal forebrain receive input from the cholinergic neurons of the mesopontine tegmentum and project diffusely to the cerebral cortex. The monoaminergic groups include the locus ceruleus (norepinephrine), raphe (serotonin), tubero-mamillary nucleus (histamine), and ventral tegmental area (dopamine). They project directly to the cerebral cortex via the median forebrain bundle.

state (sleep or wake) of the person. Because of the simultaneous effect on the thalamus and the cerebral cortex, the state-dependent changes in cholinergic and monoaminergic neuronal neurochemical groups cause global changes in cortical activity.

Cerebral Cortex

Although many specific functions, such as somatic sensation and vision, are relayed and integrated in specific areas, no single area of cerebral cortex is responsible for the maintenance of consciousness. Indeed, because of the widespread interconnections between the nonspecific thalamic nuclei and the cerebral cortex, all areas of cortex appear to participate in consciousness and therefore are considered part of the consciousness system.

Physiology of the Consciousness System

Neurophysiology of Single Cells

As described in Chapter 5, neurons generate two types of potentials: synaptic potentials and action potentials.

Synaptic Potential

The *synaptic potential* is a local potential generated in the dendrite or soma portion of the nerve cell as a result of a neurotransmitter interacting with the cell membrane of the postsynaptic neuron (Fig. 9). Synaptic potentials are localized, nonpropagated, graded fluctuations of the postsynaptic membrane potential and can be excitatory [excitatory postsynaptic potentials (EPSPs)] when the neurotransmitter causes depolarization in the cell membrane or inhibitory [inhibitory postsynaptic potentials (IPSPs)] when the neurotransmitter causes hyperpolarization of the cell membrane. The duration of these potentials is usually 15 to 20 milliseconds, and they do not have a refractory period.

Action Potential

The action potential usually arises in the initial segment (near the axon hillock) and propagates along the axon (Fig. 9). (In some instances, it can also arise from a dendrite or cell body.) The action potential occurs only when the neuronal membrane is depolarized beyond a critical (threshold) level. The spike discharge is brief (usually less than 1 millisecond). It is an all-or-none phenomenon propagated down the axon and followed by a temporary refractory period (Fig. 9).

Neurophysiology of Neuronal Aggregates

Neurons in the central nervous system and cerebral cortex do not function in isolation but as part of neuronal aggregates. These neurons have rich synaptic interconnections, and the electrical activity of the aggregate reflects the summated effect of all the dendritic po-

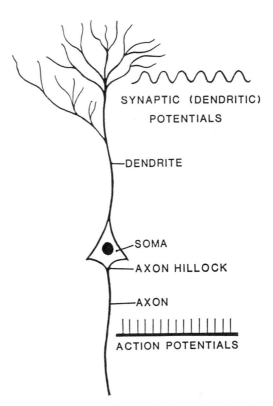

FIG. 9. Diagram of a cortical neuron showing synaptic potentials generated in a dendrite and action potentials generated in an axon.

tentials and action potentials occurring within that aggregate. This activity is recorded as complex waveforms rather than as the simple spikes of single cells. The cerebral cortex generates these electrical waves in response to local activity within the neuronal aggregate and to input from both the specific and the nonspecific nuclei of the thalamus. Because the thalamic nuclei have widespread connections with the cerebral cortex, they can exert a strong influence on cortical activity. They can act to excite, inhibit, or promote widespread synchronization and coordination of cortical neuronal activity. In addition, neurons may have spontaneous oscillations of the membrane potential at rest, in the absence of synaptic input. These oscillations allow the neuron (1) to respond only when the synaptic stimuli arrive at a particular time, (2) to serve as pacemakers, or (3) to initiate rhythmic patterns of activity transmitted to other areas of the nervous system.

Electrical activity of the cerebral cortex can be detected with the EEG, which records cortical activity from electrodes placed on the scalp. This brain-wave activity consists of continuous rhythmic or arrhythmic oscillating waveforms that vary in frequency, amplitude, polarity, and shape. These electrical potentials are usually in the range of 20 to 50 μV. The activity seen on the EEG (Fig. 10) reflects the summation of synaptic potentials of many dendrites lying near the surface of the cerebral cortex. The fluctuation of the EEG is due to varied excitatory and inhibitory synaptic potentials impinging on the dendritic membranes.

Cortical neuronal activity is modulated by synaptic input from other cortical neurons, basal forebrain, thalamus, and brainstem. Thalamic influences determine the intrinsic resting frequencies of the brain waves, because structures in the thalamus serve as the "pacemakers" in producing widespread synchronization and rhythmicity of cortical activity over the cerebral hemispheres.

Electrical stimulation of the thalamus alters the EEG pattern. A low-frequency stimulus produces a more rhythmic and synchronized

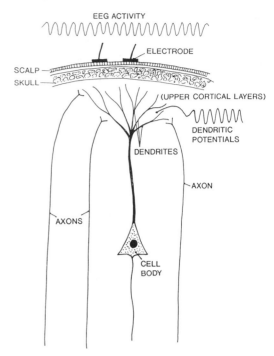

FIG. 10. The electroencephalogram (EEG) is a recording of the dendritic potentials in the upper cortical layers as they appear on the scalp.

EEG pattern, whereas a high-frequency stimulus produces a low-amplitude fast pattern that appears desynchronized on the surface recording.

Thalamic neurons projecting to the cerebral cortex have two basic modes of generating action potentials: tonic, single spike activity, and rhythmic burst activity. Single spike activity allows precise transmission of sensory information to the cerebral cortex and is typical of the states of *activation* of the cerebral cortex. By contrast, rhythmic burst firing impairs transmission of thalamocortical information because the encoding ability of the action potential frequency is lost; this is typical of states of *inactivation* of the cerebral cortex (Table 3).

Functions of the Consciousness System

The consciousness system is responsible for the maintenance of consciousness, attention, and regulation of the wake-sleep states.

TABLE 3. *Functional states of the cerebral cortex and thalamocortical circuits*

	Thalamocortical activation	Thalamocortical inactivation
Ascending input from the mesopontine reticular formation	Present	Reduced
Thalamic activity	Tonic, single spikes	Rhythmic burst firing
Sensory processing	Present	Impaired
Electroencephalogram	Low-voltage, fast activity	High-voltage, rhythmic slow activity
Examples	Wakefulness	Non-REM sleep
	REM sleep	General anesthesia
		Absence seizure
		Coma

REM, rapid eye movement.

Consciousness

Consciousness is a subjective state defined as an "awareness of environment and self." It implies an awake and alert condition in which the person is capable of perceiving his or her internal and external environments and, if the motor system is intact, of responding in an appropriate manner to stimuli. There are two aspects of consciousness: (1) the *content of consciousness,* representing cognitive mental functions that reflect the activity of the cerebral cortex; and (2) *arousal* and *wakefulness,* which are dependent on the reticular activating system and its projections and which in turn are activated by sensory stimuli or cortical influences.

Direct electrical stimulation of the reticular formation in a sleeping animal results in a state of behavioral arousal, indicated by opening of the eyes, turning of the head, and movement of the limbs. Associated with this is a change in the EEG from a synchronous non-REM sleep pattern to the low-voltage, fast pattern of the waking state.

The reticular formation receives sensory input from collaterals of every major sensory pathway, which keeps the reticular activating system in an excited state and in turn activates the cerebral cortex to maintain wakefulness. The importance of sensory influences in maintaining a wakeful state is illustrated by the progressive decrease in the degree of wakefulness that occurs with loss or reduction in sensory input. If the consciousness system is intact, stimulation of the reticular activating system results in an arousal response; however, if a portion of the consciousness system is destroyed, particularly the rostral part of the brainstem and thalamus, a permanent sleep state ensues.

Neurons of the reticular formation and basal forebrain diffusely activate the cerebral cortex directly and via the thalamus (Fig. 8). They receive input from restricted areas of the cerebral cortex, such as the orbitofrontal cortex and the superior temporal cortex; stimulation of these areas evokes an arousal response.

Cholinergic and monoaminergic inputs have a dual effect on thalamocortical circuits: (1) At the level of the thalamus, they inhibit burst activity and facilitate sensory transmission. (2) At the level of the cerebral cortex, they increase excitability and responsiveness of cortical neurons to thalamic and cortical inputs.

During wakefulness, tonic activity of cholinergic and monoaminergic neurons maintains a state of cortical excitability. Cholinergic neurons of the basal forebrain and locus ceruleus increase their activity in response to new and challenging stimuli and are involved not only in arousal but also in attention and motivation. Histaminergic neurons in the posterior lateral hypothalamus are also involved in cortical arousal and motivated behavior. Decreased activity in both cholinergic and monoaminergic inputs results in progressive decrease in excitability of thalamocortical circuits.

Attention

The consciousness system not only determines the state of alertness and wakefulness but also influences the degree of overall attentiveness to the environment and perception of specific sensory modalities. The cholinergic neurons of the basal forebrain facilitate sensory processing of cortical neurons and the response to specific sensory stimuli. The activity of basal forebrain neurons is influenced by input from the ascending pathways of the brainstem and can cause a localized or generalized activation of different cortical areas. The consciousness system also modulates cortical reactivity to stimuli by facilitating or inhibiting transmission of neural impulses of the sensory system through the thalamus. The various projections of the consciousness system act on relay nuclei in the thalamus to make them more or less receptive to sensory stimuli. Thus, the thalamus acts as a mechanism to enhance or attenuate responses to incoming stimuli and to direct attention to specific input while suppressing other incoming signals. Electrical activity reaching the cerebral cortex via specific sensory pathways is not perceived unless it is associated with activity via the diffuse projection paths. For example, reading a book, a person is absorbed by the words on the page and is not aware of body contact with the chair or outside noises. The consciousness system selectively sends alerting signals to the cerebral cortex receiving visual input and suppresses sensory input in auditory or somatic pathways. The consciousness system thus acts in an adaptive manner to prevent the cerebral cortex from being overwhelmed and to permit selective attention to specific external and internal stimuli.

Sleep States

Consciousness may be altered by several conditions. One normal physiologic alteration is that associated with sleep, which is defined as a cyclic, temporary, and physiologic loss of consciousness that is readily, promptly, and completely reversed by appropriate stimuli. Recent studies have shown that sleep is an active phenomenon in which hypnogenic areas of the brain and neurochemical substances actively promote sleep and inhibit the arousal system.

The structures implicated in the regulation of sleep include the raphe nuclei in the upper medullary and lower pontine areas of the reticular formation of the brainstem, the nucleus of the tractus solitarius in the medulla, the locus ceruleus in the lateral portion of the upper pons and lower midbrain, the lateral pontine reticular formation ventral to the locus ceruleus, the anterior portion of the hypothalamus, the reticular nucleus of the thalamus, and the basal forebrain-preoptic area (Fig. 11). These structures modulate sleep by producing excitation of other areas of the brain associated with sleep and by actively inhibiting areas of the reticular system that are responsible for maintaining a wakeful state. Destruction of these areas can result in decreased sleep.

Two distinctive patterns of sleep are seen in normal persons: REM sleep and non-REM sleep (Table 4). *REM sleep* is sleep in which there are rapid conjugate eye movements; fluctuations of body temperature, blood pressure, heart rate, and respiration; a decrease in muscle tone; muscle twitches; and penile erection. This is also the stage of sleep in which dreams occur. An EEG recorded during REM sleep shows a low-amplitude fast pattern resembling that of a person in an alert state with the eyes open (Fig. 12). Because of the above characteristics, REM sleep is also known as *paradoxical, active,* or *dream* sleep.

Non-REM sleep is sleep during which there are no rapid eye movements. There is widespread decrease in brain activity. Vital signs and autonomic activity are more stable. During non-REM sleep, the EEG shows different patterns, depending on the depth of sleep (Fig. 12). During drowsiness, the EEG shows a low-amplitude background with an attenuation of rhythmic activity. During light-to-medium levels of sleep, specific EEG waveforms (sleep spindles, V waves, and K complexes) are present. *Sleep spindles* are sinusoidal waveforms ranging from 10 to 14 Hz and are usually present over the frontal head regions. *V waves*

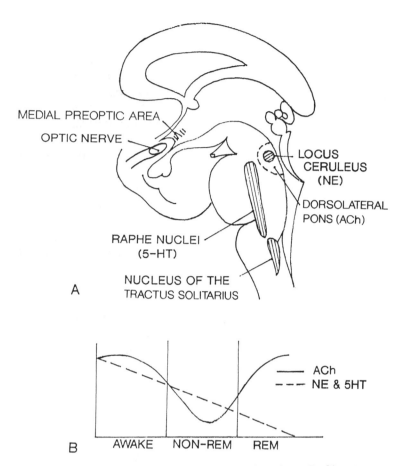

FIG. 11. **A:** Areas of the brain *(cross-hatched areas)* related to sleep. **B:** Changes in neurochemical activity during wake-sleep states. *ACh,* acetylcholine; *5-HT,* serotonin; *NE,* norepinephrine.

TABLE 4. *Characteristics of the two major patterns of sleep (REM and Non-REM)*

Sleep activity	REM sleep	Non-REM sleep
Eye movements	Rapid	Slow (during drowsiness)
Body movements	Muscle twitches	Muscle relaxation
Muscle tone	Decreased	Some tone in postural muscle groups
Vital signs	Fluctuating	Stable
Penile erection	Common	Rare
Dreams	Common	Rare
EEG	Low-voltage pattern	Spindles, V waves, K complexes, slow waves
Percentage in adults	20–25	75–80
Percentage in infants	50	50

EEG, electroencephalogram; REM, rapid eye movement.

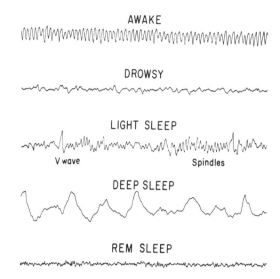

FIG. 12. EEG patterns of wakefulness and different levels of sleep. The awake EEG is recorded from occipital areas with the eyes closed. With the eyes open, the EEG resembles the rapid eye movement (REM) sleep pattern.

(vertex waves) are high-amplitude, sharp waveforms occurring over the frontal and parietal regions. *K complexes* are a combination of V waves and spindle activity and often signify a partial arousal response in the EEG. During deep levels of sleep, widespread high-amplitude slow waves are present.

Non-REM sleep is the predominant type of sleep in adults and accounts for 75% to 80% of the nocturnal sleep pattern, whereas REM sleep accounts for only 20% to 25%. In newborn infants, however, 50% of sleep is REM sleep. During a night's sleep in adults, non-REM sleep occurs first and generally lasts for 60 to 90 minutes. It is then interrupted by a REM period, which may last from several minutes to a half hour and is followed by another non-REM period. A total night's sleep usually consists of four to six cycles of alternating non-REM and REM sleep.

Experimental data indicate that non-REM and REM sleep are produced by different anatomical, physiologic, and neurohumoral systems.

Non-REM sleep is mediated by a widespread system that consists of multiple groups of neurons located in the anterior hypothalamus, the basal forebrain-preoptic area, and the brainstem, including the dorsal medullary reticular formation and the nucleus of the tractus solitarius.

REM sleep is mediated by a more discrete system in the pons and includes the dorsolateral pontine reticular formation, particularly the region just ventral and lateral to the locus ceruleus. The dorsolateral pontine neurons, interacting with other neurons in the brainstem and forebrain, are involved with the reciprocal activation and deactivation of the neuronal groups that mediate REM sleep. The norepinephrine cells in the locus ceruleus and the serotoninergic cells in the dorsal raphe nuclei become inactive during REM sleep; they are the REM-off cells. Neurons in the region just ventral and lateral to the locus ceruleus, however, fire at faster rates during REM sleep and are called the REM-on cells. This is the area most critical for REM sleep: it induces the neuronal changes mediating REM sleep.

Sleep-Wake Cycle

The mechanisms governing wake-sleep states have not been explained completely; however, they appear to involve the interaction of numerous structures and neurotransmitters. The sleep-wake cycle is only one of several circadian rhythms that occur approximately every 24 hours. The generator of sleep is not known but may involve neurons in the preoptic-anterior hypothalamic region. Many other biologic systems, such as hormonal secretion, follow a circadian pattern. The circadian rhythms are controlled by a biologic clock located in the *suprachiasmatic nucleus* of the hypothalamus. The suprachiasmatic nucleus is synchronized with the diurnal light-dark cycle through input from the retina. Among other rhythms, the suprachiasmatic nucleus controls the secretion of melatonin from the pineal gland.

The sleep-wake cycle is associated with state-specific activity of brainstem and thalamic neurons. The initiation of sleep and the transition between the various stages of sleep occur as a consequence of reciprocal activation and inhibition of these neurons.

During wakefulness, both mesopontine cholinergic neurons and monoaminergic neurons (locus ceruleus, raphe, posterior hypothalamus) are active (Table 5). This produces an active state in the thalamocortical circuits characterized by tonic activity in thalamic relay neurons and low-amplitude fast cortical oscillations (the desynchronized EEG pattern). As a consequence of this fast rhythmic oscillation, neurons in the cerebral cortex are receptive to sensory input. There is temporal synchronization of firing of separate groups of neurons located in different areas of the cerebral cortex and engaged together in a particular task. The cholinergic system is mainly responsible for thalamocortical activation, and the monoaminergic systems support the processing of external sensory information.

The onset of non-REM sleep is preceded by a decrease in the activity of both the cholinergic and monoaminergic brainstem systems, which progresses with deeper stages of non-REM sleep. The neurons that initiate non-REM sleep are widespread, and their functional organization is not completely understood. They include groups in the medial preoptic-hypothalamic region, basal forebrain, and brainstem. Output from these neurons produces deactivation or active inhibition of the cholinergic and monoaminergic reticular activating neurons. This results in progressive hyperpolarization of thalamocortical neurons, which start firing in rhythmic bursts, synchronized by the reticular thalamic nucleus and represented by sleep spindles in the EEG. With deeper stages of non-REM sleep, progressive cortical inactivation is manifested as slow rhythmic cortical activity (delta waves).

REM sleep is generated in a more restricted region of the pons and includes cholinergic neurons in the mesopontine tegmentum. The firing rate of these cholinergic neurons increases immediately before the onset of REM sleep. These neurons are responsible for the activation of thalamocortical circuits; this activation is reflected in the EEG as low-amplitude fast activity similar to that seen in the wake state. In addition to the cholinergic neurons, other neurons active during REM sleep project to the medullary reticular formation and mediate the motor inhibition and autonomic changes observed during REM sleep. Unlike in the wake state, the activity in the noradrenergic neurons in the locus ceruleus and the serotoninergic neurons in the raphe nuclei is further decreased and the firing may stop during REM sleep. Although the thalamocortical circuits are activated during REM sleep through increased activity of the cholinergic mesopontine neurons, the cerebral cortex is not able to attend to external stimuli because of the lack of monoaminergic input, and cortical activity

TABLE 5. *Comparison of wakefulness and sleep states*

State	Wakefulness	Non-REM sleep	REM sleep
Cholinergic input	Active	Reduced	Active
Monoaminergic input	Active	Reduced	Absent
Sensory processing	Present for outside information	Absent	Present for stored information (dreaming)
Attention	Present	Absent	Absent
Electroencephalogram	Alpha rhythm (8–10 Hz) with eyes closed; low-amplitude activity with eyes open	Spindles K complex High-voltage, slow rhythm (delta rhythm)	Low-voltage, fast activity

REM, rapid eye movement.

is dominated by internal stimuli (for example, from stimuli stored as memories).

Clinical Correlations   ■

Sleep Disorders

Narcolepsy is a disorder of sleep control mechanisms characterized by excessive sleepiness. The patient falls asleep spontaneously and precipitously at any time during the day. These episodes are most frequent during monotonous situations. In addition, the patient may have cataplexy, sleep paralysis, or hypnagogic hallucinations. *Cataplexy* is an abrupt loss of muscle tone that may cause the patient to fall suddenly to the ground. Cataplexy is often precipitated by emotional events such as laughter, fright, or excitement.

Sleep paralysis occurs during the transition between wakefulness and sleep and is a temporary state involving the inability to move. *Hypnagogic hallucinations* are false visual or auditory perceptions that occur just before the patient falls asleep and often in conjunction with sleep paralysis. These findings probably reflect a disorder of REM sleep. Most patients with narcolepsy have no known structural lesion, and neurologic examination reveals no abnormality.

Sleep apnea is a condition in which the patient stops breathing when asleep. This may be due to upper airway obstruction or depression of central respiratory mechanisms. After a period of apnea, which may last up to a minute, the patient with obstructive sleep apnea arouses from sleep with noisy gasping respirations. When the patient goes back to sleep, the cycle is repeated. As a result, the patient has a decreased amount of sleep and is excessively drowsy when awake.

Periodic limb movement disorder consists of periodic or repetitive stereotyped flexion-extension movements of the limbs, usually the legs, which occur during sleep and cause intermittent arousal or awakening.

Somnambulism (sleep walking) and *sleep terrors* are other types of sleep disorder. They occur predominantly during deep levels of non-REM sleep.

Prolonged sleep deprivation can cause decreased vigilance and attention span, poor performance of tasks, increased irritability, diplopia, unsteadiness, slurring of speech, hallucinations, delusions, and, occasionally, psychotic behavior.

Disorders of Consciousness

Consciousness is a function of the combined activity of the reticular activating system and the cerebral cortex. Major damage to or depression of the brainstem and/or bilateral hemispheric dysfunction results in pathologic alteration in consciousness, or *loss of consciousness*. The loss of consciousness may be transient or prolonged and may vary from mildly increased sleepiness to deep coma.

Lesions that alter consciousness are located at the supratentorial or posterior fossa level. Interruption of the reticular activating system or its projections to the cerebral cortex produces different effects on consciousness, awareness, the wake-sleep states, and life functions, depending on the level of involvement (Fig. 13).

With nonfatal destruction of the high cervical spinal cord or spinomedullary junction, the consciousness system remains intact. Therefore, the wake and sleep states are present clinically and electrographically. Arousal occurs in response either to sensory stimuli from the cranial nerves or to stimulation of the reticular formation.

If damage occurs at the midpontine pretrigeminal level, just rostral to the trigeminal nerve entry zone and above the medullary and pontine sleep centers, there will be a persistent EEG pattern of wakefulness, consisting of low-voltage fast activity characteristic of an awake state.

A lesion at the midbrain level results in a sleep state in which neither sensory stimuli nor direct stimulation of the reticular formation or thalamus will produce an arousal response.

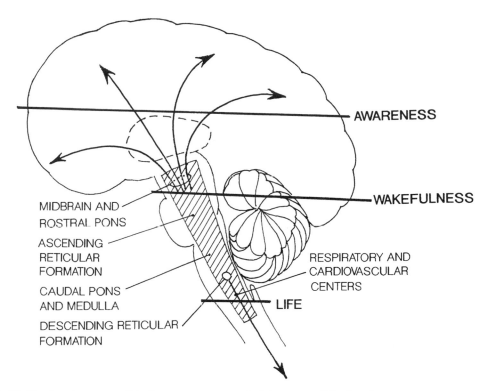

MIDBRAIN AND
ROSTRAL PONS

ASCENDING
RETICULAR
FORMATION

CAUDAL PONS
AND MEDULLA

DESCENDING RETICULAR
FORMATION

AWARENESS

WAKEFULNESS

RESPIRATORY AND
CARDIOVASCULAR
CENTERS

LIFE

FIG. 13. The levels responsible for awareness, wakefulness, and life functions.

Bilateral lesions that affect the ascending pathways in the region of the diencephalon (thalamus and hypothalamus) produce a state of sustained somnolence, with the EEG showing diffuse slow-wave activity.

Focal or unilateral lesions of the cerebral hemispheres do not result in loss of consciousness as long as the projections of the consciousness system to at least one cerebral hemisphere are intact. However, if there is bilateral destruction of the cerebral hemispheres, there is no longer a substratum for consciousness, and unconsciousness ensues.

Thus, the more rostral portions of the consciousness system, in particular the area above the trigeminal nerve entry zone, are critical for maintaining alertness and consciousness. However, portions of the reticular system of the lower pons and medulla seem to have important influences on certain stages of sleep, although they do not seem to be directly required for the maintenance of consciousness.

Degrees of Altered Consciousness

Regardless of the cause, various degrees of altered consciousness result from lesions affecting this system. *Coma* is a state of extended unconsciousness in which the patient is unarousable and shows little or no spontaneous movement and little or no alerting response to painful or noxious stimuli. Often the muscle-stretch reflexes, the plantar responses, and the pupillary and light reflexes are depressed or absent. Vital signs are usually altered, particularly with lesions affecting the brainstem; the patient has a slow and variable pulse rate and a periodic respiratory pattern.

In *stupor,* the patient often shows a moderate amount of spontaneous movement and can be aroused to respond purposefully to afferent stimuli. If sufficiently aroused, the patient can give a brief response to questions or simple commands.

Obtundation is a state in which alertness of the patient is mildly to moderately decreased. When left undisturbed, the patient falls asleep; when aroused, he or she shows a slowed or reduced response to all forms of stimuli.

In *somnolence,* the patient is easily aroused and shows appropriate verbal and motor responses to sensory stimuli. When the stimulus stops, the patient drifts back to sleep.

Confusion is a transient state, distinct from dementia, in which there is a progressive decline in cognitive functions in the presence of normal consciousness. The level of attention is decreased, and the ability to think clearly is impaired. Responses to verbal stimuli are slowed, and the patient is less able to recognize and understand what is going on in the environment.

Delirium is an agitated state of confusion associated with *illusions* (false interpretations or misrepresentations of real sensory images), *hallucinations* (false sensory perceptions for which there are not external bases), and *delusions* (false beliefs or misconceptions that cannot be corrected by reason).

Sleep, in contrast to the pathologic alterations previously described, is a normal physiologic state, but one that also can be associated with pathologic involvement of the consciousness system. A sleeping person, as compared with one in coma, is fully aroused by appropriate stimuli. During sleep, the eyes are closed, the muscles are relaxed, and cardiac output, pulse rate, blood pressure, and respiration are decreased.

Causes of Loss of Consciousness

The consciousness system may suffer either from physiologic alterations of function that produce a transient loss of consciousness or from structural lesions that result in a persistent loss of consciousness. A transient disturbance of consciousness occurs as a result of (1) concussion, (2) generalized seizure, (3) syncope, or (4) metabolic encephalopathy.

Concussion is a brief loss of consciousness, usually occurring after a sudden blow to the head. Although the patient is unconscious,

arousal by vigorous stimuli is often possible. After return of consciousness, there is some confusion and *amnesia* (loss of memory) that persist for a variable period afterward, but usually there are no permanent neurologic sequelae. Mechanisms postulated to cause the transient loss of consciousness include (1) a sudden increase in pressure in the region of neurons critical for consciousness, (2) cerebral ischemia, (3) sudden depolarization or hyperpolarization (or both) of neurons, and (4) transient alteration in neuronal functioning secondary to mechanical distortion of neurons or axons. Although no gross neuropathologic change is usually apparent, diffuse axonal injury and individual neuronal alterations have been found on microscopic examination, especially in the region of the brainstem reticular formation.

Seizures (convulsions) are transient episodes of supratentorial origin in which there is an abrupt and temporary alteration in cerebral function. Seizures may consist of abnormal movements (such as tonic or clonic movements), an abnormal sensation (such as paresthesias or visual hallucination), or a disturbance in behavior or consciousness. They are caused by a spontaneous, excessive discharge of cortical neurons, which may occur as a result of an increase in neuronal excitability, an excessive excitatory synaptic input impinging on the nerve cells, or a decrease in normal inhibitory mechanisms.

Seizures can be either focal or generalized. A *focal* seizure, also called *partial* seizure, involves only a localized area of the cerebral cortex. Partial seizures have been subdivided into simple partial seizures, in which there is no loss of consciousness, and complex partial seizures, in which there is some alteration of consciousness. A *generalized* seizure involves widespread and bilateral areas of both hemispheres simultaneously. It may have some spread to the thalamus and reticular activating system and, therefore, is associated with a loss of consciousness.

Syncope (fainting) is a transient loss of consciousness due to a decrease in cerebral blood flow and ischemia of the entire brain.

This occurs as a result of decreased cardiac output, slowing of the heart rate, or pooling of blood in the periphery. The loss of consciousness is usually brief (a matter of seconds to minutes) and is preceded by light-headedness, weakness, giddiness, sweating, and dimming of vision. During this time, the patient is pale and sweaty; pulse is weak, and blood pressure is reduced. Syncope accompanied by brief generalized tonic, clonic, or tonic-clonic movements is called *convulsive syncope.*

Several systemic disorders produce *metabolic encephalopathy,* which diffusely affects the consciousness system and causes a transient alteration in consciousness, often without localizing signs. Hypoxemia, hypoglycemia, hyponatremia, and drug overdosage are common causes of metabolic encephalopathy.

Structural lesions can result in persistent impairment of consciousness or coma. Although we use the general term *coma* in this discussion, stupor and somnolence are also produced by identical disease processes. Coma results from lesions that involve the reticular formation and its projection systems or the cerebral hemispheres bilaterally.

Direct damage or depression of the consciousness system in the posterior fossa or diencephalon may occur from infarction, hemorrhage, neoplasia, trauma, metabolic disturbances, or anesthetic agents and drugs. Unilateral lesions of the cerebral hemispheres do not cause coma if the consciousness system is intact. However, coma does result from bilateral lesions that diffusely affect the cerebral hemispheres, such as encephalitis, meningitis, subarachnoid hemorrhage, metabolic disturbances (such as hypoglycemia), hypoxia, some degenerative diseases, and certain drugs.

Indirect involvement of the consciousness system also can result in coma. This involvement is usually the result of mass lesions that, although extrinsic to the consciousness system, compress or distort the diencephalon and brainstem. Common examples are mass lesions of the posterior fossa (for example, a cerebellar neoplasm) or expanding unilateral cerebral masses that result in herniation of the brain contents and secondary compression of diencephalic or midbrain structures (see Chapter 15 for further discussion).

In summary, coma can be produced by

1. focal lesions of the posterior fossa that involve the brainstem;
2. focal supratentorial lesions, if they are of such magnitude as to directly or indirectly involve the deep midline diencephalic structures necessary for the maintenance of consciousness;
3. diffuse lesions, generally of an anoxic, toxic-metabolic, or inflammatory nature, capable of causing widespread depression.

The Electroencephalogram

The EEG is a useful adjunct to neurologic diagnosis. Electrical activity recorded by the EEG from the cerebral cortex is classified into four main types, depending on the frequency or number of waveforms per second (hertz) (Fig. 14).

1. *Beta activity* is low-amplitude fast activity occurring at a frequency of more than 13 Hz. This type of activity is usually seen over the anterior head regions.
2. *Alpha activity* is rhythmic activity at a frequency of 8 to 13 Hz. These rhythms occur in the posterior head regions and are the predominant background activity

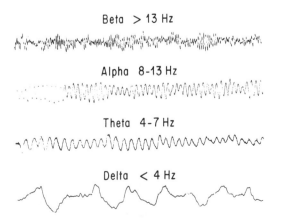

FIG. 14. Four basic EEG frequencies.

during the relaxed waking state when the eyes are closed (Fig. 15). With eye opening or with attention, there is attenuation of the rhythmic alpha background and replacement by a low-voltage pattern.

3. *Theta activity* ranges from 4 to 7 Hz and may be normal when present in a child or in an adult in a drowsy state, but when present in a fully awake adult it is abnormal.

4. *Delta activity* is the slowest waveform, occurring at a frequency of less than 4 Hz. This activity is normal when present in an infant or in a sleeping adult but is abnormal under any other circumstances.

The EEG is helpful in studying normal physiologic activity; however, it attains its greatest usefulness in detecting abnormalities of cerebral functioning. The EEG reflects the intrinsic cortical activity as modified by subcortical structures (the thalamus and the ascending projections of the ascending reticular activating system). Therefore, an EEG abnormality occurs as a result of a disturbance of (1) cortical neuronal activity, (2) subcortical structures that regulate cortical neuronal activity, and (3) the thalamocortical projection pathways.

The two main types of EEG abnormalities are slow-wave abnormalities and epileptiform abnormalities; both can be either focal or generalized (Table 6). A focal EEG abnormality indicates a localized disturbance of cerebral function, whereas a generalized EEG abnormality indicates a bilateral and diffuse disturbance of cerebral function or a disturbance that is projected to the surface from subcortical structures. Thus, the EEG helps to distinguish between a focal and a generalized disturbance of cerebral function and to determine the level of the brain involved.

In coma secondary to diffuse cerebral disease, the EEG shows widespread, generalized slowing (Fig. 16), with the degree of slowing often paralleling the degree of coma. When there is dysfunction of subcortical structures, the EEG shows different types of abnormalities, depending on the level of the neuraxis involved. With diencephalic or midbrain involvement, the EEG shows intermittent, rhythmic slow waves occurring bilaterally and synchronously over both hemispheres. If the pons or lower brainstem is involved, the EEG may contain alpha activity and resemble a normal waking record, but unlike the normal alpha rhythm in an alert person, this activity does not show normal reactivity to light,

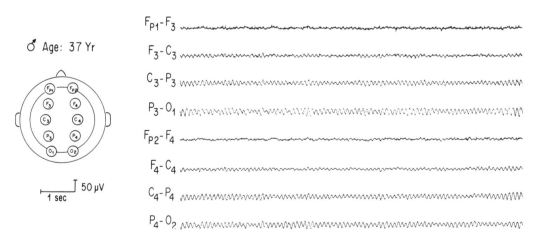

FIG. 15. Normal EEG pattern during the wakeful state, showing presence of alpha activity in the posterior head region. (In each EEG illustration, electrical activity is a bipolar recording of the potential difference between electrodes, indicated by letters and numbers to the left of each line. The location of each electrode is shown on the diagram of the head.)

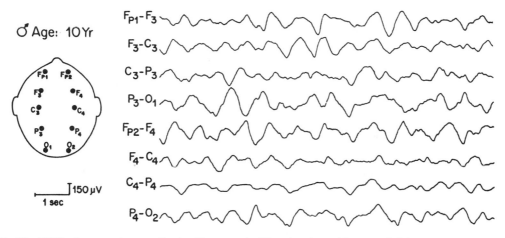

FIG. 16. EEG of a comatose patient with encephalitis, showing widespread delta slowing.

noise, or noxious stimuli. In addition, there may be cyclic sleep patterns consisting of sleep spindles, V waves, and delta waves. When there are focal cerebral lesions, focal slowing is seen on the EEG (Fig. 17). If the primary cerebral lesion is large enough to distort or to cause a pressure effect on diencephalic or mesencephalic structures, the EEG may show intermittent, widespread, rhythmic slow-wave abnormalities in addition to the focal slow-wave abnormality.

In the diagnosis of seizure disorders, the EEG shows epileptiform abnormalities consisting of sharp waves, spikes, or spike and slow-wave discharges that may occur in a focal or generalized manner (Fig. 18). During an actual seizure, these occur in a sustained, repetitive, and rhythmic fashion (Fig. 19).

Brain Death

Brain death occurs when neural damage is irreversible, and although cardiac activity may be present, there no longer is evidence of cerebral function. The patient is unresponsive and shows no spontaneous movement or behavioral response to external stimuli. The absence of brainstem function is manifested by

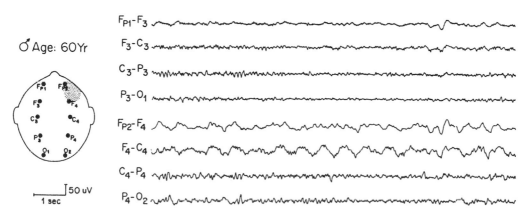

FIG. 17. EEG showing focal delta slowing over the right frontal area *(stippled)* due to right frontal tumor.

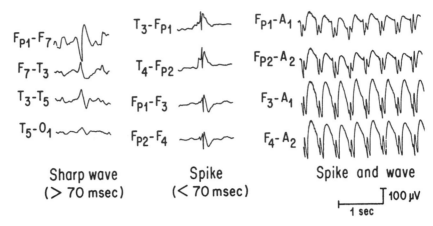

FIG. 18. Three types of epileptiform discharges. The sharp-wave discharge *(left)* was recorded from the left temporal region. The spike *(center)* and spike-and-(slow) wave discharges *(right)* were recorded from widespread areas of cortex.

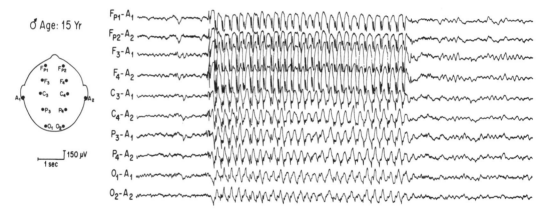

FIG. 19. Generalized 3-Hz spike-and-wave discharge with an absence seizure, during which the patient was unresponsive.

TABLE 6. *Electroencephalographic (EEG) changes in various disease processes*

Disease process	EEG changes	
	Focal	Diffuse
Infarct	Slow	
Tumor	Slow	
Focal seizure	Spikes, sharp waves	
Hypoxia		Slow
Hypoglycemia		Slow
Generalized seizure		Spikes, sharp waves
Brain death		No activity

loss of respiratory activity and all brainstem reflexes. Absence of cerebral function can be confirmed by blood flow studies that show cessation of blood flow in the brain or by the EEG, which shows a flat pattern with no sign of electrocerebral activity. Because brain function is markedly depressed by certain anesthetic agents and other drugs, they also can produce a flat EEG. This cause should be excluded before concluding that irreversible brain death is present.

Neurologic Examination of the Consciousness System ▪

Examination of a patient with altered consciousness represents a challenge to physicians. The situation is often emergent, and the patient is frequently uncooperative. Furthermore, assessment of the functions of the consciousness system alone seldom provides sufficient information for anatomicopathologic diagnosis, and one must rely on other associated clues from the history and results of physical examination to determine the location and cause of the responsible lesion.

Assessment of Consciousness System

Involvement of the consciousness system is evaluated by noting the patient's ability to perceive and attend to the external environment. The degree of coma is determined by the patient's response to stimuli, such as touch, pinprick, calling the patient's name, a hand clap, or some other form of loud noise. If the patient is unresponsive to milder forms of stimulation, then noxious or painful stimuli such as pinching or deep pressure in sensitive areas are used. The patient's response is observed to define the presence of delirium, confusion, somnolence, stupor, or coma (as described above), any of which would suggest some involvement of the consciousness system. However, from this evaluation one cannot determine the site or nature of the involvement.

Anatomicopathologic Diagnosis

Lesions affecting the consciousness system are located at the supratentorial or posterior fossa (or both) level; therefore, one must seek clues that suggest involvement at these levels by noting the vital signs (pulse, blood pressure, respiration, temperature) and examining motor, sensory, and cranial nerve functions. Precise anatomical localization is seldom necessary, but some attempt should be made to apply the general principles of anatomical diagnosis described in Chapter 3 to decide if the responsible lesion is located at the supratentorial level or the posterior fossa level, or if it is diffusely distributed at both levels.

This seemingly crude localization is actually extremely useful in the clinical setting, and when combined with information about the temporal evaluation of the illness, it is used (as described in Chapter 4) to establish a cause (vascular, inflammatory, toxic-metabolic, traumatic, neoplastic, or degenerative). Judicious selection of appropriate ancillary studies such as radiography, neuroimaging studies, blood studies, EEG, and cerebrospinal fluid examination is often required to establish a precise anatomicopathologic diagnosis.

Clinical Problems ▪

1. A 56-year-old man with diabetes mellitus became confused and then unresponsive over a period of several hours. He had given himself his usual injection of insulin on awakening in the morning. Because of an upset stomach, he failed to eat anything during the day. When brought to the emergency room, he was comatose but did not show localizing neurologic signs.
   a. What is the anatomicopathologic diagnosis?
   b. What portions of the consciousness system are involved?
   c. What is the precise etiologic diagnosis?

d. What changes might be found in the EEG?

2. A 74-year-old woman with a history of hypertension had a sudden onset of a severe, right-sided headache, followed by weakness of the left side of her face and body and somnolence. When hospitalized 1 hour later, she had severe weakness on the left side of the body and face and decreased sensation on the left side of the body and face. During the next few hours, she became progressively less responsive and finally comatose.

 a. Before the time the patient entered the hospital, what would be the most appropriate anatomicopathologic diagnosis?

 b. What is the nature of the pathologic lesion?

 c. What is the mechanism of her becoming comatose?

 d. What changes would be expected in the EEG?

3. A 38-year-old woman had a 3-year history of generalized grand mal seizures. On the day of admission to the hospital, she was found unresponsive on the floor of her living room. When brought to the emergency room, she was stuporous, with continuous bilateral convulsive movements of the face and upper and lower extremities. These subsided, and within 24 hours the results of neurologic examination were normal.

 a. What is the anatomicopathologic diagnosis?

 b. What changes might be seen in the EEG during the seizure?

 c. List six types of conditions that cause generalized seizures.

 d. If focal seizures were also present in this patient, would that influence your choice about their possible cause?

Additional Reading ■

Culebras, A. (ed.). The neurology of sleep. *Neurology* 42 (suppl 6), 1992.

Engel, J., Jr. *Seizures and Epilepsy.* Philadelphia: F. A. Davis, 1989.

Fisch, B. J. *Spehlmann's EEG Primer* (2nd ed.). Amsterdam: Elsevier, 1991.

Guilleminault, C., and Baker, T. L. Sleep and electroencephalography: Points of interest and points of controversy. *J. Clin. Neurophysiol.* 1:275, 1984.

Kandel, E. R., Schwartz, J. H., and Jessell, T. M. (eds.). *Principles of Neural Science* (3rd ed.). New York: Elsevier, 1991.

Kryger, M. H., Roth, T., and Dement, W. C (eds.). *Principles and Practice of Sleep Medicine* (2nd ed.). Philadelphia: W. B. Saunders, 1994.

Napier, T. C., Kalivas, P. W., and Hanin, I. (eds.). *The Basal Forebrain: Anatomy to Function.* New York: Plenum Press, 1991.

Plum, F., and Posner, J. B. *The Diagnosis of Stupor and Coma* (3rd ed.). Philadelphia: F. A. Davis, 1980.

Siegel, J. M. Mechanisms of sleep control. *J. Clin. Neurophysiol.* 7:49, 1990.

Steriade, M. Arousal: Revisiting the reticular activating system. *Science* 272:225, 1996.

Wijdicks, E. F. M. Determining brain death in adults. *Neurology* 45:1003, 1995.

Wijdicks, E. F. M. *Neurology of Critical Illness.* Philadelphia: F. A. Davis, 1995.

The Vascular System

◼

Objectives

1. Define ischemia, infarction, intracerebral hemorrhage, subarachnoid hemorrhage, aneurysm, arteriovenous malformation, embolus, transient ischemic attack, syncope, angiogram, and bruit.
2. Describe the methods of formation and the role of adenosine triphosphate in brain metabolism.
3. Describe the mechanisms of cell damage that occur with ischemia.
4. Define autoregulation, and discuss the factors that can alter cerebral blood flow.
5. Identify the following major vessels, and list the symptoms that might develop in a patient with a lesion of the affected artery:
   a. Vertebral artery
   b. Posterior communicating artery
   c. Common and internal carotid arteries
   d. Anterior cerebral artery
   e. Middle cerebral artery
   f. Basilar artery
   g. Posterior cerebral artery
6. Given a patient protocol:
   a. Recognize when the problem suggests cerebrovascular disease, and list those aspects of the protocol that led to this conclusion.
   b. Localize the area of abnormality to a specific area of the neuraxis, and identify whether that area of abnormality falls within the distribution of the internal carotid, vertebrobasilar, or spinal arterial systems.

c. Decide if the basic pathologic mechanism is hemorrhage or infarction, and state the reasons for your choice.

Introduction ◼

The blood vessels to an organ provide it with a relatively constant supply of oxygen and other nutrients and a means for removal of metabolic wastes. Failure to meet these vital requirements results in disease in that organ. Because of the unique structure and organization of the nervous system, localized abnormalities in blood supply may produce devastating alterations in neural function. In this chapter, the normal anatomy and physiology of the vascular supply to neural tissue and the clinical manifestations of pathologic processes affecting this system are described.

Of all neurologic diseases likely to be encountered, cerebrovascular disease (stroke) is among the most common. Cerebrovascular disease represents a major cause of disability and death throughout the world. In the United States, stroke ranks third as a cause of death (heart disease is first; cancer is second; accidents are fourth). The amount of money spent annually on diagnosis, treatment, and rehabilitation is extremely high, and because the majority of stroke victims survive the acute phase of illness and may live for years thereafter in a disabled condition, the social and economic impact of stroke is immeasurable.

Vascular disease involving cerebral vessels is no different from vascular disease involving other organ systems. The processes of athero-sclerosis and thromboembolism differ little whether they involve the cerebral, peripheral, or coronary circulation. However, understanding the clinical problems in patients with cerebrovascular disease depends on a more detailed understanding of activities that are unique to the nervous system.

In the other longitudinal systems already discussed, the manifestations of disease are a direct result of damage to neural tissue within that system. The vascular system, however, is a supporting system, and diseases of the vascular system will be manifest as secondary alterations in function in other neural systems. The vascular cause of disease is identified by the characteristic temporal profile of sudden onset and rapid evolution of symptoms involving other systems.

Overview ▪

To sustain aerobic metabolism, the brain is supplied by two major arterial systems. Much of the cerebral hemispheres is supplied by the carotid arterial system, whereas the entire posterior fossa, occipital lobes, and portions of the temporal lobes are supplied by the vertebrobasilar system. A series of anastomotic channels, including the circle of Willis located at the base of the brain, interconnect these two systems. The surface of the neuraxis receives its blood supply from large circumferential vessels, and the deep structures are supplied by smaller penetrating arteries and arterioles.

Lesions involving the carotid arterial system may alter function in the distribution of any or all of its three clinically important branches: ophthalmic artery, anterior cerebral artery, and middle cerebral artery. Therefore, the various combinations of hemiparesis, hemisensory deficit, monocular visual loss, homonymous hemianopia, and aphasia are suggestive of a lesion in this system. Lesions involving the vertebral and basilar arteries may alter function in the distribution of any or

all of their clinically important branches, which include those to the brainstem, to the cerebellum, and to the occipital and temporal lobes via the posterior cerebral artery. The various combinations of diplopia, dysarthria, dysphagia, and disequilibrium associated with hemiparesis, hemisensory deficit, or homonymous hemianopia are suggestive of a lesion in the vertebrobasilar system.

The blood supply to the spinal cord is via the anterior spinal artery and paired posterior spinal arteries (branches of the vertebral arteries and descending aorta), and the vascular supply to the peripheral nerves is usually via nutrient vessels from accompanying major arterial channels.

Cerebral blood flow is normally maintained at a relatively constant rate of approximately 50 to 55 ml/100 g brain tissue per minute by a process of *autoregulation* and can thereby compensate for fluctuations in perfusion pressure and cerebrovascular resistance. Reduction in blood flow below a critical threshold level results in ischemia and infarction. Several neurogenic, chemical, and metabolic factors interact to regulate cerebral blood flow in normal and pathologic states.

The clinical pattern seen with disease in the cerebrovascular system is distinctive. The cardinal identifying feature is its *acute* onset. The symptoms produced are a reflection of the location and nature of the pathologic process. The symptoms of vascular disease may be either focal or diffusely distributed and result from parenchymal dysfunction secondary to the primary pathologic change in the blood vessels or circulatory system. The parenchymal lesions, which are the result of either occlusive-ischemic or hemorrhagic disease processes, may be of a mass or a non-mass type (Table 1).

Occlusive-Ischemic Vascular Disease

When a portion of neural tissue is deprived of its blood supply, *ischemia* develops. If the normal protective mechanisms are insufficient to compensate for this deprivation, death of tissue, *infarction,* results. The process of

TABLE 1. *Correlation of vascular and parenchymal disease*

Type of vascular disease	Resultant parenchymal lesion	
	Focal	Diffuse
Occlusive-ischemic	Infarct (nonmass)	Anoxic encephalopathy
Hemorrhagic	Intracerebral hemorrhage (mass)	Subarachnoid hemorrhage

metabolic failure leading to cell death involves the cessation of blood flow, loss of energy, and neuronal depolarization. The resultant release of glutamate, entry of calcium ions into the cell, generation of oxygen free radicals and nitric oxide, and the activation of proteases and lipases all contribute to cell breakdown and infarction. The clinical symptoms reflect tissue damage in the regions of ischemia and infarction. Disease of a blood vessel may result in local thrombus formation, which may progress to occlusion—*thrombosis*—of the vessel, or a portion of the thrombus (embolus) may break loose and lodge in a more distal portion of the circulation. Both processes may result in localized areas of neural tissue being deprived of a blood supply, and both may produce a focal destructive lesion (infarct). Atherosclerosis is by far the most important disease process responsible for thromboembolic disease; however, it is not the only disease process responsible for it. Ischemia also may occur without occlusive disease if there is hemodynamic failure of the circulatory system (as might be seen with cardiac disease or profound hypotension). This type of ischemia also may result in infarction, but the defect is usually diffusely distributed throughout the brain as *anoxic encephalopathy.*

Hemorrhagic Vascular Disease

A diseased blood vessel may rupture and leak, producing *hemorrhage.* Depending on the site of accumulation of the blood, focal or diffuse neurologic symptoms may result. Blood that extravasates throughout the subarachnoid space is a *subarachnoid hemorrhage* and results in diffuse neurologic signs. Subarachnoid hemorrhage is commonly the result of trauma, rupture of an intracranial aneurysm, or bleeding from an arteriovenous malformation. Blood that accumulates within the substance of the brain is an *intracerebral hemorrhage* and results in signs of a focal, mass lesion. Intracerebral hemorrhage is commonly the result of hypertensive arteriolar disease or bleeding from an arteriovenous malformation.

Radiographic examination of the cerebral blood vessels by injection of a radiopaque substance into the arterial system (cerebral angiography), magnetic resonance angiography and imaging, and computed tomography are important neurodiagnostic techniques that are used to identify vascular and other intracranial disease processes.

Anatomy of the Vascular System ■

Blood Supply to the Brain

All the arteries that supply the supratentorial and posterior fossa levels arise from the aortic arch (Fig. 1). The innominate (brachiocephalic) artery divides into the right common carotid and the right subclavian arteries. The left common carotid artery arises directly from the apex of the aortic arch. The right and left common carotid arteries ascend in the neck lateral to the trachea. Slightly below the angle of the jaw, each vessel bifurcates into the internal and external carotid arteries.

The *internal carotid* artery on each side enters the skull, without branching, through the carotid canal located in the petrous portion of the temporal bone. After entering the cranium, each internal carotid artery forms an S-

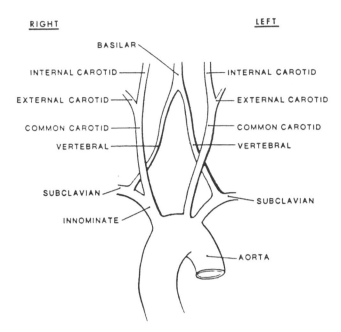

FIG. 1. Major arteries supplying the supratentorial and posterior fossa levels.

shaped curve, the carotid siphon, and lies within the cavernous sinus. As the artery leaves the cavernous sinus to enter the subarachnoid space at the base of the brain, it gives rise to the *ophthalmic artery,* which is an important anastomotic communication with branches of the external carotid artery. Each internal carotid artery then divides into an anterior cerebral artery and a middle cerebral artery (Fig. 2).

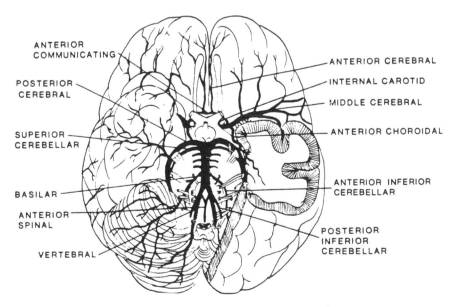

FIG. 2. Principal arterial vessels on the basal aspect of the brain. Portions of the left temporal lobe and the left cerebellar hemisphere have been removed. (Modified from Pansky, B., and House, E. L. *Review of Gross Anatomy* [3rd ed.]. New York: Macmillan, 1975. With permission.)

The *vertebral arteries* arise as the first branches of the right and left subclavian arteries. Each artery ascends through foramina in the transverse processes of the upper six cervical vertebrae, curves behind the articular process of the atlas, pierces the dura mater, and enters the subarachnoid space at the level of the upper cervical spinal cord. The vertebral arteries enter the cranial cavity through the foramen magnum. The vertebral arteries are subject to normal anatomical variations; the left vertebral artery frequently arises directly from the arch of the aorta. In addition, the two vertebral arteries are often of unequal caliber.

The vertebral arteries enter the cranium and ascend on the ventrolateral surface of the medulla oblongata (Fig. 2). At the lower border of the pons, they unite to form the *basilar artery*. At the level of the midbrain, the basilar artery divides into the right and left posterior cerebral arteries.

Circle of Willis

At the base of the brain, surrounding the optic chiasm and pituitary stalk, anastomotic connections occur between the internal carotid and vertebrobasilar arterial systems. This ring-like series of vessels is called the *circle of Willis* (Fig. 3) and consists of the *anterior communicating artery,* which unites the two anterior cerebral arteries, and the *posterior communicating arteries,* which join the internal carotid arteries with the posterior cerebral arteries. The circle of Willis is subject to frequent anatomical variation, and a normal circle is seen in only approximately 50% of the population. Common variations in the circle occur when the posterior cerebral arteries arise directly from the internal carotid via an enlarged posterior communicating artery, when one or both posterior communicating arteries are absent, and when there are multiple small anterior communicating arteries.

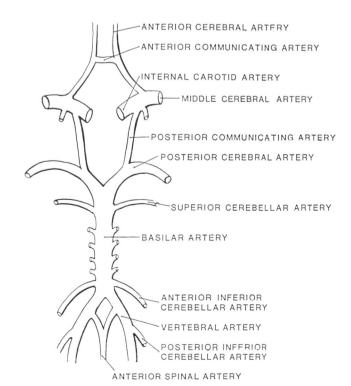

FIG. 3. The major intracranial arteries and the circle of Willis (anterior cerebral, anterior communicating, posterior communicating, and posterior cerebral arteries).

Blood Supply to the Outer Tube and Inner Tube of the Neuraxis

In developing a scheme of neural organization, the concept of an outer tube and an inner tube was presented. This concept is further reflected in the vascular supply to the brain. The cerebral cortex, involved in high-order processing in the sensory and motor systems, receives its blood supply from the large anastomotic circumferential arteries that are easily seen in the subarachnoid space. These vessels are responsive to chemical and metabolic regulation and are susceptible to the pathophysiologic processes of atherosclerosis and thromboembolism, often resulting in large areas of infarction. In contrast, the blood supply to the deep structures, including the diffuse internal regulation and consciousness systems, is from penetrating vessels and end arterioles. These vessels are less responsive to chemical and metabolic regulation and are susceptible to the pathologic changes accompanying blood pressure change, which predispose to small (*lacunar*) infarction and intracranial hemorrhage.

Blood Supply to the Cerebral Hemispheres

The supratentorial level is provided with blood from the anterior, middle, and posterior cerebral arteries (Fig. 4). The *anterior cerebral artery* supplies the medial surface of the cerebrum and the superior border of the frontal and parietal lobes. The *middle cerebral artery* supplies most of the lateral surface of the cerebral hemispheres, including the lateral portions of the frontal lobe, the superior and lateral portions of the temporal lobes, and the deep structures of the frontal and parietal lobes. The *posterior cerebral artery* supplies the entire occipital lobe and the inferior and medial portions of the temporal lobe. The deeper structures of the cerebral hemispheres are supplied by penetrating branches of the larger arteries. Of notable importance are the perforating *lenticulostriate arteries,* which supply the basal ganglia and internal capsule, and the perforating branches of the posterior cerebral artery, which supply the thalamus (Fig. 5).

Anastomoses and Collateral Circulation

Extensive communications exist between the arterial systems that supply the brain. Because of the potential for additional circulation through these alternate channels, occlusion of one or more intracranial or extracranial vessels may occur at times, with few or no resultant neurologic signs and symptoms. The major anastomotic channels

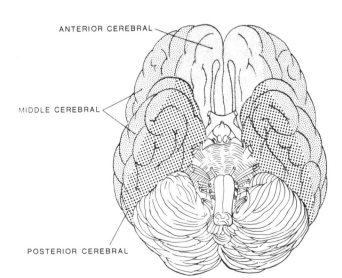

ANTERIOR CEREBRAL

MIDDLE CEREBRAL

POSTERIOR CEREBRAL

FIG. 4. Areas of distribution of the anterior, middle, and posterior cerebral arteries to the base of the cerebral hemispheres.

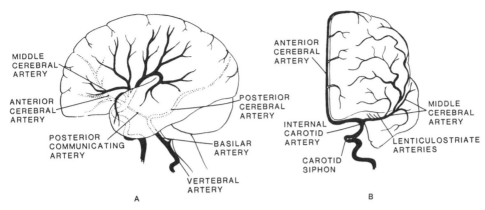

FIG. 5. Course and distribution of the major supratentorial arteries in a lateral view **(A)** and an anteroposterior view **(B)**.

are (1) the circle of Willis; (2) corticomeningcal anastomoses—communications of the three major cerebral vessels on the surface of the hemispheres at the junctional zones of the areas supplied by these vessels; and (3) anastomoses between extracranial and intracranial arteries. The most significant in the last group occur in the regions of the face and orbit, where the ophthalmic artery, a branch of the internal carotid artery, communicates with the superficial temporal and facial branches of the external carotid artery. Occasionally, anastomoses between the external carotid and vertebral arteries occur in the neck.

Blood Supply to the Posterior Fossa

The structures contained in the posterior fossa (midbrain, pons, medulla, and cerebellum) are supplied by branches of the vertebral and basilar arteries (Fig. 2). Although there are numerous branches from these vessels, the pattern of blood supply from these branches is relatively constant (Fig. 6). At each level of the brainstem, short *median* and *paramedian perforating branches* arise and supply a zone on either side of the midline. The paramedian area of the caudal medulla is supplied by the *anterior spinal artery*, which arises from the union of branches from each vertebral artery. The paramedian area at higher levels is sup-

plied by penetrating branches of the basilar artery. An intermediate zone, situated more laterally at each level, is supplied by *short circumferential branches* of the vertebrobasilar system. The lateral areas of the brainstem and the cerebellum are supplied by three pairs of *long circumferential arteries.* The *posterior inferior cerebellar arteries* arise from the vertebral arteries and supply the lateral medulla and posterior inferior aspect of the cerebellum. The *anterior inferior cerebellar artery* is a branch of the basilar artery and supplies the lateral aspect of the pons and the anterior inferior cerebellum. The *superior cerebellar artery* is a branch of the basilar artery and supplies the lateral midbrain and superior surface of the cerebellum.

Functional Anatomy of the Cerebral Vasculature

Clinically, the distribution of a presumed arterial lesion can be inferred by relating the observed signs and symptoms to the anatomy of the cerebral vessels. Although precise localization to a specific blood vessel is at times desirable, it is *essential* to be able to determine whether a lesion lies in the distribution of either the carotid or the vertebrobasilar arterial systems (Table 2).

Lesions involving the internal carotid artery may alter function in the distribution of

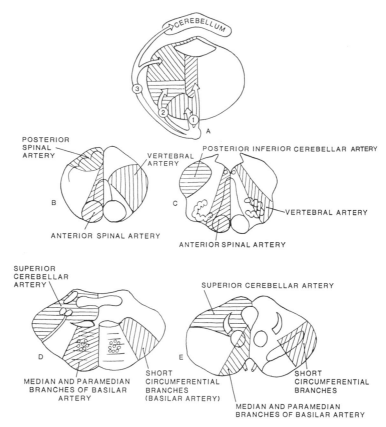

FIG. 6. Blood supply to the posterior fossa. **A:** General pattern of blood supply. Arising from the basilar artery are *(1)* short median and paramedian branches supplying blood to the medial tegmentum and base of the brainstem, *(2)* short circumferential branches supplying blood to the ventrolateral tegmentum, and *(3)* long circumferential branches supplying blood to the dorsolateral tegmentum and the cerebellum. The areas of distribution of specific arteries are shown in the caudal medulla **(B)**, medulla **(C)**, rostral pons **(D)**, and midbrain **(E)**.

any or all of its three clinically important branches: (1) the ophthalmic artery, producing ipsilateral monocular loss of vision; (2) the anterior cerebral artery, producing contralateral weakness and sensory loss primarily in the leg; and (3) the middle cerebral artery, producing contralateral weakness and sensory loss maximal in the face and arm and, to a lesser degree, in the leg. If the optic pathways are involved, a contralateral homonymous

TABLE 2. *Neurologic signs associated with lesions of the carotid and vertebrobasilar systems*

Carotid system	Vertebrobasilar system
Hemiparesis (contralateral body and face)	Hemiparesis (contralateral body, ipsilateral face)
Hemisensory loss (contralateral body and face)	Hemisensory loss (contralateral body, ipsilateral face)
Homonymous hemianopia	Diplopia
Monocular loss of vision	Dysphagia
Aphasia	Dysarthria
	Dysequilibrium

hemianopia may be produced. With dominant hemisphere lesions, there may be involvement of speech areas, which will result in aphasia.

Therefore, the various combinations of hemiparesis, hemisensory deficit, monocular loss of vision, homonymous hemianopia, and aphasia are suggestive of a lesion in the carotid arterial system.

Lesions involving vertebral and basilar arteries may alter function in the distribution of any or all of their clinically important branches: (1) branches to the brainstem itself, resulting in loss of brainstem function, cranial nerve abnormalities with or without hemiparesis, and hemisensory deficits; (2) branches to the cerebellum, resulting in ataxia and disequilibrium; and (3) posterior cerebral artery, resulting in unilateral or bilateral hemianopia.

Therefore, the various combinations of diplopia, dysarthria, dysphagia, and disequilibrium associated with hemiparesis, hemisensory deficit, and homonymous hemianopia are suggestive of a lesion in the vertebrobasilar arterial system.

Blood Supply to the Spinal Cord

The spinal cord is supplied with arterial blood by one anterior and two posterolateral vessels that run along the length of the cord and by an irregular plexus of segmentally arranged vessels that encircle the cord and interconnect the major vessels (Fig. 7). The *anterior spinal artery* is a single vessel lying in the ventral median fissure. It arises from a pair of small branches of the vertebral arteries that fuse along the caudal medulla and descend along the cervical spinal cord (Fig. 2). A series of six to eight ventral radicular arteries arising from the intercostal, lumbar, and sacral arteries connect with the anterior spinal artery at various levels along the length of the spinal cord (Fig. 8). The largest of these radicular arteries enters at the low thoracic or upper lumbar region. Because of this uneven blood supply, the spinal cord is most vulnerable to ischemia at the midthoracic and upper lumbar levels, as shown by the stippled areas in Fig. 8. Sulcal branches of the anterior spinal artery pass alternatively to the right and left at each segment to supply blood for the interior of the spinal cord (Fig. 7).

The *posterior spinal arteries* are paired structures that run along the posterolateral aspect of the cord near the dorsal roots. They receive contributions from the posterior radicular arteries (Fig. 9) and supply the dorsal funiculus and dorsal gray horns (see Fig. 7).

Vascular diseases of the spinal cord are less common than they are in the posterior fossa or cerebrum. When ischemic disease occurs, however, it is most often confined to the distribution of the anterior spinal artery, where it produces loss of motor function and loss of pain and temperature sensation below the lesion; the functions associated with the dorsal columns are spared (Fig. 7).

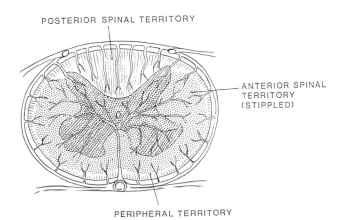

POSTERIOR SPINAL TERRITORY

ANTERIOR SPINAL TERRITORY (STIPPLED)

PERIPHERAL TERRITORY

FIG. 7. Diagram of a transverse section of the spinal cord illustrating the areas of supply of the anterior and posterior spinal arteries and the peripheral zone supplied by the circumferential vessels.

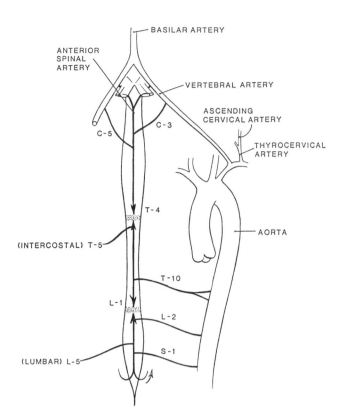

FIG. 8. Anterior spinal artery. Radicular arteries are variable in location but are shown here at C-3, C-5, T-5, T-10, L-2, and S-1. *Stippled areas* indicate zones of marginal blood supply at T-4 and L-1.

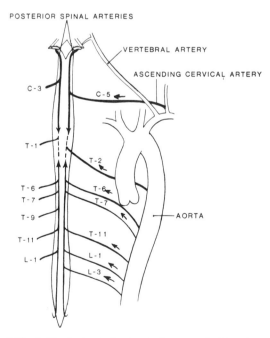

FIG. 9. Posterior spinal arteries supply blood to the posterior aspect of the spinal cord. They receive blood from radicular arteries at multiple levels.

Blood Supply to Peripheral Structures

All neural structures must receive adequate arterial blood supply in order to sustain life and to maintain their integrity. Axons traveling to the periphery are gathered into bundles or fascicles that have a connective tissue covering. Within this covering, along the entire course of the nerve, is a rich and highly anastomotic plexus of small arterioles derived from the branches of the major extremity vessels (Fig. 10). This dense anastomosis renders the peripheral nerve relatively immune to ischemic vascular disease. Such abnormality, when noted in peripheral neural structures, is usually associated with either direct compression of a nerve or with multiple segmental vascular lesions from small vessel arterial disease.

Venous Drainage of the Central Nervous System

The venous drainage of the brain is divided into superficial and deep systems. The cere-

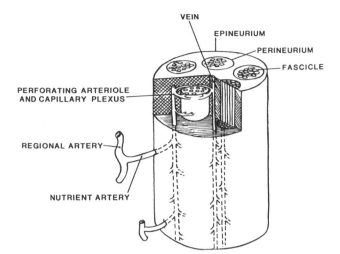

FIG. 10. Blood supply to peripheral nerve. Multiple anastomotic channels are derived from regional arteries.

bral cortex and outer half of the white matter drain into the superficial system of veins located over the convexity of the brain in the subarachnoid space. The superficial veins of the superior half of the brain drain into the *superior sagittal sinus;* those from the inferior half drain into the *lateral sinuses.* The deep white matter and deep nuclei of the brain drain into the deep venous system, which includes the *great cerebral vein of Galen, infe-*

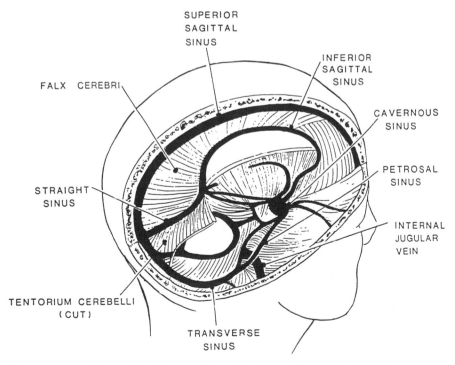

FIG. 11. Dura mater and its major sinuses. Dorsolateral view illustrating the falx cerebri, tentorium cerebelli, and dura mater lining the base of the skull. The dural venous sinuses are *stippled* or *black.*

rior sagittal sinus, and *straight sinus.* From these venous channels, blood empties into the transverse sinuses, the sigmoid sinuses, and ultimately the jugular veins (Fig. 11). Veins on the inferior surfaces of the cerebrum terminate directly or indirectly in the *cavernous sinus,* an important dural structure located on either side of the pituitary fossa containing the carotid artery; cranial nerves III, IV, and VI; and branches of cranial nerve V.

The spinal cord is drained by an anastomotic venous plexus surrounding the dural sac. Veins drain outward along both the dorsal and ventral roots into this plexus, which has numerous connections with the veins of the thoracic, abdominal, and pelvic cavities.

Physiology of the Vascular System ■

Cerebral Blood Flow

For normal neural function, adequate blood flow and oxygenation must be maintained. The normal blood flow through the brain is approximately 750 ml per minute, or about 50 to 55 ml/100 g brain tissue per minute. Although the brain constitutes only 2% of the body weight, it receives 15% of the cardiac output and utilizes 20% of the oxygen consumed in the basal state. The total oxygen consumption of the brain is approximately 50 ml per minute, or 3.7 ml/100 g brain tissue per minute. Any decrease in the amount of available oxygen provided to the brain reduces neural activity. Under normal conditions, the total oxygen consumption and blood flow to the brain are nearly constant. Cortical gray matter, with its increased metabolic demand, has about six times the blood flow of white matter. Local changes in blood flow may occur with the changing demands of varying neural activity.

In any hemodynamic system, blood flow is directly proportional to the perfusion pressures and inversely proportional to the total resistance of the system. For the brain, this can be expressed by the following equation:

Cerebral blood flow ≈

$$\frac{\text{mean arterial pressure} - \text{central venous pressure}}{\text{cerebrovascular resistance}}$$

Several factors can modify cerebral blood flow by altering different elements in the equation above. These have been arbitrarily divided into two groups: (1) extracerebral factors and (2) intracerebral factors (Table 3).

Extracerebral Factors

Factors outside the cranial cavity that modify or regulate cerebral blood flow are related primarily to the cardiovascular system and include the systemic blood pressure, the efficiency of cardiac function, and the viscosity of the blood. The principal force in maintaining the cerebral circulation is the pressure difference between the arteries and the veins. Because under normal circumstances cerebral venous pressure is low (approximately 5 mm Hg), arterial blood pressure becomes the most important factor in maintaining cerebral blood flow. Variations in systemic arterial blood pressure do not, however, ordinarily produce changes in cerebral blood flow in healthy persons if the intrinsic regulatory mechanisms are intact, unless the mean arterial pressure decreases to less than 50 to 70 mm Hg. Systemic arterial blood pressure is dependent on the efficiency of cardiac function (cardiac output) and peripheral vasomotor tone or resistance. These factors are governed principally by autonomic control from the vasomotor center in the medulla. Alterations in cardiac rhythm and myocardial function or the presence of cardiac disease may result in changes in cardiac output that may secondarily influence cerebral blood flow. Baroreceptors in the carotid sinus and aortic arch participate in reflexes that mediate cardiovascular tone and help to maintain a constant blood pressure. Advancing age, the presence of atherosclerosis, and certain drugs may alter these reflex mechanisms, and a simple physiologic act such as assuming an upright posture may result in severe orthostatic hypotension and pronounced reduction in cere-

TABLE 3. *Factors regulating cerebral blood flow (CBF)*

Factors	Increased CBF	Decreased CBF
Extracerebral		
Systemic blood pressure		Mean arterial pressure <50 to 70 mm Hg
Cardiovascular function		Cardiac arrhythmias; orthostatic hypotension; loss of carotid sinus and aortic arch reflexes
Blood viscosity	Anemia	Polycythemia
Intracerebral		
State of the cerebral vasculature	Arteriovenous malformation	Atherosclerosis
Intracranial CSF pressure		Increased intracranial pressure
Cerebral autoregulatory mechanisms		
Myogenic factors	Decreased intraluminal pressure (vasodilation)	Increased intraluminal pressure (vasoconstriction)
Neurogenic factors	Parasympathetic stimulation (vasodilation)	Sympathetic stimulation (vasoconstriction)
Biochemical-metabolic factors	Increased carbon dioxide (vasodilation)	Decreased carbon dioxide (vasoconstriction)
	Decreased oxygen (vasodilation)	Increased oxygen (vasoconstriction)
	Decreased pH (acidosis) (vasodilation)	Increased pH (alkalosis) (vasoconstriction)
	Lactic acid (vasodilation)	

CSF, cerebrospinal fluid.

bral blood flow (causing fainting or syncope). In addition, the viscosity of the blood may alter cerebral blood flow; severe anemia may increase flow as much as 30% and polycythemia may decrease it by more than 50%.

Intracerebral Factors

The state of the cerebral vasculature also can influence cerebral blood flow. Widespread intracranial arterial disease increases cerebrovascular resistance and can result in a reduction in cerebral blood flow, whereas pathologic processes that are associated with a rapid shunting of blood from arteries to veins (such as occurs with an arteriovenous malformation) may produce both an increase in total cerebral blood flow and a local reduction in tissue perfusion.

Any increase in intracranial pressure is transmitted directly to the low-pressure venous system and increases cerebral venous pressure, thus decreasing cerebral blood flow. In pathologic states that are frequently accompanied by an increase in intracranial pressure (see Chapter 6), this reduction in blood flow may further accentuate the signs and symptoms produced by the primary lesion.

Regulation of Cerebral Blood Flow

Several factors can modify cerebral blood flow: (1) metabolic regulation, (2) autoregulation, (3) chemical factors, and (4) neurogenic control (Fig. 12).

Metabolic Regulation

Under normal conditions, cerebral blood flow is coupled directly to neuronal metabolic activity, with a linear increase or decrease in cerebral blood flow resulting from a corresponding change in brain metabolic activity. This coupling of blood flow occurs with a short latency of 1 to 2 seconds and is a strictly regional effect, producing little alteration in overall total blood flow despite measurable local change. Local metabolic coupling can be demonstrated during sleep, during various sensorimotor tasks, and in pathologic conditions such as coma and seizure. The mechanism of metabolic coupling involves vasodilator metabolites such as adenosine, potassium

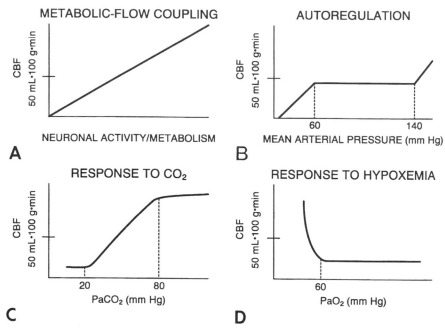

FIG. 12. Factors that regulate cerebral blood flow (CBF). **A:** There is a linear relationship between focal neuronal metabolism and blood flow. This coupling involves local factors affected by neuronal activity and ATP consumption by the sodium-potassium pump, particularly at the level of the synapses (gray matter). These local factors include extracellular acidosis, potassium, adenosine, and nitric oxide. **B:** Cerebral autoregulation maintains CBF constant despite changes in mean arterial blood pressure between approximately 60 and 140 mm Hg and depends on myogenic mechanisms. **C:** Carbon dioxide (CO_2) is a potent vasodilator even at physiologic Pa_{CO_2}, whereas hypoxemia **(D)** produces vasodilatation only when it is severe.

and hydrogen ions, prostaglandins, oxygen free radicals, and nitric oxide.

Autoregulation

The normal brain has the ability to regulate its own blood supply (*autoregulation*) in response to changes in arterial blood pressure and metabolic demand. *Autoregulation* is defined as the ability of an organ (for example, the brain) to maintain its blood flow constant for all but the widest extremes in perfusion pressure. Autoregulation of the cerebral blood flow occurs when the mean arterial blood pressure is between 60 and 150 mm Hg; below 60 mm Hg blood flow decreases, and above 150 mm Hg blood flow increases.

The brain can accomplish autoregulation by using myogenic, neurogenic, and chemical-metabolic mechanisms. Autoregulation occurs in both large and small arterioles. Cerebral vessels, like other hollow organs that contain smooth muscle, can alter their diameter in response to intraluminal pressure. This effect (known as the Bayliss effect) results in vasoconstriction with increased intraluminal pressure and in vasodilatation with a decrease in pressure. Therefore, autoregulation is primarily a pressure-controlled myogenic mechanism that operates independently but synergistically with other neurogenic and chemical-metabolic factors.

Autoregulation is a major homeostatic and protective mechanism. In normal persons, it prevents alteration in cerebral blood flow despite variations in systemic blood pressure or regional increases in metabolic demand on the brain. In the situation of regional increase in metabolism, a corresponding increase in carbon dioxide results, to produce local vasodilatation and increased blood flow, thus accommodating the increased metabolic demand. In certain disease states associated with vascular occlusion, an area of regional ischemia develops because of the reduction in available blood supply; intraluminal pressure decreases, oxygen is no longer available, carbon dioxide tension increases, lactate is produced, and the tissue becomes acidotic. All these factors produce vasodilatation of nearby vessels and may provide an increase in blood flow to an area of ischemia. In certain situations, this is sufficient to increase regional cerebral blood flow and to prevent infarction; in other situations, it may reduce the size of the resultant infarct. In a region of cerebral infarction, these protective mechanisms have reduced cerebrovascular resistance to a very low value. Because there is little acute change in the central venous pressure, the major determinant of blood flow in the region of ischemic tissue becomes the mean arterial blood pressure. The proper maintenance of systemic blood pressure, therefore, may be of prime importance in the treatment of ischemic infarcts, and any pronounced reduction in systemic pressure or the presence of cerebral edema (which will secondarily increase venous pressure) may further alter cellular function.

Chemical Factors

Chemical factors exert a strong influence on cerebral blood flow. *Carbon dioxide,* a substance that diffuses rapidly across the blood–brain barrier and an end product of cerebral metabolism, is also the most potent physiologic and pharmacologic agent that influences cerebral blood flow. Cerebral blood vessels react rapidly to any change in local carbon dioxide tension ($PaCO_2$). Any increase in $PaCO_2$ produces vasodilatation and increased cerebral blood flow, whereas a decrease in $PaCO_2$ has the opposite effect. The cerebral circulation reacts to *oxygen* in the reverse manner: a reduction in local oxygen tension (PaO_2) produces vasodilatation and increased cerebral blood flow, and an increase in PaO_2 produces vasoconstriction and a decrease in cerebral blood flow. The exact mechanism by which these agents exert their effects on cerebral blood vessels is unknown. They may act directly on the smooth muscle of the vessel wall, indirectly via neurogenic chemoreceptors, or by producing alterations in brain hydrogen ion concentration (pH). A reduction in brain pH (acidosis) from any cause produces vasodilatation and increased cerebral blood flow, whereas an increase in brain pH (alkalosis) is associated with vasoconstriction and decreased cerebral blood flow. *Lactic acid,* which is produced by the shift to anaerobic metabolism in regions of ischemia, is therefore a potent vasodilator.

Neurogenic Control

Although the extracranial and intracranial arteries are richly supplied by a neural network, neurogenic factors do not seem to have as great a role in the regulation of cerebral blood flow as chemical and metabolic factors. Neurogenic control can be viewed as composed of extrinsic, intrinsic, and local components in the brain (Table 4):

1. Extrinsic neurogenic control is provided by postganglionic fibers from the *superior cervical sympathetic ganglion* that innervate the carotid and vertebral arteries and their major intracranial branches. Norepinephrine released from these sympathetic fibers produces vasoconstriction. The main role of this neurogenic control is to protect capillaries against hyperperfusion whenever blood pressure is increased. Parasympathetic fibers travel in the *facial and superficial petrosal nerves* to innervate cerebral blood vessels of large and small diameter. These fibers use aceteylcholine as a transmitter. Fibers from the facial nerve are a source of *ni-*

TABLE 4. *The effect of neurogenic factors on arteries*

Type	Source	Neurotransmitter	Effect
Extrinsic	Sympathetic (superior cervical ganglia)	Norepinephrine	Constrict
		Neuropeptide Y	Constrict
	Parasympathetic	Acetylcholine	Dilate
	(facial and superficial petrosal nerves)	VIP	Dilate
		Nitric oxide	Dilate
	Trigeminal nerve	Substance P	Dilate
		CGRP	Dilate
Intrinsic	Locus ceruleus	Norepinephrine	Dilate (microcirculation)
	Raphe nucleus	Serotonin	Constrict
Local	Interneurons	Neuropeptide Y	Constrict
		VIP	Dilate
		Nitric oxide	Dilate

CGRP, calcitonin gene-related peptide; VIP, vasoactive intestinal peptide.

tric oxide, a potent vasodilator substance. Fibers from the *trigeminal ganglion* that use substance P and calcitonin gene-related peptide also innervate cerebral vessels and produce vasodilatation and increased permeability.

2. Intrinsic neurogenic control of the cerebral circulation is provided by pathways originating in the brainstem and by interneurons in the cerebral cortex. The major brainstem pathways are from (a) the locus ceruleus, whose neurons use norepinephrine to produce microcirculatory vasodilatation; and (b) the raphe nuclei, whose neurons use serotonin, a vasoconstrictor substance. Some cortical interneurons contain neuropeptide Y (a vasoconstrictor) or vasoactive intestinal polypeptide (a vasodilator) and, thus, could contribute to local regulation of blood flow.

Cerebral Metabolism

High metabolic activity and high oxygen consumption characterize cerebral metabolism. A constant supply of energy is necessary for the support of neuronal and neurologic functions. These vital energy-dependent processes include the establishment of membrane potentials, maintenance of transmembrane ionic gradients, membrane transport, and the synthesis of cellular constituents such as proteins, nucleic acids, lipids, and neurotransmitters. The energy needed is supplied in the form of high-energy phosphate bonds from adenosine triphosphate (ATP), which is synthesized in the brain, as in other organ systems, through the glycolytic pathway, the Krebs (citric acid) cycle, and the respiratory (electron-transport) chain (Table 5).

Under aerobic conditions, glucose is effectively metabolized through the glycolytic pathway, citric acid cycle, and respiratory chain to yield 38 moles of ATP per mole of glucose. Under anaerobic conditions, the Krebs (citric acid) cycle and respiratory chain cannot be activated (because of lack of oxygen); therefore, the pyruvate derived from glycolysis is metabolized to lactate and yields only 2 moles of ATP per mole of glucose. Another source of high-energy phosphate bonds is *creatine phosphate.* This compound, which is even more abundant than ATP in the brain, is used to regenerate ATP from adenosine disphosphate and is thus important for maintaining the level of tissue ATP. Although glycogen is present and the brain is capable of its rapid synthesis and breakdown, the role of glycogen in brain metabolism is not completely understood. Glucose is the basic substrate for brain metabolism. The astrocytes store glycogen and are the source of lactate, which can be used by the neurons to produce glucose.

TABLE 5. *Glucose metabolism*

1. Anaerobic glycolysis

$$\text{Glucose} \xrightarrow[+4\ \text{ATP}]{-2\ \text{ATP}} \text{2 pyruvate} + \text{2 NADH} \qquad (+2\ \text{ATP})$$

2. Krebs (citric acid) cycle

$$\text{2 Pyruvate} \longrightarrow \text{2 acetyl-CoA} + \text{2 NADH}$$

$$\begin{array}{l} \longrightarrow \text{oxaloacetic} \longrightarrow \quad +6\ \text{NADH} \\ \longleftarrow \alpha\text{-ketoglutarate} \longleftarrow \quad +2\ \text{FADH}_3 \end{array} \qquad (+2\ \text{ATP})$$

3. Respiratory (electron-transport) chain

10 NADH	$\longrightarrow$	10 NAD$^+$ (+30 ATP)
2 FADH$_3$	$\longrightarrow$	2 FAD (+4 ATP)
Summary: Glucose	$\longrightarrow$	CO$_2$ + H$_2$O (+38 ATP)

ATP, adenosine triphosphate; CO_2, carbon dioxide; FAD, flavin adenine dinucleotide; FADH$_3$, flavin adenine trinucleotide; NADH, reduced nicotinamide adenine dinucleotide.

Pathophysiology

Reversible alteration in cell function due to lack of oxygen results in *ischemia,* and irreversible alteration results in *infarction.* After vessel occlusion and deprivation of blood flow to the brain, a series of events unfold (the "ischemic cascade") that consist of the following alterations and lead ultimately to neuronal dysfunction and death (Fig. 13):

1. Cerebral blood flow and cerebral oxygen and glucose consumption decrease in the center of the ischemic area. These functions are less impaired at the periphery of the ischemic area (the "ischemic penumbra") where there are accompanying metabolic and electrophysiologic changes but where blood flow is sufficient to prevent irreversible cell damage (Fig. 13).
2. Local autoregulatory mechanisms are impaired and local responsivity of vessels to chemical and metabolic changes and to alterations in perfusion pressure is lost.
3. Anaerobic glycolysis is initiated as the vital substrates, oxygen and glucose, are decreased and brain glycogen content falls. Tissue lactate increases but pH decreases, and a zone of hyperemia and increased perfusion develops in the periphery of the ischemic zone.
4. Substrate depletion leads to failure of mitochondrial function and inefficient ATP generation, with leakage of potassium ions from cells and the intracellular accumulation of sodium, chloride, and calcium ions and free fatty acids. The net effect is neuronal depolarization, loss of the transmembrane potential, and increase in tissue water. This also produces impairment of ATP-dependent neurotransmitter reuptake.
5. Energy loss also results in increased release of excitatory neurotransmitters such as glutamate. The neurotoxic effect of this large accumulation of glutamate in the extracellular space is exerted through activation of N-methyl-D-aspartate (NMDA) and α-amino-3-hydroxy-5-methylisoxazole-4-propionate (AMPA) receptors, causing increased permeability to sodium ions, cellular swelling and lysis, and massive entry of calcium ions into the postsynaptic neuron. Additional calcium-induced release of excitatory neuro-

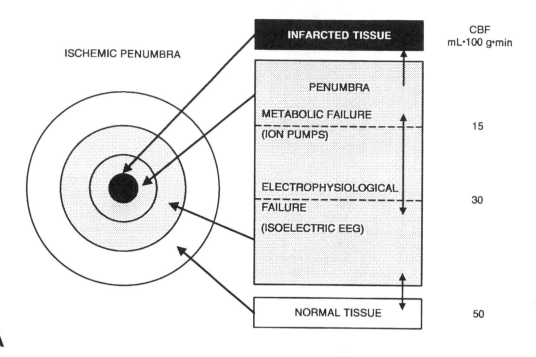

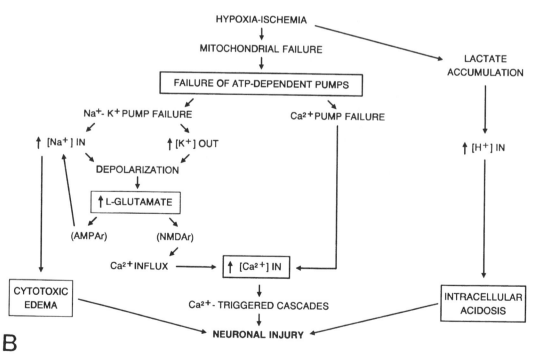

transmitters during the ischemic process heightens neuronal necrosis.

6. The increase in intracellular calcium activates phospholipases, proteases, and endonucleases and generates oxygen free radicals and nitric oxide. This leads to membrane, mitochondrial DNA, and microtubular damage and eventually cell destruction (Fig. 13B).

If the period of ischemia is short and the supply of high-energy phosphate bonds can be reestablished, neuronal function can resume. The local accumulation of adenosine, potassium, and hydrogen, which occurs in response to the production of lactic acid, produces local vasodilatation in an attempt to restore an adequate blood supply. However, if the cell continues to be deprived of its nourishment, catabolic and morphologic changes occur in the neuron. Initially, the cell begins to swell (acute cell change); if its metabolic needs are not met, the cell becomes irreversibly damaged. This is referred to as *infarction,* the morphologic correlate of which is *ischemic cell change* (described in Chapter 4). If the area of infarction is large, other cellular elements and the blood–brain barrier will be affected. In the region of maximal change, there is death and destruction of cells. With the catabolic changes and breakdown in the blood–brain barrier, the water content of the tissue increases. The associated *brain edema* may further impair the function of cells in the regions surrounding the infarction. After scavenger cells enter the area and the cellular debris is removed, a cystic cavity remains.

In conditions of partial ischemia, the decline of high-energy phosphate bonds is less precipitous, and the irreversible damage occurs only after a more prolonged period of ischemia. Thus, in *cerebral hypoxia,* because there is an abundant supply of glucose, the metabolic changes are similar to those of anoxia but lesser in extent. However, if the hypoxia is prolonged, the accumulation of lactate due to accelerated glycolysis becomes significant and ischemia and infarction may result.

In *hypoglycemia,* the brain is supplied with adequate oxygen but lacks glucose as a substrate. Hypoglycemia produces a different metabolic pattern from that seen in cerebral ischemia. In hypoglycemia, the brain can maintain high-energy phosphate bonds through the utilization of creatine phosphate and other substances. Although function is temporarily altered, if the glucose deficiency is not present for a prolonged period, then catabolic changes are not produced and recovery can occur upon reversal of the hypoglycemic state.

Pathology of the Vascular System

The symptoms and signs produced by vascular disease are a reflection of altered neuronal function in focal or diffuse areas of the ner-

---

FIG. 13. **A:** The ischemic penumbra. Decreased cerebral blood flow (CBF) produces a gradient of severity of deprivation of oxygen and glucose in brain tissue. Between the area of infarction and normal tissue is an area of jeopardized brain tissue called the ischemic penumbra. Neurons in this region have potentially reversible electrophysiologic failure due to energy deprivation but have not undergone the cascade leading to neuronal death. The ischemic penumbra is the target of neuroprotective treatment in ischemic stroke. **B:** Cascade of events leading to ischemic neuronal injury. The initial mechanism is mitochondrial failure, ATP depletion, and pump failure. This leads to neuronal depolarization due to increase of extracellular potassium (K^+), decrease in the reuptake of L-glutamate, and increase in intracellular sodium (Na^+) and calcium (Ca^{2+}). Calcium-triggered cascades, including phospholipases, proteases, and nucleases together with intracellular acidosis (due to accumulation of lactate), lead to production of oxygen free radicals, disruption of the cytoskeleton, and neuronal death. AMPAr, α-amino-3-hydroxy-5-methylisoxazole-4-proprionate receptor; NMDAr, *N*-methyl-D-aspartate receptor.

vous system. The location and nature of the underlying neural-parenchymal lesion are directly related to the abnormalities found in the blood vessels or circulatory system. Therefore, this discussion of the pathology of the vascular system considers (1) the major derangements involving blood vessels and (2) the neural-parenchymal lesions produced by these vascular abnormalities.

Vascular Pathology

Normal Arterial Histology

The normal arterial wall contains three distinct layers (Fig. 14): (1) the *intima,* a layer of endothelial cells surrounding the vessel lumen with a small amount of extracellular connective tissue, the internal elastic lamina; (2) the *media,* a layer of diagonally oriented smooth muscle cells surrounded by collagen and mucopolysaccharides; and (3) the *adventitia,* the outermost layer, containing fibroblasts and smooth muscle cells intermixed with bundles of collagen and mucopolysaccharides. An external elastic lamina generally is not found in cerebral arteries.

Intracranial Arterial Aneurysms

An *aneurysm* is an abnormal, localized dilatation of the arterial lumen. The most commonly encountered type is a round or oval-shaped, berry-like structure that arises at the bifurcation of cerebral vessels (Fig. 15). The

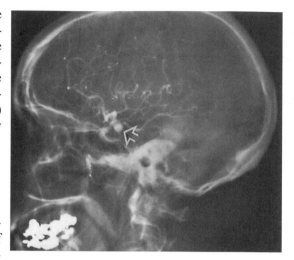

FIG. 15. Angiographic study showing aneurysm *(arrow)* that arose from the internal carotid-posterior communicating artery junction.

majority of cerebral aneurysms are located in the anterior half of the circle of Willis, with the most favored sites being the internal carotid-posterior communicating artery junction, the anterior cerebral-anterior communicating artery junction, and the middle cerebral artery bifurcation. Perhaps secondary to a developmental anomaly, a ballooning of the intima is seen associated with a defect in the media and internal elastic lamina (Fig. 16). Varying in size from 1 mm to more than 10

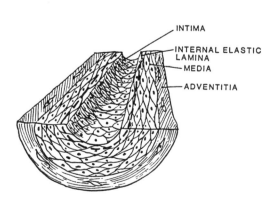

FIG. 14. Cross section of normal arterial wall; note the intima, internal elastic lamina, media, and adventitia.

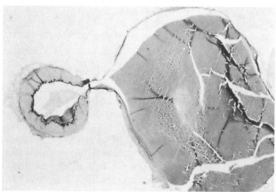

FIG. 16. Aneurysm **(right)** of internal carotid artery **(left)**. Note abrupt termination of the media and internal elastic lamina of the carotid artery at the neck of the aneurysm. (Elastic stain; ×4.)

mm, these lesions occasionally produce symptoms by exerting pressure on adjacent structures but more often present with rupture and bleeding into the subarachnoid space or brain (Fig. 17). Occasionally, aneurysms arise secondary to destruction of the arterial wall by atherosclerosis (atherosclerotic aneurysm) or to infected emboli arising from the heart (septic or mycotic aneurysm).

Arteriovenous Malformations

Arteriovenous malformations are developmental abnormalities that are often encountered in young adults. They result from defective communication between arteries, capillaries, and veins, with dilatation of one or more of the vascular elements, thus forming a variable-sized meshwork of tortuous blood vessels (Figs. 18 and 19). The walls of these abnormal vessels may be thin (and predisposed to rupture) or they may be hypertrophic. Rapid shunting of blood generally occurs and may produce a chronic ischemic state in the neighboring brain. Depending on the location and structure of the malformation, there may be associated seizures and focal neurologic deficit, infarction, or bleeding into the subarachnoid space or brain.

Atherosclerosis

A generalized vascular derangement of unknown but probably multifarious causes, atherosclerosis is the most important pathologic lesion responsible for cerebral infarction. The basic pathologic lesion is the atherosclerotic plaque. Although secondary changes may occur in other layers of the vessel wall, the intima is the layer that is principally involved in

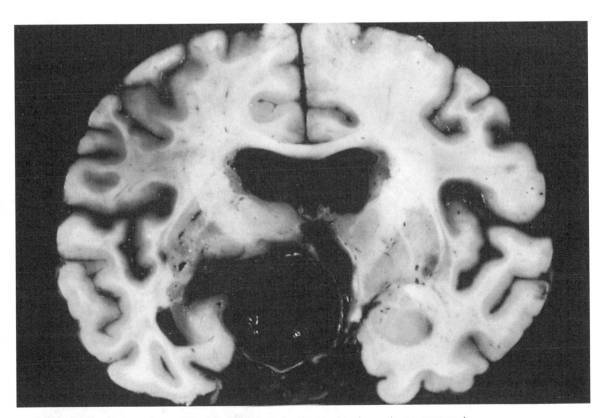

FIG. 17. Coronal section of the cerebral hemispheres showing a large ruptured aneurysm of the left internal carotid artery associated with subarachnoid and intraventricular hemorrhage.

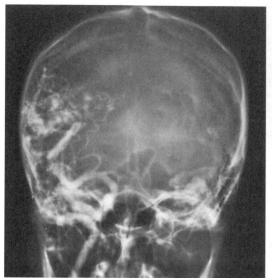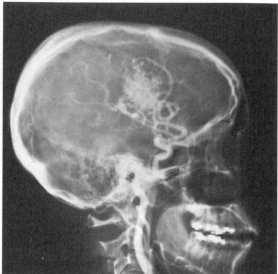

FIG. 18. Angiograms showing a large arteriovenous malformation. **Left,** antero-posterior view. **Right,** lateral view.

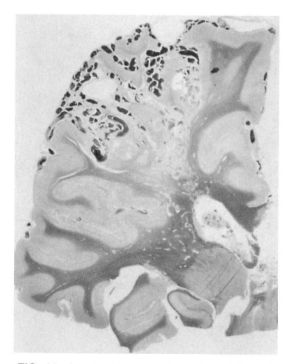

FIG. 19. Arteriovenous malformation of the left parietal lobe. Note the tangled mass of dilated vessels in a roughly wedge-shaped area pointing toward the ventricle, with degeneration of the cerebral tissue between vessels. Celloidin section. (Luxol fast-blue stain; ×1.)

atherogenesis. Injury to the arterial wall causes focal desquamation of endothelial cells and exposes subendothelial connective tissue to circulating platelets. Stimulated by the denuded surface, platelets aggregate and adhere to the arterial wall. The process of platelet aggregation releases substances that, in association with certain lipids, induce smooth muscle and endothelial proliferation to form an elevated fibrous plaque that protrudes slightly into the arterial lumen. Although these early atherogenic lesions may regress, with further arterial injury the process is repeated and the plaque becomes altered by ulceration, increased lipid content, hemorrhage, cell necrosis, mural thrombosis, and calcification to form the typical atherosclerotic plaque with narrowing (stenosis) or occlusion of the arterial lumen (Fig. 20). Clinically, many of the so-called risk factors for atherogenesis are also factors that have been shown experimentally to be capable of producing chronic injury to the arterial wall: increased shear stress, hypertension, hyperlipidemia, and diabetes mellitus.

The basic processes of platelet aggregation and release and secondary plaque formation can be inhibited by certain drugs. Platelet-ves-

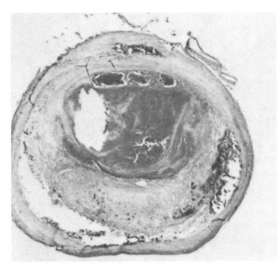

FIG. 20. Cross section of an atherosclerotic plaque in the carotid artery. Arterial wall necrosis with mural thrombosis and stenosis of the lumen is seen. (H&E; ×3.5.)

sel wall interaction is influenced by the selective oxygenation of arachidonic acid in both the platelet and the vascular endothelium. In the platelet, thromboxane synthase converts prostaglandin H_2 to thromboxane A_2, which is a potent aggregator of platelets as well as a constrictor of arterial conductance vessels. Vascular endothelium, however, metabolizes prostaglandin H_2 to prostacyclin, a compound that antagonizes platelet aggregation and dilates blood vessels. These observations suggest that pharmacologic agents that selectively inhibit thromboxane synthase or facilitate the biosynthesis of prostacyclin might be beneficial in preventing the thromboembolic complications of atherosclerosis. Although the optimal pharmacologic agent is not yet available, drugs such as acetylsalicylic acid (aspirin) are beneficial.

The vascular endothelium itself is a source of vasoactive substances. Endothelium-derived relaxing factors such as nitric oxide produce vasodilatation. Endothelium-derived constricting factors such as the endothelin group of peptides are potent vasoconstrictors.

Atherosclerosis tends chiefly to affect large-caliber blood vessels; in the cerebral circulation, both intracranial and extracranial arteries may be involved (Fig. 21). Although

minimal patchy involvement of the carotid and vertebral arteries is seen, significant stenosis or occlusion commonly occurs at selected sites. The carotid arteries, in their extracranial portion, tend to develop atherosclerotic plaques at the carotid bifurcations and in the proximal portions of the internal carotid arteries, whereas the vertebral arteries are especially likely to develop lesions at their sites of origin from the subclavian arteries. Atherosclerosis of the intracranial arteries is usually limited to the larger arteries related to the circle of Willis and is found most frequently in the internal carotid, proximal middle cerebral, vertebral, and basilar arteries. The smaller distal branches of the major cerebral arteries are seldom involved by gross atheromatous plaques.

The relative importance of the intracranial compared with the extracranial arteries in the pathogenesis of cerebral ischemia is not known. Localized atheromatous plaques may occur in either site, produce focal thrombosis, and reduce blood flow distal to the lesion. This mechanism may be responsible for producing some types of cerebral infarction.

An additional danger is the development of local intraarterial thrombosis, with subsequent *embolization* to distal vessels (Fig. 22). These

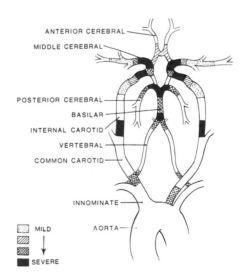

FIG. 21. Location and severity of atherosclerotic lesions in major extracranial and intracranial vessels.

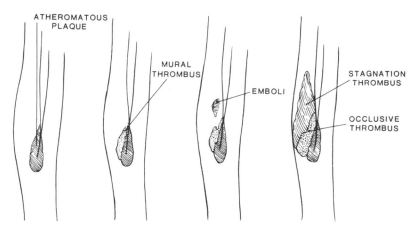

FIG. 22. Mechanism of thromboembolism secondary to atherosclerosis.

changes are frequently noted when there are lesions at the carotid bifurcation and other extracranial sites. Therefore, although it was formerly assumed that thrombosis of an intracranial artery was the most common cause of cerebral infarction, it has become evident that atherosclerotic involvement of extracranial vessels with distal embolization is probably of equal significance; in fact, this may represent the major pathogenetic mechanism for the production of transient ischemic attacks. Atherosclerotic narrowing of extracranial or cerebral vessels may lead to cerebral ischemia and infarction, with or without actual thrombosis, if there is a sudden hemodynamic reduction in cerebral blood flow in an area of the brain where the blood supply is already marginal.

Fibrinoid Necrosis

Fibrinoid necrosis (also referred to as lipohyalinosis and arteriolar sclerosis) is a segmental, nonatherosclerotic arteriopathy that involves primarily smaller intraparenchymal blood vessels and is found almost exclusively in the brains of patients with hypertension. The lesion is characterized by the presence of a fibrinoid material and lipid-laden macrophages in the subintimal layer of cerebral vessels (Fig. 23). It is postulated that sustained elevations in blood pressure result in further arterial disorganization. Some of these

lesions show progressive luminal obliteration and eventually result in small areas of infarction called *lacunae,* but others produce progressive weakening of the vessel wall and microaneurysm formation and eventually rupture and produce an intracerebral hemorrhage.

Other Types of Blood Vessel Lesions

Other pathologic processes that may result in disease of intracranial arteries and veins can produce local thrombosis and resultant infarction or hemorrhage. Common examples include (1) inflammatory involvement of cerebral blood vessels, *arteritis,* which may occur

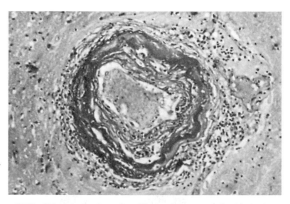

FIG. 23. Hypertensive fibrinoid necrosis. Note irregular degeneration and dilatation of wall associated with infiltration by fibrinoid material and lymphocytes. (H&E; ×100.)

secondary to infectious processes (syphilis, pyogenic meningitis) or may accompany certain systemic disorders (lupus erythematosus, periarteritis nodosa); (2) certain hematologic disorders (polycythemia, sickle cell disease); and (3) emboli of various types arising from distant sources (usually the heart).

Neural-Parenchymal Pathology

The neural-parenchymal lesions produced by the vascular lesions just discussed are of two major types: (1) hemorrhage and (2) infarction (Fig. 24). Lesions of both types are common at the supratentorial and posterior fossa levels but less frequent at the spinal level. Symptomatic vascular disease involving the peripheral level is distinctly rare and generally occurs with lesions involving smaller arteries and arterioles that secondarily alter the blood supply to peripheral nerves.

Hemorrhagic Lesions

Pathologic examination reveals that nontraumatic intracranial hemorrhagic disease may be defined by its anatomical location. It is usually found within the subarachnoid space as *subarachnoid hemorrhage* (see Chapter 6, Fig. 14), within the parenchyma of the brain as *intracerebral hemorrhage* (Fig. 25), or as a combination of the two. Hemorrhage in either of these locations may be produced by various pathophysiologic mechanisms, the most common being (1) rupture of an intracranial aneurysm, usually producing subarachnoid hemorrhage (occasionally with an associated intracerebral hemorrhage); (2) rupture of an intraparenchymal vessel, usually producing a variably sized, blood-filled mass lesion (intracerebral hemorrhage), which often has some extension of bleeding into the ventricles; and (3) bleeding

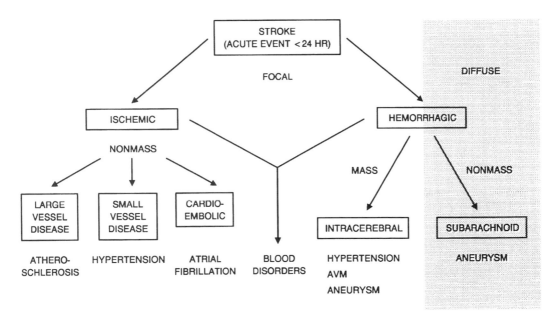

FIG. 24. Stroke, typically an acute event, can be divided into two main groups. Ischemic stroke produces focal nonmass lesions (infarction). Common causes are large-vessel disease due to atherosclerosis, small-vessel disease due to hypertension, and cardiac emboli due to atrial fibrillation. Intraparenchymal hemorrhage is a focal mass lesion. It may occur as a consequence of hypertension, amyloid angiopathy, or a coagulation disorder. Subarachnoid hemorrhage is a diffuse, nonmass lesion. The most common cause is rupture of a saccular aneurysm. Rupture of an arteriovenous malformation (AVM) can produce either an intraparenchymal or a subarachnoid hemorrhage and can be manifested by seizures or headache.

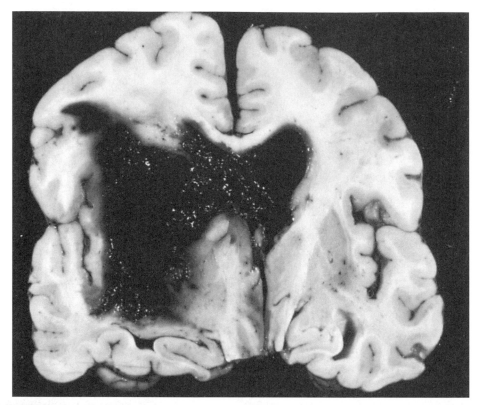

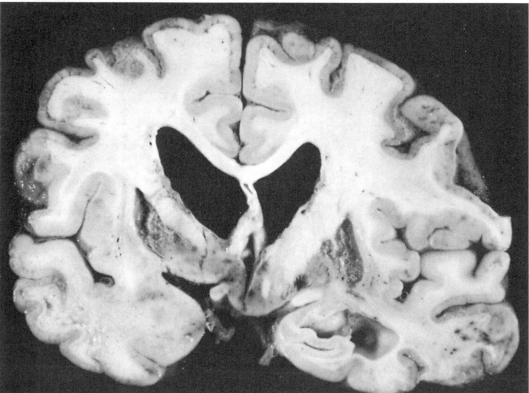

FIG. 26. Diffuse hypoxic brain damage in a patient who survived 7 months in coma after cardiac arrest. Note infarction of the cerebral cortex and basal ganglia. Cortical infarction is maximal in the arterial border zones and in the depths of the sulci.

FIG. 25. Massive left intracerebral hemorrhage with intraventricular rupture in a patient with hypertension.

from an arteriovenous malformation, commonly producing either a subarachnoid hemorrhage or an intracerebral hemorrhage, alone or in combination.

Infarction

With prolonged tissue ischemia, permanent pathologic change occurs in neuronal function and structure. In the presence of diffuse oxygen deprivation, wide areas of cerebral cortex (which is more sensitive to metabolic alteration than other cerebral structures) show evidence of necrosis and cell loss, *anoxic encephalopathy* (Fig. 26). More commonly, the

area of infarction is localized to the distribution of a diseased blood vessel (Fig. 27). In that region, softening and necrosis with *ischemic cell change* (see Chapter 4) are observed. The size of the infarct varies; smaller lesions (0.5 to 10 mm) are often referred to as *lacunar infarctions* and are common in the brains of patients with hypertension (Fig. 28). On occasion, especially with large infarctions, the original nonmass lesion may become edematous and assume the characteristics of a mass lesion. With the passage of time, the necrotic tissue in an infarcted area is removed by phagocytes and replaced by a cavity containing cystic fluid surrounded by an area of glial tissue (Fig. 29).

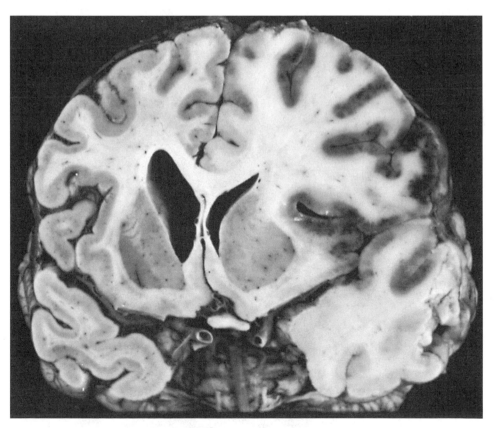

FIG. 27. Acute infarction in the middle cerebral artery distribution. Note swelling and cortical discoloration and petechial hemorrhages in the infarcted territory, with marked shift of midline structures.

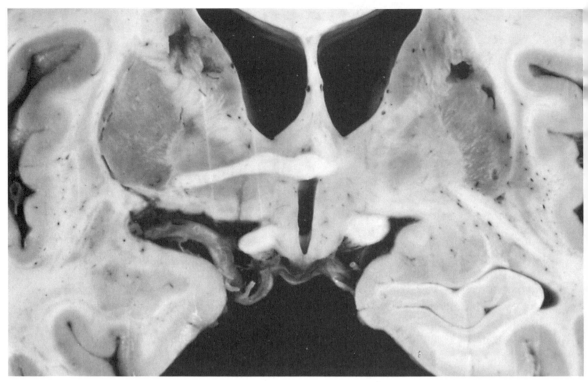

FIG. 28. Small, old cystic infarcts (lacunae) in the basal ganglia bilaterally in a patient with hypertension.

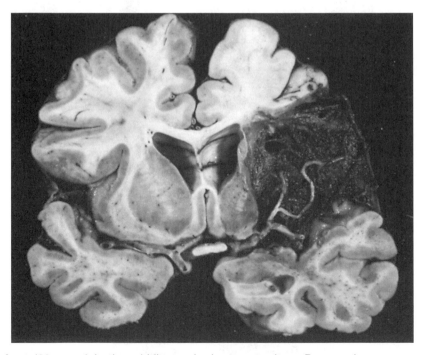

FIG. 29. Old infarct (20 years) in the middle cerebral artery territory. Damaged brain tissue has been completely absorbed, leaving a cystic area traversed by glial-vascular membranes. Note the relatively intact middle cerebral artery within the area of infarction.

Clinical Correlations   ■

Risk Factors for Stroke

The goal of medical therapy in cerebrovascular disease is prevention. Epidemiologic studies have identified numerous factors, including hyperlipidemia, obesity, diabetes mellitus, and excessive smoking, that appear to be associated with atherosclerosis. Because atherosclerosis is a major cause of stroke, many of these same factors are present in the stroke-prone profile. In addition, there are three highly specific factors that have been shown to be associated with a greatly increased risk of stroke but, more importantly, to result in a significant decrease in stroke incidence when promptly recognized and treated: (1) transient focal ischemic attacks, (2) hypertension, and (3) certain cardiac disorders.

Transient Focal Ischemic Attacks

These spells are defined as brief (less than 24 hours, usually 5 to 30 minutes) episodes of focal neurologic dysfunction of abrupt onset, which clear without permanent neurologic deficit. These episodes may occur in the distribution of either the carotid or the vertebrobasilar arterial system. There are many theories about the cause of these ischemic events, but current evidence suggests that the majority are caused by emboli that arise from a proximal ulcerated atherosclerotic plaque. Lesions in the region of the carotid bifurcation are a common source of transient ischemic attack. *Amaurosis fugax* (fleeting blindness) is a related episode consisting of transient monocular blindness that often arises from temporary alteration of the retinal blood supply caused by ipsilateral carotid artery disease. These events must be recognized because between 20% and 35% of patients experiencing these transient episodes subsequently have permanent cerebral infarction.

Hypertension

Sustained elevation in systemic blood pressure increases the risk of subsequent stroke by at least four times when compared with normotension. Hypertension of even modest degree exerts its effect on the cerebral vasculature by two distinct mechanisms: (1) acceleration of atherosclerosis—patients of any age with hypertension have a greater amount of atherosclerotic disease than those without hypertension and are at higher risk for the forms of atherothrombotic disease previously described; and (2) initiation of pathologic change in small arterioles (fibrinoid necrosis). This type of arterial degeneration is found almost exclusively in patients with hypertension and seems to be the vascular lesion that predisposes to both lacunar infarction and intracerebral hemorrhage. (Intracerebral hemorrhage in the absence of an arteriovenous malformation is seldom found in normal, nonhypertensive patients.)

Certain Forms of Cardiac Disease

Valvular heart disease of various types, endocarditis, and various cardiac arrhythmias (primarily atrial fibrillation) are associated with intracardiac thrombus formation. Because a large proportion of the cardiac output supplies the cerebrum, the nervous system remains a major target organ for all forms of cardiac emboli.

Generalized Cerebral Ischemia—Syncope

Under normal circumstances, cerebral blood flow remains relatively constant in spite of minor fluctuations in blood pressure. When systemic blood pressure decreases to extremely low levels and the cerebral autoregulatory mechanisms are no longer effective, a state of generalized cerebral ischemia develops. The momentary giddiness and light-headedness occasionally experienced when a person abruptly assumes an upright posture is an example of this. If cerebral perfusion remains inadequate, syncope results and consciousness is lost. States of decreased cardiac output, hypotension from many causes, vagal hyperactivity, and impairment of sympathetic vasomotor reflex activity are common causes of syncope, which should not be confused with a transient ischemic attack as previously defined. Transient ischemic attack is a *focal* ischemic event, syncope is a *generalized* ischemic event that occurs as a result of vastly different pathogenetic mechanisms and has a different prognosis. In the presence of severe focal intracranial vascular disease, syncope may infrequently be associated with focal neurologic signs and symptoms.

Radiographic Anatomy—Angiography

We do not have an opportunity to examine the cerebral blood vessels directly until autopsy; in patients we rely on a procedure called *angiography*. High-resolution images of the cerebrovascular anatomy are obtained by cannulation of an extracranial artery and injection of a radiopaque material. As the contrast medium is carried through the cerebral circulation, serial radiographs are obtained in both the lateral and anteroposterior projections. The contrast medium outlines the interior of the blood vessels, and the arterial, capillary, and venous phases of the circulation can be assessed.

Normal vascular anatomy as seen in a conventional cerebral angiogram is illustrated in Fig. 30. Deviations from the normal vascular pattern may be indicative of disease and should be correlated with the clinical history and examination. Images of lower resolution, primarily displaying the larger arterial vessels, can be produced by magnetic resonance imaging or by electronic enhancement of radiographs obtained after the intravenous injection of contrast medium (digital subtraction angiography). Magnetic resonance angiography, which alleviates the potential risks of an arterial puncture, is, at times, a useful alternative to conventional angiography in selected patients (Fig. 31). Three major types of changes may be seen on the angiogram: structural abnormalities of vessels, alterations in position of vessels, and alterations in flow patterns.

Structural Abnormalities of Vessels

Stenosis (narrowing) of the dye column or occlusion (nonfilling) of a vessel may be seen. Vascular malformations and aneurysms are examples of this type of change. Collections of abnormal vessels may be demonstrated within neoplasms, in particular gliomas, meningiomas, and metastatic lesions, and these collections may be responsible for a so-called tumor blush or stain seen as an area of increased dye concentration.

Alterations in Position of Vessels

Mass lesions commonly produce displacement of vessels. Such displacement may be local and result in delineation of the mass or be distant and indirect; examples of the latter include shift of the anterior cerebral artery with anteriorly placed lesions or of the internal cerebral vein with more posteriorly placed lesions. At times, such a shift or displacement of vessels is associated with a stain or blush; in other instances, as with subdural hematoma, only the shift is recognized, the lesion itself being represented by an avascular area. In hydrocephalus, the vessels may be stretched out over the dilated ventricular system.

Alterations in Flow Patterns

Changes in the circulatory pattern may be evident as an expression of abnormal vascular shunts, as with arteriovenous malformations or in some tumors. Collateral flow patterns may be identified in instances of thrombosis of major arteries as, for example, through the ophthalmic artery in instances of carotid artery occlusion; diminution or absence of flow is found distal to the site of vascular occlusion itself. A general slowing of the circulation may be noted when the intracranial pressure is elevated.

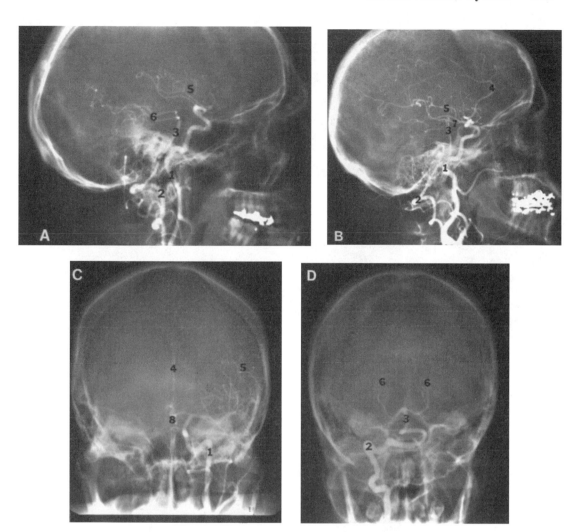

FIG. 30. Arteriographic anatomy. **A,B:** Lateral views. **C,D:** Anteroposterior views. *(1)* Internal carotid artery, *(2)* vertebral artery, *(3)* basilar artery, *(4)* branches of anterior cerebral artery, *(5)* branches of middle cerebral artery, *(6)* branches of posterior cerebral artery, *(7)* posterior communicating artery, and *(8)* anterior communicating artery.

Measurement of Ocular Arterial Pressure

Vessel stenosis must be greater than 60% or 70% before flow is reduced and distal arterial pressure is lowered. An inference can be made about the presence of such a lesion by demonstrating a reduction in blood pressure along a distal segment of that artery.

Thus, severe stenosis of the subclavian artery lowers the brachial blood pressure. Similarly, severe stenosis of the internal carotid artery lowers the ipsilateral ophthalmic or retinal artery pressure. Several simple and safe *noninvasive techniques* (ophthalmodynamometry, oculoplethysmography) are now available. Unilateral reduc-

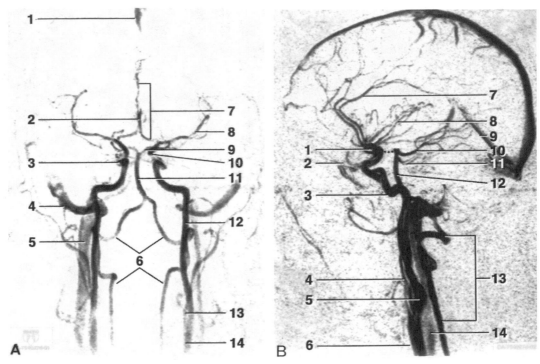

FIG. 31. Magnetic resonance angiography showing the major intracranial and extracranial arteries and veins. **A:** Anteroposterior view. *(1)* Superior sagittal sinus, *(2)* anterior communicating artery, *(3)* internal carotid artery siphon, *(4)* transverse sinus, *(5)* internal jugular vein, *(6)* vertebral arteries, *(7)* anterior cerebral artery, *(8)* middle cerebral artery, *(9)* posterior cerebral artery, *(10)* posterior communicating artery, *(11)* basilar artery, *(12)* internal carotid artery, *(13)* external carotid artery, *(14)* common carotid artery. **B:** Lateral view. *(1)* Internal carotid artery siphon, *(2)* ophthalmic artery, *(3)* internal carotid artery, *(4)* external carotid artery, *(5)* carotid bulb, *(6)* common carotid artery, *(7)* anterior cerebral artery, *(8)* middle cerebral artery, *(9)* straight sinus, *(10)* posterior cerebral artery, *(11)* superior cerebellar artery, *(12)* basilar artery, *(13)* vertebral artery, *(14)* internal jugular vein.

tion in ocular arterial pressure is a reliable indicator of the presence of a highly stenotic or occlusive lesion in the ipsilateral carotid system and may be of value in the assessment of patients with suspected carotid arterial disease.

Computed Tomography

Computed tomography is a radiographic technique capable of visualizing intracranial anatomy and pathology and has proved to be helpful in the assessment of patients with cerebrovascular disease. As shown in Fig. 32, areas of infarction (Fig. 32A) often appear as regions of reduced attenuation, whereas regions of hemorrhage (Fig. 32B) show increased attenuation. At times, after subarachnoid hemorrhage, there is sufficient blood in the subarachnoid spaces to be identified by this technique (Fig. 32C). Enhancement of the vascular structures of the brain can be achieved by the injection of intravenous contrast material and can be used to identify large vascular anomalies such as the arteriovenous malformation shown in Fig. 32D.

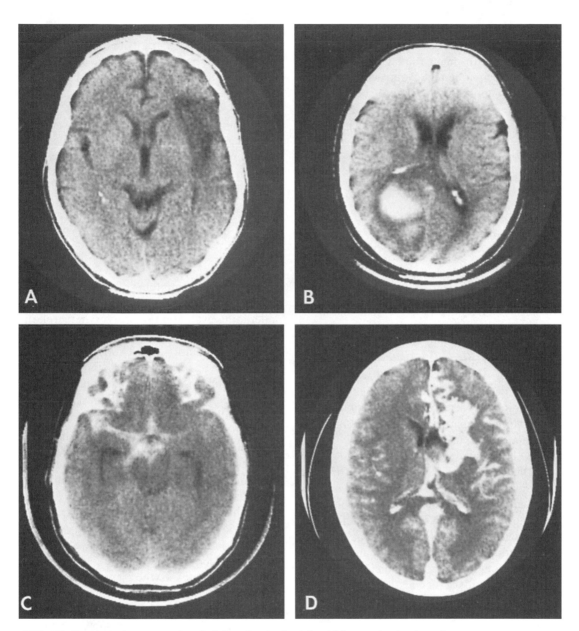

FIG. 32. Computed tomography. **A:** Infarction in the left middle cerebral artery distribution. **B:** Area of hemorrhage in the right occipital lobe. **C:** Blood in the basilar cisterns. **D:** Large, predominantly left frontal arteriovenous malformation in a contrast-enhanced scan.

Magnetic Resonance Imaging

Magnetic resonance imaging is another imaging technique that can provide useful information about the status of the cerebral vasculature and brain parenchyma. This technique is becoming more widely available for the assessment of patients with all types of neural and cerebrovascular disorders.

Examination of the Vascular System ■

Because *vascular* refers to both an anatomical system and an etiologic category, its evaluation requires both historical data and information obtained from the physical examination. Patients with cerebrovascular disease may present with a wide range of symptoms of diverse causes. The evaluation of such patients should be designed to enable the clinician to determine (1) the nature of the presenting symptoms and signs; (2) the type, location, and extent of the pathologic process in the neural parenchyma; (3) the type, location, and extent of the pathologic process in the vasculature; and (4) the pathophysiologic mechanism responsible for the observed symptoms and signs. This evaluation usually can be accomplished with reasonable accuracy through a detailed history and physical examination, aided by the judicious selection of certain ancillary diagnostic studies.

Historical Aspects

From the history, it is possible to determine if a problem is vascular and if the primary pathologic process is hemorrhage or infarction and to define the likely pathophysiologic mechanism responsible for the problem.

The judgment as to whether a problem is vascular is made almost exclusively from the *temporal profile,* with the onset, evaluation, and course of the presenting symptoms. An acute onset with rapid evolution (minutes to hours) to maximal deficit implies a vascular cause. In the absence of a history of a clearly defined acute onset, the diagnosis of nontraumatic cerebrovascular disease must remain uncertain.

Patients with symptoms of acute onset may be seen at any stage in the development of their symptoms. Some patients have symptoms that have resolved completely by the time they present for evaluation. They may describe the focal symptoms of transient ischemia attacks, but such events must be distinguished from seizures, labyrinthine disturbances, migraine, and generalized ischemic disorders (syncope).

Patients with symptoms of acute onset may progress and display increasing deficit while undergoing evaluation (a progressing stroke); but with these patients, careful historical inquiry must be undertaken to uncover the possibility of an underlying neoplasm, other mass lesions (that is, subdural hematoma), or superimposed metabolic or inflammatory encephalopathy.

Finally, the condition of some patients with symptoms of acute onset may have stabilized with residual deficit or may show some improvement at the time of evaluation. Most of these patients will have a *completed stroke.* Again, historical inquiry must be directed toward uncovering the pathophysiologic mechanism responsible for the deficit and must take into account other intracranial processes that could account for the symptoms.

The distinction between hemorrhage and infarction, although of major clinical importance and readily made in most cases, may be difficult in certain instances. The onset of symptoms in association with severe headache, though not invariably associated with hemorrhage, favors a hemorrhagic process. If the primary pathologic lesion is located at the supratentorial level (rather than posterior fossa), the presence of alteration in consciousness, stupor, or coma coincident with or shortly after the onset of symptoms favors the diagnosis of hemorrhagic disease.

When hemorrhage is suspected, a clinical determination of the location of the hemorrhage is often possible. The early absence of focal neurologic symptoms favors a subarachnoid hemorrhage and, in the absence of trauma, suggests the possibility of a ruptured intracranial aneurysm. The presence of focal neurologic symptoms suggests an intracerebral hemorrhage. In patients with suspected intracerebral hemorrhage, a history of significant, untreated hypertension renders the diagnosis more likely. In its absence, one must consider either the possibility of a ruptured aneurysm with associated intracerebral hemorrhage or a parenchymal hemorrhage secondary to an arteriovenous malformation (which also can present as a subarachnoid hemorrhage). The history of preexistent focal seizures, localized headache, or previous intracranial bleeding supports the diagnosis of an arteriovenous malformation.

When an ischemic process is suspected, it is necessary first to distinguish between carotid and vertebrobasilar arterial system disease. Although in most patients ischemic lesions are related to atherosclerosis, the patient's entire medical and neurologic history should be used to determine whether the symptoms are a result of (1) intracranial pathologic processes involving large-caliber or small-caliber arteries and arterioles, (2) thromboembolic disease in the major extracranial vessels, (3) emboli arising from distant sources (most often the heart), or (4) other systemic disorders.

The Neurovascular Examination

The physical evaluation of patients with suspected cerebrovascular disease must include, in addition to a general physical examination and more detailed study of neurologic function, an assessment of the neurovascular system. Cerebrovascular disease seldom occurs in isolation; the basic pathologic process often exerts its effect on multiple target organs, and therapeutic intervention can be planned only after consideration of the general well-being of the patient. A careful cardiac, pulmonary, and peripheral vascular examination (including recording of pulse rate and rhythm and measurement of the brachial blood pressures bilaterally and in the lying and standing positions) is particularly essential. In addition, the degree to which underlying disorders such as hypertension, diabetes mellitus, hyperlipidemia, and hematologic abnormalities may be contributing to the production of cerebrovascular symptoms must be determined.

The neurovascular examination includes examination of neck flexion for evidence of nuchal rigidity in patients with suspected hemorrhagic disease and three additional procedures designed to provide evidence of disease in the cerebrovascular system: auscultation of the head and neck, palpation of the cephalic vessels, and neuro-ophthalmologic examination.

Auscultation of the Head and Neck

The examiner should gently apply the stethoscope over the great vessels arising from the aortic arch, the carotid bifurcations, the orbits, and the skull, listening for evidence of bruits. A *bruit* is an abnormal pulsatile sound indicating turbulent blood flow through a vessel. It is usually, but not always, associated with stenosis of that vessel. A bruit may be audible over an area of abnormal arteriovenous communication and may at times be heard over an anatomically normal vessel if there is turbulent flow.

Palpation of the Cephalic Vessels

Gentle palpation of the carotid arteries in the neck and of the superficial temporal arteries anterior to the ear should be performed. Altered pulsation, especially if unilateral, is usually indicative of proximal obstructive vascular disease. Although palpation of the peripheral pulses is an important part of the assessment of the general vascular system, palpation of the carotid pulses is less reliable and carries with it the potential danger of dislodging material from an atheromatous plaque. If pulsation of a carotid artery cannot be felt on gentle palpation, vigorous compression will add little diagnostic information.

Neuro-Ophthalmologic Examination

The optic fundus should be examined in all patients, because this provides valuable information about intracranial vascular disease. Atherosclerosis, hypertension, diabetes mellitus, and other systemic disorders produce recognizable retinal and vascular changes. Subhyaloid (preretinal) hemorrhages may be seen in patients with subarachnoid hemorrhage. Evidence of retinal embolic events in the form of retinal infarcts and of cholesterol (Fig. 33), platelet-fibrin, or calcific emboli may be seen in patients with carotid occlusive disease. These intraarterial fragments are presumed to result from an ulcerated atheromatous lesion in the circulation proximal to the ophthalmic arteries, and their presence correlates well with demonstrable lesions in the ipsilateral internal carotid artery.

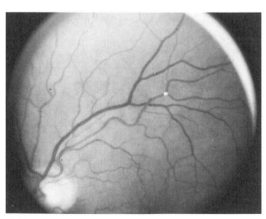

FIG. 33. Small cholesterol embolus seen in a distal arteriole of the optic fundus of a patient with atherosclerosis of the proximal internal carotid artery.

Clinical Problems ■

1. A 16-year-old boy with endocarditis noted the sudden onset of complete loss of vision; within minutes, this partially cleared, and he noted only a loss of vision in the left half of the visual field of each eye. He had improved slightly when he reached the hospital, but examination still revealed a left homonymous hemianopia.
    a. What is the anatomicopathologic nature of the lesion?
    b. What is the location of the lesion with respect to its vascular supply? Why did you make this choice?
    c. What is the pathologic term that describes the parenchymal lesion?
    d. What is the pathophysiologic mechanism responsible for the symptoms?
    e. What biochemical changes have taken place in the region of the lesion?
2. A 65-year-old woman suddenly experienced the onset of severe weakness on her left side, loss of feeling on her left side, and an inability to see in the left half of her visual fields. Examination revealed weakness of face, arm, and leg, increased reflexes with Babinski's sign on the left, sensory loss on the left side, and a left homonymous hemianopia. A right carotid bruit was noted.
    a. What is the anatomicopathologic nature of the lesion?
    b. What is the location of the lesion with respect to its vascular supply?
    c. What is the pathologic term that describes the parenchymal lesion?
    d. What is the pathophysiologic mechanism responsible for the symptoms?
    e. In the region immediately surrounding the lesion, the blood vessels are maximally dilated: true or false?
3. A 55-year-old man with hypertension noted the sudden onset of severe headache on the left side, loss of speech, and right hemiparesis. Within minutes, he became somnolent. Examination in the emergency

room 30 minutes later revealed a comatose patient with a blood pressure of 220/120 mm Hg, a dense right hemiparesis with increased reflexes on the right, and Babinski's sign bilaterally. Computed tomography of the head showed a 7-mm shift of the pineal gland from left to right.

a. What is the anatomicopathologic nature of the lesion?
b. What is the pathologic term that describes the parenchymal lesion?
c. What are three common causes of this type of parenchymal lesion?
d. What clinical signs suggest the pathologic diagnosis?
e. What other noninvasive diagnostic test would be useful in defining the pathologic lesion?

4. A 50-year-old man experienced the sudden onset of vertigo. Examination revealed dysarthria, difficulty in swallowing, left Horner's syndrome, left palatal weakness, and loss of pain sensibility over the left face and the right limbs and trunk. He had coarse ataxia and incoordination of his left arm.

a. What is the anatomicopathologic nature of the lesion?
b. What is the location of the lesion in respect to its vascular supply?
c. What is the pathologic term that describes the parenchymal lesion?
d. What is the pathophysiologic mechanism responsible for the symptoms?
e. List the tract or nucleus responsible for each of the symptoms or signs in this patient.

5. A 62-year-old man had frequent, highly stereotyped episodes. He suddenly felt giddy and light-headed, lost consciousness, and fell to the ground. A physician observed one of his spells and noted that during the episode there was no peripheral pulse, and the blood pressure was too low to be detected. Both blood pressure and peripheral pulse returned to normal coincident with the patient's regaining consciousness.

a. What is the anatomicopathologic nature of the lesion?
b. What is the pathophysiologic mechanism responsible for the symptoms?
c. Define autoregulation.
d. Under normal physiologic conditions, which of the following could be expected to produce cerebral vasodilation: inhalation of oxygen, 20% decrease in arterial blood pressure, 20% increase in arterial blood pressure, inhalation of carbon dioxide?
e. How do these spells differ from transient ischemic attacks?

6. A 38-year-old man suddenly experienced a severe headache associated with nausea, vomiting, and neck stiffness. When examined 2 hours later, he was somnolent but easily aroused. He had no focal neurologic findings but had marked nuchal rigidity. Lumbar puncture revealed grossly bloody cerebrospinal fluid.

a. What is the anatomicopathologic nature of the lesion?
b. What is the pathophysiologic mechanism responsible for the symptoms?
c. How would you determine whether the bloody cerebrospinal fluid was due to a traumatic puncture?

Additional Reading

Adams, R. D., and Victor, M. *Principles of Neurology* (5th ed.). New York: McGraw-Hill, 1993, pp. 669–748.

Barnett, H. J. M., and Hachinski, V. C. (eds.). Cerebral ischemia: Treatment and prevention. *Neurol. Clin.* 10(1), 1992.

Kety, S. S., and Schmidt, C. F. The nitrous oxide method for the quantitative determination of cerebral blood flow in man: Theory, procedure and normal values. *J. Clin. Invest.* 27:476, 1948.

Meyer, F. B., Sundt, T. M., Jr., Yanagihara, T., and Anderson, R. E. Focal cerebral ischemia: Pathophysiologic mechanisms and rationale for future avenues of treatment. *Mayo Clin. Proc.* 62:35, 1987.

Powers, W. J. Cerebral hemodynamics in ischemic cerebrovascular disease. *Ann. Neurol.* 29:231, 1991.

Scheinberg, P. The biologic basis for the treatment of acute stroke. *Neurology* 41:1867, 1991.

The Neurochemical Systems

Objectives ■

1. Name the different groups of neurochemical transmitters and the main components of each group.
2. Describe the functional and neurochemical characteristics of the relay, diffuse, and local circuit neurochemical systems.
3. Describe the distribution and functions of L-glutamate in the brain. Describe the effects of activation of different glutamate receptor subtypes. Define *long-term potentiation*. List examples of L-glutamate-induced neurotoxicity.
4. Describe the distribution and function of γ-aminobutyric acid (GABA) in the brain. Describe the function of astrocytes in GABA metabolism. Explain why GABAergic dysfunction produces seizures.
5. Describe the distribution and list the main functions of acetylcholine in the central and peripheral nervous systems.
6. Describe the biosynthesis and metabolism of catecholamines. Describe the distribution and function of dopaminergic neurons in the brain. Describe the projections and functions of the locus ceruleus and the lateral tegmental systems.
7. Describe the distribution and function of central serotoninergic and histaminergic systems.
8. Name the rate-limiting enzymes for the biosynthesis of GABA, acetylcholine, catecholamines, serotonin, and histamine. Describe the main mechanism of inactivation of amino acids, acetylcholine, catecholamines, serotonin, and neuropeptides.
9. Describe the main mechanism of synthesis, transport, release, and inactivation of neuropeptides. List the brain regions richest in neuropeptides. Give examples of neuropeptides in hypothalamic, autonomic, pain-controlling, striatal, and cortical circuits. Name the neuropeptide cotransmitters in sympathetic and parasympathetic pathways.
10. Name the primary neurotransmitter in the following: corticospinal tract, basal ganglia and cerebellar circuits, basal forebrain, locus ceruleus, substantia nigra pars compacta, raphe nuclei, skeletal neuromuscular junction, autonomic ganglion, postganglionic sympathetic neuron, postganglionic parasympathetic neuron, primary afferent (unmyelinated) nociceptive fibers, and inhibitory interneurons.

Introduction ■

The nervous system uses chemical substances for transmission of information and for maintenance of neuronal function. Transmission of information in all the systems studied involves chemical synapses that use various neurochemical mediators. On the basis of their biochemical and functional characteristics, these mediators can be classified into different groups referred to as *neurochemical systems.* Neurochemical systems include amino acid, acetylcholine, monoamine, neuropeptide, and purine systems.

This chapter provides an overview of the neurochemistry, distribution, and function of these neurochemical systems. A comprehensive review of their pharmacology is beyond the scope of this chapter. Relevant examples are discussed.

Overview ■

Neurochemical Systems

Neuroactive substances can be subdivided into several categories, according to their biochemical and functional characteristics: amino acids, acetylcholine, monoamines, neuropeptides, and purines (Table 1). These substances may produce fast neuronal excitation or inhibition, referred to as *classic neurotransmission,* or they may modulate the excitability and responsiveness of neurons to stimuli, referred to as *neuromodulation.* In addition, neurochemical systems may produce long-term effects on neuronal activity critical for neural development, learning, and response to injury. Thus, they are important for plasticity in the nervous system.

Amino acids include excitatory amino acids, such as *L-glutamate,* and inhibitory amino acids, such as *γ-aminobutyric acid* (GABA) and *glycine.* L-Glutamate is the excitatory neurotransmitter in most rapidly conducting relay pathways of the motor and sensory systems, including the corticospinal, lemniscal, spinothalamic, and special sensory pathways. L-Glutamate produces fast or prolonged synaptic excitation and triggers various calcium-dependent processes in the target cells, including production of nitric oxide. L-Glutamate also has a major role in synaptic plasticity during development and in the processes of learning and memory. *GABA* is the most common inhibitory neurotransmitter in the central nervous system and is found mainly in inhibitory interneurons and in projection neurons of the circuits of the basal ganglia and cerebellum. *Glycine* is located in inhibitory interneurons in the spinal cord and brainstem.

Acetylcholine is an important neurotransmitter in both the central and peripheral nervous systems. In the central nervous system, it is present in diffusely projecting neurons of the basal forebrain and mesopontine tegmentum, in local interneurons, and in spinal and cranial motor neurons (see Table 1). At the peripheral level, acetylcholine is the neurotransmitter of skeletal neuromuscular junctions, autonomic ganglia, and parasympathetic neu-

TABLE 1. *Main features of neuroactive agents*

Neuroactive agent	Main source	Function	Inactivation
L-Glutamate	Excitatory projection neurons	Fast excitation	Reuptake
γ-aminobutyric acid (GABA)	Inhibitory interneurons	Fast/slow inhibition	Reuptake
Acetylcholine	Basal forebrain	Modulation	Acetylcholinesterase
	Mesopontine tegmentum		
	Motor neurons	Fast excitation	
Monoamines	Brainstem and hypothalamic diffuse systems	Modulation	Reuptake
			Monoamine oxidase
			Catechol-*O*-methyltransferase
Neuropeptides	Local and diffuse systems in hypothalamus and limbic, autonomic, and pain circuits	Long-lasting modulation	Peptidases
Purines			
ATP	Autonomic and pain circuits	Fast excitation	Nucleotidase
Adenosine	Throughout the brain	Modulation	Deaminase

ATP, adenosine triphosphate.

roeffector junctions. Central cholinergic mechanisms are important for memory, arousal, and rapid eye movement sleep. Peripherally, acetylcholine mediates activation of skeletal muscles and visceral effectors.

Monoamines include *catecholamines* (dopamine, norepinephrine, epinephrine), *serotonin,* and *histamine.* These substances are present in neurons that are located in restricted areas of the brainstem and hypothalamus and that have abundant projections throughout the central nervous system. They modulate ongoing synaptic activity in the brain and spinal cord, and their effects are mediated by various subtypes of receptors, which mediate complex excitatory or inhibitory synaptic interactions.

Dopamine is located in neurons of the substantia nigra pars compacta and in other neurons of the midbrain and hypothalamus. It is important for motor control and endocrine regulation. *Norepinephrine* and epinephrine are located in the central and peripheral nervous systems. In the central nervous system, norepinephrine neurons form two systems: the *locus ceruleus system* in the pons and the *lateral tegmental system* in the lower pons and medulla. (The latter system also contains epinephrine-synthesizing neurons.) In the periphery, norepinephrine is the primary neurotransmitter of postganglionic sympathetic pathways. *Serotonin* is located in the raphe nuclei of the brainstem, and *histamine* is located in neurons of the lateral hypothalamus, specifically of the *tuberomamillary nucleus.* Central catecholaminergic, serotoninergic, and histaminergic systems are important for control of arousal, attention, emotion, and affect.

Neuropeptides include several families of genetically related substances. In the central nervous system, neuropeptides are most abundant in the hypothalamus and limbic system and in the autonomic and pain-processing pathways of the brainstem. Hypothalamic peptidergic neurons tend to project throughout the central nervous system, whereas those in other regions are primarily local circuit neurons. Peripherally, neuropeptides are present in unmyelinated nociceptive afferents, postganglionic parasympathetic and sympathetic fibers, and enteric neurons. Neuropeptides frequently coexist with other neurotransmitters and act as cotransmitters involved in presynaptic and postsynaptic modulation. They have a slow onset and produce prolonged and potent effects.

In addition to acting at the site of release, monoamines and neuropeptides may diffuse through the extracellular fluid of the central nervous system to influence neurons located at a distance, a process called *volume transmission.* Volume transmission affects not only neurons but also glial cells and blood vessels and is important for coupling neuronal activity with regional cerebral blood flow and metabolism. Also, neuropeptides may be released into the peripheral circulation and act as hormones.

Receptor Mechanisms

Classic neurotransmission and neuromodulation are mediated by two different families of receptors. Fast neurotransmission involves ion channel receptors (also referred to as *ligand-gated ion channels*) and results in a rapid and transient increase in membrane permeability to cations (sodium, calcium) or anions (chloride) (Table 2). This is the *ionotropic effect.* Neuromodulation involves *G-protein–coupled receptors,* which initiate several biochemical cascades that produce changes in the excitability and responsiveness of neurons (predominantly by affecting potassium channels), affect neurotransmitter release (by affecting presynaptic calcium channels), and initiate long-term changes in neural function important in development, learning, and response to injury. These are referred to as *metabotropic effects.* There are several families of G proteins, and they mediate a large variety of effects via different transducing mechanisms: G_s activates adenylate cyclase and synthesis of cyclic adenosine monophosphate (cAMP); $G_{i/o}$ inhibits adenylate cyclase, increases potassium currents, and decreases calcium currents; and $G_{q/11}$ is coupled to the phospholipase C-phosphatidy-

TABLE 2. *Types of receptors and synaptic effects*

Receptor	Mechanism	Synaptic effect
Ion channel receptors		
Cation channels	Increase permeability to sodium (and calcium)	Fast EPSP
Anion channels	Increase permeability to chloride	Fast IPSP
G-protein–coupled receptors		
G_s	Stimulates cAMP	Variable
$G_{q/11}$	Stimulates diacyl glycerol/IP$_3$	Slow EPSP
	Increases intracellular calcium	
	Decreases permeability to potassium	
$G_{i/o}$	Inhibits cAMP	Slow IPSP
	Increases permeability to potassium	
	Decreases permeability to calcium	Presynaptic inhibition

cAMP, cyclic adenosine monophosphate; EPSP, excitatory postsynaptic potential; IP$_3$, inositol triphosphate; IPSP, inhibitory postsynaptic potential.

linositol pathway, associated with production of diacyl glycerol and inositol triphosphate, accumulation of intracellular calcium, and inhibition of potassium currents (Table 2). All these second-messenger systems activate enzymes that either phosphorylate or dephosphorylate various neural proteins, including ion channels.

Ion currents that cause depolarization produce excitatory postsynaptic potentials (EPSPs), because they bring the membrane potential toward the threshold for triggering an action potential. Fast EPSPs result from the opening of cation channels (conducting sodium and, in some cases, calcium currents), and slow EPSPs result from a decrease in potassium currents. Fast inhibitory postsynaptic potentials (IPSPs) result from opening of chloride channels. Slow IPSPs are primarily due to an increase in potassium (see Chapter 5).

A single neurotransmitter may act on different receptor subtypes, each coupled to a distinct transduction pathway. Also, different neurotransmitters, through their respective receptors, may activate the same transduction pathway. An important final transduction mechanism is a change in the state of phosphorylation of various synaptic, cytoskeletal, and nuclear proteins. These depend on a balance between the activity of several protein kinases and protein phosphatases. Activation of immediate early genes, including c-*fos* and c-*jun,* is a critical step in the response to environmental stimuli that affect the structure and function of the neuron. Immediate early genes are rapidly induced by neural stimuli via several second messengers, including calcium and cyclic adenosine monophosphate, and encode for proteins (referred to as *transcription factors*) that control transcription of other genes. Similar mechanisms are triggered by neurotrophic factors (such as nerve growth factor) that act through a different family of receptors.

Functional and Anatomical Organization of the Neurochemical Systems

Neurochemical systems are functionally organized into three main patterns of neuronal connectivity: *relay systems, diffuse systems,* and *local circuits.*

Relay systems are located in the outer tube of the central nervous system and include the direct sensory and motor pathways (Table 3). They are involved in fast sequential transmission of precise, point-to-point information via excitatory relay neurons that use L-glutamate or other excitatory amino acids. Local interneurons contain GABA and control information processing at each relay station. Interruption of any link in a motor or sensory relay pathway incapacitates the whole system and is the basis for most focal neurologic signs.

Diffuse systems consist of neuronal groups of the inner tube of the central nervous sys-

TABLE 3. *Functional organization of the neurochemical systems*

	Relay systems (outer tube)	Diffuse systems (inner tube)
Pathway	Direct	Indirect
Type of information	Fast	Slow, modulation
	Point-to-point excitation or inhibition	
Neurotransmitter	Excitatory amino acids (L-glutamate)	Acetylcholine
	Inhibitory amino acids (GABA)	Monamines
		Neuropeptides
Receptor mechanism	Opening of neurotransmitter-linked ion channel	G-protein–mediated opening or closing of voltage-gated channels
Effect on neurons	Rapid transmission of excitatory or inhibitory signals	Modulation of neuronal excitability
Function	Sensory and motor control	Visceral control
		Arousal and attention
Systems	Motor system	Internal regulation system
	Sensory system	Consciousness system

GABA, γ-aminobutyric acid.

tem, specifically in the brainstem, basal forebrain, and hypothalamus. These neurons contain acetylcholine, monoamines, or neuropeptides and send diffuse axonal projections to modulate global excitability of neurons at all levels of the nervous system (Table 3). Diffuse systems are important for regulation of arousal-attention processes, emotion, and homeostasis via both synaptic and volume transmission. Alteration of these systems produces profound changes in the state of alertness, attention, emotion, behavior, and visceral and endocrine control.

Local circuit neurons have connections mainly within the immediate vicinity of their location and regulate the flow of information in relay systems and diffuse systems. Local neurons in the relay stations of the direct systems mainly use GABA. Local neurons may use many other transmitters, including glycine, glutamate, acetylcholine, and neuropeptides.

The neurochemical systems are involved in the pathophysiology of many neurologic diseases. Excitatory amino acids may cause neuronal injury (referred to as *excitotoxicity*), which may be responsible for neuronal death in acute conditions such as stroke and in chronic neurodegenerative disorders such as Huntington's disease and Alzheimer's disease. Impairment of GABAergic inhibition

may cause seizures and other motor disorders. Defective cholinergic transmission in the cerebral cortex produces memory deficits or confusional state. Impairment of dopamine circuits for motor control results in movement disorders. Disorders of norepinephrine and serotonin mechanisms may be involved in sleep and psychiatric disorders. Neuropeptides may be involved in neuroendocrine, autonomic, and neurogenic pain disorders.

Neurochemical Systems

The different neurochemical systems vary in their distribution, mechanism of action, and function. Amino acids are the most abundant neurotransmitters in the central nervous system and are used for fast neurotransmission in most clinically relevant pathways. Monoamines are less abundant and produce more prolonged effects that are important for modification of neural responses to amino acid neurotransmitters; their effect depends on the behavioral state. Neuropeptides are the least abundant but are very potent and produce responses that have a long latency and are prolonged.

Excitatory Amino Acids

L-Glutamate and L-aspartate are the neurotransmitters used by most excitatory neurons in the central nervous system.

Biochemistry

L-Glutamate is formed by intermediate metabolism of glucose via precursors of the Krebs cycle (particularly alpha-ketoglutarate). It may also be synthesized from glutamine. The synaptic effects of L-glutamate are terminated by its presynaptic reuptake via a sodium ion/adenosine triphosphate (ATP)-dependent pump.

Anatomical Distribution

L-Glutamate is the neurotransmitter for (1) pathways from the cerebral cortex (corticospinal, corticostriate pathways); (2) intrahemispheric and interhemispheric association pathways; (3) hippocampal circuits; (4) primary afferents and somatosensory and special sensory (visual, auditory) pathways; (5) cerebellar afferents; and (6) excitatory interneurons.

Receptor Mechanisms

Virtually all fast excitation in the central nervous system is mediated by excitatory amino acid receptors, of which there are several subtypes. The best characterized are the AMPA (α-amino-3-hydroxy-5-methylisoxazole-4-propionate) receptor, the NMDA (*N*-methyl-D-aspartate) receptor, and the metabotropic receptors. The AMPA receptor is diffusely distributed in the central nervous system and produces fast excitation, primarily through opening of sodium ion channels. The NMDA receptor is coupled to an ion channel that allows influx of calcium and sodium ions and produces prolonged bursts of depolarization. Activation of NMDA receptors is voltage-dependent, because at normal resting membrane potential the channel is blocked by magnesium ions. This blockade is removed by depolarization. In many brain regions, AMPA and NMDA receptors are coupled functionally, and AMPA receptor–mediated depolarization may remove the magnesium ion blockade of NMDA receptors, allowing NMDA channels to open and calcium ions to enter. The NMDA receptor–calcium channel is modulated by a variety of factors. Glycine is a positive modulator and is critical for activation of the receptor. Other factors include polyamines and changes in the oxidation-reduction state of the cell.

Glutamate also acts through different metabotropic receptors that are linked to different G-protein–coupled cascades. Some facilitate the release of calcium from intracellular stores, and others inhibit the calcium channel and presynaptically control glutamate release or directly inhibit their targets.

Intracellular calcium ions have a crucial role in mediating many of the effects of excitatory amino acids. The AMPA receptor–mediated depolarization opens voltage-gated calcium ion channels, the NMDA receptor allows direct influx of calcium ions through its channel, and the metabotropic receptor triggers the release of calcium ions from intracellular stores. Increased levels of intracellular calcium have important consequences, including prolonged depolarization bursts, long-lasting changes in synaptic efficacy (known as *synaptic plasticity*), and, in pathologic conditions, calcium-mediated excitotoxic neuronal injury. The effects of intracellular calcium depend on its interaction with several target proteins and its activation of several enzymatic cascades, including phospholipases and proteases. Important effects are activation of arachidonic acid cascade and synthesis of nitric oxide. Nitric oxide acts as a short-acting messenger molecule that may diffuse retrogradely to affect the presynaptic neuron and other neighboring neurons. Also, it may be critical in synaptic plasticity and mediation of neuronal injury.

Functions

L-Glutamate is the most abundant neurotransmitter and mediates rapid excitation within the central nervous system. Glutamate is critically involved in mechanisms of synaptic plasticity during development and learning. These include long-term potentiation and long-term depression. *Long-term potentiation* refers to a long-lasting facilitation of excitatory transmission after repeated activation of an excitatory amino acid pathway, particularly when co-incident with activity in the postsynaptic neuron. This effect, best characterized in hippocampal circuits, occurs throughout the brain. Long-term potentiation has been implicated in mechanisms of synaptogenesis during development, learning, and plastic changes in spinal, cortical, and other circuits. *Long-term depression,* in contrast, is a long-lasting decrease of efficacy of excitatory amino acid transmission. It has been studied primarily in the cerebellum. When the firing of a climbing fiber coincides with that of a mossy fiber, the response of the Purkinje cell to the mossy fiber is decreased (see Chapter 8). Long-term depression has been implicated in mechanisms of motor learning and adaptation. Both long-term potentiation and long-term depression involve an increase in intracellular calcium that triggers phosphorylation or dephosphorylation cascades, changes in gene transcription, and synthesis of nitric oxide. Long-term potentiation may also involve a presynaptic mechanism involving increased release of L-glutamate.

Inhibitory Amino Acids

GABA (found throughout the central nervous system) and glycine (found mainly in the spinal cord and brainstem) account for most of the inhibitory synapses in the central nervous system.

Biochemistry

The main source of GABA is glucose. The synthesis and metabolism of GABA are intimately linked with those of L-glutamate and involve interactions between GABAergic neurons and astrocytes. In GABAergic terminals, GABA is synthesized from L-glutamate by action of *glutamic acid decarboxylase.* After release, GABA undergoes reuptake both by GABAergic terminals and astrocytes and is then metabolized through the Krebs cycle to reconstitute L-glutamate. In astrocytes, glutamate is used to fixate ammonia to form glutamine by action of glutamine synthetase. This process is important for ammonia detoxification. In neurologic conditions associated with high ammonia levels, such as liver disease, there is compensatory hypertrophy of astrocytes.

Anatomical Distribution

GABA is present in two main classes of neurons: (1) inhibitory interneurons in local circuits (throughout the central nervous system), and (2) projection neurons in circuits of the basal ganglia and cerebellum.

Receptor Mechanisms

The inhibitory actions of GABA are mediated by two classes of receptor: $GABA_A$ and $GABA_B$ receptors. Activation of $GABA_A$ receptors triggers influx of chloride ions, which brings the membrane potential close to -75 mV. In most neurons, this results in fast hyperpolarization, but in primary afferents in the spinal cord it causes depolarization (*primary afferent depolarization*). $GABA_A$ mechanisms are inhibitory because they stabilize the membrane potential so that the membrane is unable to respond to stimuli, a process known as *shunting inhibition.* $GABA_A$ responses are potentiated by benzodiazepines and barbiturates, drugs commonly used for treatment of neurologic and psychiatric disorders. $GABA_B$ receptors are G-protein–linked receptors. They produce an increase in potassium ion conductance, which results in slow synaptic inhibition.

Both types of GABA receptor may mediate postsynaptic and presynaptic inhibition. Postsynaptic $GABA_A$ input to the axon initial segment (the site of spike generation) controls the global output of the neuron, whereas individual GABAergic terminals may have localized effects in dendritic microcircuits. The slow hyperpolarizing $GABA_B$ effect modulates the overall level of excitability of the neuron. Presynaptic GABA$_A$ and GABA$_B$ receptors decrease neurotransmitter release.

Functions

Inhibitory GABAergic interneurons participate in local feed-forward and feedback circuits, which are important for spatial and temporal restriction of excitation in the central nervous system. In brain regions, including the cerebral cortex, glutamatergic input produces not only monosynaptic excitation of the target neuron but also disynaptic fast inhibition through activation of local GABAergic interneurons. This excitation-inhibition sequence ensures that the transmission is extremely brief and localized. This is critical for sensory discrimination and fine motor control.

Cortical GABAergic interneurons are important both for information processing and control of excitability of pyramidal neurons. At a local level, GABA interneurons are involved in feed-forward and feedback interactions with pyramidal neurons, which are important for prevention of repetitive discharge and for lateral inhibition necessary for sensory discrimination. In addition, local GABAergic inhibition may decrease activation of NMDA receptors and dendritic voltage-dependent calcium ion channels and thus prevent *burst firing* or *epileptic neuronal discharges* (Fig. 1).

In the thalamus, cyclic activity of GABAergic neurons of the reticular nucleus imposes a rhythmic inhibition on thalamocortical relay neurons. This is reflected in the rhythmic activity of the electroencephalogram (for example, during non–rapid eye movement sleep); (see Chapter 10).

GABA is the neurotransmitter of the output neurons of the striatum and globus pallidus and of the Purkinje cells in the cerebellar cortex and thus is important in motor control.

In the basal ganglia and cerebellum, serial GABAergic inhibitory synapses are the basis of the process of *synaptic disinhibition.* In these circuits, GABAergic neurons exert a tonic inhibition on their targets. Thus,

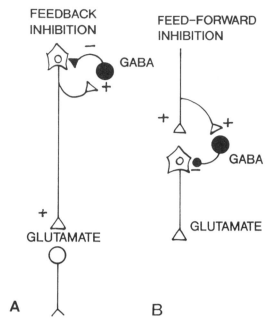

FIG. 1. Interactions between excitatory (glutamate) neurons and afferents and local inhibitory (GABA) interneurons. **A:** GABA interneurons activated by collaterals of projection neurons produce recurrent (or feedback) inhibition of neuronal output. **B:** Interneurons activated by collaterals of afferents produce feed-forward inhibition. Both mechanisms restrict discharge of the projection neuron spatially and temporally.

GABAergic input to these tonic inhibitory neurons produces transient disinhibition and increased activity of the effector neurons.

Glycine is an important inhibitory neurotransmitter in interneurons in the ventral horn of the spinal cord and in the brainstem. The actions of glycine, like those of GABA, are mediated through receptors linked to a chloride ion channel.

Acetylcholine

Acetylcholine is an important neurotransmitter in both the central and peripheral nervous systems.

Biochemistry

Acetylcholine is synthesized from acetyl coenzyme A and choline by the enzyme choline acetyltransferase. The synaptic actions of acetylcholine are rapidly terminated through hydrolysis by acetylcholinesterase (Table 4).

Choline acetyltransferase   Acetylcholinesterase

$\downarrow$ $\downarrow$

Acetyl coenzyme A + Choline → Acetylcholine → Choline + Acetate

Drugs that inhibit acetylcholinesterase (*anticholinesterase agents*) markedly potentiate cholinergic transmission.

Choline is provided by the diet and by hydrolysis of acetylcholine. An active, high-affinity presynaptic uptake of choline is the main limiting factor for the biosynthesis of acetylcholine.

Anatomical Distribution

Acetylcholine is an important neurotransmitter at synapses in the central and peripheral nervous systems. In the central nervous system, it is contained in five types of neurons: (1) projection neurons in the basal forebrain (Fig. 2); (2) projection neurons in the mesopontine tegmentum (Fig. 3); (3) interneurons in the striatum, cerebral cortex, and other areas; (4) motor neurons in the brainstem and spinal cord; and (5) preganglionic autonomic neurons in the brainstem and spinal cord.

Receptor Mechanisms

Acetylcholine acts via two classes of receptors: nicotinic and muscarinic. *Nicotinic receptors* include muscle, ganglion, and neuronal types. There are nonselective cation channel receptors that produce fast depolarization of their target cells. For example, nicotinic receptors mediate the rapid excitatory effect of acetylcholine at the skeletal neuromuscular junction (motor end plate), where it produces the end-plate potential in muscle fibers. Nicotinic receptors mediate the rapid excitatory effects of acetylcholine

---

TABLE 4. *Comparison of cholinergic and monoaminergic systems*

System	Location of neurons	Precursor	Enzyme for synthesis	Inactivation
Cholinergic				
Acetylcholine	Basal forebrain Mesopontine tegmentum Motor neurons Preganglionic and postganglionic parasympathetic neurons	Choline	Choline acetyltransferase	Acetylcholinesterase
Monoaminergic				
Dopamine	Substantia nigra Ventral tegmental area	Tyrosine	Tyrosine hydroxylase	Reuptake Monoamine oxidase Catechol-O-methyltransferase
Norepinephrine	Locus ceruleus Lateral pontomedullary tegmentum	Tyrosine	Tyrosine hydroxylase Dopamine β-hydroxylase	Reuptake Monoamine oxidase Catechol-O-methyltransferase
Epinephrine	Lateral pontomedullary tegmentum	Tyrosine	Tyrosine hydroxylase Dopamine β-hydroxylase Phenylethanolamine-N-methyltransferase	Monoamine oxidase Catechol-O-methyltransferase
Serotonin	Raphe nuclei	Tryptophan	Tryptophan hydroxylase	Monoamine oxidase
Histamine	Tuberomamillary nucleus	Histidine	Histidine decarboxylase	Monoamine oxidase Histamine-N-methyltransferase

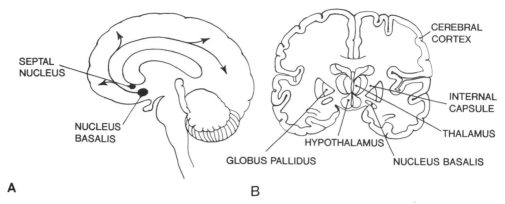

FIG. 2. Distribution of the cell bodies and projections of the cholinergic system of the basal forebrain. **A:** Sagittal view of projections from the nucleus basalis to the cerebral cortex and from the septal nuclei to the hippocampus. **B:** Coronal section showing the location of the nucleus basalis underneath the globus pallidus.

released from preganglionic autonomic neurons on sympathetic and parasympathetic ganglion cells. Nicotinic receptors are also present in the central nervous system, for example, in Renshaw cells, where they mediate activation by cholinergic collaterals of the alpha motor neuron (see Chapter 8). Nicotinic receptors are also located presynaptically and produce an increase in neurotransmitter release.

Muscarinic receptors are G-protein–coupled receptors. They include five genetic forms (M_1 to M_5), which have different distributions and different transducing mechanisms. The M_1 receptors produce a decrease in potassium conductance and have a predominantly excitatory effect, whereas M_2 receptors increase potassium conductance and are inhibitory. Muscarinic receptors mediate most of the effects of acetylcholine in the central

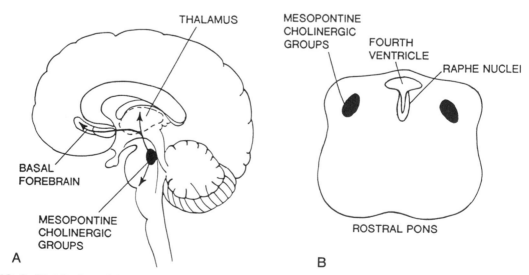

FIG. 3. Distribution of the cell bodies and projections of mesopontine cholinergic neurons. **A:** Sagittal view of projections to the thalamus. **B:** Cross section showing the location of cholinergic neurons in rostral pons.

nervous system. The main effect in the cerebral cortex is postsynaptic excitation of pyramidal neurons, mediated via M_1 receptors and involving a decrease in potassium conductance. The M_2 receptors are inhibitory autoreceptors in terminals of axons originating in the basal forebrain and the brainstem. In the periphery, muscarinic receptors are present in the targets of postganglionic parasympathetic fibers and sweat glands.

Functions

The most common effect of acetylcholine in the brain is excitation, mediated largely by muscarinic receptors. Cholinergic neurons in the basal forebrain, including the nucleus basalis, are important for cortical activation and memory processing. Cholinergic neurons in the mesopontine tegmentum project to the thalamus and activate thalamocortical circuits involved in arousal and rapid eye movement sleep. Cholinergic interneurons in the striatum may participate in the control of posture and movement. Acetylcholine is the neurotransmitter of all motor neurons of the brainstem and spinal cord, including skeletomotor neurons, branchiomotor neurons, and preganglionic autonomic neurons. The main effect of these cholinergic neurons is fast synaptic excitation mediated by nicotinic receptors. Acetylcholine is also the neurotransmitter in postganglionic parasympathetic pathways, which innervate the heart, glandular tissue, and smooth muscle of all viscera via muscarinic receptors.

Monoamines

General Characteristics

Central monoaminergic systems include neuronal groups containing catecholamines, serotonin, or histamine (Table 4). These systems have several characteristics in common: (1) restricted localization of cell bodies in specific regions of the brainstem and hypothalamus; (2) diffuse projections throughout the central nervous system via axon collaterals; (3) neurotransmitter biosynthesis dependent on specific enzymes and synaptic uptake of dietary amino acid precursors; (4) presynaptic inhibition of neuronal activity and neurotransmitter release via autoreceptors; (5) termination of neurotransmitter action by presynaptic reuptake and enzymatic degradation; (6) frequent coexistence with neuropeptides; (7) slow tonic neuronal activity dependent on the behavioral state of the person (sleep-wake cycle, attention); (8) synaptic effects mediated by various subtypes of G-protein–linked receptors; (9) modulatory, or "gain setting," influence on their neuronal targets; and (10) interaction of neurochemicals on a single target.

Catecholamine Biochemistry

Catecholamines include *dopamine, norepinephrine,* and *epinephrine.* These substances are synthesized from the amino acid L-tyrosine. The rate-limiting step is mediated by *tyrosine hydroxylase.*

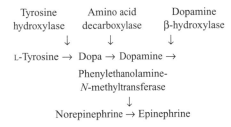

The most important mechanism for termination of the synaptic effect of catecholamines is specific sodium ion/ATP-dependent presynaptic reuptake. The enzymatic catabolism of catecholamines involves two classes of enzymes: monoamine oxidases and catechol-*O*-methyltransferase. *Monoamine oxidases* are mitochondrial enzymes that inactivate intraneuronal catecholamines that are free in the terminals after reuptake and include two classes, A and B. *Catechol-O-methyltransferase* acts on extraneuronal catecholamines. The principal metabolites of catecholamines result from the combined action of monoamine oxidase and catechol-*O*-methyltransferase. The principal metabolite of dopamine is *homovanillic acid.* The principal metabolite of norepinephrine and epinephrine in the central nervous system is *3-methoxy-4-hydroxyphenylethyleneglycol,* and in the periphery, *vanillylmandelic acid.*

Dopamine

Anatomical Distribution

Dopamine is located in two main groups of central neurons: a mesencephalic group and a hypothalamic group. The mesencephalic dopaminergic group includes the substantia nigra pars compacta and the ventral tegmental area (Fig. 4). These neurons are interdigitated and form the mesotelencephalic dopaminergic system. This system includes (1) the *nigrostriatal pathway* that projects from the substantia nigra pars compacta to the caudate and putamen; (2) the *mesolimbic pathway* that projects from the ventral tegmental area to the limbic striatum (nucleus accumbens), amygdala, and hippocampus; and (3) the *mesocortical pathway* that projects to the prefrontal and association cortices.

Hypothalamic dopaminergic neurons are located in the tuberoinfundibular area (which controls pituitary function) and the lateral hypothalamus.

Receptor Mechanisms

Dopamine receptors are G-protein–coupled receptors and can be subdivided into two main subfamilies: the *D_1-like* receptor subfamily, including the D_1 and D_5 receptors, and the *D_2-like* receptor subfamily, including the D_2, D_3, and D_4 receptors. D_1-like (D_1 and D_5) receptors stimulate adenylate cyclase and decrease potassium conductance; in many systems, they have predominantly an excitatory effect. D_1 receptors predominate in the neostriatum (caudate and putamen) and nucleus accumbens, whereas D_5 receptors are restricted mainly to the hippocampal circuit, thalamus, and hypothalamus. D_2-like receptors (D_2, D_3, and D_4) produce inhibition of adenylate cyclase, increase potassium conductance, and decrease calcium conductance. Thus, they primarily exert an inhibitory effect on their targets. D_2 receptors, like D_1 receptors, are concentrated in the neostriatum (caudate and putamen). D_2 receptors are also presynaptic inhibitory autoreceptors in

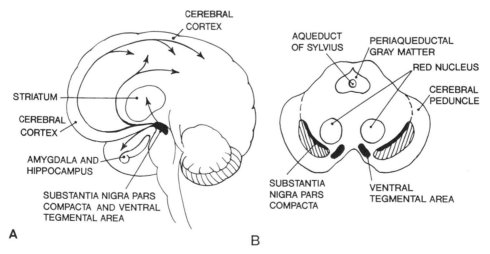

FIG. 4. Distribution of the cell bodies and projections of the mesotelencephalic dopaminergic neurons. **A:** Sagittal view of projections from the substantia nigra pars compacta and adjacent ventral tegmentum to the striatum and cerebral cortex. **B:** Cross section showing the location of dopaminergic cell bodies in the ventral tegmentum of the midbrain.

dopaminergic neurons. D_3 and D_4 receptors occur primarily in limbic regions, including the nucleus accumbens; D_4 receptors are concentrated in the frontal cortex, amygdala, and hippocampus. In the striatum (and probably other areas), neurons may contain both D_1 and D_2 receptors, and the interaction of both types may be necessary for optimal regulation of cell function.

Functions

The dopaminergic projection from the substantia nigra pars compacta to the striatum (the nigrostriatal pathway) regulates the basal ganglia circuits involved in motor planning and execution. The primary target of the dopaminergic projection is the GABAergic output neurons of the putamen, caudate, and nucleus accumbens. Dopamine exerts dual effects on neurons in the striatum according to the relative distribution of D_1 and D_2 receptors in different neuronal populations. The net effect of dopamine in the striatum is to facilitate execution of motor programs. Nigral dopaminergic fibers also synapse in the subthalamic nucleus and globus pallidus.

Dopaminergic projections from the ventral tegmental area to the nucleus accumbens (the mesolimbic pathway) modulate biologic drives and motivation and control complex, stereotypical motor behavior in response to significant external or internal stimuli. This pathway may be a "final common pathway" for the addictive effects of drugs. Drugs of addiction acutely increase dopamine levels in the nucleus accumbens, by various mechanisms. *Cocaine* directly blocks the dopamine transporter and thus increases the synaptic half-life of dopamine. *Amphetamine* prevents dopamine uptake by synaptic vesicles, triggering the nonvesicular release of dopamine. Nicotine increases dopamine release via presynaptic receptors in ventral tegmental neurons. Opioids disinhibit dopaminergic neurons by preventing the release of GABA from local inhibitory neurons in the ventral tegmental area.

Dopaminergic inputs to the prefrontal cortex, cingulate cortex, and other areas involved in higher order processing of sensory and motor mechanisms modulate the processes of attention, planning, and central executive functions.

Dopamine is important in the hypothalamic control of anterior pituitary function. The main effect is a tonic inhibition of the synthesis and release of prolactin by the anterior pituitary. Drugs that block D_2 receptors increase prolactin release. Other functions of dopamine include modulation of local circuits in the retinal and olfactory bulb. In the periphery, dopamine may be released by autonomic nerves and control cardiac, renal, and other visceral functions.

Norepinephrine and Epinephrine

Anatomical Distribution

Norepinephrine and epinephrine are neurochemical mediators in both the central and peripheral nervous systems. In the brain, norepinephrine and epinephrine neurons are restricted to two main areas: the locus ceruleus in the dorsal pons (Fig. 5) and the lateral tegmentum of the medulla and pons (Fig. 6). The locus ceruleus provides widespread innervation of the brain and spinal cord via extensive axonal collateralization. This nucleus innervates regions controlling responses to external stimuli, including sensory and motor nuclei of the brainstem and spinal cord, cerebellum, hippocampus, thalamus, and cerebral cortex.

The lateral tegmental system includes neurons that contain norepinephrine or epinephrine. These neurons are located in the ventrolateral pons and the intermediate reticular zone of the medulla. They have extensive interconnections with areas involved in autonomic and neuroendocrine control, such as preganglionic autonomic neurons, the hypothalamus, and the amygdala (see Chapter 9).

At the peripheral level, norepinephrine is the primary neurotransmitter of postganglionic sympathetic fibers. Epinephrine is released from neuroendocrine cells of the adrenal medulla and circulates in the blood as a neurohormone.

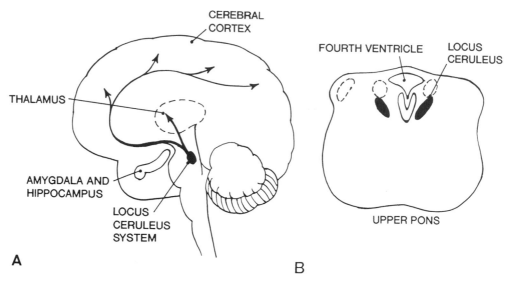

FIG. 5. Distribution of the cell bodies and projections of the locus ceruleus noradrenergic system. **A:** Sagittal view of the main projections to areas involved in sensory, associative, and motor functions in the thalamus and cerebral cortex. **B:** Cross section showing the location of the locus ceruleus in dorsal pons.

Receptor Mechanisms

Norepinephrine and epinephrine receptors constitute three main families that have various receptor subtypes. These include the α_1 (α_{1A}, α_{1B}, α_{1D}), α_2 (α_{2A}, α_{2B}, and α_{2C}), and β (β_1, β_2, and β_3) receptor families. The different subtypes of receptors have different effector mechanisms and different distributions. In general, α_1 receptors mediate excitatory responses and are abundant on the targets of catecholaminergic neurons, both in the brain and in the peripheral targets of the sympathetic system. The α_2-receptors predominantly mediate inhibitory responses and include presynaptic autoreceptors on catecholaminergic neurons. β-Receptors are distributed in supratentorial structures, the cerebellum, and the peripheral targets of the sympathetic system.

Functions

Locus ceruleus neurons provide most of the noradrenergic innervation of the cerebral cortex, thalamus, cerebellum, and sensory and motor nuclei of the brainstem and spinal cord.

The locus ceruleus has been implicated in the mechanisms of attention and response to stress and the regulation of rapid eye movement sleep (see Chapter 10). Neuronal activity in this nucleus decreases during non–rapid eye movement sleep and is suppressed during rapid eye movement sleep. The firing of locus ceruleus neurons increases markedly in response to environmental or physiologically challenging stimuli, such as stress, pain, extreme alteration of body temperature, and hypoglycemia.

Noradrenergic and adrenergic neurons of the lateral tegmental system, particularly those in the ventrolateral medulla, have a critical role in the regulation of autonomic and endocrine functions. For example, epinephrine neurons of the rostral ventrolateral medulla provide massive monosynaptic input to preganglionic sympathetic neurons, and norepinephrine neurons of the caudal ventrolateral medulla control hypothalamic function, including the secretion of vasopressin.

The functional interaction between the neurons in the locus ceruleus and the lateral tegmentum in response to challenging exter-

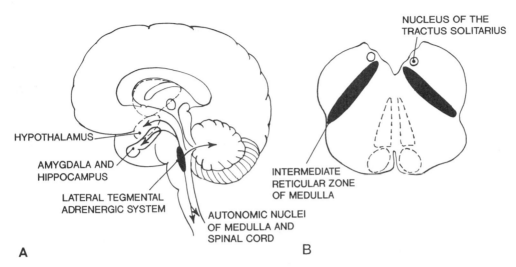

FIG. 6. Distribution of the cell bodies and projections of the lateral tegmental system of catecholaminergic neurons. **A:** Sagittal view of projections to the hypothalamus, amygdala, and autonomic nuclei of the brainstem and spinal cord. **B:** Cross section showing the distribution of norepinephrine and epinephrine neurons in the intermediate reticular zone of the medulla.

nal or internal stimuli results in simultaneous increase in alertness (locus ceruleus) and activation of the sympathetic system (the lateral tegmental system). At the peripheral level, norephinephrine and epinephrine act at sympathetic neuroeffector junctions in the heart, blood vessels, and viscera (see Chapter 9).

Serotonin

Serotonin is an important central neurotransmitter that has widespread influence.

Biochemistry

Serotonin (5-hydroxytryptamine [5-HT]) is synthesized from the amino acid L-tryptophan by tryptophan hydroxylase. The intermediate product is 5-hydroxytryptophan, which is converted to serotonin by L-amino acid decarboxylase, a nonspecific enzyme.

Tryptophan   L-Amino acid
hydroxylase   decarboxylase
↓   ↓
L-Tryptophan → 5-Hydroxytryptophan → Serotonin

Similar to catecholamines, the main mechanism of inactivation of serotonin is through reuptake by terminals of serotoninergic neurons. Serotonin is then metabolized by monoamine oxidase. The main metabolite of serotonin is *5-hydroxyindoleacetic acid.*

Anatomical Distribution

The cell bodies of central serotoninergic neurons are located in the raphe nuclei, which are in the midline reticular formation of the brainstem. The group of *raphe nuclei* includes the rostral raphe nuclei in the upper pons and midbrain and the caudal raphe nuclei in the caudal pons and medulla. Neurons in the rostral nuclei project to the basal ganglia, thalamus, hypothalamus, limbic system, and cerebral cortex, and those in the caudal group to the brainstem and spinal cord (Fig. 7).

Receptor Mechanisms

There are multiple families of serotoninergic receptors, with several receptor subtypes. With one exception, all serotoninergic recep-

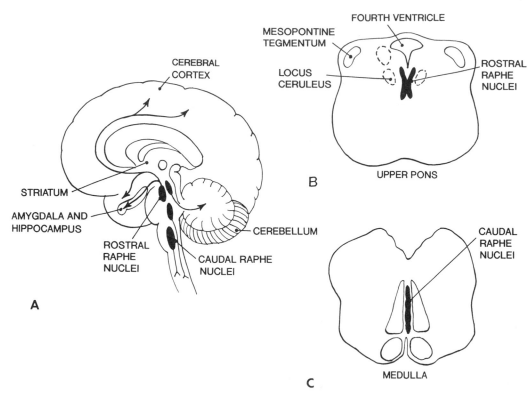

FIG. 7. Distribution of the cell bodies and projections of the serotoninergic neurons of the raphe nuclei. **A:** Sagittal view of the widespread distribution of cell bodies and pathways throughout the central nervous system. **B:** Cross section showing the location of rostral raphe neurons in rostral pons (project to supratentorial structures). **C:** Cross section showing the caudal raphe neurons of the medulla (project to posterior fossa and spinal structures).

tors that have been cloned are G-protein–coupled receptors. The main types are 5-HT$_1$ receptors, coupled to G$_{i/o}$ (inhibition of adenyl cyclase and increase in potassium conductance); 5-HT$_2$ receptors, coupled to G$_{q/11}$ (activation of the phospholipase C-phosphoinositol cascade and decrease in potassium conductance); 5-HT$_3$ receptors, which are a *ligand-gated cation channel;* and 5-HT$_4$ (and 5-HT$_6$ and 5-HT$_7$) receptors, coupled to G$_s$ (stimulation of adenyl cyclase and cyclic adenosine monophosphate formation). In general, 5-HT$_1$ receptors are inhibitory and include autoreceptors located in the soma of raphe neurons (5-HT$_{1A}$) or in their axon terminals (5-HT$_{1D}$). 5-HT$_2$ receptors are excitatory and predominate in the cerebral cortex

and hippocampus. 5-HT$_3$ receptors are excitatory and predominate in nerve terminals, including primary afferents, cerebral cortex, hippocampus, and area postrema. 5-HT$_4$, 5-HT$_6$, and 5-HT$_7$ receptors are linked to cyclic adenosine monophosphate and are present in the striatum and limbic system.

Functions

Similar to norepinephrine, serotonin exerts its influence throughout the brain via diffuse collateralization of the axons of raphe neurons. Serotoninergic systems are important in behavioral state control, pain suppression, and autonomic and endocrine regulation. Because the serotoninergic innervation of the sensory areas of the cerebral cortex is abundant, particularly in the layers that receive thalamic input, serotonin may be important in the modulation of cortical sensory (particularly visual) processing. Like locus ceruleus neurons, raphe nuclei neurons are active during wakefulness, decrease their firing during non–rapid eye movement sleep, and become silent during rapid eye movement sleep. Cerebral blood vessels and glial cells receive an abundant serotoninergic and adrenergic innervation, which indicate that these systems are important for intrinsic regulation of cerebral blood flow and metabolism.

Projections from the caudal raphe nuclei to the spinal cord are important in the central inhibition of nociceptive transmission in the dorsal horn. This projection also increases the excitability of motor neurons.

Histamine

Similar to serotonin, histamine produces widespread effects in both neural and nonneural tissues in the brain.

Biochemistry

Histamine is synthesized from the amino acid L-histidine by the enzyme histidine decarboxylase.

$$\begin{array}{c} \text{histidine decarboxylase} \\ \downarrow \\ \text{L-histidine} \rightarrow \text{histamine} \end{array}$$

Histamine is metabolized by the enzymes histamine-N-methyltransferase and monoamine oxidase to its final product *methylimidazoleacetic acid.* Unlike other monoamines, histamine does not undergo reuptake.

Anatomical Distribution

Histamine neurons are located in the lateral *tuberomamillary nucleus* of the hypothalamus and provide widely divergent pathways to the cerebral cortex, limbic system, hypothalamus, basal ganglia, brainstem, and spinal cord (Fig. 8).

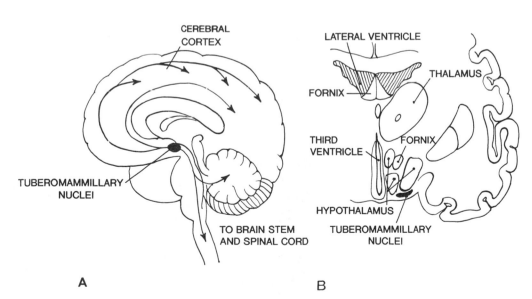

A   **B**

FIG. 8. Distribution of the cell bodies and projections of histamine neurons of the tuberomamillary nuclei. **A:** Sagittal view of widespread projections to the cerebral cortex and rest of the central nervous system. **B:** Cross section showing the location of these neurons in the lateral hypothalamic region.

Receptor Mechanisms and Functions

The effects of histamine are mediated via H_1, H_2, and H_3 receptors. The H_1 receptors are important for arousal. Histamine may play an important role in arousal mechanisms, in coupling neuronal activity with cerebral metabolism, and in neuroendocrine control (see Table 4).

Neuropeptides

Neuropeptides are abundant in the central and peripheral nervous systems. Many are also present in nonneural tissues, particularly in the tissue of the so-called gastroenteropancreatic axis and other endocrine systems.

Biochemistry

Neuropeptides form several families. The neuropeptides of each family have common gene precursors, structural homologies, and functional similarities. Unlike other neurochemicals, neuropeptides are not synthesized in nerve terminals but from messenger RNA in neuronal cell bodies. They are processed and transported to the terminals in large dense-core vesicles via fast anterograde axonal transport. Neuropeptides are synthesized first as a large precursor molecule containing several copies of the same or related peptides. This precursor undergoes cleavage to smaller peptides and posttranslational modifications as it traverses the secretory pathway from the endoplasmic reticulum to the Golgi complex and finally to the secretory granule. In many central and peripheral neurons, neuropeptides coexist with other neurotransmitters and are released preferentially during burst firing of the neuron. Unlike monoamines and amino acids, neuropeptides do not undergo presynaptic reuptake. Instead, their action is terminated by hydrolysis by extracellular peptidases.

Anatomical Distribution

Neuropeptides have a widespread but heterogeneous distribution in the central nervous system; the hypothalamus contains the highest concentration. Other neuropeptide-rich areas are the amygdala, autonomic nuclei, pain-modulating circuits of the brainstem and spinal cord, and, to a lesser extent, the basal ganglia and cerebral cortex. Neuropeptides are scarce in the cerebellum and thalamus.

Central peptidergic neurons are organized into two main systems: (1) diffuse projection systems that have cell bodies in the hypothalamus, amygdala, and nucleus of the tractus solitarius and that project diffusely throughout the brain; and (2) local or short projection neurons located throughout the central nervous system. Neuropeptides frequently coexist with other neurotransmitters, including other neuropeptides (hypothalamic neurons), acetylcholine or monoamines (diffuse brainstem systems), or GABA (striatal and cortical neurons).

Receptor Mechanisms

Neuropeptides are potent and active at low concentrations; their synaptic effects have a slow onset and long duration. Similar to monoamines, they act via G-protein–coupled receptors, mainly as synaptic modulators. Because neuropeptides frequently coexist with other, primary neurotransmitters, they participate in a complex chemical coding involving presynaptic and postsynaptic modulatory interactions. The prolonged modulatory effects of neuropeptides occur not only at the synaptic level but also at a distance, including neighboring neurons, distal neural targets via volume transmission, or peripheral targets reached via the blood stream (neuroendocrine effect).

Functions

Neuropeptides exert potent, long-lasting effects on endocrine, autonomic, sensory, motor, and behavioral functions.

Hypothalamic peptidergic neurons exert three types of influence: (1) magnocellular hypothalamic neurons release *vasopressin* and *oxytocin* into the general circulation; (2) hypophysiotropic hypothalamic neurons secrete *releasing factors* (such as corticotropin-releasing factor, gonadotropin-releasing factor, and growth hormone-releasing factor) or *inhibiting factors* (for example, somatostatin) in the median eminence to control anterior pituitary function; and (3) other neurons project diffusely, especially to autonomic and limbic areas of the brain. Hypothalamic peptides are important in the control of homeostasis, reproduction, and immune function through their effects on endocrine, autonomic, and somatic motor effectors of the internal regulation system.

The amygdala has important peptidergic connections with autonomic areas of the hypothalamus and brainstem, which may be important for modulation of autonomic responses during emotional states.

Brainstem and spinal autonomic regions, including the nucleus of the tractus solitarius, ventrolateral medulla, and preganglionic autonomic nuclei, have an abundance of neuropeptides, which frequently coexist with monoamines. For example, *neuropeptide Y* coexists with catecholamines in pathways that project from the ventrolateral medulla to the hypothalamus and spinal cord. These pathways are important for modulation of visceral reflexes and hypothalamic neuroendocrine function.

At the peripheral level, neuropeptides coexist with the primary neurotransmitters of postganglionic sympathetic and parasympathetic fibers. Postganglionic sympathetic neurons contain neuropeptide Y in addition to norepinephrine. Neuropeptide Y inhibits prejunctional release and potentiates postjunctional effects of norepinephrine. Postganglionic parasympathetic secretomotor neurons contain *vasoactive intestinal polypeptide* in addition to acetylcholine. This peptide is a potent vasodilator and potentiates the secretomotor effect of acetylcholine on exocrine glands. Neuropeptides are also important neurotransmitters in the enteric nervous system (see Chapter 9).

Neuropeptides are important in central pain-controlling pathways. Primary unmyclinated nociceptive afferents contain various neuropeptides, particularly *substance P* and *calcitonin gene-related peptide*. These peptides not only mediate central transmission of nociceptive information but are also released locally by axon terminals (axon reflex) to produce vasomotor and permeability changes in response to injury—*neurogenic inflammation* (see Chapter 7). Pain transmission is controlled by opioid peptides, which play a crucial role in spinal and supraspinal analgesia. Opioid peptides include *enkephalins, beta-endorphin,* and *dynorphin.* Enkephalins and dynorphin are contained primarily in local neurons or in short projection neurons, not only in pain-controlling circuits but also in the basal ganglia and autonomic nuclei. Beta-endorphin is produced from a large precursor called *pro-opiomelanocortin,* which also gives rise to adrenocorticotropin and melanocyte-stimulating hormone. Neurons containing beta-endorphin are restricted to a particular region of the hypothalamus but send diffuse projections throughout the central nervous system. The main effect of opioids is presynaptic and postsynaptic inhibition. Opioids play an important role in supraspinal and spinal analgesia (see Chapter 7). In addition to central analgesia, opioids have other important effects, including depression of cardiovascular and respiratory functions, pupillary constriction, changes in behavior, regulation of hormone secretion, and body temperature (hypothermia).

In the basal ganglia, neuropeptides are abundant in both local neurons (neuropeptide Y and somatostatin) and in different functional classes of GABAergic projection neurons in the striatum. In the cerebral cortex, vasoactive intestinal polypeptide, neuropeptide Y, cholecystokinin, and somatostatin are localized in intrinsic, or local circuit, GABAergic neurons. They may be important in modulation of cortical neurotransmission and in local regulation of cerebral blood flow. For example, vasoactive intestinal polypeptide is a vasodilator of cerebral blood vessels, and neuropeptide Y is a vasoconstrictor. Thus, these neuropeptides may be important in coupling neuronal activity with local cerebral blood flow (see Chapter 11).

Other Neurochemical Messengers

Purines

The *purines* adenosine triphosphate (ATP) and adenosine may act both as neurotransmitters and neuromodulators in the central and peripheral nervous systems. ATP is stored in synaptic vesicles with other neurotransmitters, including acetylcholine (as in the neuromuscular junction) and norepinephrine (as in sympathetic terminals innervating smooth muscle). It is also present in synaptic vesicles in the brain. It can be co-released with other neurotransmitters or in a nonvesicular manner during conditions such as hypoxia. At the site of release, ATP is hydrolysed by surface-bound membrane enzymes to adenosine diphosphate and adenosine monophosphate. Extracellular adenosine monophosphate is metabolized by the $5'$-nucleotidase to *adenosine.* The kinetics of the hydrolysis cascade is important in determining the ratio between ATP and adenosine-mediated transmission. ATP and adenosine act through several subtypes of *purinoreceptors.*

Purinoreceptors are subdivided into two main families: *P_1 receptors* (also called *adenosine receptors*) respond to adenosine, and *P_2 receptors* respond mainly to ATP and adenosine monophosphate.

The adenosine receptors mediate several neuromodulatory effects. *A_1 adenosine* receptors mediate the presynaptic inhibition of the release of several neurotransmitters. *A_2 receptors* produce vasodilatation and increase in energy production through glucose transport. Levels of adenosine in the extracellular fluid increase sharply under conditions of energy failure, such as hypoxia and ischemia. Adenosine is thought to exert a cytoprotective effect by inhibiting the influx of calcium, and thus the release of L-glutamate (via A_1 receptors), and producing vasodilatation (via A_2 receptors).

ATP (P_2) receptors include several subtypes. Some receptors (P_{2X} and P_{2Z}) are ion channel receptors that allow the entry of calcium and sodium and produce fast depolarization. These receptors are abundant in the peripheral endings of nociceptive neurons. Other receptors (P_{2Y} and P_{2T}) are G-protein–coupled receptors and produce presynaptic inhibition of neurotransmitter release.

Nitric Oxide

Nitric oxide is an important intercellular messenger. It is synthesized from arginine by action of *nitric oxide synthase.* There are constitutive and inducible forms of this enzyme. Constitutive forms include neuronal nitric acid synthase and endothelial nitric acid synthase, which are activated by calcium (via the calcium-binding protein *calmodulin*). The inducible form is present in macrophages and mononuclear cells and is activated during inflammation. Nitric oxide diffuses rapidly and mediates responses to several calcium-mobilizing stimuli. For example, L-glutamate, via NMDA receptors, allows the entry of calcium, which stimulates the production of nitric acid synthase and nitric oxide. Nitric oxide does not act on membrane receptors but forms complexes with transition metal ions, such as those in heme-containing proteins (like hemoglobin). One target is cytoplasmic *guanylate cyclase,* which results in increased production of cyclic guanosine monophosphate. Cyclic guanosine monophosphate in vascular smooth muscle is the basis of the potent vasodilator effect of endothelial nitric oxide.

The most significant biologic property of nitric oxide is its ability to react with the iron contained in the heme molecule and in several key enzymes, including those in the mitochondrial respiratory chain. Nitric oxide also reacts with other free radicals, for example, *superoxide, to produce peroxinitrite,* a highly reactive oxidant. This is a possible mechanism for the cytotoxic effect of nitric oxide.

Carbon monoxide is another potential intercellular messenger. It is derived from the heme molecule. Like nitric oxide, carbon monoxide acts via cytoplasmic guanylate cyclase.

Functional Organization of Central Neurochemical Systems ■

On the basis of the anatomical-functional organization, the central neurochemical systems can be divided into three main groups: (1) *relay, or direct, systems;* (2) *diffuse systems;* and (3) *local circuits.*

Relay, or Direct, Systems

Relay, or direct, systems correspond to the motor and sensory systems that occupy the outer tube of the neuraxis. Information in these systems is phasic, transmitted rapidly via large myelinated fibers that form clearly defined fiber tracts, and processed sequentially in several relay stations located along each pathway. Each relay nucleus contains projection neurons and local circuit neurons. The projection neurons form the interconnecting pathways, transmit signals over long distances, and emit collaterals close to their cell bodies. They are excitatory neurons and use excitatory amino acids, particularly L-glutamate, to provide fast, short-lasting synaptic excitation. Most of the local circuit neurons are inhibitory and use GABA as a neurotransmitter. These neurons are involved in the processes of feed-forward or feedback inhibition, which are important for sensory discrimination and for fine motor control. The neurotransmitter of inhibitory interneurons in the spinal cord and brainstem is glycine.

Relay systems provide fast, precise information necessary for sensory and motor function. Interruption of any link in a relay system incapacitates the function of the whole pathway. Virtually all major focal neurologic signs and symptoms are due to interruption of relay pathways.

Diffuse Systems

The diffuse systems include the internal regulation and the consciousness systems, which are located in the inner tube of the neuraxis. Unlike the relay systems, the diffuse systems consist of neurons located in particular nuclei of the brainstem, basal forebrain, and hypothalamus. These systems include (1) brainstem and hypothalamic neuronal groups that contain monoamines (dopamine, norepinephrine, serotonin, histamine); (2) neurons of the basal forebrain and pontomesencephalic tegmentum that contain acetylcholine; and (3) many hypothalamic neurons that contain neuropeptides. Monoamine and neuropeptide transmitters usually coexist in the neurons of the diffuse systems. The neurons have unmyelinated, slow-conducting axons that have a diffuse, multibranched, and divergent pattern. Therefore, a single neuron may simultaneously innervate several functionally different parts of the central nervous system. The axons have varicosities that contain a great number of synaptic vesicles. The neurotransmitter is released in a diffuse manner, so that the cellular targets of these systems are determined by the location of the receptors and not by the site of neurotransmitter release. Projection neurons of the diffuse systems generally have a slow, rhythmic pattern of discharge, which changes markedly according to the behavioral state (sleep, attention). This activity is influenced by local interneurons and by local feedback mechanisms (generally inhibitory) that involve somatodendritic and presynaptic autoreceptors.

The diffuse systems do not convey topographically specific information but instead are involved in global functions such as regulation of the sleep-wake cycle, attention, emotion, cognition, response to stress, and regulation of visceral, hormonal, sexual, and immune functions.

The functions of the diffuse systems are consistent with the modulatory role of their neurochemical signals, which act via G-protein–linked receptors. These receptors are involved in controlling neuronal excitability and responsiveness rather than rapid excitation or inhibition.

Pathologic alterations or pharmacologic manipulation of the diffuse systems do not produce focal neurologic deficits. Instead, they may cause various clinical manifestations, including marked changes in general motor performance, abnormal responses to pain, altered state of alertness or cognition, abnormal mood and thought processes, and abnormalities in vegetative and endocrine functions.

Local Circuits in Relay and Diffuse Systems

Local circuit neurons, or interneurons, control the flow of information and the pattern of neuronal activity in both relay and diffuse systems. Axons of local circuit neurons have short ramifications that synapse on the cell bodies and dendrites of projection neurons or on terminals of afferent axons in the immediate vicinity. Local circuit neurons may be either excitatory or inhibitory. Most inhibitory interneurons in the central nervous system use GABA. Other interneurons use excitatory amino acids, acetylcholine, or neuropeptides.

Clinical Correlations   ∎

The neurochemical systems are involved in the pathophysiology of various neurologic diseases (Table 5).

Excitatory Amino Acids

Excessive exposure to L-glutamate or other endogenous excitatory amino acids may cause neuronal injury through the mechanism of *excitotoxicity.* Excitotoxicity has been implicated in the pathogenesis of two groups of neurologic diseases: *acute metabolic crises,* such as cerebral hypoxia-ischemia, stroke, hypoglycemia, seizures, and head or spinal injury; and *chronic neurodegenerative disorders,* including those that produce dementia, movement disorders, cerebellar dysfunction, and motor neuron disease. Excessive exposure to L-glutamate may result from increased presynaptic release, impaired energy-dependent reuptake, or both. Excessive activation of AMPA and particularly NMDA receptors causes sodium and calcium ions to accumulate in neurons. Increased concentration of calcium ions in the cytoplasm activates intracellular enzymatic cascades, including proteases and lipases. This generates oxygen free radicals and other intracellular mechanisms that produce neuronal injury or death. Pharmacologic blockade of AMPA or NMDA receptors may have a "neuroprotective" effect.

TABLE 5. *Neurotransmitters and their clinical associations and pharmacologic treatment*

Neurotransmitter	Receptor	Clinical correlation	Pharmacologic treatment
Glutamate	NMDA	Stroke Trauma Epilepsy Degenerative diseases	NMDA receptor blockers
GABA	GABA$_A$	Seizures	Positive GABA$_A$ modulators (barbiturates; benzodiazepines)
	GABA$_B$	Spasticity	Agonist (baclofen)
Acetylcholine	Nicotinic	Myasthenia gravis	Cholinesterase inhibitors (pyridostigmine)
	Muscarinic	Alzheimer's disease Movement disorders	Cholinesterase inhibitors (tacrine) Antagonist (trihexyphenidyl)
Dopamine	Dopamine D$_1$D$_2$	Parkinson's disease Prolactinoma Psychosis	Agonists (L-dopa, bromocriptine, pergolide) Antagonists (haloperidol, clozapine)
5-HT	5-HT$_1$	Migraine	Agonist (sumatriptan)
	5-HT$_2$		Antagonist (methysergide)
	5-HT$_3$	Vomiting Depression	Antagonist (ondansetron) Reuptake inhibitors (tricyclics, fluoxetine)
Opioid	Mu	Pain Intoxication	Agonist (morphine, codeine) Antagonist (naloxone)

GABA, γ-aminobutyric acid; 5-HT, serotonin; NMDA, *N*-methyl-D-aspartate.

Inhibitory Amino Acids

GABA is critical in maintaining tonic inhibitory control of most neurons in the central nervous system. Decreased GABA inhibition due to loss of inhibitory interneurons or to blockade of GABA receptors may produce seizures, movement disorders, exaggerated muscle tone, and anxiety. Many drugs used to treat seizures, increased muscle tone, anxiety, or insomnia act by facilitating GABA$_A$ receptor mechanisms. Chronic exposure to drugs acting through these receptor mechanisms, including alcohol, barbiturates, and benzodiazepines, may produce downregulation of GABA$_A$ receptors. Abrupt discontinuation of these drugs results in withdrawal symptoms, including anxiety, tremor, and generalized seizures. Glycine is an important inhibitory amino acid. Impairment of glycinergic transmission by tetanus toxin or strychnine causes autonomic hyperactivity and a severe increase in muscle tone.

Stiff-man syndrome is an autoimmune disorder characterized by rigidity of axial muscles, increased lordosis, and leg spasms triggered by startle or other stimuli. A hallmark of the syndrome is the presence of antibodies to glutamic acid decarboxylase, the key enzyme for synthesis of GABA.

Drugs that affect GABAergic systems are frequently used to treat neurologic disease. *Barbiturates* (*phenobarbital*) and *benzodiazepines* are allosteric activators of the GABA$_A$ receptor-chloride channel complex. These drugs are used to treat seizures and, in the case of benzodiazepines, anxiety, insomnia, spasticity, and movement disorders. Because of the widespread distribution of GABA$_A$ receptors in brain, the use of benzodiazepines for a particular purpose (for example, muscle relaxation) is frequently associated with sedation, lassitude, and other undesirable side effects. Benzodiazepines are the primary treatment for alcohol withdrawal. Benzodiazepine overdose produces coma, muscle relaxation, hypotension, and respiratory depression. The benzodiazepine receptor antagonist *flumazenil* (in combination with

supportive measures) is used to treat overdose. Recently, several drugs have been developed to increase synaptic GABA levels in patients with seizures. These include drugs that inhibit either GABA reuptake or metabolism (for example, *vigabatrin*).

Presynaptic GABA$_B$ receptors decrease the release of neurotransmitter from both large- and small-diameter afferents in the spinal cord and trigeminal nucleus. The GABA$_B$ agonist *baclofen* is used to treat spasticity (presumably due in part to lack of presynaptic inhibition of the primary spindle afferents) and neuropathic pain.

Acetylcholine

Alzheimer's disease is a degenerative disorder of the brain that causes dementia. It is associated with loss of the cholinergic neurons that innervate the cerebral cortex. Impairment of cholinergic transmission may explain memory loss in this and other degenerative disorders. Central anticholinergic drugs are used to treat movement disorders due to dysfunction of basal ganglia circuits. Many drugs used to treat neurologic and psychiatric disorders may produce pharmacologic blockade of central muscarinic receptors. This may cause, particularly in elderly persons, confusional state or delirium, characterized by a disorder of alertness, attention, and perception (hallucinations). At the peripheral level, dysfunction of cholinergic mechanisms in skeletal muscle produces defects in neuromuscular transmission. Pharmacologic blockade of nicotinic receptors in the autonomic ganglia produces sympathetic and parasympathetic dysfunction. The blockade of muscarinic receptors abolishes parasympathetic secretomotor and visceral motor functions.

Dopamine

Parkinson's disease is a neurodegenerative disorder characterized by loss of dopaminergic neurons in the substantia nigra. Decreased dopaminergic activity in the striatum produces decreased motor activity, or *akinesia*.

Akinesia and other manifestations of Parkinson's disease may also result from the loss of dopaminergic neurons after exposure to toxins such as MPTP (1-methyl-4-phenyl-4-1,2,5,6-tetrahydropyridine) or from blockade of dopaminergic receptors in the striatum by antipsychotic or antiemetic drugs. Antiparkinsonian drugs include L-dopa (a precursor of dopamine) in combination with carbidopa (an inhibitor of peripheral decarboxylation of L-dopa) and direct dopamine receptor agonists. Products of dopamine oxidation have been implicated in toxic injury of dopaminergic neurons. A relative increase of dopaminergic activity in the striatum causes *hyperkinetic movement disorders* such as chorea.

Abnormal dopaminergic activity in limbic and prefrontal circuits may result in hallucinations. Antipsychotic drugs act via blockade of dopaminergic receptors. Their side effects include symptoms similar to those of Parkinson's disease, with the development of stereotypic movements, referred to as *tardive dyskinesia.*

Activity in the dopaminergic mesolimbic system is part of the basis of drug addiction. Dopaminergic neurons of the hypothalamus exert a tonic inhibitory control on prolactin release. Hypothalamic lesions or pharmacologic blockade that disrupts the inhibitory control causes *hyperprolactinemia.* Dopamine receptor agonists are used to treat prolactin-secreting pituitary tumors. *Neuroleptic malignant syndrome* is characterized by hyperthermia, muscle rigidity, and life-threatening autonomic hyperactivity and may be caused by blockade of dopamine receptors by neuroleptic agents or by the abrupt discontinuation of dopaminergic agonists.

Norepinephrine and Serotonin

Abnormal function of central noradrenergic and serotoninergic circuits has been implicated in disorders of arousal, attention, and affect, including anxiety and depression. Drugs that either increase α_2 receptors or block β receptors in the brain produce somnolence, depression, and hypotension. Drugs that decrease reuptake of norepinephrine or serotonin or that inhibit their metabolism are used to treat depression, panic disorder, narcolepsy, and chronic neurogenic pain. Migraine headache is treated with drugs that act via serotoninergic presynaptic receptors in the terminals of trigeminal nerve axons that synapse on blood vessels. They activate presynaptic $5-HT_{1D}$ receptors in trigeminal nerve terminals that innervate cerebral blood vessels and prevent release from the trigeminal terminals of neuropeptides implicated in the pain and vasodilatation that occur with migraine attacks. Many drugs frequently used to treat depression inhibit the presynaptic reuptake of serotonin. Antagonists of $5-HT_3$ receptors are potent antiemetics.

Neuropeptides

Hypothalamic disorders may produce abnormal secretion of circulating neuropeptides, for example, deficient or inappropriate secretion of vasopressin, or abnormal control of pituitary function, producing pituitary hyperfunction or hypofunction. Central stimulation of opioid receptors by morphine or similar drugs produces potent analgesia and marked autonomic, respiratory, endocrine, and behavioral effects. Degenerative diseases of the central nervous system may produce significant alterations in neuropeptide concentration in selected areas of the brain. For example, somatostatin is decreased in the cerebral cortex of patients with dementia but may be relatively increased in such degenerative diseases of the striatum as Huntington's disease.

Clinical Problems ◼

1. A 55-year-old man had cardiorespiratory arrest. After resuscitation, he remained comatose and the electroencephalogram showed persistent epileptiform activity.
   a. Where is the lesion?

b. What is the type of lesion?

c. What central neurochemical system is most likely to cause this type of neuronal injury?

d. What are the general mechanisms of injury?

e. What areas of the brain are most likely affected?

f. Name possible pharmacologic approaches for neural protection in this and similar cases.

2. A 44-year-old bartender with a history of alcohol abuse had been taking sleeping pills to control his anxiety and insomnia. Because of flu-like illness, with vomiting and diarrhea, he abruptly discontinued taking medication and drinking alcohol, and 24 hours later he had increased anxiety and generalized tremor. Two days later he had a generalized tonic-clonic seizure.

a. What is the location of the disorder?

b. What is the type of disorder?

c. What neurochemical system most likely is affected by alcohol and sedative agents?

d. What is the mechanism involved that explains the patient's symptoms?

3. A 65-year-old man with a 1-year history of memory loss was given a drug for treatment of depression and sleep disturbance. After the dose of medication was increased, there was a relatively rapid onset of disorientation, agitated behavior, and visual hallucinations. On physical examination, dry hot skin, dry mouth, tachycardia, and pupil dilatation were noted. Computed tomography of the head and cerebrospinal fluid examination did not reveal any abnormality. Generalized slowing was found on electroencephalography.

a. Involvement of what area of the brain explains the memory loss?

b. What type of lesion accounts for the memory loss?

c. Dysfunction of what neurochemical system most likely is responsible for the development of the abrupt change in mental status?

d. In the absence of acute confusional state, what effects would this drug have on memory and other cognitive functions of the patient?

4. A 55-year-old woman in a psychiatric ward received a drug for treatment of her bizarre behavior and auditory hallucinations. After the treatment was initiated, she had decreased facial expression and an absence of arm swing while walking. After 6 months of treatment, stereotyped, repetitive involuntary movements of the tongue, mouth, and face developed. Findings on neurologic examination were otherwise normal except for minimal piano playing–like movements of the fingers. The abnormal movements increased with attempts to discontinue treatment with the drug, and they abated temporarily with an increase in dosage. Results of computed tomography of the head, electroencephalography, and cerebrospinal fluid examination were unremarkable. She had no family history of dementia or movement disorders.

a. Involvement of what area of the brain explains the underlying psychiatric disorder?

b. What type of lesion is responsible for the movement disorder?

c. What neurochemical system most likely is involved in this patient?

d. What is the mechanism of the initial effects of the drug?

e. What is the probable mechanism of the stereotypic movements of the face and tongue?

f. What is a potentially dangerous consequence of iatrogenically induced dysfunction of this system?

5. A 25-year-old woman with a history of chronic pain was comatose when examined in the emergency room. Her boyfriend stated that she had been going to different doctors to have her prescription for pain killers refilled and had become increasingly depressed. On physical examination, she was unresponsive to noxious stimuli, had shallow respirations, slow pulse, and

low blood pressure. Her pupils were markedly constricted but reactive to light.

a. Where is the lesion?

b. What is the type of lesion?

c. What neurochemical system most likely is involved in this patient?

d. What type of drug should be used to treat the coma of this patient?

Additional Reading   ▪

Bliss, T. V., and Collingridge, G. L. A synaptic model of memory: Long-term potentiation in the hippocampus. *Nature* 361:31, 1993.

Cooper, J. R., Bloom, F. E., and Roth, R. H. *The Biochemical Basis of Neuropharmacology* (7th ed.). New York: Oxford University Press, 1996.

Kalkman, H. O., and Fozard, J. R. 5HT receptor types and their role in disease. *Curr. Opin. Neurol. Neurosurg.* 4: 560, 1991.

Koob, G. F. Drugs of abuse: Anatomy, pharmacology and function of reward pathways. *Trends Pharmacol. Sci.* 13: 177, 1992.

McGeer, E. G. Excitatory amino acid neurotransmission and its disorders. *Curr. Opin. Neurol. Neurosurg.* 4:548, 1991.

Nakanishi, S. Molecular diversity of glutamate receptors and implications for brain function. *Science* 258:597, 1992.

Schimerlik, M. I. Structure and function of muscarinic receptors. *Prog. Brain Res.* 84:11, 1990.

Weiner, N., and Molinoff, P. B. Catecholamines. In Siegel, G. J., Agranoff, B. W., Albers, R. W., and Molinoff, P. B. (eds.), *Basic Neurochemistry: Molecular, Cellular, and Medical Aspects* (5th ed.). New York: Raven Press, 1994, pp. 261–281.

THREE

HORIZONTAL LEVELS

The Peripheral Level

Objectives

1. Name the four major systems represented at the peripheral level, and describe the location, histologic features, and function of each.
2. Name the four subdivisions of the peripheral level at which lesions occur, and describe their gross anatomical location and histologic features.
3. List the neurologic deficits that would be associated with damage in each of these subdivisions of the peripheral level, and explain their mechanism of occurrence.
4. Describe the mechanism of muscle contraction.
5. Name the location of, function of, and deficit (motor, sensory, and reflex) resulting from a lesion of each of the following: spinal nerves C-5, C-6, C-7, C-8, L-4, L-5, and S-1; brachial and lumbosacral plexuses; and radial, ulnar, median, sciatic, femoral, peroneal, and tibial peripheral nerves.
6. Describe the main clinical features that distinguish large fiber neuropathies from small fiber neuropathies.
7. Describe the main electromyographic characteristics of axonal neuropathy, demyelinating neuropathy, neuromuscular transmission defect, and myopathy.
8. Describe the main clinical, electrophysiologic, laboratory, and biopsy findings that distinguish a typical neuropathy from myopathy.

Introduction

Precise anatomical localization is one of the major goals of neurologic diagnosis. The study of the major longitudinal systems and the manifestations of diseases within each system permit localization of a lesion in one or more systems. In the remaining chapters, the patterns of disease at each of the four major levels are presented. The combination of signs and symptoms resulting from damage to the systems at each major level often allows highly specific localization of the underlying disorder.

The *peripheral* level includes all neuromuscular structures outside the skull and spinal column, including peripheral nerves, sensory receptors, muscles, and the portions of cranial nerves lying outside the cranium. The anatomy, physiology, pathophysiology, and clinical disorders of these structures, which have many common characteristics, are considered in this chapter.

Overview

The peripheral level contains four of the longitudinal systems: motor, sensory, internal regulation, and vascular systems. The peripheral axon of the lower motor neuron, the neuromuscular junction, and the muscle fibers of the motor unit are found at the peripheral level. The distal axon of the primary sensory neuron and the sensory receptors are peripheral. The distal axon of the autonomic preganglionic neuron, the entire postganglionic efferent neuron, and the visceral afferent axons are peripheral. The cell bodies of motor neurons, second-order sensory neurons, and preganglionic autonomic neurons and the central processes of dorsal root ganglion cells are located in the spinal cord or brainstem. The axons of the systems travel together in the periphery, and peripheral lesions typically produce combinations of symptoms and signs from all three of the neural systems. Blood vessels of the vascular system supply all these structures.

Diseases in the periphery may be focal (for example, involving a single nerve) or diffuse (involving all peripheral nerves). A focal lesion may be a mass or a nonmass lesion. Diffuse lesions often involve only one type of structure in the periphery, as in primary disease of muscle. The temporal profile of peripheral diseases may be transient or may be that of one of the major disease types—inflammatory, neoplastic, degenerative-metabolic, vascular, or traumatic.

On the basis of gross anatomical features, the periphery can be divided into nerves and end-organs. Diseases of these subdivisions have different clinical manifestations.

Nerves

Peripheral and Cranial Nerves

These are the gross structures carrying motor, sensory, and visceral axons to the end-organs. (Some nerves contain only internal regulation fibers, for example, the vagus nerve.)

Plexus

A plexus is a complex network of axons traveling peripherally and centrally from the spinal nerves at the spinal level to the peripheral nerves.

End-Organs

Sensory Receptors

The somatic receptors for the sensations of pain, touch, position, vibration, and muscle

proprioception have been considered in detail in the chapters on sensory and motor systems and will not be discussed further. The special sensory receptors of the cranial nerves are considered in Chapters 15 and 16.

Somatic Motor Effectors

Movement is produced by muscle. Within the muscles are the neuromuscular junctions, the muscle fibers, and the contractile elements. Tendons, bones, and joints play an integral part in movement but are not considered further in this text.

Autonomic Receptors and Effectors

The widespread and diverse group of visceral structures was considered in Chapter 9. Although diseases of these structures are common in general medical practice, they will not be discussed further because they are more properly studied with other organ systems.

Nerve   ■

The major peripheral structures are nerves and muscles. Nerves are a collection of nerve fibers called *axons,* which are bound together by connective tissue. At the peripheral level, nerves form the plexuses and peripheral nerves; at the spinal level, they form the nerve roots entering or leaving the spinal cord and the spinal nerves leaving the spinal column. Nerves, whether peripheral or spinal, are made up of the axons traveling between the central nervous system and the peripheral end-organ. They are similar in their microscopic features, their physiology, and their pathophysiologic alterations with disease. The general features that are common to all types of nerves are considered first and the differences considered subsequently.

Histology

A nerve is composed of thousands of axons ranging in size from less than 1 to 20 μm in diameter. In each nerve trunk, individual fibers are surrounded by a connective tissue sheath, the *endoneurium*. Each of these is grouped with many other axons into bundles of fascicles by the *perineurium*. Groups of fascicles are bound together by an outer covering of connective tissue, the *epineurium* (Fig. 1). Nerves have their own blood supply. The nutrient arteries enter at intervals along their length and form anastomotic channels within the connective tissue framework of the nerve. These anastomoses make nerves relatively resistant to vascular disease.

Nerves are made up of afferent and efferent fibers. The axons can be differentiated histologically on the basis of their size and the presence or absence of myelin. The unmyelinated fibers are small and include autonomic fibers and fibers carrying pain and temperature. Proprioceptive and somatic motor fibers are large (Table 1). However, these characteristics do not permit the identification of the function of an individual axon, because the afferent (carrying information centrally) axons and the efferent (carrying information peripherally) axons have a similar microscopic appearance.

Each nerve fiber consists of an axon embedded in a series of Schwann cells arranged longitudinally along the axon. Each Schwann cell covers 0.5 to 1.0 mm of axon. The junctions between Schwann cells along the axon are seen as constrictions of the nerve fiber and are called the *nodes of Ranvier* (Figs. 1 and 2). A single Schwann cell surrounds either a number of unmyelinated axons or one myelinated axon. During development, either many unmyelinated axons become embedded in the Schwann cell or the Schwann cell wraps around one axon in concentric circles to form the myelin of the myelinated nerve fiber (Fig. 3). Although the fibers in a nerve are adjacent to one another, the electrical activity in each nerve fiber is independent of the activity in all the other fibers in the nerve. The action potentials are isolated from each other by the endoneurium and the myelin.

As the Schwann cell encircles an axon, layers of plasma membrane fuse to form myelin (Fig. 4). *Myelin* is thus a series of concentric layers of lipids and proteins. The lipids include cerebrosides, sulfatides, proteolipids, sphingomyelin, inositol phosphatides, phos-

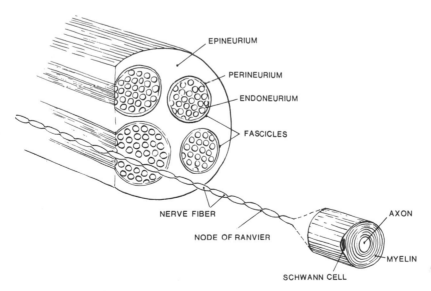

FIG. 1. Histologic features of a peripheral nerve. A nerve is subdivided into fascicles by the perineurium, with multiple motor and sensory nerve fibers intermingled in each fascicle.

TABLE 1. *Nerve fiber types*

Type	Diameter (μm)	Conduction velocity (m/s)	Function
Muscle nerve afferents			
Ia	12–20	70–120	Afferents from muscle spindle (primary endings—annulospiral)
Ib	12–20	70–120	Afferents from Golgi tendon organs
II	6–12	30–70	Afferents from muscle spindle (secondary endings—flower spray)
III	2–6	4–30	Pressure-pain afferents
IV	<2	0.5–2.0	Pain afferents
Cutaneous nerve afferents			
Aα	12–20	70–120	Joint receptor afferents
Aα	6–12	30–70	Paccinian corpuscle and touch receptor afferents
Aδ	2–6	4–30	Touch, temperature, and pain afferents
C	<2	0.5–2.0	Pain, temperature, and some mechanoreceptors
Visceral nerve afferents			
A	2–12	4–70	Internal regulation receptors
C	<2	0.2–2.0	
Efferents			
Alpha	12–20	70–120	Extrafusal skeletal muscle innervation from alpha motor neurons
Gamma	2–8	10–50	Intrafusal muscle spindle innervation from gamma motor neurons
B	<3	3–30	Preganglionic autonomic efferents
C	<1	0.5–2.0	Postganglionic autonomic efferents

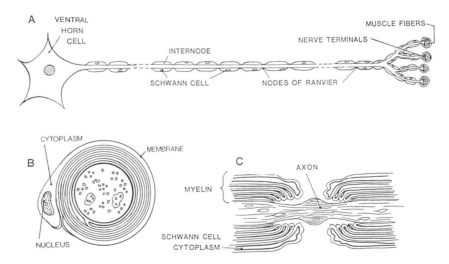

FIG. 2. Histologic features of a myelinated motor nerve fiber. **A:** Single myelinated axon extends from a ventral horn cell to nerve terminals on muscle fibers. **B:** Cross section through an internode of a nerve fiber, with layers of myelin formed by Schwann cell membrane wrapped around it. **C:** Longitudinal section of a node of Ranvier, with Schwann cell and myelin terminations abutting around continuous central axon.

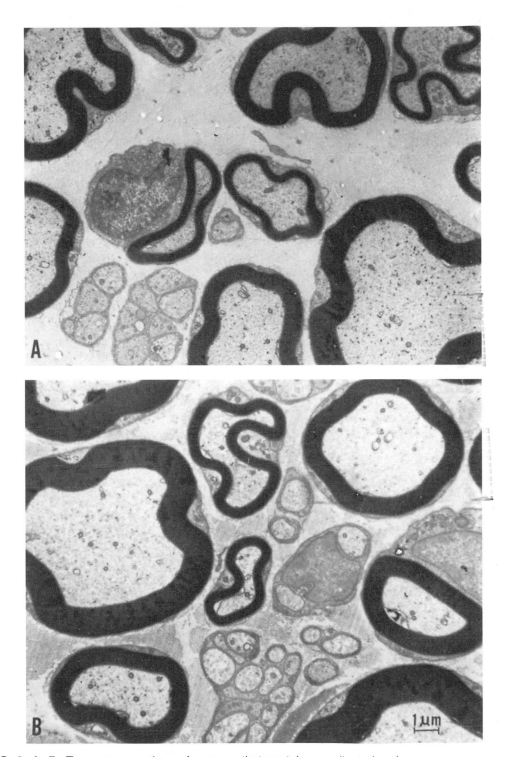

FIG. 3. A, B: Transverse sections of a nerve that contains myelinated and un-myelinated axons of various sizes. (×8,500.) (From Sugimura, K., Windebank, A. J., Natarajan, V., Lambert, E. H., Schmid, H. H. O., and Dyck, P. J. Interstitial hyperosmolarity may cause axis cylinder shrinkage in streptozotocin diabetic nerve. *J. Neuropathol. Exp. Neurol.* 39:710, 1980. With permission.)

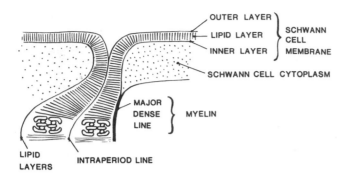

FIG. 4. Formation of myelin from layers of Schwann cell membrane. Major dense lines are formed from protein layers of membrane and are separated by the lipid layer, which contains cholesterol, cerebroside, sphingomyelin, and phospholipids.

phatidylserine, glycolipids, glycoproteins, and cholesterol.

Myelin contains specific proteins expressed in myelin-forming Schwann cells (or in oligodendrocytes in the central nervous system). These proteins are adhesion molecules involved in the processes of wrapping and *compaction* of the myelin sheath. Myelin proteins in the peripheral nervous system include *protein zero* (P_0) and *peripheral myelin protein 22* (PMP-22). The gap junction protein *connexin* is expressed in Schwann cells and is also critical for myelination. Mutations in the genes encoding for myelin proteins produce several types of *hereditary sensory and motor neuropathies.*

Although myelin is relatively inert metabolically, it has a significant turnover and responds to various disease states. For instance, myelin may be lost (demyelination) in certain immunologic disorders. When myelin is lost along a peripheral nerve, it is usually lost in the region of a single Schwann cell, which extends from one node of Ranvier to another. This loss is called *segmental demyelination* and alters the function of a nerve fiber.

Myelin also may be formed abnormally or may accumulate myelin metabolites in abnormal quantities. This condition occurs in genetic disorders due to enzyme defects, such as *metachromatic leukodystrophy* in which a deficit of arylsulfatase A results in the accumulation of metachromatic sulfatides in nerve fibers and loss of function in myelinated axons.

The axons of all nerve fibers consist of the axon membrane, or *axolemma,* and the axoplasm. The axoplasm contains mitochondria, microtubules, microfilaments, and neurofilaments. The *mitochondria* mediate the generation of energy needed to establish the concentration gradients across the axolemma. The *microtubules* participate in the transport of proteins, enzymes, and other materials down the axon from the cell body to the periphery. The function of the neurofilaments and microfilaments is related to axonal transport and axon growth.

Axonal Transport

The continuous and regulated flow of material from the cell body to the axons and synaptic terminals (and in the reverse direction) is critical for neuronal function and survival. Transport of substances along axons is not random but directed by the microtubules, which give polarity to the transport. Axonal transport includes *anterograde* transport, which allows the constant flow of material synthesized in the cell bodies and dendrites to reach the axon terminals, and *retrograde* transport, which is the transport of material from axon terminals to the cell body. Retrograde transport is a mechanism for the cell body to sample the environment around the synaptic terminals of its axons. *Fast axonal anterograde transport* occurs at a rate of 200 to 400 mm/day and is involved in the movement of proteins associated with membrane vesicles. These include glycosylated proteins that are delivered preferentially to synaptic terminals (for example, synaptic vesicles, receptors, ion channels, neuropeptides, and enzymes for neurotransmitter biosynthesis). *Slow anterograde axonal transport* occurs at a rate of 0.1 to 4 mm/day and is involved in the movement of *cytoskeletal* proteins (for example, tubulin, actin, and neurofilament proteins). *Retrograde transport* occurs at a rate of 100 to 200 mm/day and is an exaggerated manifestation of the process of endocytosis. It is involved with the incorporation and recycling of lysosomes, pinocytotic vesicles, synaptic vesicle proteins, and neurotrophic factors. Retrograde transport is the mechanism by which some viruses (for example, rabies and herpes simplex) and toxins (for example, tetanus and botulinum toxins) enter the nervous system.

Organic solvents (used in industry for cleaning, extraction, laboratory work, paint, printing ink), pesticides, and some antineoplastic drugs can produce axonal neuropathy by disrupting the normal mechanisms of axonal transport and cytoskeletal assembly. Overexposure to these toxic chemicals produces a distal symmetrical sensorimotor axonal neuropathy that affects large-diameter sensory and motor axons in peripheral nerves and, in severe cases, long tracts in the spinal cord.

Physiology

The resting potential and action potentials in single axons are described in detail in Chapter 5. In this chapter, we focus on the physiology of whole nerve trunks. The function of the axons is to carry information in the form of electrical activity from one area to another. A measure of the ability of a nerve to perform this function would be of major clinical value in the identification of disease involving a nerve. However, during normal function, the electrical activities of the fibers in a nerve are asynchronous and cancel each other out.

The action potential of a single axon can be recorded experimentally with an intracellular microelectrode, which records the action potential as a monophasic wave of depolariza-tion. The electrical activity in a single nerve fiber also can be monitored by placing electrodes in the extracellular fluid close to the nerve fiber. This method does not detect transmembrane potential changes; rather, it senses potential changes in the extracellular fluid that result from longitudinal current flow between the depolarized and nondepolarized regions of the axon. The extracellular recording is improved (a bigger voltage change is measured) if the extracellular resistance is artificially increased by recording from the nerve experimentally in air or in oil.

Extracellular recording from single axons is difficult because of their small size; however, it is possible to record from groups of axons or from whole nerve trunks, if all axons discharge synchronously. This recording is obtained experimentally and from patients by applying an electrical shock that activates all axons simultaneously. The potential recorded from a nerve activated in this way is the *compound action potential.* The configuration of the signal obtained from an extracellular recording of the nerve impulse depends on the electrode arrangement. A monophasic potential change is observed from nerve fibers conducting an impulse if only one of the electrodes is placed over an active nerve. A biphasic potential is recorded if both electrodes are placed over the active nerve (Fig. 5).

As in the stimulation of a single axon, the whole nerve trunk is activated by passing a current between the cathode (negative pole) and the anode (positive pole). The cathode depolarizes the underlying axons, and the anode hyperpolarizes them. Depolarization requires current flow inside the axons. Because large axons have lower internal resistance, the threshold for activation is lowest for the larger fibers. The *threshold stimulus* for a nerve trunk is that which just excites the large fibers. Supramaximal stimuli activate all fibers, including the small fibers, and require greater current flow. Excitability, therefore, depends on axon size.

The *excitability* of a nerve can be defined in terms of the two variables of a stimulus:

A

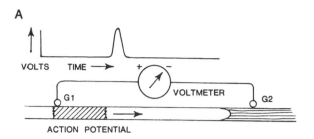

B

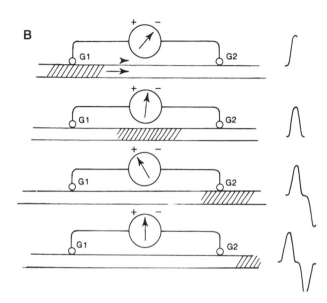

FIG. 5. Recording action potentials from a nerve trunk with electrodes (G1 and G2). **A:** With G2 over damaged nerve and G1 over active nerve, a monophasic action potential is recorded as depolarization passes under G1. **B:** If both electrodes are over active nerve fibers, potentials of opposite polarity are recorded as depolarization passes under G1 and G2, a biphasic action potential. When G1 and G2 are close together, the two potentials fuse to form a smooth biphasic response.

voltage and duration. If the strength of the current (or voltage) is plotted against the duration of a stimulus needed to produce excitation of a nerve, a curve is obtained, which is called a *strength-duration curve*. A shift in the strength-duration curve indicates a change in excitability and is seen in nerve diseases. The strength-duration curve is often characterized in terms of two points. The *rheobase* is the minimal voltage needed to produce excitation with a long stimulus duration (usually 300 milliseconds) and the *chronaxie* is the time required to excite a nerve by a stimulus with a voltage twice as large as the rheobase (Fig. 6).

The compound action potential recorded from a nerve trunk after supramaximal stimulation is the summation of action potentials from many axons. Its amplitude can be graded by varying the strength of the stimulus. A threshold stimulation evokes only a small potential resulting from activity in a few large fibers. As the stimulus strength is increased, more fibers are excited, and their activity is added to the compound action potential as each additionally activated fiber produces a small increment in the recorded voltage. When all the fibers are excited, the amplitude of the compound action potential is maximum; it will not increase in amplitude with further increases in the stimulus strength (supramaximal). The compound action potential thus can be graded in amplitude, while action potentials in single axons are not graded but fire in an all-or-nothing fashion.

Variation in axon diameter in a nerve trunk results in different conduction velocities as well as different thresholds for activation. The rate at which an axon conducts is a function of

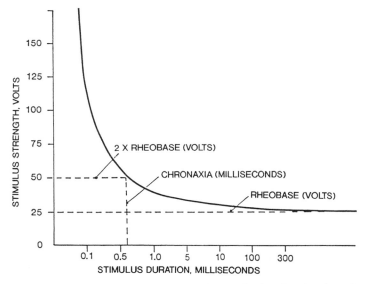

FIG. 6. Strength-duration curve. Threshold voltage for each duration is plotted. Rheobase is 25 V, and chronaxie is 0.6 millisecond.

the amount of longitudinal current flow and is greater with larger axons. The *conduction velocity* is calculated by dividing the distance a potential travels by the time it takes to travel that distance. It is approximately five times the axon's diameter in microns—for example, 5 to 100 meters per second for axons of 1 to 20 μm in diameter. If a nerve trunk is stimulated at a distance from the recording electrodes, the compound action potential exhibits several components (Fig. 7) because of the dispersion of the potentials from fibers of different diameters. The impulses in the large fibers reach the recording site first. The components of the compound action potential thus distinguish activity in groups of fibers whose diameters are within certain size ranges. The afferent fibers in cutaneous nerves (to joints and skin) are subdivided into groups named by letters (Aα, Aδ, and C). The afferent fibers in muscle nerves (nerves to muscle) are subdivided into groups designated by Roman numerals (I, II, III, IV). These are listed in Table 1.

Nerves that innervate muscle contain both sensory and motor fibers. The motor fibers arise from the alpha and gamma motor neurons and innervate the extrafusal and intrafusal muscle fibers. The sensory fibers are the group Ia and II fibers from muscle spindles and the group Ib fibers from Golgi tendon organs. Cutaneous nerves innervate joints and skin and are commonly considered sensory nerves, although both they and the muscle nerves contain efferent and afferent fibers of the internal regulation system, the "C" or group IV fibers. Table 2 lists by size the components of a mixed nerve.

In addition to transmitting action potentials, axons move proteins along their length. This process of axonal transport is important for making available the enzymes needed for the production of neurotransmitter in the nerve terminal, for maintaining the integrity of the distal parts of the axon, and for the release of trophic factors from the nerve terminal. *Trophic factors* are released from nerve terminals and are necessary for the normal function of the postsynaptic cell. Loss of these trophic factors occurs in some nerve diseases and results in physiologic and histologic abnormalities of the postsynaptic cell.

Pathophysiology

A nerve may be altered in several ways by disease processes. These can be classified as

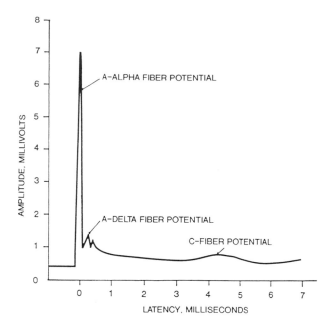

FIG. 7. Compound action potential recorded directly from a cutaneous nerve, showing peaks generated by different fiber types.

diseases of the axolemma, the axoplasm, or the myelin sheath.

Axolemmal Disorders

The axon membrane may undergo physicochemical alterations that block conduction without destruction or histologic alteration of the axon. Such alterations may occur by electrical, pharmacologic, thermal, or mechanical means. The alterations are usually transient and reversible and include the familiar phenomenon of a leg "going to sleep."

Electrical conduction blocks do not occur clinically but can be obtained by the application of steady depolarizing (cathodal block) or hyperpolarizing (anodal block) currents to a nerve fiber or nerve trunk. A depolarizing current may initially evoke an action potential and then block impulse transmission. An anodal block results from a hyperpolarization of the axon membrane, which moves the membrane potential away from threshold.

A clinically useful method of producing conduction block is the application of pharmacologic agents (local anesthetics) to a nerve. These include compounds such as procaine hydrochloride (Novocain), benzocaine, cocaine, and other esters of benzoic acid. Local anesthetics interfere with nerve conduction by preventing the membrane permeability changes that occur with depolarization (Table 3). The membrane is said to be "stabilized" by local anesthetics. Small, unmyelinated nerve fibers, such as those mediating pain, are more sensitive to local anesthetics than are the larger myelinated fibers and are blocked at low concentrations of the drug that do not appreciably affect large fibers.

A transient, reversible conduction block can be obtained by lowering the temperature of nerve fibers. This method of blocking nerve impulse transmission is accomplished

TABLE 2. *Fiber types in a mixed nerve*

Diameter (μm)	Conduction velocity (m/s)	Type
12–20	70–120	Ia, Ib, Aα, alpha efferent
6–12	30–70	II, Aα, gamma efferent, visceral afferent
2–6	4–30	III, Aδ, gamma efferent, visceral afferent
<2	0.5–2.0	IV, B, C

TABLE 3. *Sequence of events of local anesthetic block*

Displacement of calcium ions from nerve receptor site
↓
Binding of local anesthetic to receptor site
↓
Blockade of sodium channel
↓
Decrease in sodium conductance
↓
Decreased depolarization of nerve membrane
↓
Failure to achieve threshold potential level
↓
Lack of development of propagated action potential
↓
Conduction blockade

by the local application of ice or an ethyl chloride spray and is used clinically to produce superficial anesthesia. Mechanical conduction blocks occur with distortion of a nerve and may be due to alteration of the blood supply or to changes in the configuration of the membrane, with secondary changes in its ionic permeability.

Axoplasmic Disorders

Axons may be affected by acute or chronic disorders of the axoplasm. An acute lesion is one in which the axon is disrupted. This may occur with complete division of the nerve in a laceration or with a severe local crush, traction, or ischemia. In laceration, the connective tissue framework is destroyed; in the other lesions, it remains intact. In each instance, the continuity of the axons is lost, the distal axon is deprived of axonal flow from the neuron, and it undergoes dissolution in a process called wallerian degeneration. Central chromatolysis and peripheral muscle atrophy accompany *wallerian degeneration* (Fig. 8). In most lesions other than laceration, not all axons are destroyed and some function may remain. The smaller fibers are more resistant to such injuries and are more likely to be spared. After acute axonal disruption, recovery occurs only through the growth of new axons.

If a nerve is completely severed, reinnervation is poor because the axonal sprouts have no pathway to follow. Axonal sprouts may

grow in the wrong direction and produce spirals or large bulbous tips. These sprouts, with their Schwann cells and connective tissue, may form a *neuroma*. The neuroma may not only prevent proper regrowth of the nerve but may also be painful.

The activity of Schwann cells in the distal nerve stump provides an aid to reinnervation across a gap, as they divide, elongate, and migrate toward the proximal nerve stump. If axonal sprouts manage to reach this Schwann cell outgrowth, they may eventually reinnervate the denervated organs. However, the amount of functional recovery is always less than that seen in a crush injury. One reason for this is that most axonal sprouts do not find their way along the pathway followed originally by their parent fibers and reinnervate an inappropriate organ. A motor axon that establishes a connection with a sensory receptor organ will not function, and a motor axon that reinnervates a muscle different from the one it originally supplied cannot take part in the same reflex actions. *Synkinesis* is the result of such aberrant reinnervation, in which attempts to activate one group of muscles produce concomitant contraction in other muscles innervated by that nerve. The patient can no longer selectively activate a muscle. In injuries to long nerves, the end-organs may atrophy before reinnervation can occur, thus preventing normal recovery.

The rate of nerve regeneration varies with the type of injury. Recovery is quicker with crush injuries than with nerve severance. The delay in recovery depends on axonal growth, reversal of atrophy of the end-organ, reinnervation of the end-organ, and remyelinization and maturation of the axon. In humans, the overall rate of functional recovery under optimal conditions is about 1 to 3 mm per day. The recovery rate in a limb may be quicker proximally than distally.

Axoplasmic disorders may be chronic or slow in evolution and present with different findings than do acute lesions. When the process is complete, the axons degenerate just as they do in acute lesions; however, there are intermediate stages in which the axons first

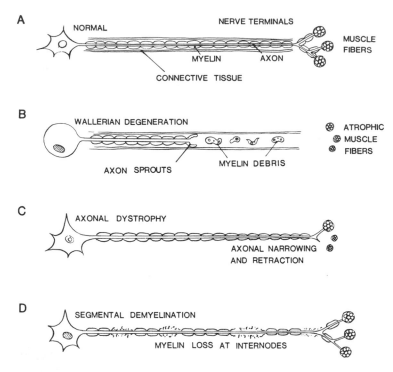

FIG. 8. Pathologic changes in peripheral nerve fibers. **A:** Normal axon. **B:** Wallerian degeneration occurs distal to local destruction of an axon and is associated with central chromatolysis and muscle fiber atrophy. Regeneration occurs along the connective tissue path. **C:** Axonal dystrophy results in distal narrowing and dying back of nerve terminals due to either intrinsic axon or motor neuron disease. **D:** Segmental demyelination destroys myelin at scattered internodes along the axon without axonal damage.

lose their integrity distally, a so-called *dying back*. This occurs first in the longest axons and results in loss of function in the most distal parts of the body. The axons also may atrophy or become narrowed in chronic disorders, referred to as axonal *atrophies* or axonal *dystrophies* (Fig. 8). In either situation, there are abnormalities of the axon before there are changes in the myelin. Therefore, unless major narrowing of an axon is present, the conduction of the axons is slowed very little. Chronic axonal disorders occur with many diseases, including genetic, toxic, and metabolic, and deficiency states.

The narrow axons seen in some axoplasmic disorders also occur with local compression of a nerve and in regenerating fibers. Moderate narrowing of an axon results in slowing of conduction velocity, but by itself it usually causes little functional impairment. A nerve with slowed conduction velocity can still transmit impulses, though not at as high rates as normal. High-frequency impulses, such as rapid vibrations, the output from muscle spindles, and motor activity in strong muscle contraction, are poorly transmitted so that vibratory sensation and reflexes are lost.

Myelin Disorders

Genetic, immunologic, and toxic disorders can produce primary damage to myelin. In these disorders, myelin is usually lost at internodes, with normal myelin remaining at other internodes. This scattered loss of myelin is *segmental demyelination* (Fig. 8). The loss of myelin results in slowing of conduction velocity, with mild impairment of vibratory sensation, loss of reflexes, some loss of proprioceptive sensation, and loss of strong muscle contractions. However, with moderate demyelination, the action potential is blocked, producing more severe deficits. Genetic disorders can be associated with a lack of myelin (hypomyelination) or abnormal myelin and can result in functional disturbances similar to those seen with segmental demyelination.

In each of these disorders, there may be varied severity of damage and selective involvement of one or another fiber type. In localized lesions, there is loss of function in the areas supplied by the nerve. In generalized nerve disease, the axons are affected randomly throughout the cross section of a nerve and randomly along the length of the nerve, so that the most likely areas to lose function are the distal regions supplied by the longest nerves. This produces a characteristic distribution of *abnormalities in the distal portions* of the extremities. This distal deficit also occurs in primary neuronal disease in which the neuron is unable to provide sufficient nutrients to the most distal portion of the nerve, with a resultant dying back of the distal portions of the long nerves.

Summary

Because the function of peripheral nerves is to conduct action potentials from one area to another, three general kinds of functional abnormality occur:

1. The excitability of axons may be increased with spontaneous or excessive firing of an axon. This occurs in many disorders, but especially in ischemic or metabolic diseases.
2. The axon may be unable to conduct an action potential, because of either transient metabolic changes or structural damage to the axon. If an axon is severed, the distal portion undergoes wallerian degeneration but is able to conduct an impulse in the distal part of the nerve for 3 to 5 days. The proximal portion of the axon continues to function normally.
3. The axon may conduct an impulse slowly or at low rates of firing. This may occur from loss of myelin or be due to narrowing and deformation of the axon. The latter may be seen in the area of compression or in regenerating fibers. Slow conduction results in mild clinical symptoms or signs except for the ability to carry high-frequency information such as vibration, which is severely impaired.

The physiologic alterations seen with diseases of the nerves are associated with two clinically important manifestations. The threshold for activation of some portion of lower motor neurons may be low, and they may discharge spontaneously. If this occurs, all the muscle fibers in the motor unit will contract simultaneously. Such a single, spontaneous contraction of a motor unit is visible as a small twitch under the skin called a *fasciculation*. It is evidence of irritability of the motor unit and occurs in normal persons and in many disorders. Similar irritability in sensory fibers is perceived as paresthesia (tingling) in large fibers or as pain in small fibers.

A second important manifestation is the result of the loss of trophic factors of the nerve acting on muscle. A denervated muscle atrophies and undergoes change in its membrane. This change includes a hypersensitivity to acetylcholine. Normally, most of the acetylcholine receptors are confined to the area immediately adjacent to the end plate. After denervation, the receptors spread along the surface, until the entire fiber responds to the drug. This is one form of denervation hypersensitivity (Table 4). Muscle fibers undergo

TABLE 4. *Examples of denervation hypersensitivity*

Site	Clinical finding	Due to destruction of	Hypersensitivity to
Striated muscle	Fibrillation	Alpha efferents	Acetylcholine
Ventral horn cell	Spasticity, clonus, hyperreflexia	Descending pathway	Local sensory input
Pupil	Miosis	Postganglionic sympathetic	Epinephrine analogues
Pupil	Mydriasis	Postganglionic parasympathetic	Acetylcholine analogues

denervation hypersensitivity and begin to discharge and twitch approximately 2 weeks after losing their innervation. Such spontaneous, regular twitching of single muscle fibers is called *fibrillation*.

Peripheral Nerves   ■

Anatomy

The peripheral nerves are the major nerve trunks in the extremities and are derived from the plexuses. They have the histologic and physiologic features described in the previous section. Each nerve has a well-defined anatomical course in an extremity, supplies a specific area of skin, and provides innervation for specific muscles (Fig. 9). The major peripheral nerves and their important areas of innervation are described in Table 5. More detailed distributions are shown in Fig. 10.

Clinical Correlations

The proximity of some nerves to bony structures makes them particularly vulnerable to lesions at those sites. The *median nerve* passes through a tunnel at the wrist (the carpal tunnel) where it is easily and often compressed, producing arm pain, sensory loss of the first three digits, and weakness of the thenar muscles—the carpal tunnel syndrome. The *ulnar nerve* is commonly compressed at the elbow, where it passes around the medial epicondyle in an exposed position (the "funny bone"). Lesions here produce sensory loss in the ring and fifth fingers, with flaccid weakness and atrophy of the intrinsic muscles of the hand. The *radial nerve* is particularly susceptible to injury where it curves around the humerus in the spiral groove in the mid-upper arm. Lesions at this site produce a weakness of wrist and finger extension. The *peroneal nerve* is in an exposed position over a bony prominence where it curves around the head of the fibula at the knee. Damage at this site produces footdrop and sensory loss of the dorsum of the foot. The deep, protected locations of the sciatic, tibial, and femoral nerves result in fewer injuries. These and all other lesions of the peripheral nerves can be recognized by an analysis of the distribution of the motor, sensory, and reflex changes. The type of lesion may be any of those previously described—with total, irreversible destruction due to wallerian degeneration or with mild, reversible changes due to membrane or myelin alterations. The use of nerve conduction studies to determine the location of slowing or block of conduction is of particular value in identifying the location and severity of such lesions.

Peripheral nerves also may be involved in *diffuse disease* of the myelin or axons. In either instance, the clinical features are similar. There is distal loss of sensation in the upper and lower extremities (more severe in the lower extremities), usually for all modalities, although in some disorders there may be selective involvement of certain fiber types and therefore of certain modalities of sensation. There may be paresthesia, dysesthesia, or hyperalgesia, usually in the same distribution. Reflexes are generally lost. Distal muscles are weak and flaccid and eventually atrophy. Atrophy of distal muscles produces deformities, for example, pes cavus and hammer toes (high arches with cocked-up toes) with loss of intrinsic foot muscles.

Some neuropathies have a predilection for large myelinated fibers involved in touch, proprioception, joint position sense, and reflexes. These large fiber neuropathies may be manifested by paresthesia; sensory ataxia (Romberg's sign); loss of tactile discrimination, joint position sense, and vibratory sensation; and areflexia. Important examples are neuropathies caused by vitamin B_{12} deficiency, immune or inflammatory demyelinating neuropathies, and paraneoplastic neuropathies. In other neuropathies, small myelinated or unmyelinated sensory and autonomic fibers are selectively affected. They are manifested by burning pain, lack of temperature and pain sensation, and autonomic manifestations including orthostatic hypotension, impaired sweating, and gastrointestinal, sex-

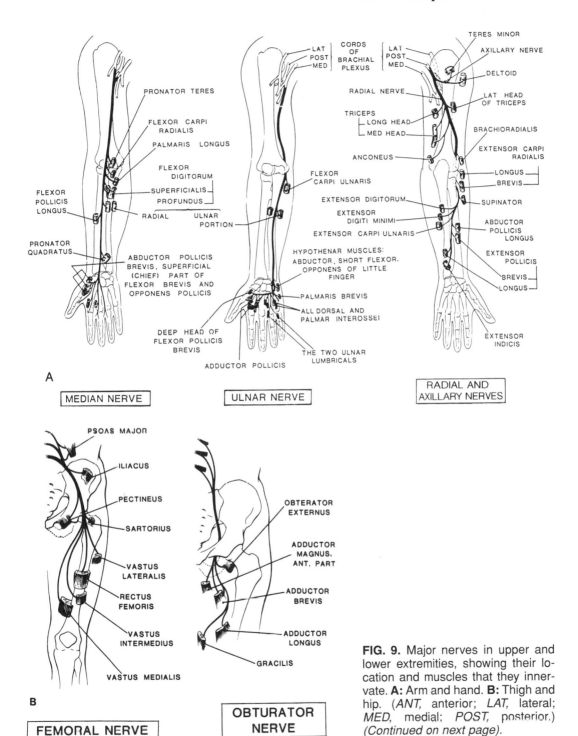

FIG. 9. Major nerves in upper and lower extremities, showing their location and muscles that they innervate. **A:** Arm and hand. **B:** Thigh and hip. (*ANT,* anterior; *LAT,* lateral; *MED,* medial; *POST,* posterior.) (*Continued on next page*).

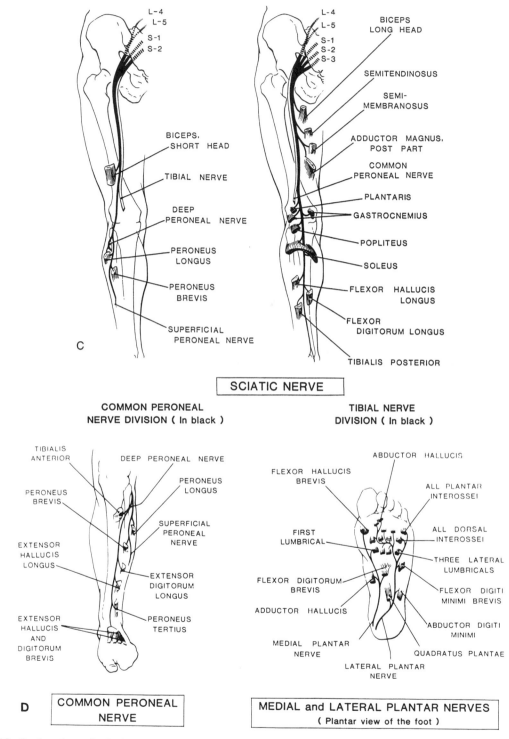

FIG. 9. *(continued):* **C:** Leg. **D:** Lower leg and foot. (*ANT,* anterior; *LAT,* lateral; *MED,* medial; *POST,* posterior.) (**A** *left* and *center,* **B–D** from Rosse, C., and Gaddum-Rosse, P., *Hollinshead's Textbook of Anatomy* [5th ed.]. Philadelphia: Lippincott-Raven, 1997. With permission. **A** *right* from Hollingshead, W. H., and Rosse, C., *Textbook of Anatomy* [4th ed.]. Philadelphia: Harper & Row, 1985.)

TABLE 5. *Peripheral nerve distributions*

Nerve	General innervation
Median	Sensory: Palmar surface of thumb and first three fingers Motor: Finger and wrist flexion
Ulnar	Sensory: Fourth and fifth fingers Motor: Intrinsic hand muscles
Radial	Sensory: Dorsum of the hand Motor: Forearm, wrist, and hand extension
Femoral	Sensory: Anterior aspect of thigh and medial part of leg Motor: Hip flexion and knee extension
Sciatic	Sensory: Posterior aspect of thigh and portion of leg below the knee Motor: Knee flexion and all ankle and foot motion
Peroneal	Sensory: Lateral aspect of leg and dorsum of foot Motor: Foot and toe dorsiflexion
Tibial	Sensory: Posterior part of leg and sole of foot Motor: Foot and toe plantar flexion

ual, or bladder dysfunction. Strength, reflexes, vibration and joint position sense, and electromyographic findings (see below) may be normal. An important example is a form of diabetic neuropathy. Most neuropathies affect both motor and sensory fibers and large and small fibers and exhibit a combination of clinical features.

Although many peripheral nerve diseases affect both axon and myelin, if the disease process primarily affects the axon, atrophy is more severe, with loss of innervation and prominent fibrillation in distal muscles. Disorders primarily producing myelin damage are associated with less atrophy, are more readily reversible, and have little or no fibrillation.

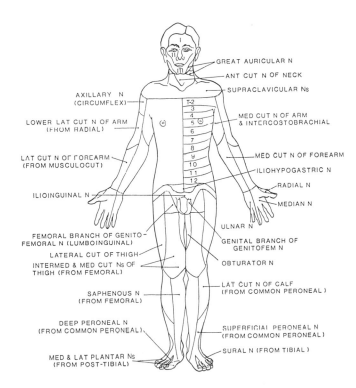

FIG. 10. Cutaneous distribution of peripheral nerves. (*ANT,* anterior; *CUT,* cutaneous; *INTERMED,* intermedial; *LAT,* lateral; *MED,* medial; *N,* nerve.) (Modified from Haymaker, W., and Woodhall, B., *Peripheral Nerve Injuries:* Principles of Diagnosis [2nd ed.]. Philadelphia: W. B. Saunders, 1953. With permission.)

Plexus   ■

Anatomy

A *plexus* is a complex recombination of axons as they rearrange themselves in passing from one area to another. There are three major somatic plexuses: the brachial, lumbar, and sacral (lumbosacral) plexuses. The *brachial plexus* is derived from spinal nerves C-5 through T-1 and gives rise to the major nerves of the upper extremity. The axons of the spinal nerves are rearranged into trunks, divisions, and cords of the plexus just beneath and behind the clavicle (Fig. 11).

The *lumbar plexus,* derived from L-2 through L-4 spinal nerves, and the *sacral*

plexus, derived from L-4 through S-3 spinal nerves, give rise to the major nerves of the lower extremity. The femoral and obturator nerves arise from the lumbar plexus, and the sciatic nerve arises from the sacral plexus. The rearrangements of the axons in the lumbosacral plexus occur in the pelvis, posteriorly, deep to the psoas major muscle (Fig. 11).

Clinical Correlations

Each of these plexuses may undergo the same physiologic or histologic alterations described previously. They are most commonly involved in trauma, tumor, or hemorrhage. The

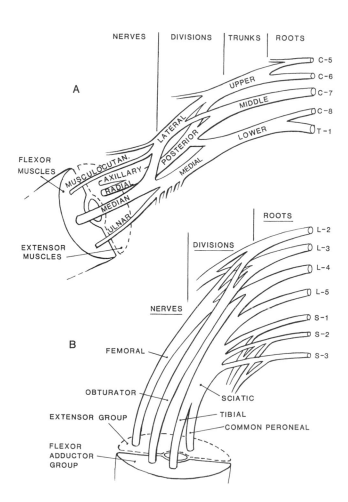

FIG. 11. Major components of plexuses. **A:** Brachial plexus, showing the origin of the three trunks, three cords, and peripheral nerves. **B:** Lumbosacral plexus divisions forming the nerves of the lower extremity. (*MUSCULOCUTAN,* musculocutaneous.)

diagnosis of disease in these regions depends on the presence of involvement of proximal muscles innervated by multiple roots, multiple dermatomal involvement, and sparing of the paraspinal muscles. The changes involve motor and sensory fibers and, when severe, result in autonomic disturbances such as loss of sweating, thinning of the skin, and trophic changes in the skin. Reflex loss also occurs.

Several major plexuses are purely visceral and are part of the internal regulation system. Although these plexuses may be involved in localized disease processes, this involvement is uncommon and not of clinical significance. The spinal nerves and nerve roots are within the spinal canal and are discussed in the next chapter.

The Neuromuscular Junction ■

The *neuromuscular junction* is the site at which the motor nerve terminal meets a muscle fiber and where the efferent nerve terminals evoke contraction of the muscle. This contraction is accomplished through the production of an excitatory synaptic potential called an *end-plate potential*. In a normal skeletal muscle fiber, the end-plate potential always reaches threshold for the production of an action potential, which then propagates along the muscle fiber. The action potential in turn triggers a contraction.

Histology

Each junction consists of a presynaptic portion derived from the nerve terminal and a postsynaptic portion derived from the muscle fiber. As an axon enters a muscle, it branches into many nerve terminals, each of which innervates one muscle fiber. As the terminal approaches the muscle fiber, the axon loses its myelin sheath and comes to lie in a depression in the muscle fiber. The nerve terminal is covered by a Schwann cell, but the inferior portion of the axolemma is directly apposed to the sarcolemma of the muscle fiber, with an

intervening synaptic cleft of 500 µm. The postsynaptic portion of the junction consists of complex folds of sarcolemma immediately beneath the nerve terminal (Fig. 12). This region can be demonstrated with histochemical techniques that stain acetylcholinesterase. The sarcolemma, with its folds, forms the subneural apparatus. The cytoplasm of the nerve terminal contains a concentration of mitochondria and many synaptic vesicles. Often, the synaptic vesicles seem to be clustered near a region of density of the presynaptic membrane. These specialized areas are located opposite the postsynaptic folds. Acetylcholine is bound to the vesicles in the nerve terminal.

There is a precise coordination between presynaptic and postsynaptic elements in the mature neuromuscular junction. Synaptic vesicles containing acetylcholine are clustered around the voltage-gated calcium chan-

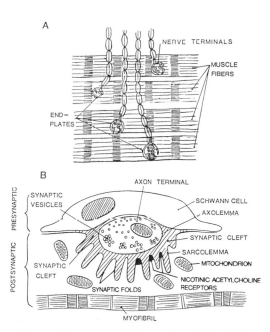

FIG. 12. Neuromuscular junction. **A:** End plates where single nerve terminals innervate single muscle fibers. **B:** Cross section of an end plate. Axon terminal lies in depression on muscle surface covered by Schwann cell. Postsynaptic sarcolemmal folds contain acetylcholine receptors. Acetylcholine is stored in synaptic vesicles in the nerve terminal.

nels in the *active zones.* The active zones are precisely apposed to the *postjunctional folds,* which contain the densely clustered nicotinic acetylcholine receptors. During development, the growth cone of a motor neuron induces a local clustering of nicotinic receptors in the muscle membrane, precisely at the site of acetylcholine release. This involves signals from the motor axon, including a protein called *agrin.* This protein, together with *dystroglycans* in the muscle basal membrane, interacts with a molecular complex related to the submembrane cytoskeleton, including a protein called *dystrophin.* This dystrophin-associated complex includes proteins that serve to anchor the nicotinic receptor at the level of the folds. Both survival of the motor neuron and stabilization of its synapses depend critically on the level of activity in the muscle.

Physiology

Small electrical potentials can be recorded from the region of the neuromuscular junction of skeletal muscle fibers, even in the absence of nerve impulses in the motor fibers. These potentials have all the electrical and pharmacologic properties of end-plate potentials, except that they are small and occur in a random fashion without the need of nerve activity. These have been called *miniature end-plate potentials.*

The miniature end-plate potentials are due to leakage of the neurotransmitter acetylcholine from the presynaptic terminals. The leakage occurs in "quanta" of transmitter; that is, the miniature end-plate potentials are produced by thousands of molecules of acetylcholine released together. The end-plate potential, in contrast, is produced by the near-synchronous release of many quanta triggered by the nerve impulse. The *synaptic vesicles* are the storage sites of quanta of acetylcholine.

When the resting potential of the motor axon terminal at a neuromuscular junction is reduced, the frequency of release of miniature end-plate potentials is increased. However, the relationship is not a linear one. There is a tenfold increase in frequency for every 15 mV of depolarization. The depolarization associated with an action potential in the motor axon terminal results in the release of a burst of several hundred acetylcholine quanta, thus accounting for the end-plate potential. The number of quanta (M) released by a presynaptic action potential can be calculated by dividing the average end-plate potential amplitude (EPP) by the average miniature end-plate potential amplitude (MEPP):

$$M = \frac{EPP}{MEPP}$$

Acetylcholine increases the permeability of the postsynaptic membrane to both sodium and potassium ions. The membrane potential is thus only partially depolarized; the synaptic currents do not flow long enough for the membrane to be depolarized to zero. Therefore, the end-plate potential is considerably smaller than the action potential; nevertheless, it is well above the threshold for generating a muscle fiber action potential. This is referred to as the *safety margin* of neuromuscular transmission. When the end-plate potential reaches threshold, it triggers the action potential of the muscle. The acetylcholine is rapidly broken down by the enzyme acetylcholinesterase after binding with the postsynaptic membrane and producing the end-plate potential.

Acetylcholine is synthesized by *choline acetyltransferase* from acetyl coenzyme A (CoA) and choline in the nerve terminal. It is stored in the vesicles and released by the action potential through calcium binding in the membrane. Acetylcholine diffuses across the synapse and binds with the cholinergic receptor until it is broken down by acetylcholinesterase. A summary of the events occurring at the neuromuscular junction is shown in Fig. 13.

Pharmacology

Many important drugs affect neuromuscular transmission. For instance, curare, the poison once used by some South American Indians on the tips of their blowgun arrows, prevents acetylcholine from reacting with the

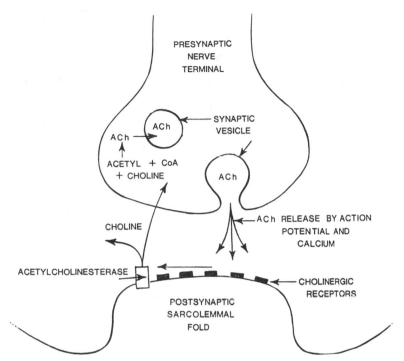

FIG. 13. Neurotransmitter action at the neuromuscular junction. Acetylcholine *(ACh)* is formed and stored in the nerve terminal. It is released by nerve terminal depolarization in the presence of calcium and binds with receptors on the postsynaptic membrane. After producing an ionic conductance charge, it is hydrolyzed by acetylcholinesterase. (*CoA,* coenzyme A.)

receptor sites of the muscle membrane by competitively binding with the sites and causes paralysis. In contrast to the effect of acetylcholine, the reaction between the curare molecule and the acetylcholine receptor molecule does not change conductance in the membrane. Curare thus blocks neuromuscular transmission.

Another substance that blocks neuromuscular transmission is botulin, the agent that causes botulism in food contaminated by *Clostridium botulinum.* Botulin blocks the release of acetylcholine from the motor nerve terminals, causes a loss of end-plate potentials, and results in paralysis.

Neuromuscular transmission is enhanced by drugs that block the action of acetylcholinesterase. In the absence of this enzyme, the acetylcholine released by nerve impulses has a greater and more prolonged action. However, if too much acetylcholine accumu-

lates, it may cause a depolarizing block of the muscle membrane. Excess acetylcholine may also desensitize the acetylcholine receptor molecules and reduce the response to acetylcholine. Normally this interaction occurs but is only transient because the acetylcholine is removed by the esterase. An example of an anticholinesterase used clinically is *physostigmine.* Some insecticides and nerve gases are also anticholinesterases. Several drugs can mimic the action of acetylcholine at the neuromuscular junction. One of these is *nicotine.* In low doses, nicotine has an excitatory effect on skeletal muscle, but in high doses it blocks neuromuscular transmission.

Clinical Correlations

Disorders of neuromuscular transmission theoretically can involve several mechanisms, including the synthesis of acetylcholine, packaging of acetylcholine in the vesicles, release of vesicles from the nerve terminal, diffusion of acetylcholine across the synaptic cleft, binding of the acetylcholine with the receptor, response of the receptor to the transmitter, and breakdown of the acetylcholine by acetylcholinesterase. Two of these disorders are well known clinically. Both are manifested as weakness without sensory loss. One of these is *myasthenia gravis,* in which there is partial receptor blockade resulting in weakness that increases after exercise. In the other disorder, *Lambert-Eaton myasthenic syndrome,* the release of acetylcholine from the nerve terminal is impaired. This also results in weakness; however, it can be partially overcome by continued activity because, with continued activation, changes in the nerve terminal membrane facilitate acetylcholine release. Thus, patients with this syndrome show increasing strength with a brief period of exercise. In myasthenia gravis, both the end-plate potentials and the miniature end-plate potentials are small. In Lambert-Eaton myasthenic syndrome, a disorder often associated with carcinoma, the miniature end-plate potentials are normal but the end-plate potentials are small because of a decrease in the number of quanta released.

Muscle ■

All body movements are produced by muscles. Through their activity, all the behavior of the organism is affected. The function of muscle is to produce force and movement and to stabilize joints. Striated muscles act through their attachment to tendons and bones, but they depend foremost on their contractile elements. They vary in size and structure, from the very tiny stapedius muscle of the ear to the large, powerful gastrocnemius muscle of the leg. Each is designed to perform specific functions, whether they be finely controlled, rapid, skilled movements, powerful, sudden contractions, or slow, continuous, steady exertion of force. The size, shape

(fusiform, unipennate, bipennate, and multipennate), and microscopic anatomy of muscles vary with their function. Muscles requiring sudden, strong, or phasic contractions are made up predominantly of *type II, white, or fast-twitch muscle fibers* that can function anaerobically; those requiring steady, continuous contractions are made up primarily of *type I, red, slow-twitch muscle fibers* that depend on aerobic metabolism. The size of motor units, the innervation ratios, and the number of motor units in a muscle also are designed to efficiently perform the appropriate activity. The extraocular muscles, which must perform rapid, quick, very finely controlled movements, have large numbers of motor units—more than a thousand per muscle. Each motor unit has a low innervation ratio, controlling only five to ten muscle fibers. In contrast, the gastrocnemius muscle is a much larger muscle with approximately the same number of motor units. However, the innervation ratio is much higher, with each lower motor neuron controlling as many as 2,000 muscle fibers.

Muscles have long been classed as red or white on the basis of their color. More recently, other biochemical and histochemical differences, such as the content of glycogen, mitochondria, and particular enzymes, have been used to identify different types of muscle fiber (Fig. 14). Type I fibers (red) contain large amounts of oxidative enzymes (lactic dehydrogenase, succinic dehydrogenase, and cytochrome oxidase), Type II fibers (white) contain little of these enzymes but relatively large amounts of phosphorylase and glycolytic enzymes [adenosine triphosphatase (ATPase)]. The fibers in any one motor unit are *uniform;* that is, all muscle fibers innervated by a single anterior horn cell are identical in their histochemical and physiologic properties. These properties are determined by the ventral horn cell. Reinnervation of muscle fibers by other anterior horn cells after denervation changes the muscle fiber type as well as the size of the muscle fiber. Some of the differences in type I and type II motor units are shown in Table 6.

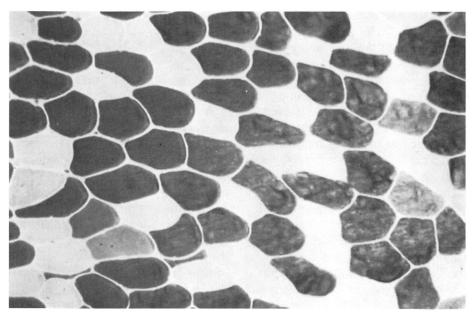

FIG. 14. Transverse section of muscle fiber treated with an adenosine triphosphatase (ATPase) stain showing normal random checkerboard pattern of the two types of muscle fibers. Type I fibers are stained lightly; type II fibers are stained darkly. (ATPase stain; ×200.) (Courtesy of Dr. Andrew G. Engel, Mayo Clinic.)

Structure

Each muscle consists of a large number of muscle fibers arranged in parallel with the longitudinal axis of the muscle. The fibers range from 2 to 15 cm in length and from 30 to 60 μm in diameter. Each is attached to the tendon of the muscle via connective tissue attachments. Individual muscle fibers are multinucleated cells containing *myofibrils*, the contractile elements, as well as mitochondria, nuclei, and other cellular constituents. Each

TABLE 6. *Characteristics of motor units*

Tonic	Phasic
Motor neuron	Motor neuron
Small alpha motor neuron	Large alpha motor neuron
Small axon	Large axon
Low firing frequency	High firing frequency
Slow-twitch fibers	Fast-twitch fibers
Muscle fibers (red) (Type I)	Muscle fibers (white) (Type II)
Aerobic oxidative enzymes (lactic and succinic dehydrogenase, cytochrome oxidase)	Anaerobic glycolytic enzymes and phosphorylase
Small quantities of glycogen	Large quantities of glycogen
Rich in myoglobin	Poor in myoglobin
Lower threshold to stretch	Higher threshold to stretch
Longer contraction time	Shorter contraction time
More mitochondria	Fewer mitochondria
Lower muscle tension	Higher muscle tension
High oxygen consumption	Low oxygen consumption
Constant good blood flow	Rapidly insufficient blood flow
Low fatigability	Pronounced fatigability

muscle fiber has a single end plate located approximately halfway along its length.

The myofibrils of the muscle are banded and give the muscle fiber a banded appearance. Each muscle contains bundles of myofibrils arranged with their bands in register (Fig. 15). The bands are due to the overlapping of the component fibrillar protein of the myofibrils. Each myofibril is approximately 1 μm in diameter and contains two types of filaments: thin filaments and thick filaments. The thick filament contains *myosin,* a large protein material of approximately 0.1 μm in diameter, with lateral projections of meromyosin. *Actin,* the thin filament, is 0.05 μm in diameter. Actin has two proteins, *troponin* and *tropomyosin,* associated with it; these can prevent the interaction of actin and myosin. The actin and myosin filaments are arranged in a hexagonal formation where they overlap (Fig. 16). The area of overlap is darker and is called the *A band.* The area that includes only thin actin filaments is lighter and is called the *I band.* The thin actin fila-

ments are attached to a crystalline structure, which is also dark and is called the *Z disk.* The region including only myosin filaments is the *H zone.* The myosin filaments are bound together at an area of darkness centrally called the *M line* within the H band.

A muscle fiber can be divided longitudinally into areas called *sarcomeres,* which extend from one Z disk to the next. The sarcomere is approximately 2 μm long and consists (in order) of I band, A band, H zone, A band, and I band between two Z disks. Running throughout the muscle and intertwined with the myofibrils is sarcoplasmic reticulum, which forms a longitudinal, anastomotic network of irregular tubular spaces surrounding the myofibrils (Fig. 17). At specific locations along the length of the myofibrils, usually at the junction of the A and I bands, are transverse tubular structures, the *T tubules,* which are near the sarcoplasmic reticulum. T tubules are hollow structures, continuous with the surface membrane (or sarcolemma) and therefore open to the extracellular fluid. They run perpendicu-

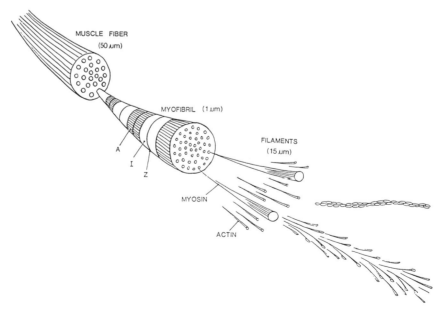

FIG. 15. Ultrastructure of a muscle fiber. Each fiber is made up of many myofibrils containing filaments of actin and myosin organized in bands A, I, and Z. (*nm,* nanometers.)

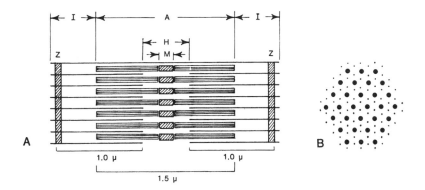

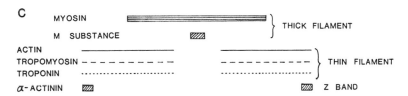

FIG. 16. Organization of protein filaments in a myofibril. **A:** Longitudinal section through one sarcomere (Z disk to Z disk) showing overlap of actin and myosin. **B:** Cross section through A band, where the thin actin filaments interdigitate with the thick myosin filaments in a hexagonal formation. **C:** Location of specific proteins in a sarcomere.

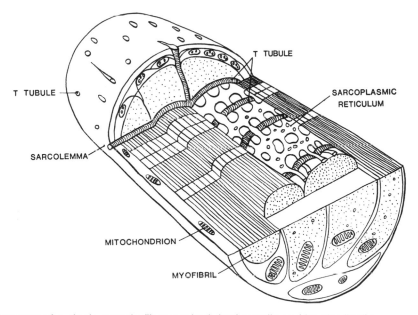

FIG. 17. Structure of a single muscle fiber cut both horizontally and longitudinally. Individual myofibrils are surrounded and separated by sarcoplasmic reticulum. T tubules are continuous with the extracellular fluid and interdigitate with the sarcoplasmic reticulum.

larly from the surface membrane into the muscle fiber, encircling the myofibrils.

Physiology

The contraction of a muscle is initiated by the action potential. When the end-plate potential reaches threshold, an action potential is initiated in the end-plate region and propagates in both directions down the length of the muscle fiber.

Depolarization of the muscle membrane is initiated by the nicotinic receptor and involves activation of voltage-gated sodium channels. As the action potential sweeps down the muscle fiber, the current flow generated by the potential passes internally into the depth of the fiber through the *T-tubule system.* The T tubule contains voltage-sensitive calcium channels and, when depolarized, triggers the release of calcium stored in the adjacent sarcoplasmic reticulum. This involves the opening of calcium-release channels in the sarcoplasmic reticulum (referred to as the *ryanodine receptors*). Calcium binds to troponin C, leading to the detachment of tropomyosin from actin. Actin then attaches to the cross-bridges provided by the myosin heads protruding from the thick filaments, which contain an ATPase site (in the relaxed state when there is no interaction between actin and myosin, these cross-bridges bind adenosine diphosphate and phosphate). When the inhibitory effect of tropomyosin is removed by calcium via troponin, the myosin cross-bridges attach to actin and tilt toward the midsarcomere, driving the thin filament toward the midsarcomere, resulting in shortening of the sarcomere. The length of the thick (myosin) filament and the thin (actin) filament does not change during muscle contraction. The interaction between actin and myosin is rapid and short lasting. In the presence of adenosine triphosphate (ATP), there is reuptake of calcium by the sarcoplasmic reticulum that terminates the active state and results in relaxation. The cross-bridges bind ATP and detach from actin; then they split ATP into adenosine diphosphate and phosphate and assume a relaxed position perpendicular to the shaft of the thick filament. If the ATP in muscle is depleted, the myosin cross-bridges remain attached to actin, and the muscle becomes rigid (*as in rigor mortis*). Mutations in the gene encoding for the calcium-release channel of the sarcoplasmic reticulum (the ryanodine receptor) produce leakage of calcium from the sarcoplasmic reticulum stores on exposure to anesthetics such as halothane. This promotes severe and prolonged muscle contraction on recovery from anesthesia, a serious condition referred to as *malignant hyperthermia.*

The generation of tension depends on overlap of actin and myosin filaments. If a muscle is stretched too far, there will be only minimal overlap and little opportunity for interaction. Therefore, the muscle has optimal lengths for contraction, as shown on a length-tension diagram (Fig. 18).

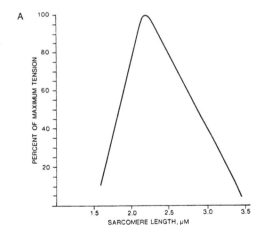

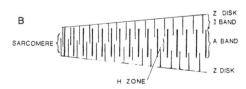

FIG. 18. Length-tension diagram of muscle fiber in relation to its sarcomere length. **A:** Tension generated at different sarcomere lengths. **B:** Extent of overlap of actin and myosin filaments at different sarcomere lengths.

The rate at which tension develops varies with muscle fiber type. In a slow-twitch muscle in which the twitch lasts 100 milliseconds, repetitive stimulation at 10 per second results in a steady contraction. The same rate of activation in a fast-twitch fiber with a twitch time of 25 milliseconds results in a series of brief distinct twitches with each impulse. The sequence of events leading to the contraction of a muscle is illustrated schematically in Fig. 19.

Clinical Correlations

A disease may damage a muscle directly, as in a *myopathy,* or indirectly by damaging nerves to cause *neurogenic atrophy.* In either instance, there are weakness and atrophy of the muscle. However, myopathy and neurogenic atrophy are histologically and physiologically distinct. If a muscle loses its innervation because of disease of the lower motor neuron, the muscle fibers fibrillate and atro-

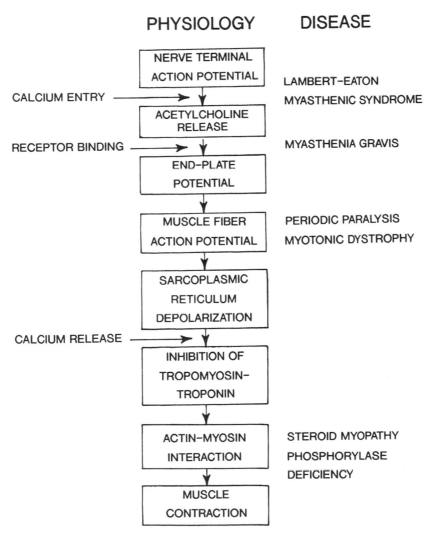

FIG. 19. Sequence of events leading to muscle contraction and the pathophysiologic correlations.

phy. In disorders with incomplete denervation, scattered muscle fibers atrophy. If the process is chronic, viable axons in the muscle reinnervate the denervated fibers, resulting in motor units with a higher innervation ratio and large motor unit potentials. If the large units are lost, the atrophy subsequently appears in large groups of fibers to produce the typical histologic pattern of neurogenic atrophy (see below).

In many myopathies, entire muscle fibers degenerate in a random process, affecting muscle fibers of many motor units, with a loss of fibers from all motor units. With this loss, a smaller force is generated when the motor units are activated. In addition to weakness, the loss of muscle fibers results in smaller motor unit potentials, a feature that can be recognized by needle electromyography. Whereas many primary muscle diseases or myopathies have specific histologic changes, some features are common to all myopathies: random variation in fiber size, internal migration of nuclei, increased connective tissue, and degenerative changes in the muscle fibers (see below).

Although these abnormalities may affect all muscles in the body, most primary muscle diseases affect the proximal muscles to a greater extent than the distal muscles. Therefore, proximal muscle weakness is characteristic of myopathy. It is associated with normal sensation and normal reflexes as long as there is muscle left to contract. The weakness is not associated with an alteration of tone.

Destruction of muscle fibers in their entirety or segmentally along their length is the most common manner for disease processes to affect a muscle. However, two other specific pathophysiologic alterations can occur:

1. Disorder of the sarcolemma, preventing it from generating normal action potentials.
2. Disorder of the excitation-contraction coupling mechanism within the muscle fiber.

Disorders of the Sarcolemma

Mutations encoding for subunits of the sodium, chloride, or calcium channel result in disorders of muscle excitability, referred to as *muscle channelopathies*. The two manifestations are (1) *periodic paralysis* due to transient inability to generate action potentials; and (2) *myotonia,* which consists of excessive muscle contraction, prolonged contraction, or the inability to stop contraction because of increased excitability of the muscle membrane. Sometimes both phenomena occur together. For example, mutations that impair inactivation of the sodium channel produce a transient increase of excitability, followed by the inability to generate new action potentials because of membrane depolarization. This may be triggered by an increase in extracellular potassium, as in *hyperkalemic periodic paralysis*. Mutations in the chloride channel result in increased excitability of the muscle membrane, as in *congenital myotonia.*

Disorders of the Contractile Mechanism

In these disorders, muscle fibers generate normal electrical activity but do not generate enough energy to support normal muscle contraction and relaxation. Muscle depends on the metabolism of glycogen and glucose for a short-term energy supply. In genetic defects of glucose metabolism (for example, muscle phosphorylase deficiency), sufficient energy cannot be produced. As the muscle runs out of energy, it *cramps* without electrical activation. Other metabolic and toxic disorders interfere with the excitation-contraction coupling and produce weakness similar in distribution and character to that described in muscle fiber degeneration.

Clinical Findings With Lesions in the Periphery

Peripheral Nerve Disease

Diseases involving the peripheral nerves have a combination of motor, sensory, and autonomic symptoms and signs. This includes flaccid weakness and atrophy and sensory loss involving all modalities of sensation in the same distribution as the motor findings. Deep tendon reflexes and superficial reflexes are absent in the distribution of the involved peripheral nerves. Damage to the sympathetic fibers traversing the peripheral nerves may result in alterations in sweating and skin temperature. Other internal regulation disturbances such as hypotension and impotence may also occur.

Diseases of the peripheral nerves are of two types: (1) symmetrical polyneuropathies, usually distal and due to a disturbance involving many nerves; and (2) localized mononeuropathies involving a single peripheral nerve, often from trauma, neoplasm, or compression. In mononeuropathy, or plexus disease, the weakness, pain, sensory deficit, and reflex loss are within the distribution of a specific peripheral nerve, for example, the sciatic, radial, median, or ulnar nerve.

Peripheral neuropathy in which there is death or destruction of a portion of the axon results in degeneration of the distal part of the axon in a process called *axonal degeneration* in diffuse disorders and *wallerian degeneration* with focal lesions (see Chapter 4). Axonal degeneration occurs in generalized disorders of peripheral nerve, such as toxic neuropathies, diabetic neuropathies, and neuropathies due to nutritional deficiencies. In these disorders, the peripheral nerves show loss of axons, fragmentation of axis cylinders, and breakdown of myelin into fragments or myelin ovoids (see Fig. 8).

Other peripheral neuropathies are characterized primarily by *segmental demyelination*. In the *Guillain-Barré syndrome* (acute inflammatory demyelinating neuropathy), there are edema and swelling of myelin and Schwann cell cytoplasm, with cellular infiltration and segmental loss of myelin. If severe, this may be associated with axonal destruction and wallerian degeneration. In the genetic hypertrophic neuropathies, such as *Charcot-Marie-Tooth disease,* there is repeated demyelination and remyelination of nerve fibers. Each episode leaves a layer of connective tissue forming concentric layers around the axon. Such nerves become very large and firm, and the axons may finally be lost, leaving only the connective tissue stroma.

Peripheral neuropathy may be only one manifestation of a widespread genetic error of metabolism. In *metachromatic leukodystrophy,* there is a deficit of arylsulfatase, an enzyme that is active in the breakdown of myelin products. The absence of the enzyme results in the accumulation of abnormal sulfatides in peripheral nerves and produces the clinical pattern of peripheral neuropathy. There is associated involvement of the white matter of the central nervous system. Pathologically, there is accumulation of metachromatically staining material along the axons as well as breakdown of myelin.

Refsum's disease is another genetically determined disease in which the metabolic defect results in an accumulation of phytanic acid, a fatty acid. The disease is characterized by a chronic, sensorimotor polyneuropathy associated with hypertrophic changes and onion-bulb formation of peripheral nerves. The patient also has ichthyosis (dry, rough, scaly skin), retinitis pigmentosa, and deafness. In the past, this was considered an untreatable degenerative neurologic disorder; however, it has now been shown that a diet low in phytanic acid is helpful in treating this condition.

Neuromuscular Junction Disease

The major symptom in patients with defects of neuromuscular transmission is weakness, usually in proximal or cranial muscles. There is no atrophy, and tone is normal. The major features differentiating neuromuscular junction disease from muscle disease are fluctuation of weakness with exertion and the response to drugs acting at the neuromuscular junction, which do not occur in myopathies.

Myasthenia gravis, a disorder affecting the neuromuscular junction, is an autoimmune disease in which antibodies are formed against acetylcholine receptors in the postsynaptic membrane at the motor end plate. The reduction in the number of receptor sites at the motor end plate results in a decrease in the response of the muscle fiber to acetylcholine. Clinically, myasthenia gravis is characterized by a fatigable weakness that is induced or increased by exercise and improved by rest or anticholinesterase agents.

Lambert-Eaton myasthenic syndrome is another immune-mediated disorder affecting neuromuscular junctions. In contrast to myasthenia gravis, it affects the presynaptic terminal and blocks the release of acetylcholine quanta. This disorder is usually a paraneoplastic one in which circulating antibodies secreted by small-cell carcinoma of the lung bind with calcium channels in the nerve terminal to prevent calcium entry and quantal release. Lambert-Eaton myasthenic syndrome is similar to myasthenia gravis in that strength fluctuates with activity, but in contrast to myasthenia gravis, strength may improve with activity because more quanta of acetylcholine are released with continued activation. In this syndrome, the associated findings of muscle weakness and reduced reflexes are due to the neuromuscular junction effects; the dry mouth is due to involvement of parasympathetic junctions.

Muscle Disease

Patients with primary myopathy have weakness often accompanied by significant atrophy. Voluntary movement is otherwise normal, with no involuntary movements or spasticity. The common types of myopathy, such as muscular dystrophy and polymyositis, involve proximal muscles. There is relative preservation of reflexes because the neural apparatus is intact. Fasciculations (twitching of the muscles), which are indicative of disease of the lower motor neuron, are not present. Patients with disease of muscle show no evidence of damage to the longitudinal systems of the central nervous system. They do not have involvement of mental function, and they do not have sensory symptoms or signs.

Muscular dystrophy is a disease primarily affecting muscle. It is of genetic origin, with one form (Duchenne) due to a defect in the protein, dystrophin, needed to maintain intact sarcolemma. There are several forms of muscular dystrophy with different clinical patterns. The three major types are Duchenne, fascioscapulohumeral, and limb-girdle. Each of these shows the histologic alterations typical of myopathy, with random, patchy degeneration of muscle fibers, central nuclei, and connective tissue proliferation. *Polymyositis,* a connective tissue disease, is an immunologic disorder. It shows pathologic changes similar to those of dystrophy but with inflammatory cell infiltrates, particularly in and around blood vessels. These changes are more prominent in the peripheral areas of the muscle. Muscular dystrophies have the characteristic temporal profile of degenerative disorders; that is, they are diffuse, chronic, and progressive. However, polymyositis has the histologic features of an inflammatory disorder and often shows a subacute temporal profile.

Laboratory Studies in the Identification of Lesions in the Periphery   ∎

In addition to the clinical features previously listed, a number of laboratory tests are helpful in differentiating diseases involving the peripheral structures. These include biochemical, electrophysiologic, and histologic studies.

General Medical Tests

Peripheral neuromuscular disorders are often found with, or secondary to, systemic disease processes. For example, neuropathies occur with diabetes mellitus, nutritional deficiencies, kidney diseases, carcinoma, and poisonings. Myopathies occur with endocrine diseases, connective tissue diseases, metabolic disorders, and neoplasm. Therefore, a general medical assessment is important in the evaluation of peripheral disease.

Muscle Enzymes

Muscle contains several enzymes that are important in their metabolism, such as aldolase, serum glutamic-oxaloacetic transaminase, and lactic dehydrogenase. Muscle damage from any disease that results in destruction or degeneration of muscle fibers releases these enzymes into the general circulation. Thus, their levels are commonly increased in the blood of patients with active primary muscle diseases. However, these enzymes are also found in many other tissues, and their levels can be increased with other diseases, especially those that damage the heart or liver. *Creatine kinase* is an enzyme that transfers a phosphate group from creatine phosphate to adenosine diphosphate to form creatine and adenosine triphosphate. This enzyme is found mainly in muscle and therefore is a more specific indicator of muscle disease. Creatine kinase levels may be increased in the serum of patients with early or mild myopathy who have minimal clinical evidence of disease and in persons who are carriers of the abnormal gene in recessively inherited muscle disease.

Nerve Conduction Studies

Often, it is not possible to be certain, on the basis of clinical findings, whether a patient has a peripheral disorder. To help in this differentiation, the function of peripheral nerves can be evaluated by nerve conduction studies that quantitatively measure their responses to stimulation. Nerve conduction studies are of particular value in localizing disease in peripheral nerves, in assessing the severity of the disease, and in characterizing nerve disease.

The natural activity in individual axons of a peripheral nerve is random and cannot be recorded readily; however, with the application of an electrical stimulus, all the large myelinated fibers can be discharged simultaneously and the resulting compound action potential can be recorded and measured. If an electrical stimulus (20 to 100 V for 0.1 millisecond) is applied to a mixed peripheral nerve, action potentials will be initiated that travel in both directions along the nerve. Action potentials traveling centrally will be perceived by the patient as a shock in the distribution of the nerve stimulated. Those traveling peripherally will invade each of the terminal branches of the nerve, where they can be recorded either from cutaneous sensory branches or from muscles innervated by motor branches. Thus, either the motor or the sensory components of the peripheral nerves can be selectively studied.

These two types of potentials, the compound sensory nerve action potential and the compound muscle action potential, are measured on an oscilloscope. The *amplitude* of the potential is a function of the number of axons that can carry activity from the point of stimulation to the recording site. The *latency* is a function of the rate at which the largest fibers in the nerve propagate action potentials down the axon. By measuring the distance traveled and dividing this value by the time, the *conduction velocity* can be determined (Fig. 20). Conduction velocity depends on the diameter of the axon and the extent of myelination of the axons. If a nerve is stimulated repetitively at rates of 2 to 40 per second, a normal muscle can respond with the same number of fibers, and the compound action potential with each stimulus will be identical.

The presence of peripheral nerve disease is reflected in nerve conduction studies. In an axolemmal disorder, the action potential is blocked in the region of the abnormality. Stimulation distal to this point results in normal responses, but proximal stimulation produces either no response or only a reduced amplitude response. Axoplasmic disorders with axonal narrowing result in slowing of conduction, whereas those with axonal degeneration result in a reduced amplitude or absence of response to stimulation. In myelin disorders, there is slowing of conduction, with progressive loss of amplitude on more proximal stimulation.

Localized lesions of a peripheral nerve produce a local block or a slowing of conduction in the region of the damage. The block results

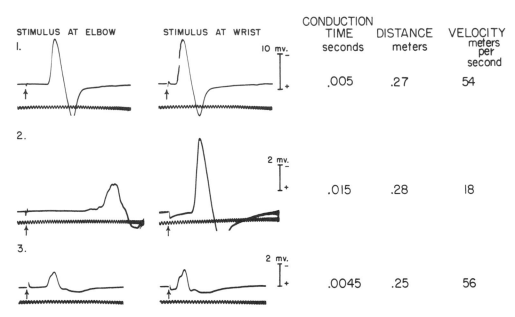

FIG. 20. Measurement of conduction velocity. *1,* normal; *2,* neuropathy: conduction velocity is slowed along entire nerve, and amplitude is reduced with proximal stimulation because of dispersion of the response; *3,* myopathy: conduction velocity is normal, but amplitude is reduced because of muscle atrophy. (From Department of Neurology, Mayo Clinic and Mayo Foundation, *Clinical Examinations in Neurology* [6th ed.]. St. Louis: Mosby-Year Book, 1991. With permission.)

in a smaller evoked response with proximal rather than with distal stimulation (Fig. 21). In generalized disorders of peripheral nerves, there may be a generalized slowing of conduction in segmental demyelinating disorders (Fig. 22), a loss of amplitude of responses, especially distally in axonal dystrophies, or a combination of both.

Disorders of neuromuscular transmission are characterized by progressive loss of amplitude of an evoked motor response with *repetitive stimulation,* especially at rates of 2 to 5 per second. The evoked responses in primary muscle disease with atrophy are low amplitude but are without other changes in nerve conduction. In upper motor neuron lesions, results of nerve conduction studies are normal.

Nerve conduction studies are usually performed in conjunction with electromyography because they use similar techniques and complement each other in arriving at diagnoses of peripheral nerve and muscle disease.

Electromyography

Muscle function can be evaluated by measuring the electrical activity by electromyography (EMG) or needle examination (Fig. 23). EMG provides information about the presence and type of disease involving muscle. Because nerve disorders produce secondary changes in muscle, EMG is valuable not only in diagnostic primary muscle diseases but also in differentiating neurogenic disorders, diseases of neuromuscular transmission, and diseases of the central nervous system.

In EMG, a needle electrode is inserted into a muscle, and the electrical activity is recorded on an oscilloscope and a loudspeaker. The recorded potentials are characterized by their amplitude, duration, and firing patterns (Fig. 24). Recordings are made in multiple muscles in three states: at rest, with needle movement, and with voluntary activity.

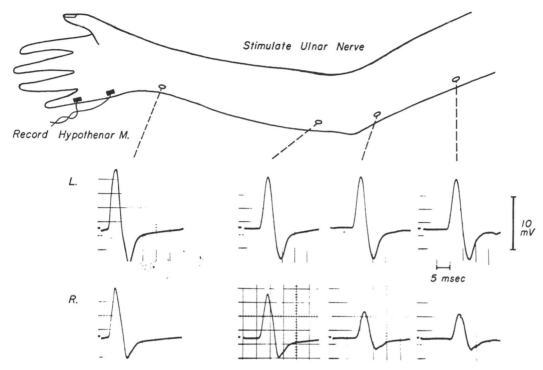

FIG. 21. Nerve conduction studies in a patient with ulnar neuropathy at the elbow. Normal responses from left arm *(L)*; abnormal on right *(R)*. Note the localized partial block of conduction (decreased amplitude above the elbow) and localized slowing of conduction velocity at the elbow. (Courtesy of Dr. E. H. Lambert, Mayo Clinic.)

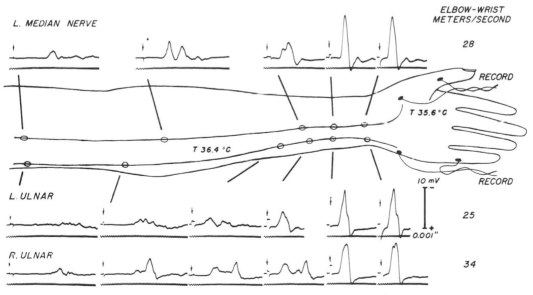

FIG. 22. Nerve conduction studies in generalized demyelinating neuropathy. The evoked muscle action potentials with nerve stimulation are shown. Conduction velocity is listed at *right*. All nerves are affected, with slowing of conduction and dispersion of potentials along their entire length. (*L*, left; *R*, right.) (Courtesy of Dr. E. H. Lambert, Mayo Clinic.)

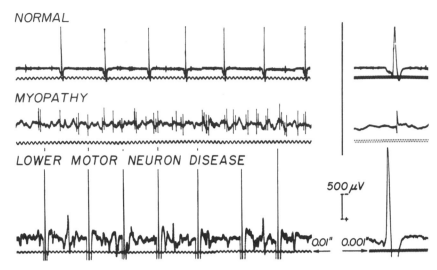

FIG. 23. Potentials recorded in electromyography. Motor unit potentials during voluntary contraction in a normal person, muscular dystrophy (myopathy), and amyotrophic lateral sclerosis (lower motor neuron disease). Potentials on *left* are displayed with a slow time base; on *right,* with a fast time base.

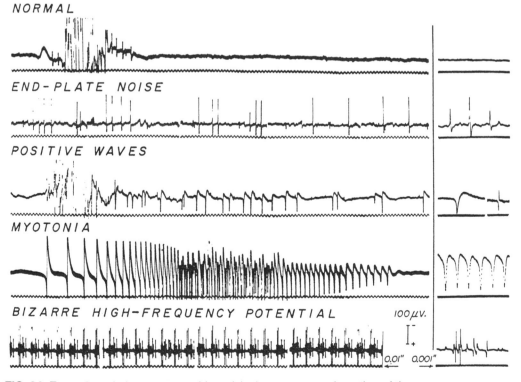

FIG. 24. Examples of electromyographic activity in response to insertion of the needle into the muscle. The top segment shows a normal discharge; the second segment shows biphasic spikes arising in the end-plate region; the third segment shows abnormal positive waves (downward deflections) from denervated muscle; the fourth segment shows a rapid burst of potentials that is characteristic of myotonia; the bottom segment shows a complex repetitive discharge in a chronic neurogenic atrophy.

At rest, there is electrical silence in a normal muscle, except in the region of motor end plates where end-plate potentials or other small potentials may be recorded (Fig. 24). If the needle is moved in the muscle, the mechanical stimulation produces a discharge of the muscle fibers in a characteristic brief burst called *insertional activity* (Fig. 24). With voluntary contraction of the muscle, the motor units fire repetitively, in an orderly fashion, with a frequency and number proportional to the effort exerted. The motor unit potentials are measured to determine their amplitude, duration, and firing rate.

If there is a primary myopathy with random degeneration of muscle fibers, each motor unit will have a reduced innervation ratio and the motor unit potential will be of short duration and low amplitude (see Fig. 23). Because of the reduction in power of each motor unit, many more will fire for any given strength than in a normal muscle. If there is partial destruction of some muscle fibers, the still-viable portions may fire spontaneously (fibrillate). In sarcolemmal disorders, there is an overall reduction in activity, with small motor unit potentials. In disorders of excitation-contraction coupling, no abnormality is recorded on EMG.

In contrast to the changes in myopathy, a neurogenic disorder produces primarily a loss of a number of motor unit potentials and is seen as poor recruitment with increasing effort and a small number of units firing rapidly with maximal effort. In addition, if there has been a chronic denervation with opportunity for reinnervation and resultant increase in innervation ratio, the motor unit potentials will be of long duration and high amplitude (Fig. 25). Any muscle fibers that are denervated because of axonal degeneration will fibrillate. If

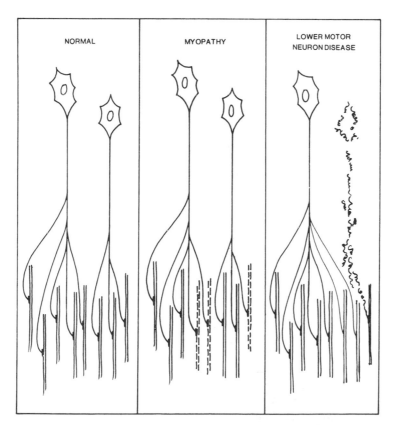

FIG. 25. Alteration in innervation patterns in peripheral disease. Myopathy shows random loss of muscle fibers from all motor units. Neurogenic atrophy shows loss of innervation of all fibers in motor unit, with partial reinnervation by surviving axons.

a motor unit is irritable, single brief twitches or fasciculation of the motor units will occur.

Diseases of neuromuscular transmission are characterized by variable conduction blocks across individual neuromuscular junctions and result in variations in the amplitude of the motor unit potentials with voluntary contraction. In upper motor neuron disease, the motor units appear normal and recruit normally but fire slowly (poor activation).

By combining the findings from EMG and nerve conduction studies, it is often possible to localize the disease in the periphery and at times to specific sites, to characterize the general type of disorder, and to assist in determining the severity or prognosis in the disorder.

Nerve Biopsy

In some peripheral nerve diseases, the clinical, biochemical, and electrophysiologic studies do not reveal the nature of the abnormality. For these patients, a nerve biopsy specimen, usually of a fascicle of the sural nerve, is studied. Nerve biopsy specimens are best studied in three ways: by light microscopy of nerve bundles, teased fiber studies, and cross-sectional fiber counts. For ordinary light microscopy, a piece of nerve is fixed and stained with standard histologic stains and special stains for specific diseases. For instance, in leprosy, *Mycobacterium leprae* can be stained with acid-fast stains. In metachromatic leukodystrophy or amyloid, other specific stains demonstrate the accumulation of the abnormal materials.

If another portion of the nerve is fixed and stained for myelin, it can be teased or pulled apart into single fibers. These single fibers then can be examined for the presence of segmental demyelination, paranodal loss of myelin, or other characteristic changes such as the presence of linear rows of myelin ovoids after axonal degeneration (Fig. 26). In addition, the diameter and the length of the internodes can be measured. Plots of the internodal length compared with the axon diameter can give quantitative estimates of the presence of myelin disorders.

Cross sections of a portion of the nerve also can be stained with myelin stains, and the diameters of the fibers can be measured and plotted as density of fibers. The presence of selective loss of certain fiber types then can be quantitatively determined.

Muscle Biopsy

Although at times the clinical history or pattern of muscle impairment in a patient can permit the diagnosis of a myopathy, often neither the clinical nor the electrophysiologic findings can provide a specific diagnosis. In these situations, muscle biopsy is of clinical diagnostic value (Fig. 27). It, like EMG and nerve conduction studies, can differentiate muscle abnormalities due to neurogenic disorders (neurogenic atrophy) (Figs. 28 and 29) from those due to primary myopathy. In the latter case, a muscle biopsy can often provide an even more specific diagnosis.

Muscle biopsy specimens are taken from a muscle that shows moderate (but not severe) weakness. In severe weakness, there may be so much replacement of muscle by fat or connective tissue that a diagnosis cannot be made. The specimen is stained with routine stains such as hematoxylin and eosin or trichrome and with various histochemical stains that permit the identification of different fiber types. It is also stained for specific abnormalities, such as glycogen in glycogen-storage diseases or lipid in lipid-storage diseases. Fiber-type grouping provides evidence of neurogenic disease, and the presence of specific materials may allow the diagnosis of a specific myopathy.

Special Studies

Both prejunctional (with impairment of acetylcholine release) and postjunctional (due to abnormalities in the number or function of nicotinic receptors) disorders of neuromuscular transmission may result from immune, toxic, or congenital mechanisms. The diagnosis of immune neuromuscular transmission disorders is supported by the presence of cir-

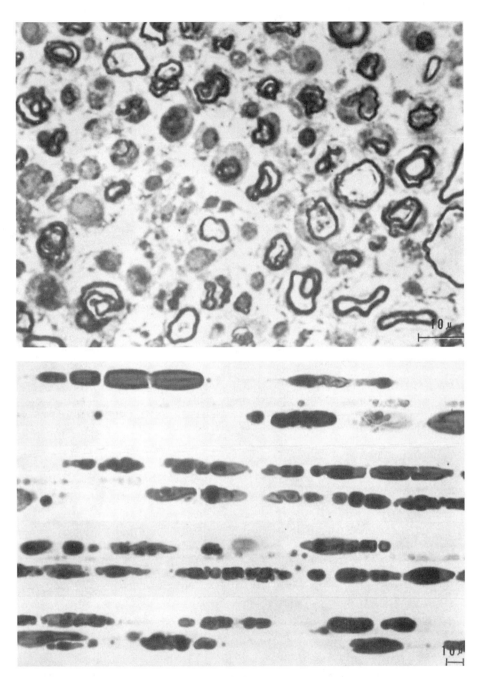

FIG. 26. Phase microscopy of a damaged nerve fiber caused by a crush injury. The upper segment is a transverse section of the nerve showing dilatation, fragmentation, and collapse of the myelin sheaths and an increase in the number of nuclei. The lower segment is a longitudinal section of the nerve showing rows of myelin ovoids, indicating disintegration of the myelin. (From Dyck, P. J. Ultrastructural alterations in myelinated fibers. In Desmedt, J. E. [ed.], *New Developments in Electromyography and Clinical Neurophysiology,* vol 2. Basel: Karger, 1973. With permission.)

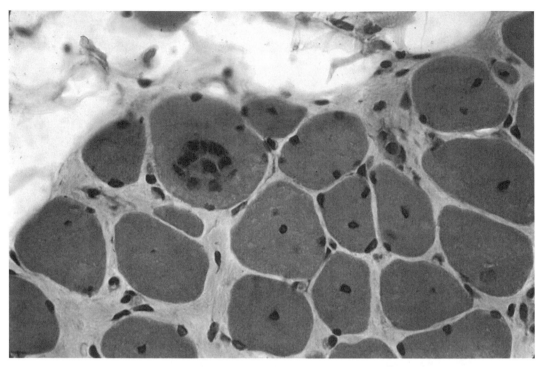

FIG. 27. Transverse section of muscle showing the general histologic features of myopathy. There is random variation in fiber diameter, with both large and small fibers. Many fibers have internal migration of nuclei, some are splitting or degenerating, and there is an increase in connective tissue. (H&E; ×200.)

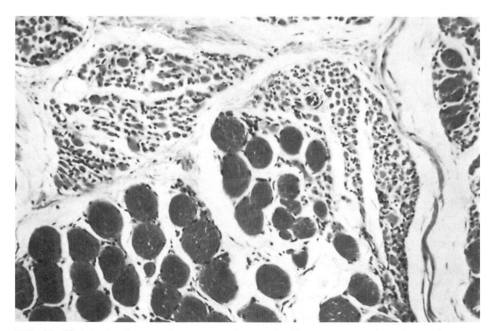

FIG. 28. Histologic changes in neurogenic atrophy. Transverse section of muscle fibers showing groups of atrophic fibers and increased connective tissue where many axons have degenerated. (H&E; ×200.) (Courtesy of Dr. Andrew G. Engel, Mayo Clinic.)

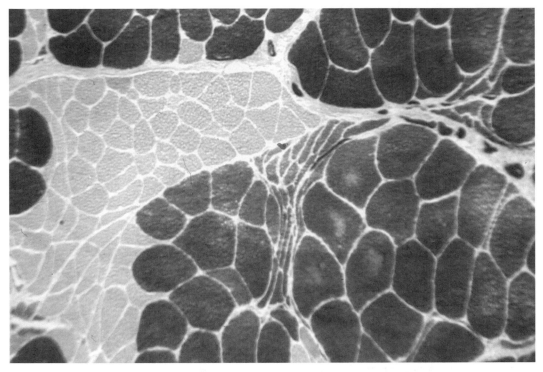

FIG. 29. Transverse section of reinnervated muscle fibers. Type I fibers are stained lightly and type II darkly. Note the loss of the normal checkerboard pattern; instead there is a grouping of the same type of fibers. (ATPase stain; ×200.)

culating autoantibodies against the ion channels involved in the release and junctional effects of acetylcholine. Myasthenia gravis, a postjunctional disorder, is characterized by the presence of *acetylcholine receptor antibodies. Lambert-Eaton myasthenic syndrome,* a prejunctional disorder, is associated with the presence of *antibodies against voltage-gated calcium channels.* Circulating antibodies can be used to confirm the diagnosis of some peripheral neuropathies. For example, the presence of *antineuronal nuclear antibodies* is associated with paraneoplastic sensory neuropathy due to involvement of the dorsal root ganglion cell and *GM₁ ganglioside antibodies* with multifocal motor neuropathies with conduction block.

Important advances have been made in the detection of the genetic defect underlying various neuromuscular disorders. For example, deletions in the *dystrophin* gene are the hallmark of X-linked *Duchenne's muscular dys-*

trophy, and expanded *trinucleotide repeats* occur in *myotonic dystrophy.*

Summary

Diagnosis of diseases at the peripheral level is based on the medical history, clinical features, and electrophysiologic and biopsy findings. Peripheral lesions that affect the motor unit and produce a lower motor neuron type of weakness can be differentiated from central lesions that involve the alpha motor neuron or ventral root (Fig. 30). Involvement of sensory and autonomic functions as well as motor function suggests peripheral neuropathy. Some clinical and electrophysiologic features indicate whether the pathologic process is demyelination, axonal loss, or both (Table 7). Fluctuating weakness (fatigability) is typical of a neuromuscular transmission defect. In prejunctional disorders with impaired release of acetylcholine (Lambert-

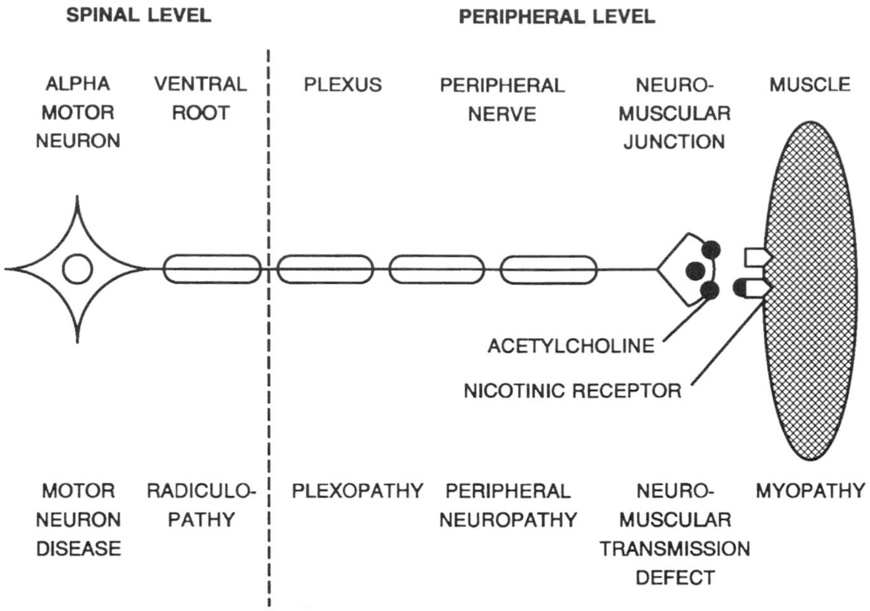

SPINAL LEVEL   PERIPHERAL LEVEL

| ALPHA MOTOR NEURON | VENTRAL ROOT | PLEXUS | PERIPHERAL NERVE | NEURO-MUSCULAR JUNCTION | MUSCLE |

ACETYLCHOLINE

NICOTINIC RECEPTOR

| MOTOR NEURON DISEASE | RADICULO-PATHY | PLEXOPATHY | PERIPHERAL NEUROPATHY | NEURO-MUSCULAR TRANSMISSION DEFECT | MYOPATHY |

FIG. 30. Localization of lesions producing lower motor neuron syndrome at the central and peripheral levels. Disorders of the roots, plexus, or peripheral nerves may produce demyelination, axonal loss, or both. They generally are associated with sensory and autonomic manifestations because of the involvement of several types of axons. Disorders of neuromuscular transmission may be prejunctional (due to impaired release of acetylcholine) or postjunctional (disorders involving the nicotinic acetylcholine receptor). Muscle disorders may produce muscle fiber loss or affect membrane excitability or force of muscle contraction.

Eaton myasthenic syndrome), there is also hyporeflexia or areflexia and cholinergic autonomic impairment (dry mouth, impotence). In postjunctional disorders such as myasthenia gravis, reflexes and autonomic function are normal. Muscle weakness and atrophy in association with normal sensation and relative preservation of reflexes suggest muscle disease. The main clinical and pathophysiologic features that typically differentiate neuropathy from myopathy are summarized in Table 8 and Fig. 31.

TABLE 7. *Differences between demyelinating and axonal neuropathies*

| Feature | Neuropathy type | |
	Demyelinating	Axonal
Mechanism of weakness	Conduction block	Axonal loss
Atrophy	No or late (disuse)	Yes
Fasciculations	No	Yes
Mechanism of recovery	Remyelination	Axonal sprouting (reinnervation)
Nerve conduction velocities	Slow	Normal or slightly decreased
Motor action potential amplitudes	Normal or smaller distally than proximally, with temporal dispersion	Equally small distally and proximally
Fibrillation potentials	No	Yes
Recruitment	Poor	Poor
Motor unit potentials	Normal	Large, long duration, polyphasic

TABLE 8. *Differences between neuropathy and myopathy (typical cases)*

Feature	Neuropathy	Myopathy
Distribution of weakness	Distal more than proximal	Proximal more than distal
Atrophy	Yes (mostly distal)	Yes (generally proximal)
Fasciculations	Yes	No
Reflexes	Decreased	Normal or decreased (late)
Sensory loss	Yes	No
Autonomic dysfunction	Sometimes	No
Creatine kinase	Normal	Increased levels (in most cases)
Electromyography		
Conduction velocity	Decreased	Normal
Sensory action potential amplitude	Decreased	Normal
Fibrillation potentials	Yes	Occasionally
Recruitment	Decreased	Increased
Motor unit potential	Long duration, large amplitude, polyphasic	Short duration, low amplitude, polyphasic
Muscle biopsy	Group atrophy	Variable muscle fiber size
	Fiber type grouping	Inclusions

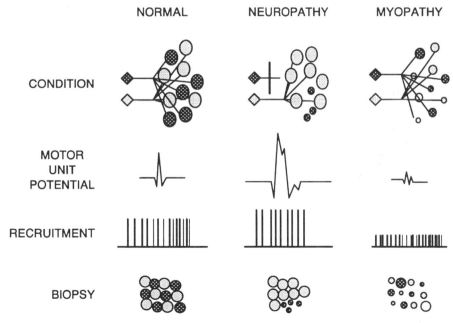

FIG. 31. Organization of the motor unit in normal conditions, neuropathy, and myopathy. In neuropathy, there is loss of motor units and axonal sprouting, with reinnervation of the muscle fibers by surviving axons. This is characterized by reduced motor unit recruitment during increased effort, long duration, large amplitude polyphasic motor unit potentials, and group atrophy, with fiber type grouping in muscle biopsy. In myopathy, there is a loss of muscle fibers in the motor units, but the total number of motor units is preserved. This is characterized by increased motor unit recruitment with increased effort, short duration, small amplitude polyphasic motor unit potentials, and variable size and intermingling of normal and atrophic muscle fibers in muscle biopsy.

Clinical Problems ▪

1. A 47-year-old bank manager has had diabetes mellitus for 14 years. The diabetes is controlled by insulin. He complains of impotence of 6 months' duration. He has had 2 to 3 years of gradually progressive burning sensations and numbness, first of his feet and recently of his hands. He has occasional dizzy spells on arising. On examination, his blood pressure is 115/75 mm Hg supine but decreases to 80/40 mm Hg, with no change in pulse, when he arises. He has mild weakness of his toe and foot dorsiflexors but no other weakness. His ankle reflexes are absent. Other reflexes are hypoactive. He has moderate loss of all modalities of sensation in a glove-and-stocking distribution. There is an absence of hair on his legs, and his skin is very dry. On nerve conduction studies, no sensory potentials could be obtained, and motor responses were of low amplitude, with a mild slowing of conduction velocity. Electromyography showed fibrillation in distal muscles bilaterally.
   a. What are the localization and type of disease?
   b. What is this disorder called?
   c. What is the significance of low-amplitude evoked potentials?
   d. What is the significance of fibrillation?
   e. How is fibrillation differentiated from fasciculation?
   f. What elements of the history and physical examination indicate involvement of small myelinated or unmyelinated fibers?
   g. What would electromyography demonstrate in a pure small fiber neuropathy?

2. A 35-year-old farmer awoke with numbness and weakness in his feet. Five hours later, the numbness ascended to involve the whole extent of the lower extremities as well as the hands, and he noticed he was unable to climb stairs. Three hours later, he was unable to raise his arms and there was a decrease in handgrip strength. The next day, he was unable to stand or walk and had difficulty lifting his head off the pillow. Neurologic examination revealed severe proximal and distal weakness in all limbs, areflexia, and loss of vibration and position sense in the fingers and toes. He also complained of shortness of breath. Electromyography showed marked reduction in nerve conduction velocities, with evidence of conduction block. Needle examination findings were normal.
   a. What are the level, side, and nature of the lesion?
   b. What type of fibers are predominantly affected?
   c. What pathologic mechanism is suggested by the electromyographic findings?
   d. What would a sural nerve biopsy reveal?
   e. What would be the mechanism of recovery?

3. A 57-year-old man has been in good health except for a chronic "smoker's cough." During the past 6 months, he has noted gradually increased difficulty in climbing steps and more recently has had trouble in arising from chairs. He has had some dryness of his mouth. Examination revealed no abnormalities other than weakness of proximal muscles and very hypoactive reflexes. Both the strength and the reflexes appear to improve somewhat with exercise. Results of laboratory studies are unremarkable other than for changes in the electromyogram suggesting the presence of a defect of neuromuscular transmission. Chest radiography revealed a mass in the right hilum of the lung. An intercostal muscle biopsy was performed, and electrophysiologic recordings were made from the muscle. The following data were obtained:

	Patient	Normal
Average resting potential (mV)	75.6	74.7
Average miniature end-plate potential amplitude (mV)	0.3 ± 0.3	0.3 ± 0.4
Average end-plate potential amplitude (mV)	3.2 ± 0.9	15+
Average single fiber action potential amplitude (mV)	97 ± 3	98 ± 3
Threshold (mV)	60	60

a. What two factors determine the size of the end-plate potential?

b. Which of these is abnormal in this patient?

c. What is the quantum content in this patient?

d. How could this produce weakness?

e. What is this disorder?

4. A 55-year-old woman developed proximal symmetric weakness during a 2-week period, with mild muscle soreness. On examination, reflexes, sensation, and mentation were normal. All proximal muscles were moderately weak, distal muscles mildly so. There was no fatigue with exercise.

a. What specific disease is this likely to be?

b. What are the location and cause of this disorder?

Results of motor and sensory nerve conduction studies were normal, except for a borderline low-amplitude compound muscle action potential. A needle electrode (electromyography) was inserted in a weak muscle, and recordings were made of the motor unit potentials. Two abnormalities were noted: the potentials were small, and they fired rapidly with minimal contraction.

c. With disease of the motor unit, if neuromuscular transmission is normal, weakness is due to either of two losses. What are they?

d. What are the two mechanisms used to increase force of contraction?

e. In what way will scattered loss of some muscle fibers alter the firing pattern and size of motor unit potentials?

f. What pattern of histologic change would you expect in this patient?

g. Would muscle fibers innervated by a single ventral horn cell be grouped together?

h. In what general situation does fiber type grouping occur?

i. How could a person with moderately severe motor neuron disease have no weakness?

j. What do T tubules, sarcoplasmic reticulum, and calcium have in common?

k. This patient had an increased serum level of creatine kinase. Why did this occur?

Additional Reading

Dyck, P. J., Thomas, P. K., Griffin, J. W., Low, P. A., and Poduslo, J. F. (eds.), *Peripheral Neuropathy* (3rd ed.). Philadelphia: W. B: Saunders, 1993.

Engel, A. G., and Franzini-Armstrong, C. (eds.), *Myology: Basic and Clinical* (2nd ed.). New York: McGraw-Hill, 1994.

Waxman, S. G., Kocsis, J. D., and Stys, P. K. (eds.), *The Axon: Structure, Function and Pathophysiology*. New York: Oxford University Press, 1995.

The Spinal Level

Objectives

1. Name and identify the four major longitudinal subdivisions and the six major horizontal subdivisions at the spinal level.
2. Describe the differences in the horizontal components at the four longitudinal subdivisions.
3. Describe the relationship of cord segment to spinal nerve and vertebrae.
4. Name the longitudinal systems found at the spinal level, and describe the location of each.
5. Describe the different types of cells in the spinal cord, their distribution, and their function.
6. Describe reciprocal inhibition, recurrent inhibition, presynaptic inhibition, and spinal shock.
7. Describe with examples the stretch reflexes and flexion reflexes.
8. List the symptoms and signs associated with lesions of the spinal cord at C-6, T-6, L-5, and S-2.
9. List the features that differentiate an extramedullary lesion from an intramedullary lesion.
10. List the major clinicopathologic features of multiple sclerosis and pernicious anemia.
11. List the spinal nerves and cord segments that mediate the biceps, triceps, knee, and ankle reflexes.

Introduction

The spinal level includes the vertebral column and its contents. The spinal canal within the vertebral column is the passage formed by the vertebrae, extending from the foramen magnum of the skull through the sacrum of the spinal column. It contains the spinal cord, nerve roots, spinal nerves, meninges, and the vascular supply of the spinal cord. Five of the major systems are represented in the spinal canal: the sensory, motor, internal regulation, vascular, and cerebrospinal fluid systems. The vascular and cerebrospinal fluid structures are the support systems of the spinal cord. Therefore, diseases of the spinal canal involve one or more of these systems to produce patterns of disease distinctive to this level. The anatomical and physiologic characteristics of the spinal cord and spinal nerves that permit identification and localization of diseases in the spinal canal are presented in this chapter.

Overview

Two distinct patterns of abnormality occur with disease of the nervous system: segmental and longitudinal. Damage to segmental structures, as already noted for peripheral lesions, produces signs localized in a single segment of the body. These signs include flaccid weakness, atrophy, loss of reflexes, and loss of all modalities of sensation in a focal distribution. Lesions in the spinal cord usually damage longitudinal systems in addition to segmental structures. Damage to a longitudinal system produces deficit in that system for all functions below the level of the lesion. It is the combination of these patterns of involvement that permits a precise definition of the location of a disease process.

Localized lesions at the spinal level may produce only segmental signs by damage to the spinal nerves and roots within the spinal column. Segmental signs can occur with spinal level lesions because of the origin and termination of primary sensory neurons and lower motor neurons in the spinal cord. The primary sensory endings in the cord distribute information widely within the cord but in an organized fashion. For example, muscle spindle afferents send excitatory fibers to motor neurons of synergistic muscles and inhibitory fibers to antagonistic muscles. Such connections result in complex reflexes mediated at the spinal cord level. The motor neurons of the somatic and visceral efferent pathways, located in the ventral and intermediolateral gray matter of the spinal cord, are the origin of the peripheral motor axons. These motor neurons integrate information from numerous sources in determining the activity of the peripheral muscles and glands.

Lesions at the spinal level can damage these central components of the primary sensory neurons or lower motor neurons and result in disorders of the peripheral structures manifested as

1. atrophy, fasciculation, and weakness, occurring with death or damage of the motor neurons in the ventral horns;
2. preganglionic sympathetic disturbances, occurring with damage to the neurons in the intermediolateral cell column;
3. loss of sensation with destruction of the central processes of the primary sensory neurons;
4. absence of segmental reflexes.

These segmental signs permit the localization of disease along the length of the spinal cord. They are recognized as originating at the spinal level by the associated involvement of ascending or descending tracts, which produces intersegmental signs. The location of a lesion within the spinal canal often can be defined further by the pattern of involvement among the structures in the cross section of the cord. The spinal cord, therefore, is subdivided both along its length and in cross section to aid in the recognition of disease.

Spinal Cord Subdivisions

The segments along the length of the spinal cord are named to correspond to the vertebrae related to the spinal nerve roots. Nerve roots may be located above or below the corresponding vertebra, according to the longitudinal level of the spinal cord:

1. Cervical: The cephalad portion of the spinal cord from which eight pairs of ventral and seven pairs of dorsal roots arise to form the cervical spinal nerves.
2. Thoracic: The middle portion of the spinal cord from which 12 pairs of nerve roots arise to form the thoracic spinal nerves.
3. Lumbar: The upper caudal portion of the spinal cord from which five lumbar nerve roots arise to form the lumbar spinal nerves.
4. Sacral: The caudal end of the cord from which five pairs of sacral nerve roots arise. The conus medullaris is the termination of the cord from which sacral nerve roots arise.

The cross section of the spinal canal is subdivided into major structures from the center to the periphery:

1. Central canal: The central remnant of the ependymal lining of the neural tube.
2. Gray matter: Accumulations of neurons in columns and clusters surrounding the central canal.
3. White matter: Longitudinal fiber tracts in the periphery of the spinal cord.
4. Blood vessels: Vascular supply of the spinal cord located on its external surface.

5. Nerve roots and spinal nerves: The segmental axons of motor and sensory fibers leaving or entering the cord bilaterally along its entire length.
6. Meninges and subarachnoid space: The connective tissue coverings of the spinal cord in the spinal canal and the space they surround.

Spinal Cord Anatomy

External Morphology

The spinal cord lies within the vertebral canal and, in the adult, extends from the foramen magnum to the lower border of the first lumbar vertebra (L-1). The spinal cord is roughly cylindrical, with a slight anteroposterior flattening. It has two wider areas, the *cervical* and *lumbar enlargements,* from which the innervation of the upper and lower extremities arises. The caudal end of the spinal cord tapers to form the *conus medullaris* (Fig. 1).

Nerve fibers enter the spinal cord and exit from it via the *spinal nerve roots.* These roots form from the union of smaller rootlets and leave the cord dorsolaterally and ventrolaterally. The dorsal and ventral roots join laterally at the intervertebral foramina to form the *spinal nerves.* Thirty-one pairs of spinal nerves are formed and divide the cord into 8

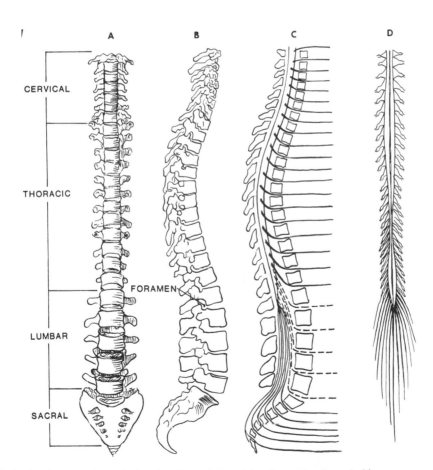

FIG. 1. Spinal column and cord showing the relationships to each other. **A:** Ventral view of the spine. **B:** Lateral view of the spine. **C:** Lateral view of the spinal cord and roots in the spine. **D:** Dorsal view of the spinal cord.

cervical, 12 thoracic, 5 lumbar, and 5 sacral segments, and 1 coccygeal segment. Each spinal segment except the first and last has a dorsal (afferent) root and a ventral (efferent) root, which emerge on each side of a spinal segment and become ensheathed by dura mater as they unite to form a spinal nerve. The *dorsal root ganglion,* which contains the cell bodies of the nerve fibers in the dorsal root, is an enlargement of the dorsal root at the intervertebral foramen. In the intervertebral foramen, the dura mater merges with the perineurium of the peripheral nerve.

Thus, four nerve roots arise from each *spinal cord segment,* a dorsal and ventral root on each side. They are contained entirely within the spinal canal and are bathed in cerebrospinal fluid. They follow a lateral or, in the lower portions of the spinal canal, a descending course to the intervertebral foramen, where the dorsal and ventral roots join to form a spinal nerve (Fig. 1). The ventral roots carry the myelinated axons of the alpha and gamma motor neurons to the somatic musculature and the myelinated

axons of the preganglionic neurons of the sympathetic (parasympathetic in the sacral region) nerves to viscera. The dorsal roots carry sensory input from cutaneous, somatic, muscular, and visceral receptors. The cell bodies of these axons are in the dorsal root ganglia.

Spinal nerves are very short nerves in which the motor, sensory, and autonomic components of a single cord segment are united in a single structure as they exit from the spinal canal through the intervertebral foramen (Fig. 2). The *foramen* is the bony canal formed by two adjacent vertebrae. Because the nerve is surrounded by this bony structure, it is particularly vulnerable to local compression by a tumor, a herniated nucleus pulposus, or arthritic changes in the bones. Each of the spinal nerves is derived from a segment of the spinal cord, and the names of the nerves correspond to the names of the segments. Because there are only seven cervical vertebrae, the C-1 through C-7 spinal nerves exit *above* the pedicle of the vertebra of the same number, and the C-8 spinal nerves emerge *between* the C-7 and T-1 vertebrae. Caudal to

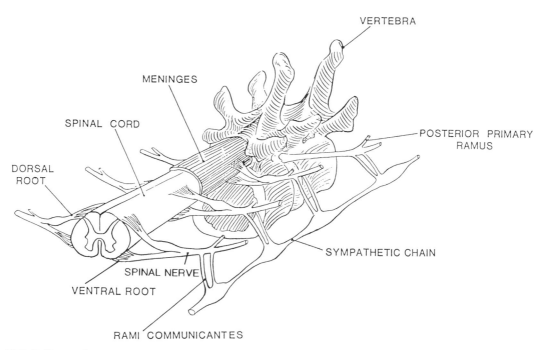

FIG. 2. Formation of a spinal nerve as it leaves the spinal canal through the intervertebral foramen.

T-1, a spinal nerve exits below the vertebra of the same number.

Each spinal nerve is distributed to a well-defined area of skin called a *dermatome* (Fig. 3). Dermatomes of adjacent spinal nerves overlap. This overlap accounts for the variation in sensory loss seen in patients with spinal nerve lesions. The spinal nerves are also distributed to specific groups of muscles called *myotomes* (Table 1).

The nerve roots are anchored in the intervertebral foramina at the point where their dural sleeves terminate. Flexion of the spinal cord or traction on a peripheral nerve (for example, with disk herniation or local tumor) can stretch and irritate a spinal nerve and cause pain.

Early in development, each spinal cord segment is at the same level as the corresponding vertebra. With growth, the vertebral column elongates more than the spinal cord does, and the spinal roots are displaced caudally. The roots of rostral cord segments are displaced less than those of caudal segments. Therefore, the lumbar and sacral nerves have long spinal roots that descend within the dural sac to reach their appropriate vertebral level of exit. These roots are called the *cauda equina* because they resemble a horse's tail. Because of the difference in length between the vertebral column and the spinal cord, care must be taken to specify vertebral level or spinal segment level in indicating the location of a lesion. Generally in a neurologic problem, the affected spinal segment is defined first, and then an attempt is made to correlate that with the appropriate vertebral level. However, in cases of vertebral lesions, the level of vertebral involvement is often seen on the radiograph, and then the level of a possible spinal injury is determined.

The general guidelines for locating the level of a spinal cord injury with respect to the vertebrae are as follows:

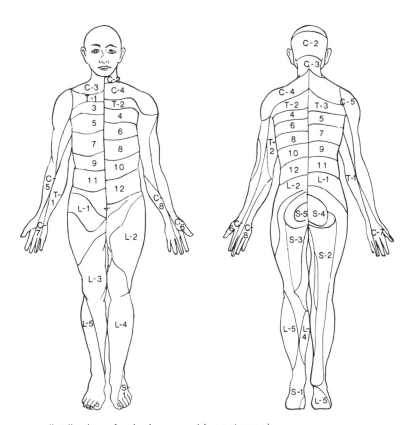

FIG. 3. Cutaneous distribution of spinal nerves (dermatomes).

TABLE 1. *Myotomes listed by spinal nerve and muscle*

Spinal nerve	Muscles
C-5	Biceps, deltoid, infraspinatus
C-6	Biceps, deltoid infraspinatus, wrist flexors, wrist extensors, forearm pronators
C-7	Wrist extensors, wrist flexors, finger flexors, finger extensors, triceps
C-8	Intrinsic hand muscles
L-4	Iliopsoas, quadriceps, anterior tibial
L-5	Anterior tibial, toe dorsiflexors, hamstrings, posterior tibial
S-1	Gluteus maximus, hamstring, gastrocnemius, intrinsic foot muscles

Muscles	Spinal nerves[a]
Neck flexors	C-1 to C-6
Neck extensors	C-1 to C-6
Shoulder external rotator	C-5, C-6
Deltoid	C-5, C-6
Biceps brachii	C-5, C-6
Triceps	C-6, *C-7*, C-8
Wrist extensors	C-6, C-7, C-8
Wrist flexors	C-6, C-7, C-8, T-1
Digit extensors	*C-7*, C-8
Digit flexors	C-7, C-8, T-1
Thenar	C-8, T-1
Hypothenar	C-8, T-1
Interossei	C-8, T-1
Abdomen	T-6 to L-1
Rectal sphincter	S-3, S-4
Iliopsoas	*L-3*, L-4
Thigh adductor	L-2, L-3, L-4
Quadriceps	L-2, L-3, L-4
Thigh abductor	L-4, *L-5*, S-1
Gluteus maximus	*S-1*, S-2
Hamstrings	L-4, *L-5*, *S-1*
Anterior tibial	L-4, L-5
Toe extensors	L-4, *L-5*, S-1
Peronei	*L-5*, S-1
Posterior tibial	*L-5*, S-1
Toe flexors	L-5, S-1
Gastrocnemius	L-5, *S-1*, S-2

[a]The spinal nerves in italics provide the major innervation for that muscle.

1. Between T-1 and T-10, add 2 to the number of the vertebral spine to determine the spinal cord segment at the same location.
2. The lumbar segments of the cord are approximately at the level of the spinous processes of T-11 and T-12.
3. Sacral and coccygeal segments are at the level of the L-1 spinous process.
4. There are eight cervical segments and only seven cervical vertebrae, so that the cervical enlargement at the C-7 cord segment is centered at the C-7 vertebral level.

The surface of the spinal cord shows several longitudinal furrows. The ventral (anterior) surface is indented by the deep ventral median fissure. The dorsal (posterior) surface contains a shallow dorsal median sulcus. The dorsal spinal roots enter each side of the spinal cord along the dorsolateral sulci. Dorsal intermediate sulci extend from the rostral cervical to the midthoracic spinal cord, between the dorsal root entry zone and the midline.

Meninges

The spinal cord is ensheathed by three membranous coverings, the *meninges* (Fig. 4). The outer membrane is the *dura mater.* The inner two membranes, or *leptomeninges,* are the *arachnoid* and the *pia mater.* The arachnoid is a nonvascular membrane separated from the pia mater by the *subarachnoid space* containing cerebrospinal fluid.

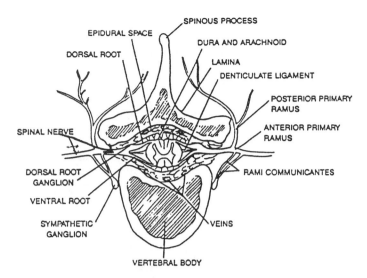

FIG. 4. Cross section of the spinal canal showing the spinal cord, its meningeal coverings, and the manner of exit of the spinal nerves.

The spinal cord is anchored to the inner surface of the dura mater by a series of lateral collagenous bands called *denticulate ligaments,* derived from the pia mater. From 18 to 24 of these ligaments firmly attach the pia mater midway between the dorsal and ventral roots to the arachnoid and the dura mater on each side of the spinal cord. The dural sheath terminates at the level of the second sacral vertebra. A pial extension, the *filum terminale,* arises from the caudal tip of the conus medullaris and pierces the end of the dural sac. It continues as connective tissue, the *coccygeal ligament,* to attach to the periosteum of the coccyx.

Blood Supply

One anterior and two posterolateral arteries run the length of the spinal cord and form an irregular plexus around it. The *spinal arteries* receive their supply from the vertebral arteries and from the intercostal, lumbar, and sacral arteries through six to eight *radicular arteries,* the largest usually entering at the lower thoracic or upper lumbar region of the cord (Fig. 5). The spinal arteries are interconnected by anastomoses circling the surface of the cord and sending short branches inside the cord. Sulcal branches from the *anterior spinal artery* in the anterior median fissure

go alternatively right and left. The *posterior spinal arteries* provide the blood supply for the posterior columns. The rest of the cord is supplied by the anterior spinal artery.

The venous plexus is irregular, and there may be six or seven longitudinal veins at the surface of the cord. This plexus communicates with the occipital and marginal sinuses and with the basal plexus of veins above the level of the foramen magnum.

Internal Morphology

A cross section of the spinal cord reveals a central H-shaped gray area surrounded by white matter.

The spinal cord is organized into four concentric zones: two zones constitute the gray matter, and two zones constitute the white matter. The gray matter occupies the central region and is divided into the *intermediate zone,* containing interneurons and propriospinal neurons, and the *dorsal* and *ventral horns,* containing sensory and motor neurons, respectively. White matter surrounds the gray matter and is divided into two zones: the *pericentral zone* consisting of intersegmental (propriospinal) fibers, and the *peripheral zone* consisting of suprasegmental projection fibers (Fig. 6).

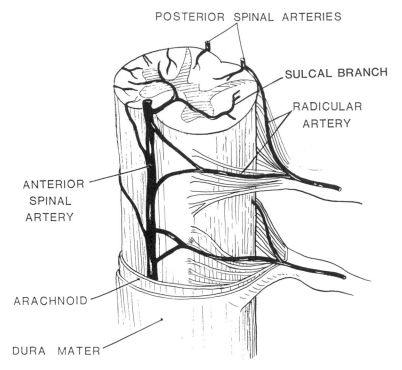

FIG. 5. The arterial supply of a spinal cord segment enters via radicular arteries.

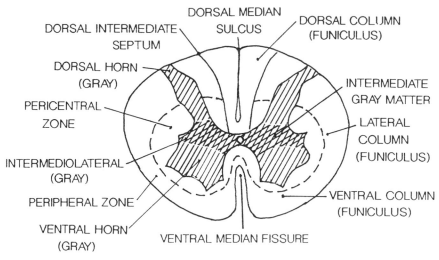

FIG. 6. Major horizontal subdivisions of the spinal cord.

Gray Matter

The gray matter consists of a longitudinally continuous matrix of neuronal cell bodies, dendrites, myelinated and unmyelinated axons, and glial cells. The gray matter is divided into *dorsal horns, intermediate gray,* and *ventral horns.* The interconnecting gray in the midline is separated into a *dorsal gray commissure* and a *ventral gray commissure* by the central canal. A lateral projection of the intermediate gray, the *lateral horn,* is present in the first thoracic (T-1) through the second lumbar (L-2) spinal cord segments.

The two main types of neurons in the gray matter are projection neurons and interneurons (Table 2). The *projection neurons* are divided into sensory projection neurons, which send axons to supraspinal centers, and motor projection neurons, which send axons out of the central nervous system via the ventral spinal roots to muscles. Sensory projection neurons consist of *nociceptive (pain)-specific neurons, nonnociceptive (low-threshold mechanoreceptive) neurons,* and *wide dynamic range (multireceptive) neurons.* They are located in the dorsal horn. The motor projection neurons consist of *alpha and gamma motor neurons;* they are located in the ventral horn. *Preganglionic* projection neurons send their axons via the ventral root to innervate autonomic ganglia.

The *interneurons* have axonal projections that remain in the spinal cord. These neurons are located throughout the spinal cord, particularly in the intermediate gray matter, and constitute the bulk of spinal neurons.

Many interneurons have axonal terminations within the cord segment where they originate. Others have axonal projections that course in a rostral or caudal direction for several spinal segments before terminating. Intersegmental axonal projections may course along several segments in the surrounding white matter before reentering the gray matter to terminate. These are termed *propriospinal* fibers and form the *fasciculi proprii,* which surround the spinal gray matter. The dorsolateral fasciculus (Lissauer's tract) is located at the apex of the dorsal horn (Fig. 7) and contains many propriospinal fibers. The axons may remain on the same side of the cord (ipsilateral) or cross the midline to terminate in the contralateral gray matter. Interneurons that send projections across the midline are termed *commissural neurons.* Such cells are found in abundance in the medial portion of the ventral horn. An interneuron is not restricted to a single pattern of axonal projection; instead, it may have several collaterals with different areas of termination. For example, a commissural neuron may also have an axon collateral that terminates ipsilaterally. Thus, spinal cord interneurons integrate seg-

TABLE 2. *Cell types in the spinal cord*

Cell type	Location	Neurotransmitter
Sensory projection neurons		
Nociceptive, nonnociceptive, wide dynamic range	Dorsal horn	Glutamate
Motor projection neurons		
Alpha motor neurons and gamma motor neurons	Ventral horn	Acetylcholine
Autonomic		
Sympathetic preganglionic	Intermediolateral cell column (T-1 to L-2)	Acetylcholine
Parasympathetic preganglionic	Intermediolateral cell column (S-2 to S-4)	Acetylcholine
Interneurons		
Inhibitory	Diffuse	GABA
Renshaw cell	Ventral horn	Glycine
Excitatory	Diffuse	Glutamate

GABA, γ-aminobutyric acid.

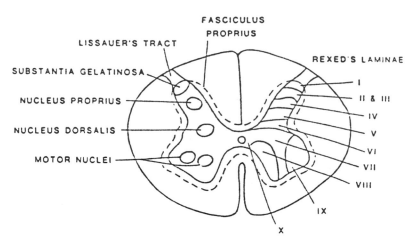

FIG. 7. Groups of nuclei in the spinal cord **(left)** and the laminae of the spinal cord **(right)**.

mental and intersegmental activity, both ipsilaterally and contralaterally.

The distribution of neurons in the spinal gray matter is not random. Scattered throughout the gray matter are clusters of neurons that extend longitudinally for varied distances along the spinal cord as cell columns (Fig. 7).

The spinal cord gray matter is organized into ten cell layers, or laminae (*Rexed's laminae*), based on neuronal size, cell density, and staining characteristics. The neurons in each lamina have specific patterns of connectivity (Table 3). Laminae I through V are located in the dorsal horn and subserve sensory functions; laminae VI and VII are located in the intermediate gray matter and are involved with reflex activity; laminae VIII and IX are in the ventral horn and are involved with motor function; and lamina X surrounds the central canal (Fig. 7):

Lamina I, the most dorsal layer, receives input from propriospinal neurons, nociceptors, and thermoreceptors. It contains *marginal cells,* important cells of the dorsal horn that project to the other segments of the spinal cord, the cervical area, the nuclei of the dorsal columns, the reticular formation, and the thalamus (forming part of the spinothalamic tracts).

Lamina II is the *substantia gelatinosa.* It contains interneurons and receives input from unmyelinated nociceptive C fibers. The *substantia gelatinosa* forms the prominent caplike portion of the dorsal horn. It consists of small cells (6 to 20 μm) with axonal projections that remain in the substantia gelatinosa. This column of cells processes sensory information entering via dorsal root fibers.

Lamina III represents the dorsal part of the nucleus proprius and receives input from mechanoreceptors.

Lamina IV represents the ventral part of the nucleus proprius. It contains several types of sensory cells. It receives input from mechanoreceptors and group II fibers from muscle spindles and gives rise to spinothalamic tract fibers.

Lamina V forms the base of the dorsal horn, is continuous with the reticular formation, and receives input from the reticulospinal tract, lamina IV, mechanoreceptors, nociceptors, group II fibers, and group Ib fibers from Golgi tendon organs.

Lamina VI contains exteroceptive and proprioceptive sensory cells with a large receptive field.

Lamina VII contains interneurons and spinocerebellar neurons of *Clarke's column.* A

TABLE 3. *Spinal cord laminae*

Lamina	Cells	Input (fiber type)	Output
I (marginal zone)	Nociceptive Thermoceptive	Nociceptors (Aδ) Warm and cold receptors (Aδ, C)	Spinothalamic tract
II (substantia gelatinosa)	Inhibitory and excitatory interneurons	Nociceptors (C)	Local Propriospinal
III–IV	Low-threshold mechanoreceptive	Low-threshold mechanoreceptors (Aβ)	Spinothalamic Postsynaptic dorsal column Spinocervical
V–VI	Wide dynamic range	Nociceptors (C) Low-threshold mechanoreceptors (Aβ) Visceral receptors	Spinothalamic Spinoreticular Spinomesencephalic
VII	Motor interneurons and propriospinal neurons	Descending motor pathways	
	Clarke's column (T-1 to L-2)	Low-threshold mechanoreceptors (Aα) Muscle receptors (Ia, Ib)	Dorsal spinocerebellar tract
	Preganglionic sympathetic neurons (T-1 to L-2)	Visceral afferents Descending autonomic pathways	Preganglionic axons to autonomic ganglia
VIII	Motor interneurons and long propriospinal neurons	Ia and Ib afferents Flexor reflex afferents Medial motor pathways	
IX	Motor neurons	Ia afferents Interneurons	
	Ventral and medial groups	Long propriospinal neurons Medial motor pathways	Axial and proximal limb muscles
	Dorsal and lateral groups	Short propriospinal neurons Lateral motor pathways	Distal limb muscles
X	Wide dynamic range Preganglionic	Visceral receptors Nociceptors	Spinoreticular Propriospinal Preganglionic axons

lateral extension of lamina VII at the thoracic levels constitutes the lateral horn. The *nucleus dorsalis (Clarke's column)* is a distinct group of cells located in the medial portion of the base of the dorsal horn. This nucleus extends from the eighth cervical (C-8) to the second lumbar (L-2) spinal segment. The cells of the nucleus dorsalis are tract cells that send axons to the cerebellum via the dorsal spinocerebellar tracts. Clarke's column receives large-diameter afferents from muscle spindles, Golgi tendon organs, and low-threshold cutaneous mechanoreceptors. Afferents from the lower limb ascend in the dorsal horn (fasciculus gracilis) to reach Clarke's column. Preganglionic efferent fibers, exiting from the cord via the ventral root, arise from a distinct column of cells located in the lateral aspect of the intermediate gray matter

(lateral horn). These cells form the *intermediolateral cell column,* which extends from the first thoracic spinal segment (T-1) to the second lumbar spinal segment (L-2). The axons of these neurons synapse with ganglion cells of the sympathetic (thoracolumbar) division of the visceral nervous system. Therefore, the intermediolateral cell column is termed a *visceral efferent nucleus.* The parasympathetic motor (efferent) neurons are in the sacral cord. However, they do not form a well-defined cell group but are located throughout the ventral horn of S-2 to S-4. The reflex center for micturition is in this area of the cord. Preganglionic sympathetic and parasympathetic neurons receive input from primary visceral afferents and from the hypothalamus and brainstem. Lamina VII extends up to the ventral border of the ventral horn at

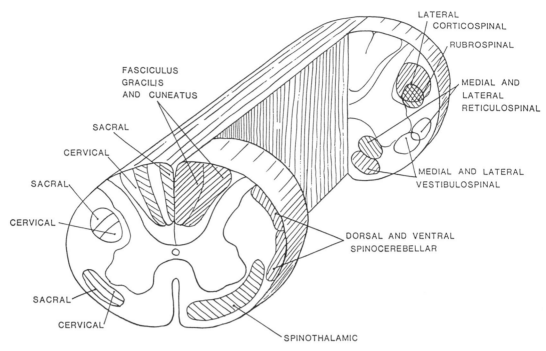

FIG. 8. Principal tracts of the spinal cord. The lamination in the dorsal columns and corticospinal and spinothalamic tracts is shown *(left).* The location of the sensory pathways is shown at the same level on the *right,* and the location of the motor pathways is shown at another level on the *far right.*

the levels of the cervical and lumbar enlargements, between laminae VIII and IX. Lamina VII interneurons contain widely ramified dendrites that extend in a ventromedial to dorsolateral direction and receive massive supraspinal and propriospinal inputs as well as a small input from primary afferents from muscle and joint receptors.

Lamina VIII contains motor interneurons and propriospinal neurons with long axons. These neurons receive input from primary afferents and vestibulospinal and reticulospinal fibers.

Lamina IX contains the motor neurons. The axons of these cells emerge from the spinal cord in the ventral root and innervate skeletal muscle fibers. The large *alpha motor neurons* innervate the extrafusal muscle fibers (responsible for muscle contraction) (see Chapter 8). Alpha motor neurons are up to 80 μm in diameter and are among the largest neurons in the nervous system. The smaller *gamma motor neurons* innervate the

intrafusal muscle fibers in the muscle spindle. The motor neurons are organized in columns that represent *somatic motor (efferent) nuclei.* Motor neurons that innervate the trunk and proximal muscles are located ventromedially and those that innervate distal muscles are located dorsolaterally in the ventral horn.

The gray matter consists of multiple interacting cell groups that process inputs from the periphery, spinal cord, and descending pathways from the brain; mediate reflexes; and give rise to ascending spinal tracts.

The nerve roots and spinal nerves are made up of myelinated and unmyelinated axons that have the same histologic and physiologic characteristics as the peripheral axons described in Chapter 13. Therefore, the pathophysiologic alterations of nerve roots are also the same.

The cell bodies of primary afferent fibers are located in the dorsal root ganglia. These cells have a distal axon segment that terminates in a sensory receptor and a central axon segment that enters the spinal cord via the dorsal root. The central, or proximal, axon segment may take several courses on entering the spinal cord. It may turn rostrally and join the dorsal columns to ascend to supraspinal centers or it may divide into ascending and descending collaterals, which course over several segments in the white matter while sending collaterals into the gray matter. The collaterals of the different types of receptors in turn synapse with cells in specific areas of the gray matter of the spinal cord, predominantly with the projection neurons in the dorsal horn. These in turn send projections to supraspinal structures. The *nociceptive-specific* cells that mediate pain send projections via the spinothalamic and spinoreticular tracts; the *low-threshold nonnociceptive mechanoreceptors* that mediate touch send projections via the dorsal columns, the dorsolateral quadrant, and spinothalamic tract; and the *wide dynamic range neurons* that mediate both pain and touch send projections via the spinothalamic tract, the dorsal columns, and the spinoreticular pathways (Table 4).

White Matter

The spinal cord white matter is subdivided into three columns, or funiculi, called the dorsal (or posterior), lateral, and ventral (or anterior) columns. Each lateral column includes a dorsolateral and a ventrolateral quadrant. The spinal white matter contains (1) ascending ax-

ons from first-order neuron of the dorsal root ganglion (direct dorsal column pathway) or second-order neurons of the dorsal horn or intermediate gray matter (for example, the spinothalamic, postsynaptic dorsal column, and spinocerebellar tracts); (2) descending axons from the motor cortex (corticospinal tract) and several brainstem motor nuclei (rubrospinal, tectospinal, vestibulospinal, and reticulospinal tracts) that innervate motor neurons and interneurons; (3) descending axons from the hypothalamus and brainstem autonomic nuclei that innervate preganglionic sympathetic and parasympathetic neurons; and (4) propriospinal pathways that interconnect several segments of the spinal cord (Table 4). The dorsal column, spinothalamic, spinocerebellar, corticospinal, rubrospinal, and vestibulospinal pathways have a somatotopic organization; the reticulospinal and propriospinal pathways do not (Fig. 8).

The white matter is composed of longitudinally arranged myelinated and unmyelinated nerve fibers, with an abundance of myelin that gives it a glistening white appearance. The white matter is also divided into longitudinal columns. The large bundle of fibers between the dorsal gray horns is divided into two posterior funiculi, or dorsal columns, by the *dorsal median septum*. This septum is composed of glial elements and pia mater and extends from the dorsal median sulcus to the dorsal gray commissure. From the first cervical spinal segment (C-1) to about the sixth thoracic segment

TABLE 4. *Ascending and descending tracts in the spinal cord*

Column (funiculus)	Ventral	Lateral (ventrolateral)	Lateral (dorsolateral)	Dorsal
Sensory tracts		Spinothalamic Spinoreticular Spinomesencephalic Ventral spinocerebellar	Spinomedullary Dorsal spinocerebellar	Fasciculi gracilis and cuneatus
Motor tracts	Vestibulospinal Reticulospinal Medial longitudinal fasciculus Anterior corticospinal	Vestibulospinal Reticulospinal	Lateral corticospinal Rubrospinal	
Autonomic tracts		Descending tracts controlling respiration, circulation, micturition, pupil, and sweating Ascending pathways for visceral pain (spinothalamic and spinoreticular)		Ascending tract for sensation of bladder fullness
Propriospinal tracts	Anterior ground bundle	Lateral ground bundle	Lateral ground bundle	Posterior ground bundle Lissauer's tract

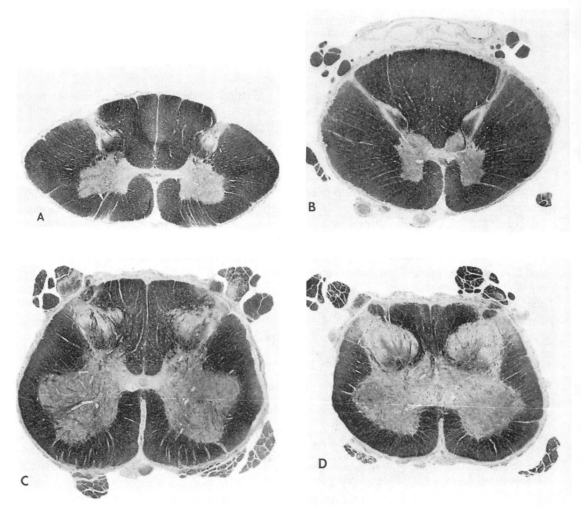

FIG. 9. Myelin-stained cross sections of spinal cord showing the relative proportions of white matter *(dark areas)* and gray matter *(light areas)* at various levels. **A:** Cervical. **B:** Thoracic. **C:** Lumbar. **D:** Sacral.

(T-6), each dorsal white column, or dorsal funiculus, is divided by the dorsal intermediate septum into a laterally located fasciculus cuneatus and a medially located fasciculus gracilis. The rest of the white matter constitutes the ventral and lateral funiculi. The ventral white commissure consists of a band of transversely oriented axons located between the ventral gray commissure and the ventral median fissure.

TABLE 5. *Configuration characteristics of the spinal cord*

Shape of cord	Oval at cervical segments, nearly circular at lumbar segments, and almost quadrangular at sacral segments
Proportion of white to gray matter	Progressively increasing from below up
Size of anterior horn	Enlargement at cervical and lumbar segments
Posterior intermediate sulcus	Present in cervical and upper thoracic segments
Lateral horn	Well marked at thoracic segments
Nerve roots	Many are present around cord at lumbar and sacral segments

The variations in the configuration of the gray and white matter at diffcrent segments of the spinal cord help in identifying the level of a section of the cord (Fig. 9 and Table 5).

Spinal Cord Physiology

The major functions of the spinal cord are the transmission of activity via the longitudinal pathways and the mediation of local reflexes. The reflex activity of the spinal cord depends on the neuronal activity of the cells in its gray matter.

A neuron does not merely relay information; rather, it processes information by the integration of its total synaptic input. The excitability of a neuron changes from moment to moment, depending on the relative effectiveness of the excitatory and inhibitory inputs in altering the state of polarization of the postsynaptic membrane.

Neurons of the spinal cord are responsible for (1) processing, modulating, and transmitting sensory input from the periphery; (2) controlling neck, trunk, and limb muscles during reflex, automatic, and voluntary movements; (3) controlling sympathetic activity throughout the body and parasympathetic outflow to the pelvic organs; and (4) integrating afferent, local, and descending influences on sensory, motor, and autonomic functions.

Sensory Functions

Afferent Input to the Spinal Cord

Information from somatic receptors is transmitted to the spinal cord by first-order sensory neurons that have cell bodies in the dorsal root (or spinal) ganglia. These primary afferent fibers enter the spinal cord at the dorsal root entry zone, with larger myelinated fibers located medially and smaller myelinated and unmyelinated fibers located laterally. From this common entry, the dorsal root fibers branch to ascend and descend in the white matter and to arborize in the gray mat-

ter. The pathways for the different sensory modalities diverge as they ascend in the spinal cord to higher centers (Table 6).

The medially located large myelinated axons relay input from low-threshold skin mechanoreceptors, muscle spindles, Golgi tendon organs, and joint receptors. They bifurcate and the branches may (1) ascend directly in the ipsilateral dorsal columns, without synapse in the spinal cord (direct dorsal column pathway); (2) synapse on dorsal horn neurons in laminae III and IV, which send axons into the dorsal column (postsynaptic dorsal column pathway), dorsolateral funiculus, and spinothalamic tract; (3) synapse on neurons in the intermediate gray matter whose axons form the spinocerebellar tracts; (4) synapse on interneurons and motor neurons in the ventral horn to trigger segmental reflexes, and (5) synapse on interneurons in the dorsal horn for segmental modulation of pain transmission.

The laterally located small myelinated and unmyelinated axons originate from high-threshold skin mechanoreceptors, polymodal nociccptors, thermoreceptors, and visceral receptors. They bifurcate and have ascending and descending branches that run longitudinally in the posterolateral funiculus as Lissauer's tract. Within two or three segments of their entry zone, these axons leave the tract to enter the dorsal horn and intermediate gray matter of the spinal cord. In the gray matter, they may (1) synapse on different groups of neurons in laminae I and V/VI that send axons into the spinothalamic and other tracts ascending in the contralateral ventrolateral quadrant; (2) synapse on dorsal horn interneurons in lamina II (substantia gelatinosa) involved in segmental modulation of pain and propriospinal pathways; and (3) activate, via interneurons, somatic and preganglionic autonomic motor neurons to initiate segmental visceral and somatic reflexes.

Somatosensory Neurons in the Dorsal Horn

The second-order somatosensory neurons in the spinal cord are located in the dorsal

TABLE 6. *Somatosensory channels in the spinal cord*

	Modality					
	Touch-pressure	Stereognosis	Vibration	Proprioception	Pain	Temperature
Receptor (afferent)	Slowly adapting receptor	Fast-adapting receptors (Meissner corpuscles) (Aβ)	Deep, fast-adapting receptors (Paccinian corpuscle) (Aα)	Muscle spindles (Ia) Golgi tendon organ (Ib) Distal joint afferents (II)	HTM (Aδ) polymodal nociceptor (C)	Cold receptors (Aδ) Warmth receptors (Aδ, C)
Dorsal horn synapse, lamina (cell type)	None—DDC III–IV (LTM)	None—DDC III–IV (LTM)	None—DDC III–VI (LTM)	None—DDC III–VIII Clarke's column	I (HTM) V (WDR, HTM)	I
Pathway	Dorsal columns Dorsolateral funiculus Spinothalamic tract	Dorsal columns Dorsolateral funiculus	Dorsal columns	Dorsal column (upper limb) Dorsolateral funiculus (lower limb)	Spinothalamic tract Spinoreticular tract Spinomesencephalic tract	Spinothalamic tract
Function	Touch Edge detection Two-point discrimination Precision grip	Active touch Spatiotemporal discrimination Stereognosia Graphesthesia Precision grip	Vibration	Join position Kinesthesia Precision grip Active touch	Pain (discriminative and affective components) Visceral pain and sexual sensation	Cold and heat sensation

DDC, direct dorsal column; HTM, high-threshold mechanoreceptors; LTM, low-threshold mechanoreceptors; WDR, wide dynamic range.

horn and intermediate gray matter (laminae I to VII). They contribute axons to all the somatosensory pathways except for the direct dorsal column pathway. These neurons include (1) nociceptive-specific cells (mainly in lamina I), (2) low-threshold mechanoreceptive cells (laminae III and IV), (3) wide dynamic range neurons (concentrated in laminae V and VI), and (4) thermoreceptive (lamina I) and other cells.

Ascending Somatosensory Pathways

The somatosensory pathways ascend in the dorsal columns and in the dorsolateral and ventrolateral quadrants of the spinal cord (Table 6).

The *dorsal columns* contain the *direct* (first-order axons from large dorsal root ganglion neurons) and the *postsynaptic* (second-order axons from neurons in laminae III and IV) dorsal column pathways. These pathways ascend ipsilaterally as the *fasciculus gracilis* (carrying low-threshold mechanoceptive and, to a lesser extent, proprioceptive input from the lower limb and lower trunk) and the *fasciculus cuneatus* (carrying low-threshold mechanoceptive and proprioceptive input from the upper limb and upper trunk). They are responsible for discriminative touch, vibratory sensation, and joint position sense. The sensory functions most affected by dorsal column lesions are two-point discrimination, stereognosis, and graphesthesia. Other effects include poor ability to detect repeated stimuli, to recognize gradation of pressure stimuli, tactile and positional hallucinations, and increase in pain and temperature sensation. Instances in which there is a loss of position sense but not vibration sense indicate that the axons transmitting these sensations are segregated. The effects occur predominantly in the distal limbs. Electrical stimulation of the dorsal columns in humans produces a buzzing sensation.

The *dorsolateral funiculus* contains the spinocervical and spinomedullary tracts. The function of these pathways in humans is not known. Lesions of this area do not affect touch, vibration, or joint position sense. These functions may be shared by the dorsolateral funiculus and dorsal columns, that is, parallel routes for the transfer of somatosensory information. Stimulation of the posterolateral funiculus evokes pain that is referred ipsilaterally. In animals, the pathways in the dorsolateral quadrant transmit information similar to that conveyed by the dorsal column and ventrolateral quadrant.

The *ventrolateral quadrant* contains the *spinothalamic tract,* which is crucial for pain and temperature sensation and for itch, visceral pain, and sexual sensation. The spinothalamic tract is functionally heterogeneous and includes second-order axons of nociceptive-specific, low-threshold mechanoreceptive, and, particularly, wide dynamic range neurons. Most of these axons cross the midline near the segment of their cell body. The tract is organized somatotopically. Stimulation of the ventrolateral quadrant in humans evokes pain sensation; less intense stimulation produces thermal sensation. Other parallel pathways include the spinoreticular and spinomesencephalic tracts. Anterolateral cordotomy causes the loss of these sensations contralateral to the lesion. The recurrence of pain after cordotomy indicates the presence of parallel pathways for the transmission of pain sensation, including pathways in the ipsilateral anterolateral and posterolateral quadrants and propriospinal pathways.

The different receptors, afferents, and pathways form specific somatosensory channels that are represented in different thalamic nuclei and different areas of cerebral cortex (see Chapter 7). These are summarized in Table 6.

Relay and Modulation of Nociceptive Information

The spinothalamic tract is a complex and heterogeneous pathway. It originates from neurons in laminae I, V, and VI in the dorsal horn and from neurons in the ventral horn. These different neurons have different functional properties and different connections. Nociceptive afferents terminate in several laminae of the dorsal horn. Lamina I contains predominantly nociceptive-specific and thermoreceptive neurons that receive input from small myelinated (Aδ) and unmyelinated (C) afferents. Neurons in lamina V are predominantly wide dynamic range neurons and receive nociceptive input directly from primary afferents and through excitatory interneurons in more superficial laminae. Wide dynamic range neurons also receive nonnociceptive (low-threshold mechanoreceptive) input from Aβ afferents and from inhibitory interneurons.

The neurotransmitter of primary nociceptive afferents is L-glutamate, which generally produces a fast excitatory potential via activation of non-NMDA (*N*-methyl-D-aspartate) receptors. In response to repetitive stimulation by primary nociceptive afferents, spinothalamic tract neurons exhibit the so-called *windup phenomenon*. This consists of an increase in spontaneous activity, decreased threshold, increased responsiveness, and the enlargement of their receptive fields to noxious stimulation. The mechanism of the windup phenomenon is complex and involves the release of neuropeptides in addition to glutamate from nociceptive afferents and the activation of NMDA receptors and calcium-triggered biochemical cascades in spinothalamic neurons. Repetitive firing of C afferents allows the release of substance P, calcitonin gene-related peptide, and other nociceptive neuropeptides. Substance P reduces potassium conductance and thus produces slow depolarization of spinothalamic neurons. Depolarization relieves the magnesium blockade of the NMDA receptor in these neurons, and this allows the influx of calcium, which activates the phosphorylation cascade and the synthesis of nitric oxide.

Transmission of nociceptive information in the spinal cord is modulated by segmental, intersegmental, and suprasegmental influences. Many interactions among these different influences occur at the level of the substantia gelatinosa (lamina II). Lamina II contains several different types of interneurons and propriospinal neurons, including local inhibitory interneurons containing γ-aminobutyric acid (GABA), enkephalin, or other neu-

rochemicals in various combinations. Segmental control of nociception is the basis for the *gate control theory,* according to which transmission of nociceptive input to the dorsal horn may be inhibited segmentally by activity of large myelinated fibers. These may activate local inhibitory mechanisms that reduce the discharge of spinothalamic neurons. These effects may be mediated by GABA. GABA-containing axons make axoaxonic contact with primary nociceptive afferents and inhibit the release of neurotransmitter from these primary afferents, via GABA$_A$ and GABA$_B$ receptors (see Chapter 12). Suprasegmental influences may either inhibit or facilitate transmission of nociceptive input in the dorsal horn. Descending inhibitory influences originate from different groups of neurons at all levels of the neuraxis, including the thalamus, hypothalamus, *periaqueductal gray matter* of the midbrain, raphe nuclei, and catecholaminergic neurons in the pons and medulla (see Chapter 7). All these regions are reciprocally interconnected, receive nociceptive and visceroceptive inputs, contain opioid neurons and receptors, and produce analgesia by selectively inhibiting transmission in Aδ or C afferents and excitability of nociceptive neurons in the dorsal horn, without affecting transmission of tactile or other nonnoxious stimuli. The descending monoaminergic pathways involved in the control of nociception include a serotoninergic pathway from the nucleus raphe magnus and several noradrenergic pathways from ventrolateral medulla and the locus ceruleus. These pathways descend predominantly in the dorsolateral fasciculus, and their potential targets include local, propriospinal, and spinothalamic tract neurons.

Central Sensitization in Peripheral and Central Lesions Involving the Spinothalamic System

Lesions affecting the somatosensory system at the peripheral, spinal, posterior fossa, or supratentorial level may produce *neurogenic pain.* This involves spontaneous activity, decreased threshold, increased receptive field size, and abnormal sensitivity of nociceptive neurons. This process is called *sensitization.* Peripheral sensitization occurs in lesions affecting a peripheral nerve, for example, in painful peripheral neuropathies (see Chapter 13). The mechanisms underlying central sensitization at the level of the dorsal horn and the thalamic relay nuclei are thought to be similar to those of the windup phenomenon, including increased firing of nociceptive afferents, release of neuropeptides, and activation of NMDA receptors and calcium-triggered cascades (phospholipids, nitric oxide) in spinothalamic neurons. Central sensitization is thought to be the mechanism of *allodynia,* which is the evocation of pain sensation by a nonnoxious stimulus (for example, touch). Allodynia is thought to be mediated by Aβ fibers, which normally evoke nonnociceptive responses in spinothalamic neurons and trigger segmental inhibition of nociceptive neurons via interneurons. However, in central sensitization, nonnoxious stimuli transmitted by Aβ fibers activate hyperexcitable spinothalamic neurons, particularly if there is impairment of local inhibition. Thus, the innocuous stimulus increases the firing of spinothalamic neurons and evokes pain sensation.

Motor Functions

The segmental motor apparatus of the spinal cord is involved in two types of activity: reflex activity, including phasic and tonic stretch reflexes; and complex motor synergies, such as locomotion. The segmental motor apparatus includes (1) topographically organized groups of motor neurons in the ventral horn, (2) local interneurons, (3) propriospinal neurons, (4) peripheral afferents, and (5) descending motor control pathways. At the segmental level, there is a high degree of sensorimotor integration, largely via interneurons that receive multiple segmental and suprasegmental inputs.

Motor Neurons

Motor neurons are arranged somatotopically into functionally distinct groups in lam-

ina IX—those innervating axial muscles are located ventromedially, those innervating intrinsic muscles of the limbs are located dorsolaterally, and those innervating girdle muscles are located in an intermediate position. Motor neurons that innervate extensor muscles are called *extensor motor neurons,* and those innervating flexor muscles are *flexor motor neurons.* Muscles that functionally aid one another are called *synergists,* and those that functionally act in opposition are *antagonists.* For example, both the gastrocnemius and soleus muscles are responsible for plantar flexion of the foot; therefore, they are synergists. The anterior tibial muscle is responsible for dorsiflexion of the foot and is an antagonist of the gastrocnemius and soleus muscles.

The motor functions are mediated by the motor projection neurons in the ventral horn: the alpha motor neurons and the gamma motor neurons.

Alpha motor neurons have large dendritic surfaces, and their discharge depends both on their intrinsic electrophysiologic properties and on the spatial and temporal summation of multiple excitatory and inhibitory postsynaptic potentials. These potentials spread electrotonically to the initial segment of the axon, where action potentials are generated. Motor neurons generally do not generate high-frequency bursts except in certain cases, for example, in response to descending catecholaminergic or serotoninergic input.

The alpha motor neuron, its axon, and all the muscle fibers that it innervates constitute a *motor unit.* The function of the motor unit, including the biochemical and contractile properties of the muscle, depends on the type of motor neuron.

The size of an alpha motor neuron and its firing pattern are related. Smaller cells have a lower threshold for firing and fire at lower frequencies; larger cells have a high threshold and fire at faster frequencies.

During reflex or voluntary muscle contraction, an increase in force is attained by two mechanisms: (1) increased firing of individual motor units (temporal summation), and (2) recruitment of other motor units (spatial summation). Normally, a second motor unit is recruited when the firing of the first unit attains approximately 10 to 15 Hz (recruitment frequency). During muscle contractions of increasing force, alpha motor neurons are recruited according to the *size principle:* small, slow-twitch units are recruited earlier than large, fast-twitch units (see Chapter 8).

On the basis of the size and firing characteristics of alpha motor neurons, motor units can be divided into two types: slow-twitch motor unit and fast-twitch motor unit. The slow-twitch motor unit is supplied by small alpha motor neurons with small diameter axons that innervate type I muscle fibers, which are slow to contract, produce smaller amounts of force, and are resistant to fatigue. The fast-twitch motor unit is supplied by large alpha motor neurons with large and more rapidly conducting axons that innervate type II muscle fibers, which contract rapidly, develop large twitch tensions, and fatigue easily. Thus, the force generated by muscle contraction depends on the number and type of motor neurons recruited and their discharge rate.

Gamma motor neurons are smaller than alpha motor neurons and innervate the intrafusal muscle fibers of muscle spindles. A muscle spindle is a complex proprioceptive stretch receptor that responds selectively to changes in muscle length. The two functional types of muscle spindle are static spindles, which respond to stretching of the muscle, and dynamic spindles, which respond to the rate of change of muscle stretch.

Control of Motor Neuron Activity

The activity of an alpha motor neuron depends on the integration of various excitatory and inhibitory synaptic inputs acting on its cell body and dendrites. Motor neurons receive three types of input: segmental, intersegmental, and suprasegmental. *Segmental* influences include afferents from muscle and skin receptors that generate local reflexes. The most important segmental input is from muscle spindles, Golgi tendon organs, and skin and muscle nociceptors. *Intersegmental*

influences are mediated via *propriospinal neurons* that coordinate the activity of different motor neuron pools to generate complex patterns of movement involving different limbs, for example, during walking. *Suprasegmental* influences include the descending motor pathways from motor cortex (corticospinal, or direct activation pathway) and brainstem (indirect activation pathways). These descending influences affect motor neurons directly or, more commonly, excitatory or inhibitory *interneurons*. These interneurons control the excitability of motor neurons directly or through presynaptic inhibition of neurotransmitter release from the primary afferents.

Spinal Reflexes

The simplest level of motor control is a reflex, in which a specific sensory input induces a specific motor response. Such reflex responses can either promote movement (phasic muscle contractions promote repositioning of the limbs) or maintain posture (tonic muscle contractions counteract gravity and maintain the body in an upright position). The segmental circuits mediating movement reflexes primarily involve excitation of flexor motor neurons, whereas those mediating posture involve excitation of extensor and axial motor neurons. Spinal reflex patterns are subjected to increasing amounts of control from supraspinal levels during the course of development. The magnitude of this reflex subordination in adults is indicated by the initial complete areflexia and flaccidity that follow spinal cord transection (see below).

A reflex arc consists of a receptor, an effector, and interconnecting neural elements. The simplest reflex, a *monosynaptic reflex,* involves only two neural elements—an afferent neuron and a motor neuron that are in synaptic contact. *Polysynaptic reflexes* involve one or more interneurons interposed between the afferent and efferent neurons.

The four main types of segmental inputs to motor neurons are (1) primary spindle endings with group Ia afferents; (2) secondary spindle endings with group II afferents; (3) Golgi tendon organs with group Ib afferents; and (4) groups III and IV muscle afferents and cutaneous receptor afferents, which together with group II spindle afferents constitute the so-called flexion reflex afferent system. The different classes of afferents converge on the same interneuronal pools; excitability of these interneurons provides flexibility of reflex responses in the spinal cord.

Segmental reflexes include the *stretch, or muscle spindle, reflex,* the *Golgi tendon organ reflex,* and the *flexion reflex* (Table 7). There is a great degree of input convergence, mediated largely by the interneuronal pool. Spinal reflexes are not stereotyped but depend on moment-to-moment integration of segmental and suprasegmental influences. This integration occurs primarily through local interneurons.

Stretch Reflex

The response initiated by an afferent discharge from the muscle spindles is a *stretch reflex* (Fig. 10). This reflex continuously activates extensor and axial muscles and results in stabilization of the trunk and limbs to counteract the downward force of gravity and to maintain upright posture. This reflex is not clearly functional in humans until approximately the 17th week of gestation. Subsequently, it becomes integrated with other postural influences that descend from pontomedullary levels. The stretch reflex is of two types: phasic and tonic.

The *phasic stretch reflex* is elicited by muscle stretch sufficient to discharge the primary spindle afferents (group Ia). These large, myelinated, primary afferent fibers enter the dorsomedial portion of the spinal cord dorsal horn and project directly onto homonymous motor neurons (neurons innervating the muscle from which the spindle discharge originated) to produce contraction of the homonymous muscle; concurrent monosynaptic reflex activation of the synergistic muscles results in stabilization of the joint across which the synergists attach.

The classic monosynaptic stretch reflex is mediated by Ia afferents. Lengthening of the spindle increases the discharge of a Ia afferent, which releases L-glutamate and monosynaptically stimulates the alpha motor neurons innervating the agonist and synergistic muscles. The Ia afferent acts via an inhibitory interneuron, the *Ia inhibitory neuron,* to inhibit the alpha motor neurons innervating the antagonistic muscles. This mechanism is referred to as *reciprocal inhibition.*

The stretch reflex mediated by Ia fibers elicits a *dynamic, or phasic,* response initiated by a rapid rate of change in muscle length and produces a burst of excitatory synaptic input to alpha motor neurons supplying the muscle and its synergists. If the change in muscle length is sufficiently sudden, a brisk contraction of the muscle occurs.

TABLE 7. *Spinal reflexes*

| | Reflex | | |
	Stretch	Golgi tendon	Flexion
Receptor	Muscle spindle (type I and type II receptors)	Golgi tendon organ	Muscle spindle type II receptors, skin, muscle and joint nociceptors
Stimulus	Change in muscle length	Tension generated by active contraction	Various mechanical inputs, particularly noxious
Afferent	Ia (phasic), II (tonic)	Ib	II, III–IV
Interneuron	Ia inhibitory	Ib inhibitory	Interneuronal pool
Effect on agonist	Monosynaptic (and polysynaptic) excitation	Disynaptic inhibition via Ib inhibitory interneuron	Polysynaptic excitation at multiple levels, predominantly of flexor muscles
Effect on antagonist	Disynaptic inhibition via Ia inhibitory interneuron	Di- or trisynaptic excitation	Contralateral excitation of extensors (crossed extensor reflex)
Function	Length servomechanism	Tension servomechanism	Withdrawal

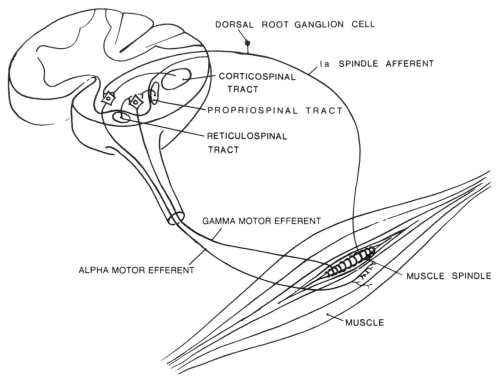

FIG. 10. Pathways for a monosynaptic reflex and the gamma loop. Group Ia afferent fibers from a muscle spindle make monosynaptic contact with the alpha motor neuron supplying that muscle. A gamma motor neuron sends an efferent fiber, via the ventral root, to innervate intrafusal muscle fibers of the muscle spindle. Input to gamma motor neurons is from segmental and supraspinal sources (corticospinal, reticulospinal, propriospinal tracts).

The gain of the Ia monosynaptic reflex is controlled by *fusimotor activity of gamma motor neurons* innervating the corresponding muscle and by *presynaptic inhibition* of neurotransmitter release from the Ia afferent.

Gamma motor neurons receive the same inputs that alpha motor neurons do, except that primary spindle afferents do not project to gamma motor neurons. In general, gamma and alpha motor neurons innervating the same muscle are activated in the same way by an incoming stimulus. However, compared with alpha motor neurons, gamma motor neurons respond at lower thresholds to segmental influences and descending activity, especially that from indirect pathways.

Contraction of the whole muscle would cause the length of muscle spindles to shorten and stop firing, unless a mechanism were available to regulate the length of the muscle spindle. Regulation is achieved by the gamma motor neurons that innervate the muscle spindles (Fig. 10). The muscle spindle consists of sensory receptors on the center of specialized muscle fibers, the *intrafusal fibers*. Gamma motor neurons activate the intrafusal fibers, causing contraction and shortening of the intrafusal fibers on either side of the central noncontractile region. Contraction of the ends of the intrafusal fibers stretches the central region and activates the sensory receptors and the afferent nerve terminals. Thus, an afferent spindle discharge may occur as a direct effect of gamma motor neuron excitation of the intrafusal fibers. When the gamma motor neurons are active during muscle contraction, the resultant intrafusal fiber contractions are sufficient to overcome the slack in the spindle that would result from the whole muscle contraction. This allows the spindle to maintain a high degree of sensitivity over a wide range of different lengths during voluntary and reflex movements.

Gamma motor neurons innervate both primary (dynamic) receptors with Ia afferents and secondary (static) receptors with group II afferents. There are two types of gamma motor neurons: dynamic and static. Dynamic fusimotor fibers enhance the responsiveness of primary spindle endings to small, rapid changes in muscle length; static fibers rapidly shorten the intrafusal muscle fibers and maintain sensitivity of the muscle spindle during unloading of the spindle as a result of the contraction of extrafusal fibers. In relaxed muscles, spindles have little background fusimotor activity and, therefore, do not contribute significantly to muscle tone.

In addition to producing monosynaptic excitatory postsynaptic potentials in homonymous and synergistic alpha motor neurons, group Ia afferents have collaterals that simultaneously inhibit motor neurons innervating antagonistic muscles. This occurs via a disynaptic pathway that involves a *Ia inhibitory interneuron* (Fig. 11). These inhibitory interneurons not only mediate reciprocal inhibition of antagonistic muscles but are an important integrating center for various inputs. Ia inhibitory neurons receive convergent excitatory input from other afferents and from descending pathways and are inhibited by collaterals of homonymous Renshaw cells.

During complete relaxation, fusimotor activity is low or absent, and there is little contribution of muscle spindle reflexes to muscle tone in most normal persons. Dorsal rhizotomy (section of the dorsal roots) interrupts the afferent limb of the tonic stretch reflex, producing a dramatic decrease in muscle tone. This procedure also abolishes the phasic stretch reflex.

Clinically, a monosynaptic reflex is elicited by tapping on a tendon to produce a sudden

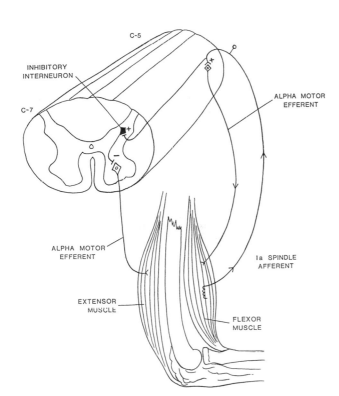

FIG. 11. Pathways for a monosynaptic reflex and reciprocal inhibition. A flexor Ia afferent is shown making monosynaptic contact with a flexor motor neuron and an inhibitory interneuron. The interneuron sends axonal projections to an extensor motor neuron, providing the pathway for reciprocal inhibition.

stretch of a muscle. A commonly observed monosynaptic reflex is that involving the contraction of the quadriceps muscle (knee jerk), elicited by tapping on the patellar tendon. The monosynaptic reflex has been given many names (*myotatic reflex,* stretch reflex, tendon-jerk reflex, and deep tendon reflex). The last term, *deep tendon reflex,* is used extensively and may be misleading. It implies that the receptors for the reflex reside in the tendon, which they do not. The tap on the tendon stretches the muscle and produces a phasic, synchronous discharge of primary spindle afferents, which triggers the monosynaptic stretch reflex.

A second type of response to muscle stretch is the *static,* or *tonic,* response, initiated by a change in the length of the muscle. It provides a continuous background of excitatory input to alpha motor neurons via group II and Ia spindle afferents. This activity contributes to clinical muscle tone and is described as the *tonic stretch reflex.*

Golgi Tendon Organ Reflex

Golgi tendon organs, innervated by group Ib afferents, provide a tension-feedback mechanism during muscle contraction. They are in series with the extrafusal fibers and are located in muscle aponeurosis at the site of tendon insertions, well positioned for monitoring tension generated by muscle contraction. They are silent in relaxed muscles but are very sensitive to increases in tension produced by contraction of their in-series motor units. Golgi tendon organs respond selectively to active tension produced by contraction of the extrafusal fibers that insert in the tendon bearing the receptor. The large Ib afferents from Golgi tendon organs located in muscles that act at the same and at different joints converge onto single interneurons, called *Ib inhibitory interneurons.* These inhibitory interneurons in turn form widespread inhibitory synapses with alpha motor neurons.

The motor neuron output of a spinal segment is determined by the balance between afferents from the length and tension receptors. Together, muscle spindles and Golgi tendon organs, which have opposite effects on the motor neuron pool, provide the central nervous system with the types of information required to control muscle length, tone, force, and movement. Their functions are complementary in the programming and reflex control of movement. In the absence of muscle tone, there is no resistance to passive movement, and the muscle is *flaccid.*

Flexion Reflex

The term *flexion reflex* is a general one encompassing various polysynaptic reflexes. These can range from reflex withdrawal of a portion of the body from a noxious stimulus to flexion of the lower extremities during walking. The flexion reflex afferents include secondary group II muscle spindle afferents; small-diameter muscle afferents (groups III and IV); and joint, touch, pressure, and nociceptive afferents. These afferents have access to motor neurons through various interneurons that receive convergent proprioceptive and descending supraspinal control.

The flexion reflex response is known by several names, including withdrawal reflex, nociceptive reflex, and cutaneous reflex. This reflex results in limb movement mediated by flexor muscle contraction away from the source of stimulation. Both ontogenetically and phylogenetically, the flexion reflex is one of the most primitive reflexes of the central nervous system. It is found in all vertebrates, and in humans it is present by the seventh to eighth week of gestation. In the adult, the circuit underlying this reflex is incorporated into the more complex volitional movements initiated by motor cortex.

Stimuli that evoke the flexion reflex cause a discharge of cutaneous receptors, which in turn triggers action potential discharges along unmyelinated and finely myelinated fibers that enter the dorsolateral portion of the dorsal horn of the spinal cord. This input is then transmitted through short, multisynaptic relays to the ventral motor neuronal pool (Fig. 12).

During flexion reflex activation, there is ipsilateral flexor motor neuron excitation and extensor inhibition (reciprocal innervation). Contralateral to the side of stimulation, there is flexor motor neuron inhibition and extensor excitation (double reciprocal innervation). This *crossed extension reflex* stabilizes the body as the ipsilateral limb is flexed. Even though flexion reflex afferents initially were thought to selectively inhibit extensor motor neurons and facilitate flexor motor neurons (hence, their name), they may also excite ipsilateral extensor motor neurons.

Because the flexion reflex is polysynaptic, there is afterdischarge in the interneuronal relays, and the motor response outlasts the stimulus. Activation of the flexor motor neurons is typically widespread so that flexor muscles at the ankle, knee, and hip contract to withdraw the whole limb (Fig. 13).

The flexion reflex circuits receive important supraspinal control, including inhibition by descending monoaminergic and dorsal reticulospinal pathways and facilitation by corticospinal and rubrospinal pathways. A function of the corticospinal tract may be to choose the synaptic actions of the flexion reflex afferents appropriate to a particular task.

Several cutaneous, or superficial, reflexes are included in a neurologic examination. In general, these reflexes are mediated by polysynaptic segmental circuits similar to those of the cutaneous flexion reflex. Abnormalities in specific superficial reflexes can be diagnostic of central nervous system lesions. For example, in a normal person, plantar flexion of the toes occurs with noxious stimulation of the sole of the foot. In the presence of corticospinal tract disease, however, these local cord reflexes are altered and a more primitive form of flexion reflex occurs—*Babinski's sign,* in which the great toe responds to plantar stimulation with dorsiflexion. The abdominal contractions normally induced by cuta-

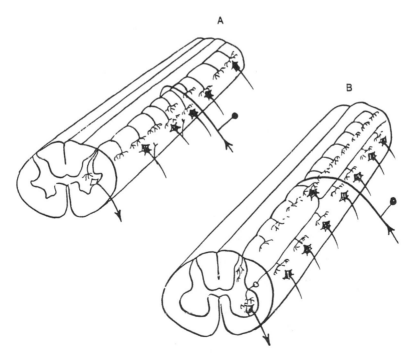

FIG. 12. Reflex connections of primary afferents. **A:** Monosynaptic (no interneurons). **B:** Polysynaptic (one or more interneurons). Note the longitudinal spread of connections in both types of reflex.

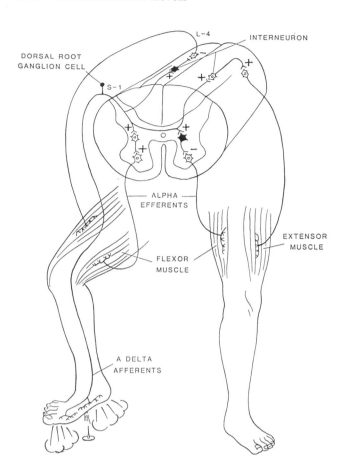

FIG. 13. Flexion reflex pathway. The afferent supply and interneuronal connections for a flexion reflex in the lower extremity are illustrated in a spinal cord section. Noxious stimulus applied to the lower extremity results in ipsilateral flexion (withdrawal) and, provided that stimulus strength is sufficiently high, extension of the contralateral limb (crossed extension reflex).

neous stimulation of the abdomen and the cremasteric contractions normally induced by cutaneous stimulation along the inner side of the thigh (both forms of flexion reflex) are no longer elicitable after a corticospinal tract (direct activation pathway) lesion.

Interneurons and Propriospinal Neurons

The two intrinsic neuronal populations that control the motor output of the spinal cord are the local interneurons and propriospinal neurons. They occupy the intermediate gray matter (laminae V–VIII).

Interneurons, including the Ia, Ib, and presynaptic inhibitory interneurons and the Renshaw cells, are interposed between incoming (afferent) and outgoing (efferent) fibers in the spinal cord. Interneurons receive input from the periphery, local spinal segments, and descending pathways from higher centers; they form multisynaptic, divergent, or convergent connections with motor neurons, afferent neurons, and other neuronal groups in the spinal cord. This convergence of input and divergence of output allow individual interneurons to receive input from many sources and to influence the activity of several neurons. The interneurons thus serve as links among the peripheral nervous system, descending pathways from the brain, local neuronal groups, and motor neurons. The interneurons (1) regulate voluntary and reflex motor acts, (2) coordinate the activity in muscle groups with the appropriate degree of contraction and relaxation of agonists and antagonists, (3) transmit information from the periphery and higher centers to motor neurons, (4) modulate afferent impulses by allowing or preventing transmission of afferent impulses from the periphery and local spinal circuits, and (5) provide a background of spontaneous activity and readiness to respond.

The excitability of alpha and gamma motor neurons and the gain of the multiple segmental and intersegmental reflexes are controlled by various local inhibitory neurons. These include the Ia and Ib inhibitory neurons described above, presynaptic inhibitory neurons, and Renshaw cells. All these interneurons use GABA or glycine or both. They receive input from primary afferents, descending pathways, and, in the case of Renshaw cells, collaterals from alpha motor neurons.

The *presynaptic inhibitory interneuron* makes axoaxonic synapses with Ia afferents. Via activation of presynaptic GABA$_A$ receptors, they bring the membrane potential of the primary afferent toward the chloride equilibrium potential, which is less negative than the resting potential in the primary afferent (primary afferent depolarization). This change in membrane potential reduces the amplitude of the action potential and prevents opening of the voltage-gated calcium channel necessary for the release of L-glutamate from the primary afferent. This process is referred to as *presynaptic inhibition* (Fig. 14).

Renshaw cells control the output of motor neurons, and hence the efferent arm of spinal reflexes, via *recurrent inhibition*. Renshaw cells are inhibitory interneurons that contain glycine or GABA and are excited by recurrent collaterals of alpha motor neuron axons (Fig. 15). Axons of Renshaw cells, after a short course in the white matter, produce inhibitory synapses on homonymous alpha motor neurons and on synergistic motor neurons located in their proximity. They also inhibit gamma motor neurons, Ia inhibitory interneurons, and other Renshaw cells. In addition to excitatory input from alpha motor neurons, Renshaw cells receive complex afferent and descending inputs. The negative feedback circuit of the alpha motor neuron–Renshaw

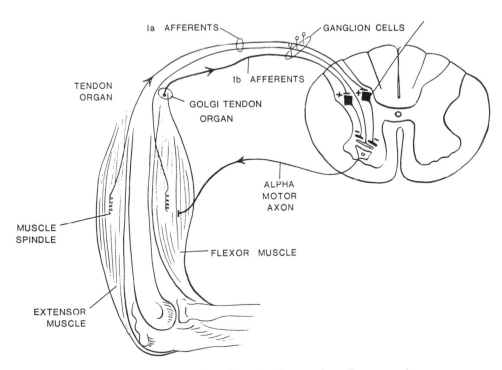

FIG. 14. Mechanism of presynaptic inhibition. Type Ia afferents from flexors are inhibited by Golgi tendon organ and antagonistic spindle afferents.

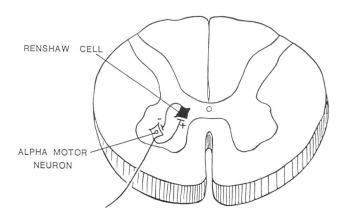

RENSHAW CELL

ALPHA MOTOR
NEURON

FIG. 15. Pathways for recurrent inhibition. Recurrent collateral of the axon of an alpha motor neuron making excitatory synaptic contact with a Renshaw cell. Excitation of the Renshaw cell produces inhibition of the alpha motor neuron.

cell–alpha motor neuron pathway stabilizes discharge of the alpha motor neuron; however, Renshaw cells may also have a role in integrating motor neuron discharge with the firing of gamma motor neurons and Ia inhibitory interneurons.

Loss or functional impairment of spinal inhibitory interneurons results in exaggerated excitability of the motor neurons and their response to afferent input. Lack of supraspinal activation of inhibitory interneurons is thought to underlie the changes in muscle tone and reflexes typical of spasticity (see below). In addition, lack of spinal inhibition produces other types of motor hyperactivity. *Tetanus toxin* impairs the release of GABA and glycine from inhibitory interneurons, causing hyperactivity of spinal cord neurons. This hyperactivity results in generalized muscle spasms, both spontaneous and in response to sensory stimuli. Similar effects are caused by the blockade of glycine receptors by *strychnine* and by antibodies against the enzyme synthesizing GABA in patients with *stiff-man syndrome*.

Pattern Generation in the Spinal Cord

Neurons that are interconnected by synapses constitute *neuronal networks*. Networks that produce specific motor patterns are referred to as *central pattern generators*. The production of motor patterns depends on the membrane properties of the neurons (for example, expression of specific ionic conductances) and on the strength of the synapses (electrical, chemical, or both) between neurons in the pattern generator network.

Suprasegmental Input to Motor Neurons, Interneurons, and Propriospinal Neurons

Motor neurons and interneurons receive input from several descending pathways from the motor cortex and brainstem (Table 8). These pathways include the corticospinal tract (direct activation pathway) and the rubrospinal, tectospinal, vestibulospinal, and reticulospinal pathways (indirect activation pathways). These pathways are discussed in detail in Chapter 8. Only a few of the concepts are emphasized again here. First, most descending axons contain the excitatory neurotransmitter L-glutamate and provide a tonic facilitatory effect on segmental motor neurons and interneurons. Second, with few exceptions, the descending pathways terminate on interneurons and propriospinal neurons and influence alpha motor neurons indirectly. For example, the inhibitory influence of the medullary reticulospinal pathway is mediated via inhibitory interneurons. Third, pathways involved in the control of postural reflexes descend ipsilaterally or bilaterally in the ventral and ventrolateral quadrants of the spinal cord, synapse on long propriospinal neurons in lamina VIII, and control trunk and proximal limb motor neurons. These me-

TABLE 8. *Descending motor tracts in the spinal cord*

	Medial group	Lateral group
Tracts	Lateral vestibulospinal Reticulospinal Medial longitudinal fasciculus (medial vestibulospinal and tectospinal) Anterior corticospinal	Lateral corticospinal Rubrospinal
Location in cord	Ventral and ventrolateral white matter	Dorsolateral white matter
Lateralization	Ipsilateral or bilateral	Contralateral
Collaterals	Extensive	Few
Termination	Ventral and medial gray matter neurons Long propriospinal neurons Few direct connection with axial and proximal limb motor neurons	Dorsal and lateral gray matter Short propriospinal neurons Direct connections with distal limb motor neurons
Function	Control of posture Synergistic whole limb movements Orientation of body and head	Independent, flexion-biased movements of extremities, particularly elbow and hand

dial pathways include the vestibulospinal and reticulospinal tracts; they exert their influence at many segments via propriospinal pathways. In comparison, the lateral corticospinal tract and the rubrospinal tract are contralateral and descend in the dorsolateral quadrant to control flexor movements of the distal portion of the limbs. Fourth, lesions in the lateral columns interrupt the lateral corticospinal tract and the reticulospinal pathways in the ventrolateral quadrant, ventral to the lateral corticospinal tract and rubrospinal tract. These lesions affect projections from the dorsolateral medullary reticular formation that are thought to inhibit flexion reflexes. Lesions that involve the lateral columns spare the vestibulospinal and excitatory reticulospinal pathways. The main descending motor pathways are summarized in Table 8.

Long-Latency Reflexes

Reflex responses to disturbance of voluntary movement or to electrical stimulation have been found in the human arm at approximately 60 milliseconds. These long-latency reflexes involve supraspinal pathways and areas and reflect higher levels of control of motor function.

Long-latency reflexes are transcortical reflexes. Input from muscle spindles is relayed via the dorsal column–lemniscal system to sensorimotor cortex, and corticospinal output to spinal motor neurons results in generation of the late responses of muscle. These responses, also called *long-loop reflexes,* supplement segmental monosynaptic stretch reflexes in their ability to compensate for changes in the mechanical load imposed on a muscle and may be altered by voluntary control.

Muscle Tone

The excitation of motor units in a muscle in response to muscle stretching provides a normal level of resistance to passive movement of a joint, which is called *muscle tone.* Muscle tone is defined clinically as the resistance to passive movements of the limbs when the patient is in a state of voluntary relaxation. It is defined physiologically as a state of tension or steady contraction of the muscle. Muscle tone depends not only on monosynaptic spindle reflex pathways but also on various other mechanisms, including (1) mechanical properties of the muscle, (2) short-latency spinal reflexes mediated by muscle spindle pathways, (3) feedback reflexes mediated by Golgi tendon organ pathways, (4) long-latency reflexes, and (5) voluntary influences.

454   III. Horizontal Levels

Effects of Interruption of Supraspinal Input to Motor Neurons

The interruption of supraspinal input to motor neurons produces two types of effects, according to the temporal profile. Acute lesions, most commonly traumatic or vascular, initially produce loss of excitability of alpha motor neurons, which results in the loss of all reflex, automatic, and voluntary motor function. This constitutes the motor component of *spinal shock* (see below). After recovery from spinal shock or with lesions that evolve more slowly, manifestations typical of upper motor neuron syndrome develop. These reflect increased excitability of motor neuron pools, which is thought to be due mainly to impairment of segmental inhibitory mechanisms. The consequences include spasticity, increased stretch reflexes, flexor or extensor spasms, and the Babinski response.

Spasticity is characterized by a velocity-dependent increase in tonic stretch reflexes (muscle tone); it generally is associated with exaggeration of stretch reflexes and clonus (repeated jerking of a muscle that occurs when stretch reflexes occur in series). Spasticity and hyperreflexia are thought to be the consequence of the loss of activity of inhibitory interneurons, including presynaptic, Ia, and Ib inhibitory interneurons (but not Renshaw cells). Activity in these neurons depends on descending input from the brainstem, particularly the medullary reticulospinal tract. In the absence of medullary reticulospinal inhibition, the lateral vestibulospinal tract (and pontine reticulospinal tract) contribute to increased motor neuron excitability. When tonic stretch reflexes are exaggerated, there is exaggerated activation of the antigravity muscles, particularly the adductors and extensors in the lower limb.

Spasticity is commonly associated with the *clasp-knife phenomenon,* in which the increased resistance to passive movement present with initial stretch subsides with continuous stretch. The genesis of the clasp-knife phenomenon is complex. The buildup of reflex resistance is a consequence of the veloc-

ity-dependent stretch reflex and can occur in any muscle, particularly in the quadriceps and hamstring. The clasp-knife response may reflect a disinhibition of local spinal cord interneurons involved in flexion reflexes. Candidates for triggering this response are flexion reflex afferents, including the secondary muscle spindles (group II) and group II, III, and IV muscle afferents and joint mechanoreceptors.

Interruption of the descending inhibitory medullary reticulospinal pathways that control the interneurons of flexion reflex afferents occurs most frequently with spinal lesions. Thus, the spasticity associated with spinal lesions differs from that associated with supratentorial or posterior fossa lesions by the presence of *flexor spasms.* These are triggered by various stimuli, including noxious somatic and visceral stimuli. In general, patients with complete transection of the spinal cord pass from a phase of alternating flexor and extensor spasms into a phase of predominantly extensor spasms. Extensor spasms may be precipitated by either cutaneous stimulation or body movements, and reflex extension of a limb commonly accompanies the withdrawal of the opposite limb.

The plantar response to noxious stimulation of the sole of the foot is part of a reflex that involves all muscles that flex the leg. In a newborn, this *triple flexion reflex* includes the toe extensors (physiologic flexors). After the age of 2 years, this flexion synergy is less brisk because of myelination of the corticospinal tract. Thus, in normal subjects, the toe extensors are no longer part of the reflex, and in response to noxious stimulation of the sole, the toes may curl down, as a result of a segmental reflex involving the small flexor muscles of the foot. When function of the corticospinal tract is impaired, as in lesions of the lateral columns of the spinal cord, the response to noxious stimulation of the sole is extension (dorsiflexion) of the great toe. This is the extensor plantar response, or *Babinski's sign.* This exaggeration of the intersegmental flexion reflex response is in sharp contrast to the inhibition of segmental nociceptive reflexes. Thus, the abdominal reflexes (elicited by stimulation of the skin of the abdomen) and the cremasteric reflex (normally induced by cutaneous stimulation along the inner side of the thigh) can no longer be elicited with lesion of the corticospinal tract (direct activation pathway).

Autonomic Functions

Preganglionic sympathetic neurons are organized into different sympathetic functional units in the intermediolateral cell column of the spinal cord. These include skin vasomotor, muscle vasomotor, visceromotor, pilomotor, and sudomotor units. These neurons do not discharge massively but instead control specific targets. There is not a generalized sympathetic tone but coordinated activity of specific subsets of sympathetic neurons.

In humans, sympathetic nerve activity in skeletal muscles is finely regulated by baroreflex activity, whereas in the skin it is regulated mainly by environmental temperature and emotional state. Several parallel pathways descending from the hypothalamus and brainstem and containing various neurotransmitters differentially modulate preganglionic neurons; this is critical for their coordinated action. Preganglionic neurons are the effectors of segmental somatosympathetic and viscerosympathetic reflexes triggered by skin, muscle, or visceral afferents in the dorsal root. In general, these afferents stimulate preganglionic neurons via local interneurons. The segmental reflexes are controlled by suprasegmental inputs. For example, innocuous stimulation of the skin or bladder distention produces minimal change in preganglionic activity. Patients with cervical cord lesions that interrupt descending pathways cannot maintain arterial pressure when they are tilted and do not have thermoregulatory responses below the level of the lesion. Also, bladder distention or innocuous skin stimulation in these patients may trigger massive sympathetic excitation, including intense sweating, muscle and skin vasoconstriction, tachycardia, and hypertension. This phenomenon is known as *autonomic dysreflexia*.

Micturition

Preganglionic parasympathetic neurons are restricted to segments S-2 to S-4 and innervate the colon, bladder, and organs of reproduction. Their function involves reciprocal interactions with sacral somatic motor neurons innervating the sphincters and pelvic floor muscles. Parasympathetic neurons are *excited*, whereas somatic sphincter motor neurons are *inhibited* during micturition and defecation; the opposite occurs during storage of urine and feces. Sacral parasympathetic inputs to the bladder are carried in the pelvic nerve; sacral somatic inputs to external sphincter muscles are carried in the pudendal nerve.

As the bladder fills, a constant low intravesical pressure is maintained because of the inherent properties of the smooth muscle. Urine is retained in the bladder by both the changes in configuration of the internal urethral sphincter and the contraction of the external urethral sphincters. This continence system involves lumbar sympathetic and sacral sphincter motor neurons activated by afferents from the bladder and pelvic floor; these neurons favor urine storage by producing relaxation of the bladder detrusor and contraction of the external sphincter. With increased stretch of the smooth muscle of the bladder, proprioceptive information, which gives rise to the feeling of bladder fullness, is carried to pontine micturition centers and to sacral reflex centers.

Normally, the coordinated activity of the bladder detrusor and external sphincter during micturition depends on supraspinal input from pontine micturition centers. Activity in these centers causes excitation of the sacral parasympathetic neurons innervating the bladder detrusor and inhibition of the sacral motor neurons innervating the external sphincter. This coordination of bladder detrusor contraction and external sphincter relaxation allows complete bladder emptying. Interruption of descending pathways from the pontine centers leads to reflex but incoordinated activity of the sacral preganglionic and sphincter motor neurons, a condition called *detrusor-sphincter dyssynergia.*

Clinical Correlations ■

Diseases at the spinal level, like those at other levels, can be classified as focal or diffuse. *Focal disease* at the spinal level may be *segmental,* with symptoms and signs at only one level, as in lesions of the spinal nerve in the intervertebral foramen, or it may present with a combination of *segmental* and *longitudinal* symptoms and signs if the ascending or descending pathways in the spinal cord are involved together with the segmental structures.

Diffuse disease in the spinal level may involve only a *single system,* for example, the motor system in motor neuron disease or the ventriculosubarachnoid system in meningitis, or it may involve *multiple systems,* as in some degenerative and inflammatory disorders.

Focal Disorders at the Spinal Level

Focal lesions at the spinal level are characterized by segmental signs or symptoms specific for a particular level of the spinal canal. These may be due to damage to a spinal nerve, a dorsal or ventral nerve root, a single vertebra, or a spinal cord function found only at a single level.

Segmental Localization

Lesions of the spinal nerves are often due to (or related to) disease of the vertebral column and are at the spinal level. However, many of their clinical features are similar to those of peripheral nerve lesions. Lesions of the spinal nerves are recognized by their pattern of distribution. They are associated with motor, sensory, autonomic, and reflex changes.

1. *Motor involvement.* There are findings of lower motor neuron damage, that is, lesions affecting the final common pathway (Table 9). There is flaccid weakness in a myotomal distribution. When present for sufficient duration, there is associated atrophy. There also may be fasciculation and fibrillation in muscles in the appropriate myotome. Because the lesion is proximal to the origin of the posterior branch of the spinal nerve innervating the paraspinal muscles, the paraspinal muscles are involved as well as other proximal muscles (see Table 1). This involvement is in contrast to lesions that involve the peripheral nerve.

2. *Sensory involvement.* There is sensory loss in a dermatomal distribution, a loss usually best recognized in regard to pain, temperature, or touch. There may be paresthesia from spontaneous firing of the larger axons or dysesthesia from abnormal firing of large and small axons. Spontaneous pain in a dermatomal distri-

TABLE 9. *Summary of findings in upper and lower motor neuron lesions*

Finding	Upper motor neuron[a]	Lower motor neuron[b]
Strength	Decreased	Decreased
Tone	Increased	Decreased
Stretch reflexes	Increased	Decreased
Superficial reflexes	Decreased	Decreased
Babinski's sign	Present	Absent
Clonus	Present	Absent
Fasciculations	Absent	Present
Atrophy	Absent	Present

[a]Involves direct and indirect activation pathways.
[b]Involves final common pathway.

bution is common and is probably due to local swelling, edema, and ionic changes in the spinal nerve, with spontaneous firing of small pain fibers. The pain is often perceived beyond the distribution of the spinal nerve because of intraspinal spread of electrical activity (referred pain). Irritable spinal nerves are more sensitive to stretch, and pain is produced when the extremities are put in certain positions, as for example, when a leg is put through a straight leg raising test.

3. *Autonomic involvement.* Autonomic fibers also are involved, but because of their more extensive overlapping, autonomic disturbances do not occur with lesions of single spinal nerves. Bilateral sacral spinal nerve or cauda equina damage, however, may result in abnormalities of bladder function.

4. *Reflex involvement.* Peripheral reflexes may be lost if either the motor or the sensory component of the reflex arc is damaged. Therefore, they are an important sign of spinal nerve disease (Table 10).

The term *radiculopathy* refers specifically to disease of the nerve root that is located within the vertebral column and spinal canal. Localized nerve root disease produces purely motor or purely sensory deficits, depending on whether the ventral or dorsal root is affected. However, the nerve roots have the same segmental derivation as the spinal nerves, and it is common usage to refer to disease of the spinal nerve (in which the dorsal and ventral roots have joined) as radiculopathy.

Localization to a specific spinal level may be on the basis of

1. local anterior root or anterior horn signs such as segmental atrophy, flaccid weakness, hypotonia, or some combination of these;
2. local sensory abnormalities such as segmental (radicular) loss of all modalities of sensation;
3. local segmental loss or depression of stretch reflexes due to interruption of the stretch reflex arc, which may occur because of damage to efferent or afferent limbs of the reflex arc;
4. segmental signs of vertebral column involvement, which occasionally may be seen as localized pain and tenderness of a vertebra, but more commonly depends on radiographic visualization of a structural abnormality at one level;
5. segmental signs of bladder involvement, such as evidence of a nuclear lesion in the conus of the spinal cord or an infranuclear lesion in the cauda equina with an autonomous (nonreflex) bladder, loss of voluntary control, loss of anal reflex, and large residual urine.

In the absence of specific signs of spinal cord involvement, it may be difficult to distinguish a purely segmental lesion at the spinal level from a more peripheral disorder. However, if the lesion is in the distribution of a single spinal nerve, it can be assumed to be at the spinal level or within the vertebral column (see Chapter 13). Other clues to a lesion at this level are the presence of bilateral abnormalities, the presence of proximal involvement such as in the paraspinal muscles, and signs of meningeal or subarachnoid involvement such as Brudzinski's sign (in which neck flexion with leg extension produces pain).

TABLE 10. *Stretch reflexes*

Reflex	Spinal nerves[a]	Plexus	Peripheral nerves
Biceps jerk	C-5, C-6	Brachial	Musculocutaneous
Triceps jerk	*C-7*, C-8	Brachial	Radial
Knee jerk	L-3, L-4	Lumbar	Femoral
Ankle jerk	L-5, *S-1*	Sacral	Sciatic, tibial

[a]Spinal nerves in italics provide the major innervation.

Intersegmental Localization

The most convincing evidence of a focal lesion at the spinal level is the combined presence of segmental signs of the type previously described in association with *intersegmental signs* due to involvement of the long ascending or descending pathways of the spinal cord. There are three major types of intersegmental signs that appear with focal diseases in the spinal canal:

1. A long tract motor level. These findings are those of an upper motor neuron lesion that involves the direct and indirect activation pathways (see Table 9). They are spastic paralysis, increased stretch reflexes, and Babinski's sign below the level of the lesion. Other abnormal reflexes due to damage of the direct and indirect activation pathways also may be seen, such as loss of the abdominal reflexes, flexion reflexes, and crossed extension reflexes.
2. A long tract sensory level. This level is indicated by posterior column or lateral spinothalamic tract deficits on the appropriate side below the level of the lesion.
3. Autonomic disturbances below the level of the lesion. The most striking is reflex (upper motor neuron or spastic) neurogenic bladder dysfunction, with incontinence due to contractions of a spastic bladder (Table 11). There also may be other evidence of autonomic disturbances, such as loss of blood pressure control, abnormalities of sweating, and loss of rectal control.

Combinations of segmental and long tract signs permit the identification of the site of cord disease with some accuracy. Some characteristic patterns of abnormality are as follows:

1. Upper cervical: This pattern includes long tract signs in the upper and lower extremities for motor and sensory modalities and a reflex bladder dysfunction.
2. Middle and lower cervical: Segmental signs of motor and sensory dysfunction appear in the upper extremities, along with long tract signs in the lower extremities and reflex bladder dysfunction.
3. Thoracic: Long tract signs in the lower extremities appear with a segmental sensory finding (level of sensation) in the trunk and a reflex bladder dysfunction.
4. Lumbar and upper sacral: This pattern includes segmental motor and sensory signs in the lower extremities with a reflex bladder dysfunction.
5. Conus medullaris: Segmental signs appear in the lower extremities with a non-

TABLE 11. *Neurogenic bladder*

	Type	
	Reflex (upper motor neuron or automatic)	Nonreflex (lower motor neuron or autonomous)
Anal and bulbocavernous reflexes	Present	Absent
Clinical features		
Urgency	Yes	No
Incontinence	Yes	Yes
Retention	Yes[a]	Yes
Detrusor-sphincter dyssynergia	Yes	No
Urodynamics		
Tone	Increased	Decreased
Uninhibited contractions	Yes	No
Capacity	Decreased	Increased
Denervation supersensitivity	No	Yes
Examples of lesions	Spinal cord lesion above the conus medullaris	Conus medullaris or cauda equina lesion

[a]If there is a detrusor-sphincter dyssynergia, it prevents complete bladder emptying.

reflex (lower motor neuron) bladder disturbance.

6. Cauda equina: There is pain and asymmetric motor and sensory involvement of multiple roots with or without a nonreflex bladder.

Spinal Shock

Focal lesions may be acute, subacute, or chronic. An acute lesion of the spinal cord may be accompanied by *spinal shock,* which may mask some of the signs previously outlined. Spinal shock occurs when the spinal cord is suddenly severely damaged or there is an acute transection of the spinal cord, after which all cord functions and reflexes below the level of the transection become depressed or lost. The normal activity of spinal cord neurons depends to a great extent on continual tonic discharges from higher centers, particularly discharges transmitted through the vestibulospinal tract and the excitatory portion of the reticulospinal tracts. The acute loss of this input results in loss of neuronal activity.

After a few days to a few weeks, the spinal neurons gradually regain their excitability. This is characteristic of neurons; that is, after loss of facilitatory impulses, they increase in excitability. In most nonprimates, the excitability of the cord centers returns to normal within a few hours to a few weeks, but in humans the return often may be delayed for several months and occasionally is never complete. However, in some patients, the recovery of excitability is excessive, with hyperexcitability of reflexes.

Some major functions are affected by spinal shock. The arterial blood pressure rapidly decreases, sometimes to as low as 40 mm Hg, with loss of sympathetic activity. The pressure ordinarily returns to normal within a few days. All muscle reflexes are blocked during the initial stages of shock. Some reflexes eventually become hyperexcitable, particularly if a few facilitatory pathways remain intact between the brain and the cord. The sacral reflexes for control of bladder and colon evacuation are suppressed in humans for the first few weeks after cord transection, but eventually they return.

The first reflexes to reappear are flexion reflexes, especially in response to stimulation of the plantar surface of the foot (Babinski's sign). After 3 to 4 weeks, flexion reflexes can be triggered from a broader area and are more generalized. After several months, hyperexcitability has developed to the point that plantar stimulation may induce flexion responses on both sides of the body as well as profuse autonomic discharge, for example, sweating and contractions of the bladder and rectum (autonomic dysreflexia). Such mass reflexes may occur even with no obvious source of stimulation. Even after flexion reflexes reappear, the limbs remain flaccid in the absence of tonic stretch reflex activation. After several months, a return of muscle tone and tendon reflexes may occur.

After recovery from spinal shock, a patient who has suffered a major spinal cord injury is left with major deficits that are a function of the level of the lesion. The primary task of the physician, after localizing a lesion and minimizing the damage, is to enable the patient to achieve maximal use of whatever residual function remains. Some of the effects of spinal cord lesions are listed in Table 12.

Transverse lesions of the spinal cord can be further localized in a cross section of the cord. In chronic or subacute lesions, it is often necessary to localize a lesion in this manner in order to identify the most likely type of lesion. It is of particular importance to determine if a lesion is *extrinsic* (extramedullary) or *intrinsic* (intramedullary). Extrinsic lesions arise outside the substance of the spinal cord and compress it. These are more common than intrinsic lesions and often can be removed surgically, with recovery of some or all functions.

Extrinsic lesions commonly damage the dorsal or ventral roots and are therefore usually associated with radicular pain. Because the dorsal root ganglion contains the cell bodies that maintain the axons traveling both peripherally and centrally in the sensory system, its destruction can result in wallerian degen-

TABLE 12. *Effects of lesions at spinal cord segments*

Segment	Deficit	Independence	Aids required
C-4, C-5	Quadriplegia Impaired respiration Reflex bladder	None	Wheelchair Constant care
C-6, C-7	Quadriplegia	Minimal	Wheelchair Hand splints
C-8, T-1	Impaired respiration Reflex bladder Paraplegia Hand weakness	Personal care Drives car	Wheelchair Special braces
T-2, T-3	Impaired respiration Reflex bladder Paraplegia	Complete	Wheelchair Leg braces
T-12, L-1	Paraplegia Reflex bladder	Complete	Wheelchair Leg braces
L-4, L-5	Paraplegia Reflex bladder	Complete	Foot braces
S-2, S-3	Nonreflex bladder	Complete	Catheter

eration in both the peripheral nerves and the central pathways. In contrast, a lesion that destroys the dorsal root proximal to the ganglion produces sensory loss and reflex loss, with degeneration in the central processes but not in the peripheral nerve. Destruction of the root distal to the ganglion produces the same clinical symptoms and signs but is associated with peripheral but not central wallerian degeneration. The presence or absence of peripheral wallerian degeneration often can be determined by electrical studies of patients. Ventral root damage produces degeneration of the peripheral nerves, with associated reflex loss, atrophy, and weakness.

Intrinsic lesions arise within the substance of the spinal cord and often spare the more peripheral pathways of the spinal cord. Although sensory symptoms are prominent, they are often painless. A review of Fig. 8 shows that the pathways of the lumbar and sacral segments in the spinothalamic and corticospinal tracts are more superficial. Intrinsic lesions preferentially damage the pathways from higher levels and may manifest sacral sparing, in which the long tract signs spare the most caudal segments because they are more laterally placed in the cord. A syrinx or tumor in the cervical cord gray matter may produce sacral sparing.

Localization is aided by knowledge of the decussations of the pathways. Because the spinothalamic pathways cross to the opposite side within two or three segments of their entry, a lesion of one side of the spinal cord produces dissociation of the sensations of pain and temperature (lost contralaterally below the lesion) from position sense and vibratory sensation (lost ipsilaterally below the lesion). Similarly, a lesion in the region of the central canal destroys the spinothalamic fibers decussating in the anterior commissure and gives segmental loss of pain and temperature, with segmental signs of motor neuron destruction if the lesion extends into the ventral horns, but sparing of other modalities of sensation.

Focal disorders of the spinal cord may be either mass or nonmass in type. The same criteria applied at other levels can be used to differentiate a mass from a nonmass. In the clinical history, progression favors a mass, as does the presence of distortion, destruction of tissue, or obstruction of the subarachnoid spaces on special studies (myelography). The pathologic changes can be identified by the temporal profile and may include vascular lesions (infarct of the cord, arteriovenous malformations, hematomas) (Fig. 16), neoplastic diseases (tumors of the nerve roots, intramedullary or extramedullary cord tumors), inflammatory disease (poliomyelitis, abscess, arachnoiditis), and traumatic lesions (cord transection, ruptured intervertebral disks) (Fig. 17). Focal lesions are typically single. However, in multiple sclerosis, there are multifocal lesions that can produce complex findings.

Multiple Sclerosis

Multiple sclerosis is a disorder associated with localized areas of demyelination in the white matter of the central nervous system (Fig. 18). Although spinal cord involvement is common, the lesions also may appear in the white matter of the brainstem, cerebellum, and cerebral hemispheres. The focal lesions develop over a few days, and the symptoms may resolve over a few days to weeks or leave a persistent deficit. They occur in scattered areas to produce a *multifocal* disorder. The disease is of unknown cause, but its subacute course, some of the histologic features, and laboratory findings suggest that it may be an autoimmune disorder with inflammatory features. The areas of demyelination vary in size from a few millimeters to several centimeters in diameter and show myelin breakdown, with preservation of the axons. In acute lesions, there may be perivascular infiltrations of lymphocytes. Later during the course of a lesion, there are predominantly macrophages phagocytosing the myelin products. As the lesion resolves, it becomes gliotic. Severe lesions may be associated with axonal destruction, and the disorder may clinically appear to be degenerative late in the course as remissions no longer occur. The clinical history of multiple sclerosis is one of recurrent episodes of deficit in widespread areas, corresponding to the intermittent occurrence of such lesions in disseminated areas. Any single such lesion in the spinal cord could be associated with segmental signs at the level of the lesion, or with longitudinal tract deficits below the level, or with both.

Diffuse Disorders at the Spinal Level

Diffuse disorders of the spinal canal are generally chronic and progressive, thus suggesting a degenerative cause. These may involve a single system or multiple systems.

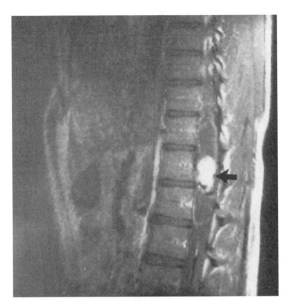

FIG. 16. Magnetic resonance image (lateral view) of the spinal cord showing a tumor *(arrow)* (hemangioblastoma of the thoracic cord).

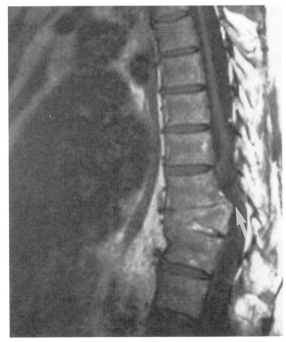

FIG. 17. Magnetic resonance image of the thoracic cord showing traumatic transection of the cord *(arrow)*.

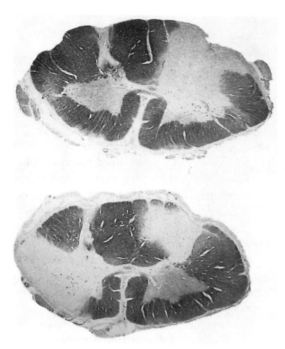

FIG. 18. Sections of the spinal cord showing multifocal areas of demyelination in a patient with multiple sclerosis.

Motor neuron diseases (amyotrophic lateral sclerosis or progressive muscular atrophy) are examples of diffuse single system disorders in the spinal cord. In motor neuron disease, there is progressive destruction of the motor neurons in the anterior horn of the spinal cord, with or without degeneration of the corticospinal tract (see Chapter 8).

However, not all diffuse, progressive system diseases of the spinal level (or elsewhere) are degenerative. *Combined system disease* is a motor and sensory system degeneration affecting the posterior and lateral columns that is due to vitamin B_{12} deficiency. The major pathologic change is that of demyelination of these regions. If the metabolic defect persists, the process becomes more severe, with axonal destruction and necrosis but little gliosis initially. In patients with long-duration progressive disease that is not treated, gliosis also develops. There is often peripheral nerve and cerebral involvement as well. These lesions result in the clinical pattern of a slowly pro-

gressive sensory ataxia, with upper motor neuron signs, some lower motor neuron signs (depressed ankle reflexes), paresthesia, and occasionally dementia. The disorder is also often associated with macrocytic anemia (pernicious anemia) that is also due to vitamin B_{12} deficiency (Fig. 19) The reclassification of this degenerative disease as a metabolic disorder due to a nutritional deficiency was a major medical advance. It can be hoped that other degenerative disorders seen in neurologic practice will soon have their causes determined in the same way, to permit appropriate treatment.

Spinal nerve lesions as described thus far have been lesions of single spinal nerves. There also may be diffuse involvement of spinal nerves in *polyradiculopathy*. Although polyradiculopathy may be difficult to recognize clinically, demonstrating the involvement of paraspinal muscles at multiple levels by electromyography is strong evidence of it. Proximal weakness, which is more commonly seen in muscle disease, may also occur in polyradiculopathy, but usually there are additional abnormalities such as reflex and sensory loss. One form of polyradiculopathy is Guillain-Barré syndrome, a subacute, inflammatory disorder that produces segmental demyelination predominantly in nerve roots.

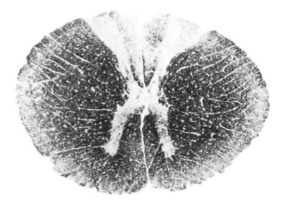

FIG. 19. Section of thoracic spinal cord showing demyelination of posterior columns secondary to pernicious anemia.

Clinical Problems ■

1. A 55-year-old man had an operation for carcinoma of the prostate 1 year ago. Six days ago, while watching TV after a big meal, he found that he was unable to walk when he tried to arise from the couch. There was no pain or trauma.

   On examination, mental status, cranial nerves, and upper extremities were normal. There was severe flaccid paralysis with hypotonia of the lower abdominal muscles, hip flexors, hip adductors, and knee extensors. There was moderate weakness of other muscles of the lower extremities but with some increase in tone (spastic). Reflexes were normal in the arms, absent at the abdomen and knees, and hyperactive at the ankles. He had Babinski's sign bilaterally and loss of sensation for pain and temperature over both lower extremities. Position, vibration, and two-point discrimination were normal. All findings were symmetric.
   a. What is the level, side, and type of lesion?
   b. What is the longitudinal and horizontal location of the lesion?
   c. Is the conus medullaris involved in the lesion?
   d. What type of bladder dysfunction would occur with lesions of the lumbar cord and sacral cord?
   e. What is the most likely cause?

2. A 60-year-old woman first noted numbness of all fingers of the right hand 2½ years ago. Clumsiness of the right hand developed shortly thereafter. Defective appreciation of temperature with the right hand had been noted 1½ years ago, and 7 months before her admission a similar numbness of all fingers of the left hand developed. At the same time, stiffness of both lower extremities was noted, accompanied by unsteadiness on rapid turning.

   On neurologic examination, mental status and cranial nerves were intact. Fasciculations and a minor degree of atrophy were present in muscles of both shoulders. Fasciculations were not present in the lower extremities. Strength was decreased bilaterally as follows: There was moderate weakness in shoulder abductors and elbow flexors and extensors. There was marked weakness of intrinsic hand muscles. The lower extremities had minimal weakness. Spasticity was noted on passive motion in the lower extremities and her gait was spastic. The triceps, quadriceps, and Achilles reflexes were increased bilaterally. Plantar responses were extensor bilaterally. Abdominal reflexes were absent. Pain and temperature were decreased at the C-4 to T-1 segments bilaterally, with total loss in her right hand and lower arm. In these segments, touch sensation was intact.
   a. What is the level and type of lesion?
   b. Which systems and which subdivisions of each are involved?
   c. Which cord segments are involved and at what horizontal location?
   d. What is the most likely cause?

3. A 52-year-old woman is hospitalized because of ataxia and mental symptoms. She is unable to give a history, but her husband relates that for the last 3 years she has complained of a pins-and-needles sensation in her feet and hands that gradually spread to her knees and elbows. For the last 18 months, she has had progressive gait ataxia and weakness of the legs. For about the same length of time, she has had mental symptoms. At first, she was irritable and uncooperative. At present, she has impaired memory, thinks her husband is trying to poison her, and is confused at night. She is also incontinent of urine and stool.

   On examination, she is demented and ataxic when she walks. Romberg's sign is present. Both legs are moderately and symmetrically weak. Tendon reflexes are normal in the arms and absent in the legs. Babinski's sign is present bilaterally. Position sense is impaired in her toes. Vibration sense is absent in her legs. Touch, pain, and temperature sensations are not significantly impaired. She has a bladder catheter in place.

  a. What is the location and type of lesion?

  b. Which sensory pathways are involved?

  c. Why are tendon reflexes absent and Babinski's sign present?

  d. What is one identifiable cause for certain neurologic disorders previously classified as degenerative diseases?

4. A 30-year-old man had acute onset of severe back and right leg pain after falling while carrying a sack of bagels. His symptoms have worsened over the 4 weeks since onset. On examination, there is slight hypalgesia on the lateral aspect of his leg. Reflexes are normal. There is mild weakness of hip abductors, hamstrings, ankle dorsiflexors, and toe extensors on the right. He experiences severe pain when he coughs or when his leg is elevated.

  a. What is the site and type of lesion?

  b. What neural structure is involved?

  c. In a patient with footdrop, at what sites could the lesion be located?

  d. What produces pain on straight leg raising?

Additional Reading

Burke, D. Spasticity as an adaptation to pyramidal tract injury. *Adv. Neurol.* 47:401, 1988.

Burke, R. E. Spinal cord: ventral horn. In Shepherd, G. M. (ed.), *The Synaptic Organization of the Brain* (4th ed.). New York: Oxford University Press, 1998, pp. 77–120.

Davidoff, R. A. Skeletal muscle tone and the misunderstood stretch reflex. *Neurology* 42:951, 1992.

Dietz, V. Human neuronal control of automatic functional movements: Interaction between central programs and afferent input. *Physiol. Rev.* 72:33, 1992.

Schoenen, J., and Faull, R. L. M. Spinal cord: Cytoarchitectural, dendroarchitectural, and myeloarchitectural organization. In Paxinos, C. (ed.), *The Human Nervous System.* San Diego: Academic Press, 1990, pp. 19–53.

Willis, W. D., Jr., and Coggeshall, R. E. *Sensory Mechanisms of the Spinal Cord* (3rd ed.). New York: Plenum Press, 1995.

Woolsey, R. M., and Young, R. R. The clinical diagnosis of disorders of the spinal cord. *Neurol. Clin.* 9:573, 1991.

The Posterior Fossa Level

Objectives ■

1. Name and identify the nuclei and peripheral portions of cranial nerves III through XII. Describe their functions, clinical examination, and the signs and symptoms that indicate their dysfunction.
2. Identify the major anatomical features of the medulla, pons, midbrain, and cerebellum as described in the text, and state their function.
3. Outline the physiologic and anatomical features of the auditory and vestibular systems, and identify the signs and symptoms of their dysfunction.
4. Describe the actions of the ocular muscles, the significance of diplopia, the anatomy of the pupillary light reflex, and the significance of nystagmus, the oculocephalic reflex (doll's eye phenomenon), and ptosis.
5. List the major herniations of the brain, and briefly describe their mechanisms of symptom production.

Introduction ■

The posterior fossa level contains all the structures located within the skull below the tentorium cerebelli and above the foramen magnum (Fig. 1). These structures are derivatives of the embryonic mesencephalon, metencephalon, and myelencephalon, and include portions of all the systems discussed earlier.

The major structures of this level are the brainstem (medulla, pons, and midbrain), the cerebellum, and segments of cranial nerves III through XII, before their emergence from the skull. The brainstem, the central core of the posterior fossa level, is a specialized rostral extension of the embryonic neural tube that preserves, even in the mature state, many of the longitudinal or intersegmental features found in the spinal cord and also provides for the segmental functions of the head.

This chapter describes the general features of each major longitudinal system as they relate to the posterior fossa level and discusses in further detail the cranial nerves and internal anatomy of the medulla, pons, midbrain, and cerebellum. Three additional systems (oculomotor, auditory, and vestibular) that are located primarily at this level are introduced and described.

Overview ■

The brainstem contains ascending and descending pathways traveling to the thalamus, hypothalamus, cerebral cortex, cerebellum, cranial nerve nuclei, and spinal cord. The main sensory pathways include those that originate in the spinal cord (the spinothalamic tracts, dorsal column–lemniscal system, and the spinocerebellar pathways), as well as those that arise from the cranial nerve nuclei (the descending tract of the trigeminal nerve, the trigeminothalamic tract, and the lateral lemnis-

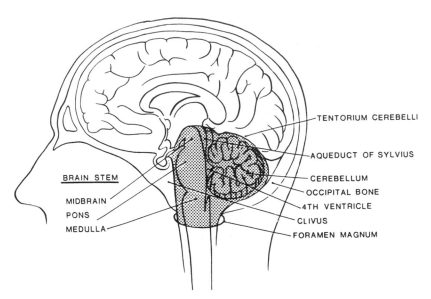

FIG. 1. The posterior fossa *(stippled area)* is bordered by the foramen magnum, tentorium cerebelli, clivus, and occipital bones.

cus). The main motor pathways include the direct activation pathways (the corticospinal and corticobulbar pathways) and the indirect activation pathways (reticulospinal, rubrospinal, and vestibulospinal pathways). Additional important intersegmental pathways found at this level include the medial longitudinal fasciculus, the ascending and descending fibers of the consciousness and internal regulation systems, and many of the structures of the oculomotor, auditory, and vestibular systems.

It is traditional to subdivide the brainstem into three parts: the medulla (derived from myelencephalon), which contains the motor neurons for swallowing, tongue movement, talking, and certain visceral motor functions; the pons (derived from metencephalon), which contains the nuclei associated with motor, sensory, and parasympathetic innervation of the face and abduction of the eye; and the midbrain (derived from mesencephalon), which contains the nuclei of the ascending reticular activating system, the nuclei that govern eye movements (except abduction), and the fibers involved in pupillary constriction and accommodation.

Although the tubular configuration of the central nervous system is greatly altered in the brainstem, the general relationships described above between systems developing in the inner tube region (primitive, indirect, diffuse) and the outer tube region (newer, direct, discrete) can still be discerned. The anatomical structure that typifies the former is the reticular formation, a complex group of nuclei and interconnections that extends throughout the core of the brainstem. In each of the three major subdivisions of the brainstem, the reticular formation is divided into medial, intermediate, and lateral zones. The relative importance of these zones and the functions they subserve differs at each level. The major functional components of the reticular formation are discussed in the following sections that deal with each of the subdivisions of the brainstem.

The brainstem has ten pairs of cranial nerves (Fig. 2), which perform segmental functions comparable to the functions of the spinal nerves. The portions of these nerves contained within the cranium are considered part of the posterior fossa level, and the segments distal to

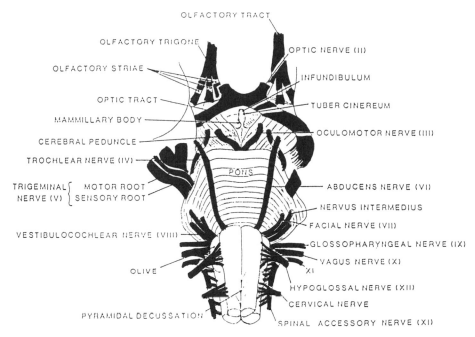

FIG. 2. Ventral (anterior) view of the brainstem showing the cranial nerves. (Only cranial nerves III through XII are at the posterior fossa level.)

the bones of the skull are considered part of the peripheral level. The location and general function of the cranial nerves at the posterior fossa level are summarized in Table 1.

The *cerebellum* (a derivative of metencephalon) lies dorsal to the pons and medulla and consists of a midline vermis and two lateral hemispheres. The cerebellum is functionally and anatomically divided into three lobes: the flocculonodular lobe, responsible for equilibration and balance; the anterior lobe, responsible for gait and posture; and the large

TABLE 1. *Location and general function of cranial nerves at the posterior fossa level*

Level	Cranial nerve	General function
Medulla	XII Hypoglossal	Motor to muscles of tongue
	XI Spinal accessory	Motor to sternocleidomastoid and trapezius muscles
	X Vagus	Motor to muscles of soft palate, pharynx, and larynx; parasympathetic fibers to thoracic and abdominal viscera; sensory fibers from pharynx and external auditory meatus; visceral sensory fibers from thoracic and abdominal cavities
	IX Glossopharyngeal	Motor to stylopharyngeus muscle; sensory from pharynx and tongue; taste from posterior tongue
Pons	VIII Vestibulocochlear	Hearing and equilibration
	VII Facial	Motor to muscles of facial expression; parasympathetic to salivary glands; taste from anterior tongue
	VI Abducens	Motor to lateral rectus muscle of eye
	V Trigeminal	Sensory from face; motor to muscles of mastication
Midbrain	IV Trochlear	Motor to superior oblique muscle of eye
	III Oculomotor	Motor to medial, superior, and inferior recti, and inferior oblique muscles of eye, and levator palpebrae of eyelid; parasympathetic to constrictors of pupil

posterior lobe, responsible for coordinated movements of the extremities.

The cerebrospinal fluid system is represented at the posterior fossa level by the aqueduct of Sylvius, the fourth ventricle, the meninges, the extraventricular subarachnoid cisterns, and the cerebrospinal fluid itself. The entire blood supply to the posterior fossa level is derived from the vertebrobasilar arterial system, which supplies paramedian arteries and short and long circumferential arteries to the brainstem and cerebellum. The major long circumferential arteries are the posterior inferior cerebellar arteries at the medullary level, the anterior inferior cerebellar arteries at the pontine level, and the superior cerebellar artery at the midbrain level.

The major components of three additional systems are also found at this level. The oculomotor system is represented by cranial nerve nuclei III, IV, and VI; their axons traveling toward the extraocular muscles; the medial longitudinal fasciculus; and the fibers for supranuclear control of eye movement descending from the cerebral cortex. The auditory system is represented by the auditory nerves, cochlear nuclei, trapezoid bodies, and multiple bilateral pathways that ascend to the inferior colliculi en route to the thalamus and temporal cortex. The vestibular system is represented by the vestibular nerves, vestibular nuclei, and their multiple connections with the cerebellum, spinal cord, medial longitudinal fasciculus, and structures at the supratentorial level.

Lesions can be localized precisely at the posterior fossa level when there is a combination of intersegmental and segmental involvement. Lesions at the posterior fossa level are unique in that unilateral brainstem lesions may produce involvement of the ipsilateral side of the face and the contralateral side of the body. Other types of neurologic dysfunction that help localize a lesion at the posterior fossa level are disturbances of cerebellar function or involvement of the intracranial portions of cranial nerves III through XII.

General Anatomy of the Posterior Fossa Level

Posterior Cranial Fossa and Tentorium

The posterior cranial fossa is formed by the occipital bones at the base of the skull and the temporal bones anteriorly and laterally (Fig. 3). The inferior limit of the posterior fossa is the foramen magnum, where the cervical cord merges with the medulla. The rostral limit of the posterior fossa is the tentorium cerebelli, which lies between the cerebellum and the occipital lobe. The tentorium is attached posteriorly and posterolaterally to the transverse sinus and anterolaterally to the petrous ridge. The anterior border is not attached to bone but forms the tentorial notch, through which the midbrain passes to merge with the diencephalon.

Systems Contained in the Posterior Fossa Level

The neural structures of the posterior fossa level consist of cranial nerves III through XII, midbrain, pons, medulla, and cerebellum. Each of the previously studied systems is represented at the posterior fossa level.

The Cerebrospinal Fluid System

Cerebrospinal fluid flows into the posterior fossa through the *aqueduct of Sylvius,* a narrow canal in the midbrain between the third and fourth ventricles. The fourth ventricle is located at the level of the medulla and pons, which form the ventricular floor. The roof of the fourth ventricle is the ventral midline portion of the cerebellum. Cerebrospinal fluid leaves the fourth ventricle through the foramen of Magendie (at the caudal end of the ventricle) and through the two foramina of Luschka (at each lateral angle of the ventricle) to enter the subarachnoid space, where it circulates through the cisterna magna, cerebellopontine, prepontine, interpeduncular, and ambient cisterns.

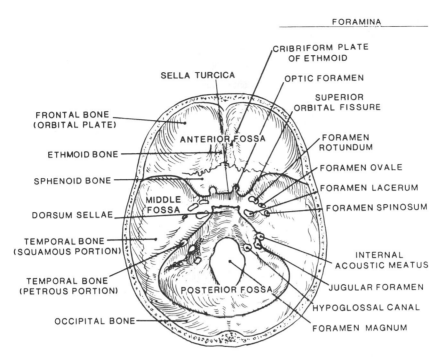

FORAMINA

CRIBRIFORM PLATE
OF ETHMOID

OPTIC FORAMEN

SELLA TURCICA

SUPERIOR
ORBITAL FISSURE

FRONTAL BONE
(ORBITAL PLATE)

ANTERIOR FOSSA

FORAMEN
ROTUNDUM

ETHMOID BONE

FORAMEN OVALE

SPHENOID BONE

FORAMEN LACERUM

MIDDLE
FOSSA

FORAMEN SPINOSUM

DORSUM SELLAE

TEMPORAL BONE
(SQUAMOUS PORTION)

INTERNAL
ACOUSTIC MEATUS

TEMPORAL BONE
(PETROUS PORTION)

JUGULAR FORAMEN

POSTERIOR FOSSA

HYPOGLOSSAL CANAL

OCCIPITAL BONE

FORAMEN MAGNUM

FIG. 3. Base of the skull with major bones and foramina.

The Sensory System

The brainstem contains ascending pathways mediating (1) pain and temperature (spinothalamic), (2) conscious proprioception and discriminative sensation (dorsal column–lemniscal), (3) unconscious proprioception (ventral and dorsal spinocerebellar), and (4) touch (spinothalamic and dorsal column–lemniscal). In addition, sensory input from the face and head enters at this level.

The Consciousness System

The central core of the brainstem contains the reticular formation and its ascending projection pathways. The brainstem, along with other areas of the nervous system, thus serves the important function of mediating consciousness, attention, and the wake-sleep cycle.

The Motor System

All subdivisions of the motor system are represented at the posterior fossa level. The lower motor neurons of several of the cranial nerves contain the final common pathway to muscles of the head and neck. The direct activation pathways are represented by the corticospinal tracts, which descend through the brainstem and decussate at the lower medulla en route to the spinal cord, and the corticobulbar pathways, which provide supranuclear innervation to brainstem motor nuclei. The indirect activation pathways in the brainstem consist of short multineuronal descending pathways of the reticulospinal, rubrospinal, and vestibulospinal tracts arising in the brainstem. Much of the cerebellar control circuit is located at this level, and portions of the basal ganglia control circuit (substantia nigra and red nucleus) are present in the midbrain.

Internal Regulation System

The posterior fossa contains visceral sensory relay nuclei (particularly the nucleus of the tractus solitarius), the reticular formation, and preganglionic parasympathetic neurons.

The intermediate zone of the medullary reticular formation contains interneurons and neurons that project to preganglionic sympathetic neurons and to spinal motor neurons controlling respiration. The lateral zone contains the central pattern generator that integrates complex motor patterns involving multiple cranial nerves to produce such actions as swallowing and vomiting. In addition to the reticular formation and the ascending and descending pathways that regulate visceral function, the posterior fossa level contains the preganglionic parasympathetic fibers carried in cranial nerves III, VII, IX, and X.

The Vascular System

The structures in the posterior fossa receive their blood supply from the vertebrobasilar arterial system (Fig. 4). The vertebral arteries enter the cranial cavity through the foramen magnum and then course rostrally along the ventrolateral surface of the medulla, where they give off branches to form the anterior spinal artery, which descends on the ventral aspect of the lower medulla to the cervical spinal cord. At the level of the pons, the two vertebral arteries merge to form the basilar artery, which continues rostrally to the upper midbrain level, where it branches to form the posterior cerebral arteries.

Branches of the vertebral and basilar arteries are subdivided into three groups that supply each level of the brainstem and the cerebellum. The paramedian zone on either side of the midline is supplied by paramedian branches, the *intermediate zone* is supplied by short circumferential branches, and the lateral zone is supplied by long circumferential branches (Fig. 5). The *paramedian* and *lateral*

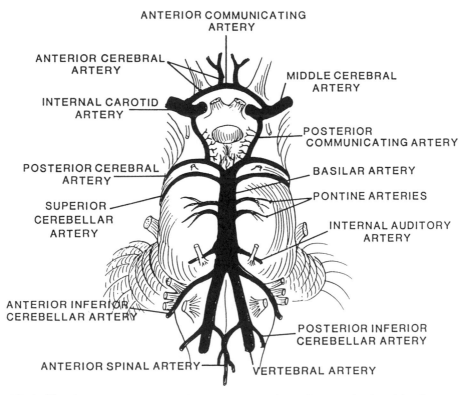

FIG. 4. Blood supply of posterior fossa structures from the vertebral and basilar arteries.

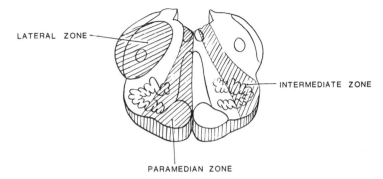

FIG. 5. Blood supply of the medulla. The lateral zone is from the posterior inferior cerebellar artery, the paramedian zone is from the anterior spinal artery, and the intermediate zone is from the vertebral artery.

zones are often involved by vascular lesions, with significant clinical deficit. The paramedian area of the medulla is supplied by paramedian branches of the anterior spinal artery, and the intermediate zone is supplied by the vertebral arteries. The paramedian areas of the pons and midbrain are supplied by the paramedian branches of the basilar artery. The lateral areas of the brainstem are supplied by three pairs of long circumferential arteries: the *posterior inferior cerebellar artery,* a branch of the vertebral artery that supplies the lateral area of the medulla and the posterior inferior aspect of the cerebellum; the *anterior inferior cerebellar artery,* a branch of the basilar artery that supplies the lateral area of the pons and the anterior inferior aspect of the cerebellum; and the *superior cerebellar artery,* a branch of the basilar artery that supplies the lateral area of the midbrain and the superior surface of the cerebellum.

Three additional special systems are found primarily at the posterior fossa level: (1) the oculomotor system, which mediates eye movement; (2) the auditory system, which mediates hearing; and (3) the vestibular system, which mediates balance and equilibrium.

Embryologic Organization of the Brainstem

The primitive neural tube displays an anatomical organization similar to that of the spinal cord, with functional areas for sensation (alar plate) and motor activity (basal plate) separated by the sulcus limitans. Within these sensory and motor areas, the brainstem is divided further into somatic and visceral regions (Fig. 6). This organizational framework

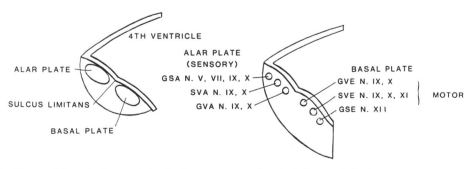

FIG. 6. Alar and basal plates of the brainstem at the level of the medulla in a 5-week *(left)* and 10-week *(right)* embryo (see Table 2).

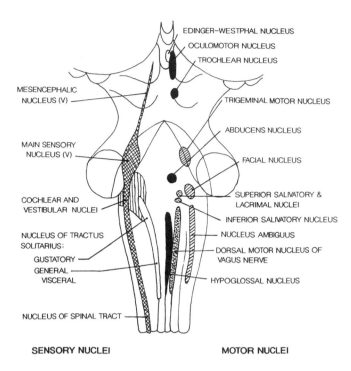

FIG. 7. Location of cell columns in the brainstem. Sensory nuclei are shown on the *left* and motor nuclei on the *right*.

is grafted onto the concepts developed above that relate older, more diffuse pathways to the inner tube of the brainstem and newer, more direct, and discrete pathways to the outer tube of the brainstem.

These functional divisions exist as rostrocaudal cell columns from which cranial nerve nuclei are derived. Some cranial nerves contain components from more than one of these columns. The appearance of new structures in the brainstem and the enlargement of the embryonic neural canal into the fourth ventricle displace some of these nuclear columns from their embryonic position. The location of the cell columns in the adult brainstem and the cranial nerves arising from each is shown in Fig. 7. These functionally oriented cell columns provide an important framework for learning the intrinsic anatomy of each of the major subdivisions of the posterior fossa. The components of each of these cell columns, found in each of the cranial nerves, are listed in Table 2.

TABLE 2. *Components of the cranial nerves*

Component	Function	Cranial nerve
Efferent	Motor	
General somatic efferent (GSE)	Somatic striated muscles	III, IV, VI, XII
General visceral efferent (GVE)	Parasympathetic glands and smooth muscles	III, VII, IX, X
Special visceral efferent (SVE)	Branchial arch muscles	V, VII, IX, X, XI
Afferent	Sensory	
General somatic afferent (GSA)	Somatesthetic senses	V, IX, X
Special somatic afferent (SSA)	Vision, hearing, and balance	II, VIII
General visceral afferent (GVA)	Pharynx and viscera	IX, X
Special visceral afferent (SVA)	Smell, taste	I, VII, IX, X

The Medulla

The medulla oblongata is that portion of the brainstem extending from the level of the foramen magnum to the caudal border of the base of the pons. Many of the features of the medulla are similar to those of the spinal cord (Fig. 8). The major ascending and descending pathways present in the spinal cord are also present in this area; however, there are several important changes that occur in this region, including (1) the location of the corticospinal tracts in the ventromedial portion of the medulla (the medullary pyramids), (2) the termination of the fasciculus gracilis and cuneatus in their respective nuclei and the subsequent course of the second-order neurons in the *medial lemniscus*, (3) the replacement of the zone of Lissauer by the *descending tract of the trigeminal nerve*, (4) the replacement of the central gray portion of the spinal cord by the reticular formation, (5) the entrance of the dorsal spinocerebellar tracts into the inferior cerebellar peduncle, and (6) the replacement of the central canal of the spinal cord by the fourth ventricle.

Anatomical Features

Additional important anatomical features of the medulla include the following:

Decussation of the Pyramids

At the lower end of the medulla, most of the fibers in the descending corticospinal pathways cross to the opposite side of the brainstem before descending in the spinal cord as the lateral corticospinal tracts (Fig. 8).

Decussation of the Medial Lemniscus

In the caudal medulla rostral to the pyramidal decussation, second-order axons originating from the nucleus gracilis and cuneatus sweep ventromedially around the central gray matter as the *internal arcuate fibers*. These fibers then cross the midline to the opposite side and continue rostrally as the medial lemniscus (Fig. 9).

Inferior Olivary Nuclei

The convoluted bands of the cells located in the ventrolateral portion of the medulla are the inferior olivary nuclei, which receive fibers from the dentate nucleus of the cerebellum, red nuclei, basal ganglia, and cerebral cortex. Axons from the inferior olivary nuclei form the olivocerebellar tract, which travels through the inferior cerebellar peduncle to the opposite cerebellar hemisphere. The inferior olive is a major relay station in the cerebellar pathways. It provides tonic cerebellar support for reflex movements and triggers phasic motor programs in the cerebellum.

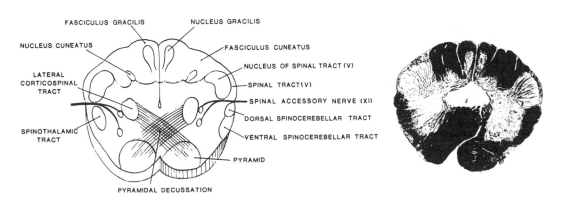

FIG. 8. Cross section of caudal medulla at the decussation of the pyramids. Myelin-stained section on the *right*.

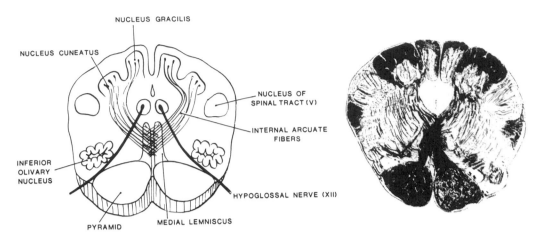

FIG. 9. Cross section of caudal medulla at the decussation of the medial lemnisci. Myelin-stained section on the *right*.

Medial Longitudinal Fasciculus

This fiber tract is located in the paramedian regions of the brainstem dorsal to the medial lemniscus (Fig. 10). The medial longitudinal fasciculus extends rostrally from the cervical cord to the upper midbrain level and transmits information for the coordination of head and eye movements.

Inferior Cerebellar Peduncle (Restiform Body)

The inferior cerebellar peduncle is one of the three major connections between the cere-

bellum and brainstem. It is located in the dorsolateral portion of the medulla and contains dorsal spinocerebellar, olivocerebellar, vestibulocerebellar, and reticulocerebellar fibers as well as cerebellovestibular fibers (Fig. 10).

Hypoglossal Nerve (Cranial Nerve XII)

Function

The hypoglossal nerve supplies motor innervation to the intrinsic muscles of the tongue. It is a motor nerve whose nucleus is part of the general somatic efferent (GSE) group of cranial nerve nuclei.

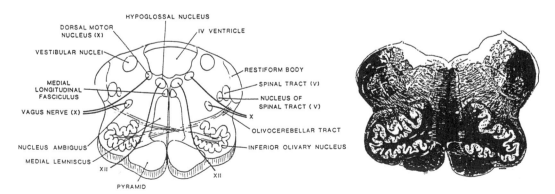

FIG. 10. Cross section of middle medulla at the origin of the hypoglossal and vagus nerves. Myelin-stained section on the *right*.

Anatomy

The hypoglossal nucleus is located in the paramedian area of the caudal medulla in the floor of the fourth ventricle (Figs. 9 and 10). The fibers course ventrally and exit from the ventral aspect of the medulla, between the medullary pyramids and the olive. After exiting from the brainstem, the fibers pass through the hypoglossal canal in the occipital condyle and innervate the striated muscles of the tongue (Fig. 11).

Pathophysiology

Diseases involving the hypoglossal nucleus or cranial nerve XII are associated with atrophy, paresis, and fasciculations of tongue muscles. Unilateral weakness causes the tongue to deviate toward the side of the weakness on protrusion of the tongue. Involvement of upper motor neuron pathways innervating the hypoglossal nuclei produces slowing of alternating movements of the tongue and weakness, without atrophy. The structure and function of the hypoglossal nerve are summarized in Table 3.

Spinal Accessory Nerve (Cranial Nerve XI)

Function

The spinal accessory nerve is a motor nerve that innervates the sternocleidomastoid and trapezius muscles. It is a special visceral efferent (SVE) nerve innervating striated muscles derived from branchial arches.

Anatomy

Cranial nerve XI arises mainly from cell bodies in the ventral gray horn of the upper five cervical cord segments (Fig. 12). The nerve ascends in the spinal canal lateral to the spinal cord, enters the skull through the foramen magnum, where it is joined by the minor accessory component that originates in the nucleus ambiguus, and leaves the cranial cavity via the jugular foramen to innervate the sternocleidomastoid and trapezius muscles. The accessory component passes to the vagus nerve below the jugular foramen and innervates the larynx and pharynx.

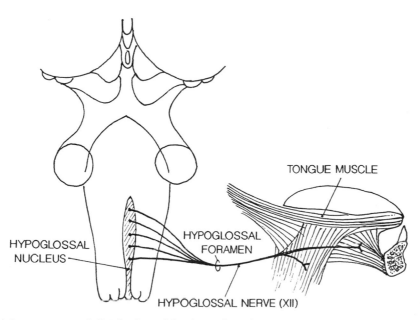

FIG. 11. Origin, course, and distribution of the hypoglossal nerve.

TABLE 3. *Structure and function of the hypoglossal nerve*

Component	Function	Nucleus of origin or termination	Ganglion	Foramen	Signs of dysfunction
GSE	Motor innervation of tongue	Hypoglossal		Hypoglossal	Weakness of tongue movement

GSE, general somatic efferent.

Pathophysiology

The spinal accessory nerve may be compressed by lesions in the region of the foramen magnum (where the nerve enters the skull) or in the region of the jugular foramen as it exits from the skull. Signs of dysfunction of cranial nerve XI include weakness of head rotation (sternocleidomastoid muscle) and inability to elevate or shrug the shoulder (trapezius muscle) on the side of the lesion. The sternocleidomastoid muscle rotates the face to the opposite side so that damage to the spinal accessory nerve results in weakness in turning the head toward the side contralateral to the lesion. The structure and function of the spinal accessory nerve are summarized in Table 4.

Vagus Nerve (Cranial Nerve X)

Function

The vagus nerve is a mixed nerve with SVE, general visceral efferent (GVE), general somatic afferent (GSA), general visceral afferent (GVA), and special visceral afferent (SVA) functions. The functions of cranial nerve X are innervation of the striated muscles of the soft palate, pharynx, and larynx derived from branchial arches (SVE); parasympathetic innervation of the thoracic

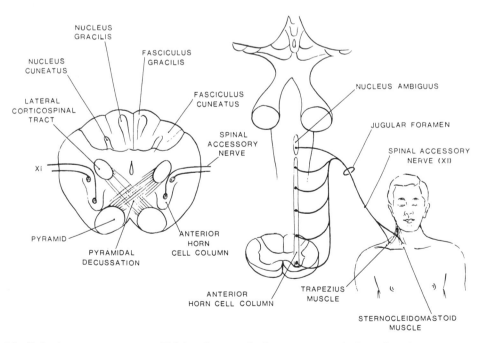

FIG. 12. Spinal accessory nerve. Origin of axons in the upper cervical cord and their course to the trapezius and sternocleidomastoid muscles are shown on the *right*. Nuclei of origin in the medulla are shown in the cross section on the *left*.

TABLE 4. *Structure and function of the spinal accessory nerve*

Component	Function	Nucleus of origin or termination	Ganglion	Foramen	Signs of dysfunction
SVE					
Spinal	Motor to sternocleidomastoid and trapezius muscles	Anterior horn cells of cervical cord		Jugular	Weakness and head rotation and shoulder elevation
Bulbar	Motor to pharyngeal and laryngeal muscles	Nucleus ambiguus		Jugular	Joins vagus below jugular foramen (see Table 5)

SVE, special visceral efferent.

and abdominal viscera (GVE); sensory innervation of the external auditory meatus (GSA); sensory innervation of the pharynx, larynx, and thoracic and abdominal viscera (GVA); and innervation of taste receptors on the posterior pharynx (SVA).

Anatomy

The SVE fibers of the vagus nerve innervating the striated muscles of the soft palate, pharynx, and larynx arise from the *nucleus ambiguus* located in the lateral medullary region dorsal to the inferior olive (Fig. 13). The GVE components of the vagus nerve contain preganglionic parasympathetic fibers arising in the *dorsal motor nucleus* to supply the thoracic and abdominal viscera. Preganglionic vagal neurons innervating the heart are located in the area of the nucleus ambiguus. These preganglionic fibers synapse with postganglionic neurons in the cardiac, pulmonary, esophageal, or celiac plexuses or within the visceral organs themselves.

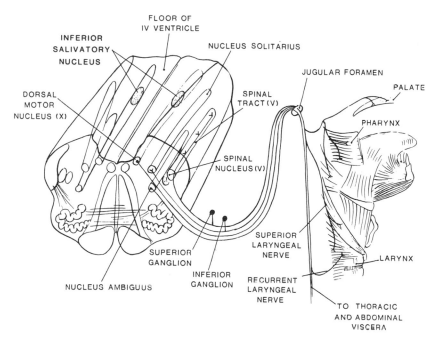

FIG. 13. Motor and sensory nuclei of the vagus nerve in the medulla and the course and distribution of some of its SVE fibers.

The afferent fibers carried in the vagus nerve arise from three different sources: (1) GSA fibers carrying general sensation from the external auditory meatus have their cell bodies in the *superior (jugular) ganglion,* and central processes from this ganglion enter the medulla with the vagus and terminate in the spinal nucleus of the trigeminal nerve; (2) GVA fibers carrying information from abdominal and thoracic viscera have their cell bodies in the *inferior (nodose) ganglion,* and the central processes terminate in the *nucleus of the tractus solitarius;* and (3) SVA fibers in the vagus nerve carrying taste from the posterior pharynx also have their cell bodies located in the *inferior (nodose) ganglion,* and the central processes terminate in the nucleus of the tractus solitarius.

The vagus nerve emerges from the lateral aspect of the medulla, dorsal to the olives, and leaves the skull through the jugular foramen. The superior and inferior ganglia of the vagus nerve are located in (or just below) the jugular foramen. The vagus nerve then passes down the neck near the carotid artery and the jugular vein. At the base of the neck, the vagus nerve passes in front of the subclavian artery. At this point on the right side, the right vagus nerve gives off the *right recurrent laryngeal nerve,* which loops below and behind the subclavian artery and runs upward to the larynx to innervate most of the laryngeal muscles on the right side. On the left side, the vagus nerve descends in front of the arch of the aorta and gives off the *left recurrent laryngeal nerve,* which loops under the arch of the aorta and then runs upward to the larynx to provide innervation of most of the laryngeal muscles on the left side. After giving off the recurrent laryngeal nerves, the vagus nerve descends into the thoracic and abdominal cavities to supply the esophagus, heart, lungs, and abdominal viscera.

Pathophysiology

Because of the dual innervation of many viscera and their ability to function within certain limits independently of innervation, unilateral disease processes that involve the vagus nerve do not produce symptoms involving the viscera. Instead, the neurologic signs usually consist of weakness of the striated muscles of the larynx and pharynx and difficulty in swallowing and speaking. Injury to the recurrent laryngeal nerves results in vocal cord paresis and a hoarse voice. The structure and function of cranial nerve X are summarized in Table 5.

Glossopharyngeal Nerve (Cranial Nerve IX)

Function

The glossopharyngeal nerve is also a mixed nerve, with SVE, GVE, GSA, GVA, and SVA

TABLE 5. *Structure and function of the vagus nerve*

Component	Function	Nucleus of origin or termination	Ganglion	Foramen	Signs of dysfunction
SVE	Motor to muscles of soft palate, pharynx, and larynx	Nucleus ambiguus		Jugular	Hoarseness, dysphagia, decreased gag reflex
GVE	Parasympathetic to thoracic and abdominal viscera	Dorsal motor nucleus of nerve X		Jugular	Visceral disturbance, tachycardia
GSA	Sensation: external auditory meatus	Spinal nucleus of nerve V	Superior (jugular)	Jugular	Decreased sensation: external auditory meatus
GVA	Sensation: pharynx, larynx, and thoracic and abdominal viscera	Nucleus of tractus solitarius	Inferior (nodose)	Jugular	Decreased sensation: pharynx
SVA	Taste: posterior pharynx	Nucleus of tractus solitarius	Inferior (nodose)	Jugular	Not clinically significant

See Table 2 for definition of abbreviations.

components. The functions of cranial nerve IX are innervation of the stylopharyngeus muscle of the pharynx (SVE); parasympathetic innervation of the parotid gland (GVE); sensory innervation of the back of the ear (GSA); sensory innervation of the pharynx, tongue, eustachian tube, carotid body, and carotid sinus (GVA); and innervation of taste receptors on the posterior one-third of the tongue (SVA).

Anatomy

The SVE fibers to the stylopharyngeus muscle originate in the nucleus ambiguus (Fig. 14). The GVE components of the glossopharyngeal nerve carry preganglionic parasympathetic fibers that arise in the inferior salivatory nucleus and terminate in the otic ganglion. Postganglionic fibers from this ganglion supply the parotid salivary gland; stimulation increases salivary flow.

The afferent fibers carried in the glossopharyngeal nerve arise from three sources: (1) GSA fibers, carrying general sensation from behind the ear, have their cell bodies in the superior ganglion; their central processes terminate in the spinal nucleus of the trigeminal nerve; (2) GVA fibers carrying sensation from the pharynx; and (3) SVA fibers carrying taste sensation from the posterior tongue. The latter two arise from cell bodies in the inferior (petrosal) ganglion and have central processes that terminate in the nucleus of the tractus solitarius. Within the medulla, there are segmental reflex connections between the pharyngeal sensory fibers and the motor neurons supplying the muscles of the pharynx to mediate the gag reflex.

The glossopharyngeal nerve emerges from the medulla, dorsal to the inferior olivary nuclei, and passes through the jugular foramen (which is also the location of its ganglia) to innervate peripheral structures. The components and structure of the glossopharyngeal nerve are thus similar to those of the vagus (Table 6).

Pathophysiology

Isolated lesions of the glossopharyngeal nerve are rare but, with or without vagus

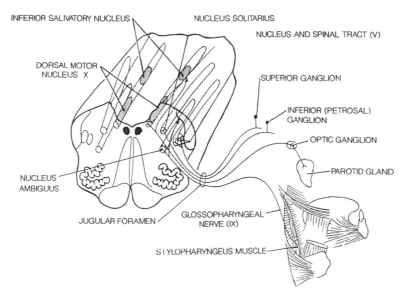

FIG. 14. Motor and sensory nuclei of the glossopharyngeal nerve in the medulla and the course and distribution of SVE fibers to the stylopharyngeus muscle and GVE fibers to the parotid gland.

TABLE 6. *Structure and function of the glossopharyngeal nerve*

Component	Function	Nucleus of origin or termination	Ganglion	Foramen	Signs of dysfunction
SVE	Motor to stylopharyngeus muscle	Nucleus ambiguus		Jugular	Not clinically significant
GVE	Parasympathetic to parotid gland	Inferior salivatory nucleus	Otic	Jugular	Decreased salivation
GSA	Sensation: back of ear	Spinal nucleus of nerve V	Superior	Jugular	Decreased sensation: back of ear
GVA	Sensation: pharynx, tongue, carotid receptors	Nucleus of tractus solitarius	Inferior (petrosal)	Jugular	Decreased gag reflex
SVA	Taste: posterior one-third of tongue	Nucleus of tractus solitarius	Inferior (petrosal)	Jugular	Decreased taste

See Table 2 for definition of abbreviations.

damage, result in loss of pharyngeal sensation and of the gag reflex. Occasionally, lesions give rise to a paroxysmal pain syndrome of unknown cause (*glossopharyngeal neuralgia*). In this disorder, the patient experiences brief attacks of severe pain that usually begin in the throat and radiate down the side of the neck in front of the ear and to the back of the lower jaw. On occasion, the pain may begin deep in the ear. Attacks of discomfort may be precipitated by swallowing or protrusion of the tongue.

Reticular Formation

The reticular formation of the medulla occupies much of the core area, in which it is dispersed among the tracts and nuclei described above. This location reflects its primitive, indirect, diffuse organization as opposed to the phylogenetically newer direct, discrete motor and sensory pathways occupying the ventral and lateral surfaces of the medulla. In transverse (transaxial) sections, the medullary reticular formation can be divided into three zones: medial, intermediate, and lateral. The medial zone projects to spinal motor neurons, predominantly via the ipsilateral lateral reticulospinal tract (an indirect activation pathway). The intermediate zone projects to preganglionic sympathetic neurons in the spinal cord to influence vasomotor tone. It also projects to spinal motor neurons supplying respiratory muscles and is one of several brainstem centers involved in control of respiration. The lateral zone contains the central pattern generator concerned with coordination of complex reflexes involving multiple cranial nerves important in swallowing and vomiting.

Vomiting

Vomiting is a complex stereotyped motor behavior integrated at the level of the medulla; it involves coordinated activation of neurons controlling gastrointestinal, respiratory, upper airway, and postural muscles. The neuronal network coordinating vomiting is located in the dorsolateral reticular formation of the medulla and has connections with the area postrema, nucleus of the tractus solitarius, nucleus ambiguus, dorsal motor nucleus of the vagus, and respiratory neurons. These neuronal networks in the dorsolateral medullary reticular formation, referred to as *central pattern generators,* can be involved in more than one physiologic function, including breathing and vomiting as well as coughing and sneezing. Vomiting is primarily the result of changes in intraabdominal and intrathoracic pressures generated by synergistic activation of the diaphragm (inspiratory) and abdominal (expiratory) muscles. Relaxation of the stomach and retrograde contraction of the proximal small intestine serve as a buffer to dilute the acidic contents of the stomach before it passes through the esophagus and mouth. Vomiting can be triggered by input to the vomiting center from the gut, oral cavity, blood, vestibular system, and higher brain centers. Vagal afferents detect emetic stimuli in the gut, including stimuli that activate mechanoreceptors and chemoreceptors in the distal stomach and proximal small intestine. These vagal afferents project primarily to the nucleus of the tractus solitarius and the area postrema. The *area postrema,* located in the walls of the fourth ventricle, lacks the blood–brain barrier and functions as a *chemoreceptor trigger zone.* Its neurons detect emetic substances in the blood and cerebrospinal fluid. Antineoplastic drugs and dopamine agonists activate the area postrema, and this is the basis for the vomiting induced by these agents. Posterior fossa lesions, particularly neoplasms involving the dorsal medulla, may present with vomiting, even in the absence of signs of increased intracranial pressure.

Clinical Correlations: Medulla and Lower Cranial Nerves

Jugular Foramen Syndrome

Cranial nerves IX, X, and XI leave the skull with the jugular vein through the jugular foramen (Fig. 15). A lesion (usually a mass lesion) in or adjacent to the jugular foramen may affect all three cranial nerves and cause ipsilateral weakness of the pharyngeal and laryngeal muscles (nerve X), decreased sensation of the ipsilateral pharynx (nerve IX), and weakness of the ipsilateral trapezius and sternocleidomastoid muscles (nerve XI). One cause of this syndrome is chemodectoma arising in chemoreceptors along the jugular vein.

Bulbar and Pseudobulbar Palsy

Dysfunction of the motor components of the cranial nerves of the lower portion of the brainstem (particularly the medulla, or "bulb") occurs with either upper or lower mo-

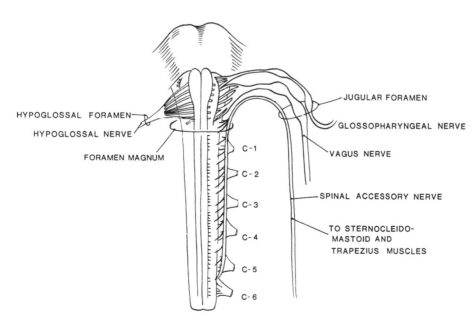

FIG. 15. Ventral view of the medulla and cranial nerves IX, X, and XI exiting together through the jugular foramen. Spinal roots of C-1 through C-6 in the upper cervical spinal cord are also shown.

tor neuron lesions. Lesions affecting lower motor neurons (final common pathway) produce *bulbar palsy,* which is manifested as flaccid weakness of the muscles associated with talking, chewing, swallowing, and movement of the tongue and lips. Supranuclear lesions, involving cortical or subcortical components of the direct or indirect activation pathways, produce upper motor neuron dysfunction of the bulbar musculature, manifested as slow movements and a harsh, strained speech pattern. Because most bulbar motor nuclei receive bilateral cortical innervation, unilateral supranuclear lesions do not usually produce significant bulbar dysfunction. However, bilateral supranuclear lesions result in severe paresis of bulbar muscles characterized by spastic weakness with dysarthria, dysphagia, and reduced mouth and tongue movements. This involvement of bulbar function by bilateral supranuclear lesions is called *pseudobulbar palsy.*

The Pons

The pons is that portion of the brainstem bounded ventrally by the rostral and caudal borders of the basis pontis (see Fig. 2). In transaxial sections, it is divided into two general areas. The ventral area is called the *basis pontis,* formed by transversely oriented crossing (pontocerebellar) fibers of the middle cerebellar peduncle and bundles of rostrocaudally running fibers of the corticospinal, corticobulbar, and corticopontine tracts. Small collections of neurons, the *pontine nuclei,* are dispersed in the basis pontis and are the origin of the axons that make up the *pontocerebellar fibers* that congregate laterally as the *middle cerebellar peduncle.*

The area of the pons dorsal to the basis pontis and ventral to the fourth ventricle is the *tegmentum,* within which are the spinothalamic tracts, medial lemnisci, and the medial longitudinal fasciculi. The reticular formation and the pathways related to the consciousness and internal regulation systems are concentrated in the core of the pontine tegmentum. The tegmentum also contains structures related to the following cranial nerves: acoustic and vestibular divisions of cranial nerve VIII, facial (cranial nerve VII), abducens (cranial nerve VI), and trigeminal (cranial nerve V). The location of many of these structures is shown in Fig. 16.

Auditory Nerve (Cranial Nerve VIII)

Cranial nerve VIII (also called the auditory, vestibulocochlear, or statoacoustic nerve) is made up of two divisions: one mediates hearing, and the other mediates vestibular input.

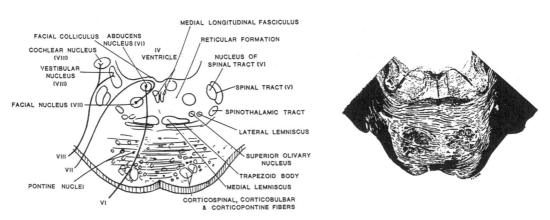

FIG. 16. Cross section of caudal pons at the level of cranial nerves VI and VII. Myelin-stained section on the *right.*

Because they are grossly inseparable in their course from the brainstem to the *internal auditory meatus,* they traditionally are considered a single nerve (Fig. 17). However, these two divisions represent the peripheral connections of two functionally distinct subsystems of the sensory system and have separate peripheral receptors and central connections and pathways. Therefore, the two divisions are discussed separately.

Acoustic Division of Cranial Nerve VIII

Function

The acoustic division of cranial nerve VIII is an afferent nerve that conducts impulses from the inner ear structures related to hearing. Hearing is a special somatic afferent (SSA) function.

Anatomy

Fibers in this division of cranial nerve VIII arise from cell bodies in the *spiral ganglion* of

the cochlea in the inner ear (Fig. 17). The nerve, composed of the central axons of these first-order neurons, enters the dorsolateral medulla at the pontomedullary junction. The axons bifurcate on entering the brainstem and synapse in both the *dorsal* and *ventral cochlear nuclei* located at that level. The subarachnoid space from the internal auditory meatus to the dorsolateral medulla, through which cranial nerve VIII courses, is bordered by the base of the pons and the ventral surface of the cerebellar hemisphere and is called the *cerebellopontine angle cistern.* Pathways arising from the cochlear nuclei relay auditory information through the brainstem to the medial geniculate body of the thalamus bilaterally and from there to the auditory cortex of the temporal lobes (see The Auditory System, below).

Pathophysiology

Lesions of the acoustic division of cranial nerve VIII produce unilateral loss of hearing. The physiology and pathophysiology of hear-

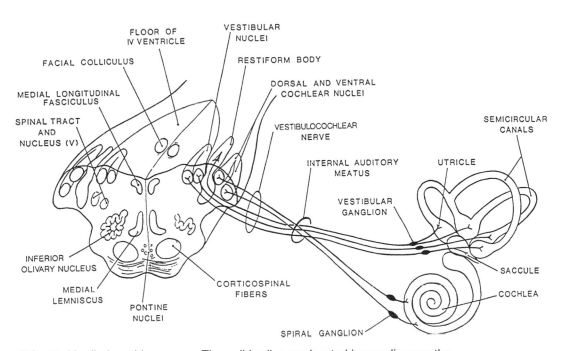

FIG. 17. Vestibulocochlear nerve. The cell bodies are located in ganglia near the cochlea and semicircular canals, with primary afferent terminations in lateral pons.

ing are discussed below (see The Auditory System). The structure and function of the auditory division of cranial nerve VIII are summarized in Table 7.

Vestibular Division of Cranial Nerve VIII

Function

The vestibular division of cranial nerve VIII is an afferent nerve that conducts gravitational and rotational information from the inner ear. This information is necessary for maintaining proper balance and equilibrium, which are SSA functions.

Anatomy

Fibers in this division of cranial nerve VIII arise from bipolar cells in the *vestibular (Scarpa's) ganglion* located in the internal auditory canal. The peripheral axons of these ganglion cells innervate sensory receptors located in the organs of balance (utricle, saccule, and semicircular canals) in the inner ear. Their central axons travel to the brainstem with the auditory division of nerve VIII and synapse in the vestibular nuclei located beneath the floor of the fourth ventricle in the rostral medulla and caudal pons (Fig. 17). Pathways arising from the vestibular nuclei conduct information to the cerebellum, spinal cord, reticular formation, and, via the medial longitudinal fasciculus, to the nuclei of cranial nerves III, IV, and VI (see The Vestibular System, below).

Pathophysiology

Lesions of the vestibular division of cranial nerve VIII cause the sensation of vertigo (hallucination of rotatory movement) or dysequilibrium. The physiology and pathophysiology of equilibrium are discussed below (see The Vestibular System). The structure and function of the vestibular division of cranial nerve VIII are summarized in Table 8.

Facial Nerve (Cranial Nerve VII)

Function

The facial nerve innervates the muscles of facial expression, which are derived from branchial arch mesoderm. This is the SVE component of the nerve. The facial nerve also has a GVE component, consisting of parasympathetic fibers to the lacrimal, submaxillary, and submandibular glands, and an SVA component that innervates taste receptors on the anterior two-thirds of the tongue.

Anatomy

The SVE fibers innervating the striated muscles of the face arise in the *facial nucleus* located in the lateral tegmentum of the pons (Figs. 16 and 18). Axons from this nucleus first course medially and then arch dorsally, forming a loop, or genu, around the abducens nucleus before proceeding to the lateral surface of the caudal pons, where they emerge medial to cranial nerve VIII. The looping of the facial nerve fibers around the abducens nucleus causes a slight bulge, called the *facial colliculus*, on each side of the midline in the floor of the fourth ventricle.

As the facial nerve leaves the pons, two separate nerve roots are apparent: the larger division carries the SVE component supply-

TABLE 7. *Structure and function of the acoustic division of cranial nerve VIII*

Component	Function	Nucleus of origin or termination	Ganglion	Foramen	Signs of dysfunction
SSA	Hearing	Dorsal and ventral cochlear nuclei	Spiral	Internal auditory meatus	Decreased hearing

SSA, special somatic afferent.

TABLE 8. *Structure and function of the vestibular division of cranial nerve VIII*

Component	Function	Nucleus of origin or termination	Ganglion	Foramen	Signs of dysfunction
SSA	Balance and equilibrium	Vestibular nuclei	Vestibular	Internal auditory meatus	Dysequilibrium, vertigo

SSA, special somatic afferent.

ing the facial muscles, and the smaller division, the *nervus intermedius,* carries the GVE and SVA components. The parasympathetic (GVE) fibers of the facial nerve originate in the superior salivatory nucleus and, after joining the SVE fibers, emerge from the pons to innervate the lacrimal, sublingual, and submandibular glands (Fig. 19).

The SVA component of the facial nerve mediates taste from the anterior two-thirds of the tongue. The cell bodies of the first-order neurons of this component are located in the *geniculate ganglion,* a name derived from its position at a bend in the facial canal. The cen-

tral axons from this ganglion enter the pons as part of the nervus intermedius. In the pons, these axons turn caudally to synapse, along with other taste fibers, in the *nucleus of the tractus solitarius.*

Both divisions pass through the cerebello-pontine angle cistern and leave the cranial cavity through the internal auditory meatus and enter the facial canal of the temporal bone. The SVE fibers to the face continue through the horizontal and then vertical parts of the canal, exiting at the stylomastoid foramen below the ear (Fig. 19). In addition to innervating the muscles of facial expression, a

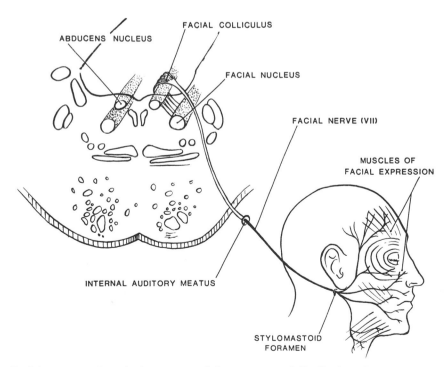

FIG. 18. Facial nerve nucleus in the pons and the course and distribution of motor axons. The loop of the facial nerve over the abducens nucleus forms the facial colliculus in the floor of the fourth ventricle.

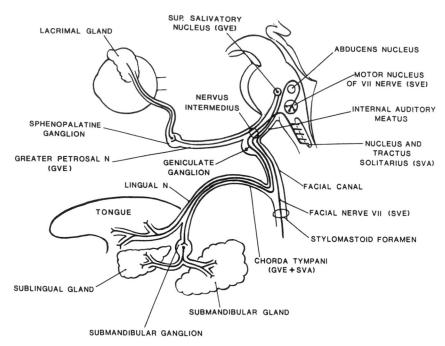

FIG. 19. Course of visceral efferent and afferent divisions of the facial nerve. (*N*, nerve; *SUP*, superior.) (Modified from Parent, A. *Carpenter's Human Neuroanatomy* [9th ed.]. Baltimore: Williams & Wilkins, 1996. With permission.)

small branch is given off to the stapedius, a tiny striated muscle in the middle ear. The nervus intermedius does not traverse the entire facial canal. In the region of the geniculate ganglion, it splits into two branches: the *greater superficial petrosal nerve* (GVE fibers for the lacrimal gland) and the *chorda tympani* (GVE fibers for the salivary glands and SVA fibers for taste).

Preganglionic parasympathetic fibers carried in the greater superficial petrosal nerve synapse in the *sphenopalatine ganglion*. Postganglionic cholinergic fibers from this ganglion proceed to the lacrimal gland. The chorda tympani nerve leaves the facial canal in its vertical segment, enters the middle ear cavity, arches over the tympanic membrane, and emerges from the petrous bone to join the lingual branch of cranial nerve V on its way to the tongue. The preganglionic parasympathetic fibers leave the lingual nerve and synapse in the *submandibular ganglion*. Postganglionic cholinergic fibers supply the sublingual and submandibular salivary glands.

Pathophysiology

The most conspicuous result of disorders of the facial nerve is weakness of the muscles of facial expression. Loss of taste on the anterior two-thirds of the tongue may also occur. Facial weakness, however, may also result from lesions involving the direct activation pathway descending from the cerebral cortex to the facial nucleus. It is clinically important to distinguish between *upper motor neuron (central) facial weakness* involving the lower half of the face and *lower motor neuron (peripheral) facial weakness* involving both the upper and lower halves of the face.

Bell's palsy is a relatively common disorder that produces peripheral facial weakness. Although the cause is usually unproved, it is thought to result from inflammation of the facial nerve in the facial canal. Patients with this condition exhibit weakness of both upper and lower facial muscles, including weakness of eye closure, a feature not seen in upper motor neuron facial weakness. Also, depending on the site of involvement of the nerve in the facial canal, patients may have decreased lacrimation and salivation, decreased taste sensation, and hyperacusis (increased sensitivity to noise due to weakness of the stapedius muscle).

The structure and function of the facial nerve are summarized in Table 9.

Abducens Nerve (Cranial Nerve VI)

Function

The abducens nerve is a GSE nerve that innervates the *lateral rectus muscle* of the eye. Contraction of this muscle produces lateral movement (abduction) of the eyeball.

Anatomy

The abducens nuclei are located in the GSE cell column at the midpontine level, beneath the floor of the fourth ventricle and near the midline (see Fig. 16). Axons take a ventral and slightly caudal course through the tegmentum and basis pontis to emerge on the ventral surface near the pontomedullary junction. The nerve then ascends ventral to the base of the pons, traverses the lateral wall of the cavernous sinus (along with cranial nerves III, IV, and the first division of V), and leaves the cranial cavity through the superior orbital fissure to supply the lateral rectus muscle of the eye (Fig. 20).

Pathophysiology

Lesions affecting the abducens nerve produce weakness of the lateral rectus muscle, with inability to abduct the eye, causing double vision (diplopia) (see The Oculomotor System, below). Because the intracranial course of cranial nerve VI is unusually long, the nerve may be affected by many pathologic processes involving the pons, the base of the skull (clivus), the cavernous sinus, the superior orbital fissure, or the orbit. The structure and function of the abducens nerve are summarized in Table 10).

Trigeminal Nerve (Cranial Nerve V)

Function

The trigeminal nerve is the sensory nerve to the face. It is a mixed nerve containing GSA and SVE components. In addition to carrying touch, pain, temperature, and proprioceptive information (GSA) from the face, cranial nerve V provides motor innervation (SVE) to the muscles of mastication, which are derived from branchial arches.

Anatomy

The GSA fibers mediating touch, pain, and temperature sense arise from cell bodies in the trigeminal (gasserian, semilunar) ganglion that lies in a dural fold called *Meckel's cave* on the medial petrous ridge (Fig. 21). Axons travel

TABLE 9. *Structure and function of the facial nerve*

Component	Function	Nucleus of origin or termination	Ganglion	Foramen	Signs of dysfunction
SVE	Motor to muscles of facial expression	Facial nucleus		Internal auditory meatus, stylomastoid	Facial weakness, hyperacusis
GVE	Parasympathetic				
	Lacrimal gland	Superior salivatory nucleus	Sphenopalatine	Internal auditory meatus	Decreased tearing
	Salivary glands	Superior salivatory nucleus	Submandibular	Internal auditory meatus	Decreased salivation
SVA	Taste: anterior two-thirds of tongue	Nucleus of tractus solitarius	Geniculate	Internal auditory meatus	Decreased taste

See Table 2 for definition of abbreviations.

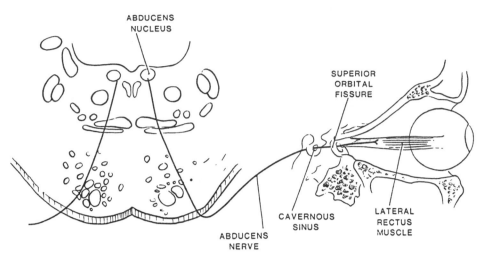

FIG. 20. The abducens nerve arises from the abducens nucleus in the pons and has a long intracranial course to the lateral rectus muscle via the cavernous sinus and superior orbital fissure.

centrally from the ganglion to enter the lateral aspect of the pons. Fibers mediating touch synapse directly in the *main (chief) sensory nucleus of V* located in the dorsolateral tegmentum of the pons. Second-order neurons from this nucleus ascend via both crossed and uncrossed pathways, the trigeminothalamic tracts, to synapse in the ventral posteromedial nucleus of the thalamus.

Pain and temperature fibers do not synapse in the main sensory nucleus but turn caudally to descend through the dorsolateral medulla and upper three or four segments of the cervical spinal cord as the *spinal (descending) tract of the trigeminal nerve* (Fig. 21). Axons in this tract synapse on cell bodies of second-order neurons in the underlying *nucleus of the spinal (descending) tract of the trigeminal nerve.* The GSA components carried in cranial nerves IX and X, from the skin of the external ear, join the spinal tract of V where they enter the medulla. The topography of the spinal tract of the trigeminal nerve is such that the fibers from the mandibular division are most dorsal and those from the ophthalmic division are most ventral as the tract descends through the caudal pons and medulla. The pattern of termination of these axons in the spinal nucleus is controversial, although some authors suggest a concentric pattern in which fibers representing the central (perioral) region of the face terminate in the most rostral part of the spinal nucleus and those representing the most peripheral areas of the face (bordering dermatomes C-2 and C-3) terminate caudally. Second-order fibers from the spinal nucleus of V cross to the opposite side of the medulla and ascend to the thalamus as the *ventral trigeminothalamic tract,* which is near the medial lemniscus. These fibers synapse in the ventral posteromedial nucleus of the thalamus, where third-order neurons send axons to the parietal lobe.

TABLE 10. *Structure and function of the abducens nerve*

Component	Function	Nucleus of origin or termination	Ganglion	Foramen	Signs of dysfunction
GSE	Motor to lateral rectus muscle	Abducens		Superior orbital fissure	Diplopia, medial deviation of eye

GSE, general somatic efferent.

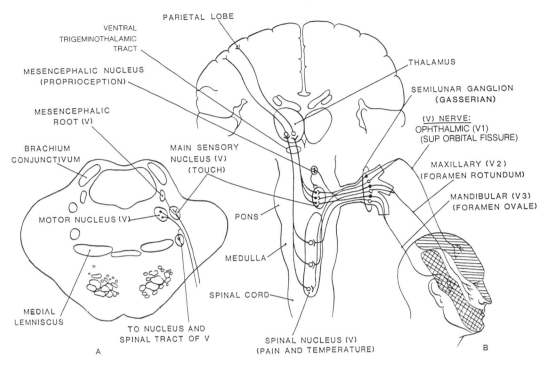

FIG. 21. Trigeminal nerve. **A:** Midpontine cross section. **B:** Horizontal section with the course and distribution of sensory axons. (*SUP,* superior.)

Proprioceptive fibers in the trigeminal nerve, unlike all other first-order sensory neurons, arise from cell bodies *located in the central nervous system.* These cell bodies form the mesencephalic nucleus of the trigeminal nerve and lie along the lateral border of the rostral fourth ventricle and aqueduct of Sylvius (Fig. 21). The peripheral axons of these unique first-order neurons innervate receptors in the muscles of mastication (and perhaps other muscles) and travel without synapse through the trigeminal ganglion to enter the lateral pons along with the rest of the nerve. Central axons from the mesencephalic nucleus synapse directly in the motor nucleus of V to mediate the monosynaptic jaw reflex.

The SVE fibers that innervate the muscles of mastication arise from cell bodies in the *motor nucleus of V,* located medial to the main sensory nucleus (Fig. 22). Axons course ventrolaterally and exit from the lateral surface of the pons as the motor root, medial to the sensory root. These fibers run along the ventral aspect of the trigeminal ganglion and join the mandibular (third) division of the trigeminal nerve to exit the skull through the foramen ovale. They innervate the temporalis, masseter, medial and lateral pterygoid, and tensor tympani muscles. The temporalis, masseter, and medial pterygoid muscles close the jaw, the lateral pterygoid muscles open and facilitate lateral movement of the jaw, and the tensor tympani, a small muscle in the middle ear, dampens vibration of the eardrum.

From the trigeminal ganglion, sensory fibers of nerve V course peripherally via three major divisions: the ophthalmic division (V_1) passes through the superior orbital fissure to innervate the upper face; the maxillary division (V_2) exits the skull via the foramen rotundum to innervate the midface; and the mandibular division (V_3), joined by the motor root, exits via the foramen ovale to innervate the lower face.

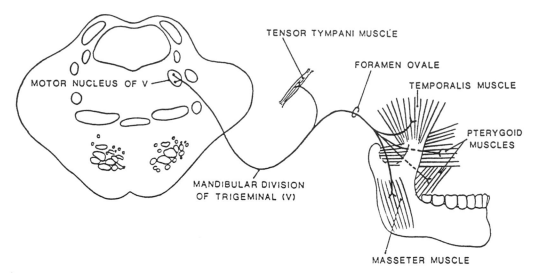

FIG. 22. Motor division of the trigeminal nerve with its nucleus in the pons and the course of the axons to the muscles of mastication.

Pathophysiology

Lesions involving cranial nerve V produce loss of facial sensation and, if the motor fibers are involved, weakness of the masticatory muscles, which causes the jaw to deviate to the side of the weakened muscles when the jaw is opened.

Trigeminal neuralgia (tic douloureux) is a disorder characterized by transient, brief, repetitive paroxysms of pain in the distribution of one or more branches of nerve V. The pain is severe and either occurs spontaneously or is triggered by relatively minor sensory stimulation of the face. Although various pathologic changes have been noted in the trigeminal ganglion, nerve, or root entry zone in the pons, the cause of the syndrome is unknown.

Two reflexes tested as part of the neurologic examination involve cranial nerve V. The *jaw jerk* is the only muscle stretch reflex that can be elicited in the head. It is mediated entirely by the mandibular branch of nerve V. Tapping the jaw briefly stretches the muscles of mastication. Proprioceptive impulses travel centrally, synapse in the motor nucleus of V, and activate reflex contraction of the jaw muscles. The clinical usefulness of this reflex in detecting lesions affecting the reflex arc is limited by the frequent difficulty in eliciting it in healthy persons. Therefore, it is regarded as abnormal only when it is hyperactive, which occurs with bilateral upper motor neuron lesions affecting the direct and indirect activation pathways to the motor nucleus of V.

The *corneal reflex* is elicited by touching the cornea of one eye with a piece of cotton. The afferent limb of this reflex is the ophthalmic division of nerve V. The observed result of this maneuver is an apparently simultaneous blink of both eyes, both the side stimulated (direct reflex) and the side not stimulated (consensual reflex). This response implies bilateral activation of facial nucleus neurons related to the orbicularis oculi muscles through complex central connections. Lesions involving the ophthalmic division of nerve V, the tegmentum of the pons, or the facial nerve alter this reflex. The structure and function of the trigeminal nerve are summarized in Table 11.

Reticular Formation

The pontine reticular formation, located in the core of the tegmentum, is continuous with the reticular formation of the medulla cau-

TABLE 11. *Structure and function of the trigeminal nerve*

Division of trigeminal nerve V	Component	Function	Nucleus of origin or termination	Ganglion	Foramen	Signs of dysfunction
Ophthalmic (V₁)	GSA	Sensation: forehead pain	Spinal nucleus of V	Gasserian (semilunar)	Superior orbital fissure	Decreased forehead pain Decreased corneal reflex
		Touch: forehead	Main sensory nucleus of V	Gasserian (semilunar)	Superior orbital fissure	Decreased forehead touch Decreased corneal reflex
Maxillary (V₂)	GSA	Sensation: cheek pain	Spinal nucleus of V	Gasserian (semilunar)	Rotundum	Decreased cheek pain
		Touch: cheek	Main sensory nucleus of V	Gasserian (semilunar)	Rotundum	Decreased cheek touch
Mandibular (V₃)	GSA	Sensation: jaw pain	Spinal nucleus of V	Gasserian (semilunar)	Ovale	Decreased jaw pain
		Touch: jaw	Main sensory nucleus of V	Gasserian (semilunar)	Ovale	Decreased jaw touch
		Proprioception	Mesencephalic nucleus		Ovale	Decreased jaw jerk
	SVE	Motor to muscles of mastication	Motor nucleus of V		Ovale	Weakness of muscles of mastication, decreased jaw jerk

See Table 2 for definition of abbreviations.

dally and of the midbrain rostrally. As in the medullary reticular formation, different functional zones can be distinguished in transverse section. The medial zone at this level is concerned primarily with the oculomotor system and the reticulospinal system. The role of the paramedian pontine reticular formation and the coordination of eye movements are discussed below. The lateral pontine reticular formation contains neurons of the internal regulation system, including those that modulate the micturition reflex. The pontine reticular formation also contains several neuronal groups of the consciousness system, including the raphe nuclei and the locus ceruleus.

The Midbrain

The midbrain is that portion of the brainstem located between the pons and the dien-

cephalon. The major external anatomical features that mark its boundaries are the cerebral peduncles ventrally and the quadrigeminal plate, featuring the paired inferior and superior colliculi, dorsally. In transverse section, the midbrain is divided dorsoventrally into three main regions: the *tectum* (dorsal), the *tegmentum,* and the *base* (ventral) (Fig. 23). Its derivation from the primitive neural tube is most clearly highlighted by its tubular cavity, the aqueduct of Sylvius.

The *tectum,* or roof, of the midbrain lies above the transverse plane of the aqueduct of Sylvius. The tectum is made up of two paired structures, the *inferior* and *superior colliculi,* collectively called the *corpora quadrigemina.* The inferior colliculi act as a relay station for auditory fibers that pass to the thalamus via the brachium of the inferior colliculus. The superior colliculi are associated with oculomotor control. The aqueduct of Sylvius, a

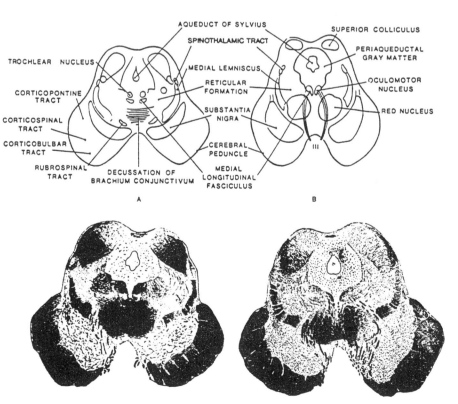

FIG. 23. Cross section of the midbrain. **A:** Caudal midbrain (level of the inferior colliculus). **B:** Rostral midbrain (level of the superior colliculus). Myelin-stained sections are shown below.

remnant of the neural canal, is surrounded by a zone of periaqueductal gray matter.

The *tegmentum* is the area lying ventral to the aqueduct and dorsal to the substantia nigra. The major longitudinal pathways in the tegmentum of the midbrain are the lateral lemniscus, spinothalamic tract, medial lemniscus, medial longitudinal fasciculus, indirect activation pathways of the motor system, descending pathways of the internal regulation system, and projection pathways of the reticular formation. In addition, it contains the nuclei of cranial nerves III and IV and their axons, the red nuclei, and the decussation of the superior cerebellar peduncles (Fig. 23A).

At the midbrain level, perhaps more clearly than at other brainstem levels, the primitive concentric organization of the neural tube can be recognized. The phylogenetically older multisynaptic pathways concerned with internal regulation, consciousness, and other primitive functions occupy the inner regions close to the aqueduct; the newer, more direct and functionally discrete pathways concerned with somatic motor and sensory functions lie more peripherally.

The Superior Cerebellar Peduncle (Brachium Conjunctivum)

Efferent fibers from the dentate nucleus of the cerebellum pass rostrally, and near the dorsal surface of the midbrain, just caudal to the inferior colliculi, they can be identified grossly as the *superior cerebellar peduncles*. From this point, they pass ventrally into the tegmentum of the midbrain. In caudal midbrain (level of the inferior colliculus), they cross to the opposite side, forming the *decussation of the brachium conjunctivum* (Fig. 23A). The fibers then proceed to the red nucleus and thalamus.

The Red Nucleus

The red nucleus is a large oval mass of gray matter in the central portion of the tegmentum on each side at the level of the superior col-liculus (Fig. 23B). When viewed in a freshly cut brain, this nucleus is slightly red because of its density of capillaries and high iron content. The red nuclei receive fibers from the cerebellum and the cerebral cortex and give rise to (1) descending fibers that synapse in the ipsilateral inferior olivary nucleus, from which fibers project to the contralateral cerebellar cortex; and (2) the rubrospinal tract, which crosses in the ventral tegmental decussation caudal to the red nucleus and descends to the spinal cord.

The Basis Pedunculi

The base of the midbrain, also called the *basis pedunculi,* consists of the cerebral peduncles (containing the corticospinal, corticobulbar, and corticopontine tracts) and the substantia nigra, which is dorsal to each cerebral peduncle (Fig. 23). The substantia nigra is dark because of its melanin-containing neurons. It is functionally related to the basal ganglia as part of the indirect activation pathway of the motor system.

Trochlear Nerve (Cranial Nerve IV)

Function

The trochlear nerve is a GSE nerve that innervates the superior oblique muscle of the eye. Contraction of this muscle causes downward movement of the eye when it is in the adducted position.

Anatomy

The trochlear nucleus lies at the level of the inferior colliculus just ventral to the periaqueductal gray matter and dorsal to the medial longitudinal fasciculus. Its axons pass dorsolaterally and caudally around the periaqueductal gray matter. They cross caudal to the tectum and emerge from the dorsal aspect of the midbrain on the side contralateral to their origin. This is the only completely crossed cranial nerve and the only cranial nerve to emerge from the dorsal surface of the brainstem (Fig. 24). The nerve then passes around

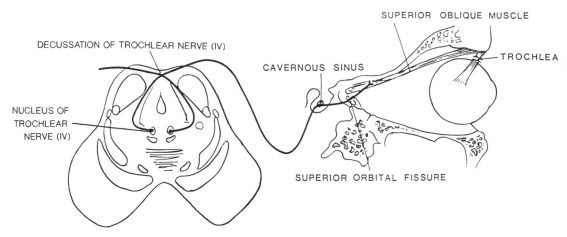

FIG. 24. Trochlear nerve. Cross section of caudal midbrain showing the trochlear nucleus and the course and distribution of axons to the superior oblique muscle of the opposite eye.

the midbrain to enter the lateral wall of the cavernous sinus. It enters the orbit through the superior orbital fissure to innervate the superior oblique muscle.

Pathophysiology

Lesions of the trochlear nerve cause weakness of the superior oblique muscle, causing diplopia on downward and inward gaze. The patient may compensate for the torsional imbalance caused by the unopposed action of the inferior oblique muscle by tilting the head to the opposite side. Isolated injury to the trochlear nerve may occur where it runs along the edge of the tentorium toward the cavernous sinus. This often results from head trauma. Otherwise, the nerve is usually involved along with cranial nerves III, V, and VI by lesions of the cavernous sinus, superior orbital fissure, or orbit. The structure and function of the trochlear nerve are summarized in Table 12.

Oculomotor Nerve (Cranial Nerve III)

Function

The oculomotor nerve is a mixed motor nerve that provides GSE innervation to the following muscles of the eye: superior rectus, inferior rectus, medial rectus, inferior oblique, and levator palpebrae superioris. Cranial nerve III also supplies GVE (parasympathetic) fibers to the pupil and to the ciliary muscle controlling the lens of the eye.

Anatomy

The GSE fibers of cranial nerve III arise from the oculomotor nucleus, which is ventral to the aqueduct at the level of the superior colliculus (Fig. 25). The nucleus is composed of subnuclei for each of the muscles innervated. All the projections are ipsilateral except for those to the superior rectus muscle (which are crossed) and those to the levator palpebrae superioris muscle (which are crossed and un-

TABLE 12. *Structure and function of the trochlear nerve*

Component	Function	Nucleus of origin or termination	Ganglion	Foramen	Signs of dysfunction
GSE	Motor to superior oblique muscle	Trochlear nucleus on opposite side		Superior orbital fissure	Diplopia

GSE, general somatic efferent.

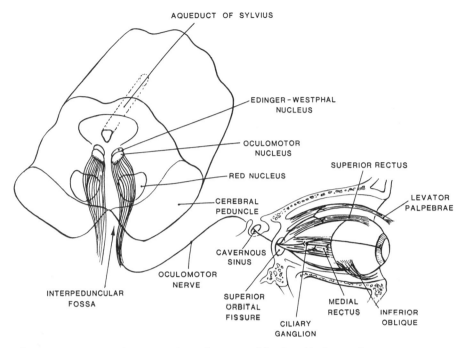

FIG. 25. Oculomotor nerve. Cross section of upper midbrain with the oculomotor nucleus and course and distribution of axons to the eye.

crossed). The crossing occurs in the nucleus itself. Axons pass ventrally through the tegmentum and base of the midbrain and emerge in the interpeduncular fossa.

The GVE fibers that provide preganglionic parasympathetic innervation to the pupil arise in a small subnucleus, the *Edinger-Westphal nucleus,* at the rostral end of each oculomotor nucleus. These GVE fibers join the GSE fibers and, after emerging from the interpeduncular fossa, pass through the lateral wall of the cavernous sinus and superior orbital fissure to enter the orbit (Fig. 25). The GSE fibers continue directly to the extraocular muscles and innervate them, and the GVE fibers synapse in the ciliary ganglion. Postganglionic fibers from this ganglion proceed to the pupilloconstrictor muscle of the iris and to the ciliary body.

Pathophysiology

Lesions involving the GSE component of nerve III produce weakness of all voluntary eye muscles, except the lateral rectus and superior oblique, and cause diplopia. The eye tends to deviate downward and outward because of the unopposed action of the lateral rectus and superior oblique muscles, and ptosis is often present because of weakness of the levator palpebrae superioris muscle. In rare cases in which the nucleus itself is the site of the lesion, there is weakness of the contralateral superior rectus and bilateral ptosis.

Ptosis caused by weakness of the levator palpebrae superioris must be distinguished from ptosis due to lesions affecting the sympathetic innervation of the eye. These postganglionic sympathetic fibers are from the superior cervical sympathetic ganglion, ascend into the cranial cavity along the internal carotid artery, and join cranial nerve III in the cavernous sinus. Damage to these sympathetic fibers causes mild ptosis because of loss of innervation of the smooth muscle in the upper lid (Müller's muscle); the damage also causes *miosis* (pupillary constriction). In contrast, lesions of the GVE component of cranial nerve III cause loss of the parasympathetic innervation of the eye and produce *mydriasis* (pupillary dilatation).

Observation of pupillary size and testing of the pupillary light reflex are an integral part of the neurologic examination. The size of the pupil is influenced by many factors, primarily by the intensity of light falling on the retina. The afferent pathway of the pupillary light reflex is conducted by the optic nerve (cranial nerve II). The fibers from each retina partially decussate in the optic chiasm and proceed via the optic tracts and brachium of the superior colliculus to the *pretectal area* (Fig. 26), from which fibers pass to the *Edinger-Westphal nucleus* on both sides. From the Edinger-Westphal nucleus, the efferent limb of the pupillary light reflex continues in the oculomotor nerve.

The normal pupil constricts briskly when light is shown on the ipsilateral retina. This is the *direct light reflex*. Because of the partial decussation of the optic pathway in the optic chiasm and again in the pretectal area, the contralateral pupil also constricts; this is the *consensual light reflex*. Unilateral lesions of the optic nerve do not produce anisocoria (unequal pupils) but diminish both the direct and the consensual light reflex when the involved eye is tested. However, moving the light source rapidly from the normal eye (with a strong direct and consensual light reflex) to the involved eye (with a diminished reflex) can make it appear as if the pupils actually dilate in response to light. Of course, they are only moving to a less constricted state due to decreased detection of light in the involved eye. Both pupils will again constrict briskly

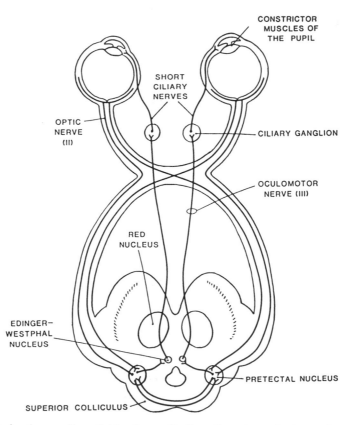

FIG. 26. Pathways for the pupillary light reflex, with the afferent arm in the optic nerve and the efferent arm in the oculomotor nerve.

when the light source is moved back to the normal eye. This phenomenon can be demonstrated repeatedly by moving the light source back and forth from the involved to the uninvolved eye. This response identifies the so-called *afferent pupillary defect,* which is due to decreased conduction in the afferent limb of the pupillary light reflex.

Lesions that involve the parasympathetic innervation of the eye cause ipsilateral mydriasis and loss of the direct pupillary light reflex with preservation of the consensual reflex on testing the involved eye (and the reverse on testing the uninvolved eye). Anisocoria also occurs with lesions involving the sympathetic innervation of the pupil, resulting in ipsilateral miosis with normal pupillary light reflexes. This pupillary abnormality is usually accompanied by other features of Horner's syndrome, including mild ptosis due to denervation of Müller's muscle (see above) and decreased sweating on the ipsilateral face due to loss of sympathetic innervation of sweat glands. The structure and function of the oculomotor nerve are summarized in Table 13.

Reticular Formation

Perhaps more clearly than at other levels of the brainstem, the reticular formation in the midbrain is concentrated around the inner tube, which surrounds the neural canal derivative, the aqueduct of Sylvius. Its most conspicuous component is the *periaqueductal gray matter,* which is concerned predominantly with the central modulation and control of pain and with integrating responses to

stress. The rostral interstitial nucleus of the medial longitudinal fasciculus (important in the coordination of vertical eye movements), the raphe nuclei and mesopontine cholinergic nuclei (important in the consciousness system), and other specific nuclei in the midbrain reticular formation are discussed in connection with the systems in which they perform important functions.

The Cerebellum

The cerebellum is the largest structure in the posterior fossa. It lies dorsal to the pons and medulla and forms the roof of the fourth ventricle. The cerebellum is an embryonic derivative of the metencephalon, and although it is derived from the alar plate (rhombic lip) and is important in the integration of unconscious proprioception, it is closely related functionally to the motor system and is the central structure in the cerebellar control circuit (see Chapter 8).

Gross Anatomy

The cerebellum is composed of two lateral lobes, the *cerebellar hemispheres,* and a midline portion called the vermis (Fig. 27). The cerebellum is also divided transversely into three lobes, with each one containing a portion of the vermis and the adjacent hemisphere.

1. The *anterior lobe* consists of the vermis and cerebellar hemispheres anterior to the primary fissure.

TABLE 13. *Structure and function of the oculomotor nerve*

Component	Function	Nucleus of origin or termination	Ganglion	Foramen	Signs of dysfunction
GSE	Motor to medial rectus, superior rectus, inferior rectus, inferior oblique, and levator palpebrae	Oculomotor		Superior orbital fissure	Diplopia, ptosis
GVE	Parasympathetic pupilloconstrictor muscles, ciliary muscle	Edinger-Westphal	Ciliary	Superior orbital fissure	Mydriasis, loss of direct pupillary reflex, loss of lens accommodation

See Table 2 for definition of abbreviations.

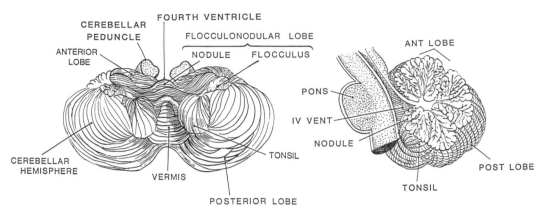

FIG. 27. Lobes of the cerebellum from the inferior surface. (*ANT,* anterior; *POST,* posterior; *VENT,* ventricle.)

2. The *flocculonodular lobe* consists of the most caudal lobule of the vermis, the nodulus (in the roof of the fourth ventricle), and the flocculus.
3. The *posterior lobe* consists of the rest of the cerebellum and includes the cerebellar tonsils, which are apparent on the inferomedial aspect of the cerebellar hemispheres just above the foramen magnum.

Functional Anatomy

Clinically, it is convenient to discuss the cerebellum in terms of its functional anatomy. The vermis of the anterior and posterior lobes forms the *midline cerebellar zone,* which receives the spinocerebellar afferents and is concerned mainly with the muscle synergies involved in walking. The terms *paleocerebellum,* reflecting its phylogenetic origin, and *spinocerebellum,* reflecting its major functional connections, roughly correspond to this zone. The *lateral zone* corresponds to most of the cerebellar hemisphere including the major part of the posterior lobe. It receives the corticopontocerebellar afferents and is also referred to as the *neocerebellum* or *corticocerebellum.* The lateral zone is involved in the coordination of ipsilateral limb movement. Between the midline zone and the lateral zone of each hemisphere, anatomists recognize an intermediate zone, which projects via the globose and emboliform nuclei to the nuclei of

the indirect activation pathways; the clinical relevance of this region in humans is unknown. The *flocculonodular lobe* receives input from the vestibular system and is also referred to as the *archicerebellum* or *vestibulocerebellum.* It is concerned primarily with coordination of head and eye movements and the maintenance of equilibrium.

The Cerebellar Peduncles

The cerebellum is connected to the brainstem by three pairs of peduncles that carry cerebellar afferents and efferents (Fig. 28).

The *inferior cerebellar peduncle* (restiform body) contains both afferent and efferent fibers. It carries most of the information the cerebellum receives from the spinal cord and medulla. The most important afferent pathways reaching the cerebellum through this peduncle are the dorsal spinocerebellar and cuneocerebellar tracts (carrying proprioceptive input that does not reach consciousness) and the vestibulocerebellar, reticulocerebellar, and olivocerebellar pathways. The main efferent fibers are the cerebellovestibular and cerebelloreticular pathways.

The *middle cerebellar peduncle* (brachium pontis) contains only afferent fibers, which originate in the contralateral pontine nuclei. The pontine nuclei receive afferents from the ipsilateral cerebral cortex via the corticopontine tract. The corticopontocerebellar connec-

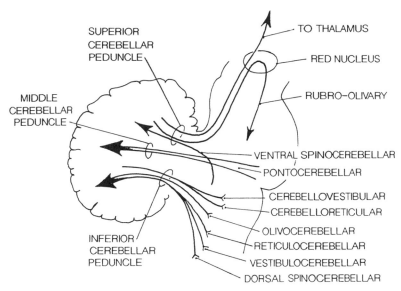

FIG. 28. Afferent and efferent fibers in the cerebellar peduncles.

tions establish a pathway whereby each cerebellar hemisphere is influenced by the contralateral cerebral hemisphere.

The *superior cerebellar peduncle* (brachium conjunctivum) contains both afferent and efferent fibers and is the main outflow pathway from the cerebellum. The only afferent component in this peduncle is the ventral spinocerebellar tract. Efferent fibers originating in the dentate nucleus constitute the bulk of the superior cerebellar peduncle. In caudal midbrain, these fibers cross as the decussation of the brachium conjunctivum and proceed to the contralateral red nucleus, thalamus, and inferior olivary nucleus. The fibers descending to the inferior olivary nucleus are in the central tegmental tract. As a result of the connections described above, two loops are established: the cortico-ponto-cerebello-dentato-thalamo-cortical pathway and the cerebello-dentato-rubro-olivo-cerebellar pathway. Their roles in monitoring and modulating the activity of the motor system are not completely understood.

Internal Anatomy

The cerebellar cortex is a highly convoluted structure. The individual convolutions are referred to as *folia* rather than gyri. Deep to the cerebellar cortex is white matter that is made up of the fiber tracts entering and leaving the cortex. Four paired nuclei lie within the deep cerebellar white matter: the dentate, emboliform, globose, and fastigial nuclei. They are relay stations for efferent fibers from the cerebellar cortex and are the origin of most of the efferent pathways from the cerebellum (Fig. 29).

Histologically, the cerebellar cortex consists of three layers: the *molecular layer,* the *Purkinje cell layer,* and the *granule cell layer* (Fig. 30). The outermost is the molecular layer; it consists mainly of axons and dendrites, among which are a small number of neurons called *basket cells* and *stellate cells.* The middle layer consists of a single layer of large goblet-shaped *Purkinje cells.* The innermost (granular cell) layer is composed of densely packed small neurons called *granule cells* and scattered larger neurons called *Golgi cells.*

Afferent fibers entering the cerebellar cortex terminate as either *mossy fibers* or *climbing fibers.* The mossy fibers represent the cerebellar afferent fibers from all sources except the inferior olivary nucleus. They synapse on the dendrites of granule cells and Golgi cells. Axons of the granule cells, in turn, enter the molecular layer and synapse on

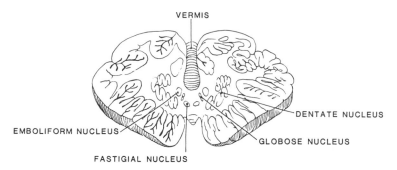

FIG. 29. Cerebellar nuclei in horizontal section.

Purkinje cell dendrites. Purkinje cell dendrites arborize in a fan-like fashion perpendicular to the long axis of the folium. Granule cell axons enter the molecular layer and bifurcate to run, as *parallel fibers,* 2 to 3 mm in each direction in the long axis of the folium. Thus, each parallel fiber can synapse with the dendrites of up to 500 Purkinje cells as well as with dendrites of basket cells and stellate cells. The Golgi cell dendrites also ramify in the molecular layer and are excited by the parallel fibers of the granule cells. Golgi cell axons end in the granule cell layer and form inhibitory synapses on granule cells. Activation of a single incoming mossy fiber can produce excitation of a small, rectangular array of Purkinje cells, because the mossy fiber contacts multiple granule cells whose parallel fibers contact multiple Purkinje cells. The mossy fiber synapses and parallel fiber synapses are excitatory. All the other neurons activated by parallel fibers (Golgi, basket, and stellate cells) are inhibitory to Purkinje cells. Because of the spatial organization of the cerebellar cortex, these inhibitory neurons create a simultaneous intense inhibition of Purkinje cells surrounding the activated zone. The mossy fiber system constantly modulates cerebellar activity during voluntary movement.

Climbing fibers are the axons of the olivocerebellar pathway; they synapse directly on Purkinje cells via an array of terminal axon branches that wind around and "climb" the Purkinje cell body and dendritic tree. The climbing fiber input to Purkinje cells, like the granule cell input, is excitatory. The climbing fiber system signals errors in motor perfor-

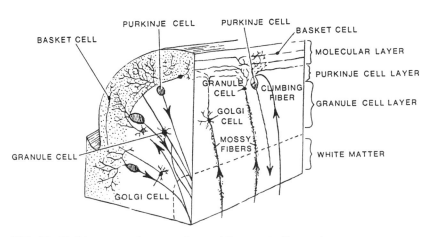

FIG. 30. Cell layers and connections of the cerebellar cortex.

mance and adapts Purkinje cell firing to the new circumstance. It is important in motor learning.

All output from the cerebellar cortex is via the axons of the Purkinje cells, which project to the deep cerebellar nuclei and form inhibitory synapses. A few Purkinje cell axons go directly to the vestibular nuclei.

Pathophysiology

As described in Chapter 8, disturbances of cerebellar function are manifested as loss of balance and equilibrium or as a disorder in the modulation of the range, force, rate, and direction of movement. The flocculonodular lobe is primarily responsible for balance and equilibrium, and lesions in this region of the cerebellum result in an inability to sit or stand without swaying or falling (*truncal ataxia*). The anterior lobe is primarily responsible for posture and coordination of gait. Lesions involving this region result in an unsteady, staggering gait (*gait ataxia*). The posterior lobe is primarily responsible for coordination of ipsilateral voluntary movements of the extremities. Lesions of this region result in loss of motor coordination of the extremities, dysmetria, and, if the dentate nucleus or its outflow pathway (the brachium conjunctivum) is involved, intention tremor (*limb ataxia*).

New Systems at the Posterior Fossa Level

In addition to the major longitudinal systems discussed in other chapters, three additional special systems—oculomotor, auditory, and vestibular—are found at the posterior fossa level.

The Oculomotor System

The oculomotor system controls eye movements and is part of the motor system. Its major components, particularly the final common pathway (lower motor neurons), are located at the posterior fossa level, although, as in other parts of the motor system, the pathways for supranuclear control originate at the supratentorial level. Vision itself is exclusively a supratentorial function. The anatomy and physiology of the visual system are discussed with that level (see Chapter 16).

Eye movement is accomplished through the action of the extraocular muscles, which are activated by cranial nerves III, IV, and VI. Most of the input to the nuclei of these cranial nerves is through the paramedian reticular formation of the brainstem, which determines the activity of lower motor neurons for both reflex and voluntary eye movements. Input to the reticular formation for voluntary and pursuit movements comes via descending supranuclear pathways from the frontal eye fields and parieto-occipital visual cortex, respectively. Reflex movements are mediated by input from the vestibular nuclei in the medulla to the abducens nucleus (nerve VI) and then via the medial longitudinal fasciculus to the trochlear (nerve IV) and oculomotor (nerve III) nuclei. Input from the retina travels to the superior colliculus and the pretectal region and then to the brainstem reticular formation.

Lesions at the supratentorial, posterior fossa, or peripheral levels can produce oculomotor disorders such as paresis of one or more extraocular muscles, with *diplopia, gaze paresis,* or *nystagmus.*

Physiology

Different neural mechanisms are used for eye movements that subserve different functions. *Saccadic eye movements* are rapid reflex movements that bring a visual image to the fovea. *Smooth pursuit* movements keep the fovea focused on a moving target. *Vergence* movements maintain the visual image on the fovea when objects move toward the eyes (convergence) or away from them (divergence). *Vestibulo-ocular reflexes* hold images steady on the retina during brief head rotations. *Optokinetic movements* hold stable images on the retina as long as possible when object-filled space is moving past the eyes and then quickly refixates on the next available target.

Each of these eye movements is mediated via the nuclei of cranial nerves III, IV, and VI and coordinated through neurons in the brainstem *paramedian reticular formation.* The different pathways acting on the reticular formation to produce these movements have not been fully clarified, but some of the anatomical features of the various control systems are well defined.

Anatomy

The five major areas of oculomotor control are (1) the nuclei of cranial nerves III, IV, and VI, described above; (2) the brainstem paramedian reticular formation; (3) the superior colliculus and pretectal region; (4) vestibular connections via the abducens nucleus and the medial longitudinal fasciculus; and (5) the cortical eye fields.

The anatomy of the oculomotor, trochlear, and abducens nuclei and nerves forming the final common pathway of the oculomotor system is described above. The medial and lateral recti muscles turn the eye inward and outward, respectively. The superior and inferior recti muscles move the eye up and down when it is turned outward, and the inferior and superior oblique muscles move the eye up and down when it is turned inward (Table 14). The muscles that turn the two eyeballs are yoked in pairs so that the eyes move conjugately in exactly the same direction with exactly the same velocity and force. This principle of equal innervation of yoked pairs of extraocular muscles is known as *Hering's law.* For example, the left medial rectus and right lateral rectus muscles are the yoked pair for right lateral gaze, and when looking to the right, the right superior rectus and left inferior oblique are the yoked pair for upward gaze. When the eye is turned outward, the oblique muscles produce more torsion than up and down movement. Similarly, when the eye is turned inward, the action of the superior and inferior recti becomes primarily torsional (Fig. 31A). Ocular movements are tested by asking the patient to look in the six cardinal directions of gaze, as depicted in Fig. 31B.

The brainstem paramedian reticular formation is located along the midline and paramedian core of the brainstem from the midbrain to the medulla and receives input from all prenuclear areas concerned with eye movements, including the vestibular nuclei, superior colliculi, pretectal region, cerebellum, and cortical eye fields. This region is made up of small scattered nuclei that show different firing patterns with different types of eye movement. On the basis of their effect on the firing pattern of the neurons of cranial nerve nuclei III, IV, and VI, the neurons in these cell groups are classified as *pause cells, burst cells,* and *tonic cells* (Table 15).

The control of conjugate horizontal eye movements is integrated primarily at the level of the pons; the control of vertical eye movements is integrated at the level of the midbrain (Table 15). The abducens nucleus of the pons contains not only the motor neurons innervating the ipsilateral lateral rectus muscle but also commissural neurons. Axons of the com-

TABLE 14. *Functions of the ocular nerves*

Nerve	Muscles	Function (deviation of the eye)	Signs of dysfunction
III	Medial rectus	Medially	Eye is deviated down and out with complete paralysis of nerve III (usually associated with ptosis and mydriasis)
	Superior rectus	Up and out	
	Inferior rectus	Down and out	
	Inferior oblique	Up and in	
IV	Superior oblique	Down and in	Limitation of downward gaze when eye is looking medially, extorsion of eye
VI	Lateral rectus	Laterally	Eye is deviated medially

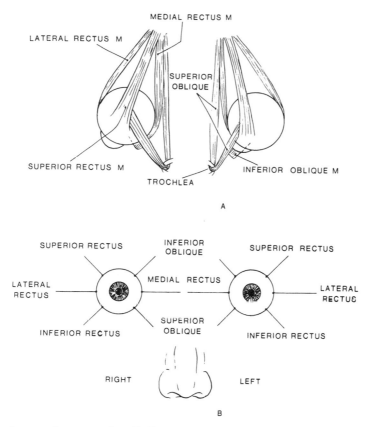

FIG. 31. A: Attachment of eye muscles. **B:** Eye movement produced by each muscle. (*M,* muscle.)

missural neurons cross the midline at the level of the pons and ascend in the contralateral *medial longitudinal fasciculus* to innervate the motor neurons in the midbrain oculomotor nucleus that innervate the medial rectus muscle. Thus, excitation of the abducens nucleus produces ipsilateral deviation of gaze by direct activation of ipsilateral lateral rectus motor neurons and indirect activation of contralateral medial rectus motor neurons via the medial longitudinal fasciculus. Conjugate vertical gaze is integrated by connections between different neurons in the oculomotor nucleus in rostral midbrain (innervating the superior and inferior recti and inferior oblique muscle) and the trochlear nucleus in caudal

TABLE 15. *Location of control cells for horizontal and vertical conjugate eye movements*

Movement	Level of integration (cranial nerve nucleus)	Saccadic burst cells	Tonic cells	Pause cells
Horizontal	Pons (abducens)	Pontine paramedian reticular formation	Flocculonodular lobe Medial vestibular nucleus Nucleus prepositus hypoglossi (rostral medulla)	Raphe nuclei
Vertical	Midbrain (oculomotor, trochlear)	Rostral interstitial nucleus of the medial longitudinal fasciculus	Flocculonodular lobe Medial vestibular nucleus Interstitial nucleus of Cajal	Raphe nuclei

midbrain (innervating the superior oblique muscle). Upward gaze depends on activation of the superior rectus and inferior oblique muscles, and downward gaze depends on activation of the inferior rectus and superior oblique muscles. Some of the interconnections between the corresponding motor neurons cross the midline in the *posterior commissure.*

These basic circuits for conjugate horizontal and vertical gaze are activated by different gaze control systems, including the *vestibulo-ocular reflex,* the *saccadic system,* the *smooth pursuit-optokinetic system,* and the *convergence system* (Table 16). Maintenance of the eyes in a particular position in the orbit depends on tonic input from neurons located in the vestibulocerebellum and other components of a central network referred to as the neural integrator. This *neural integrator* includes neurons in the vestibulocerebellum and medial vestibular nucleus as well as in the *nucleus prepositus hypoglossi* in rostral medulla (containing tonic neurons for hori-

zontal eye movements) and the *interstitial nucleus of Cajal* in the midbrain (containing tonic neurons for vertical eye movements). These groups of tonic neurons are located in the dorsal midline reticular formation (see Table 15).

The *vestibulo-ocular reflex* maintains the image on the fovea during rapid head movement. This involves conjugate movement of the eyes in the direction opposite to that of head movement. Also, the velocity of eye movement is equal to that of head movement. The receptors for this reflex are in the vestibular organs (see below). For example, in the horizontal vestibulo-ocular reflex, rotation of the head to the right produces slow conjugate rotation of the eyes to the left. This reflex involves vestibular input from the right ear that relays in the ipsilateral vestibular nucleus and crossed excitatory connections of the vestibular nucleus with the contralateral abducens nucleus (Fig. 32A).

The vestibular and optokinetic systems control compensatory eye movements to head

TABLE 16. *Systems controlling conjugate gaze*

Type of eye movement	Main function	Control mechanism	Effect
Vestibular (vestibulo-ocular reflex)	Holds images steady on the fovea during brief head rotations	Semicircular canals and vestibular nuclei	Conjugate deviation of eyes opposite to direction of head rotation
Smooth pursuit	Holds image of a moving target on the fovea	Visual pathway and parieto-occipital cortex Vestibulocerebellum	Conjugated deviation toward direction of movement of object (ipsilateral to parieto-occipital cortex)
Optokinetic	Holds images of the target steady on the retina during sustained head rotation	Visual pathway and parieto-occipital cortex, vestibulocerebellum, vestibular nuclei	Maintains deviation of eyes initiated by the vestibulo-ocular reflex
Saccade	Brings the image of an object of interest onto the fovea	Frontal eye fields Superior colliculus Pontine paramedian reticular formation	Rapid conjugate deviation toward opposite side
Nystagmus quick phase	Directs the fovea toward the oncoming visual scene during self-rotation; resets the eyes during prolonged rotation	Cortical	Quick deviation toward stimulated labyrinth (vestibular) Quick deviation toward inhibited cerebellum (cerebellar)
Vergence	Moves the eyes in opposite directions (disconjugate) so that images of a single object are placed on both fovae	Unknown direct input to oculomotor neurons, likely via interneurons	Accommodation to near targets

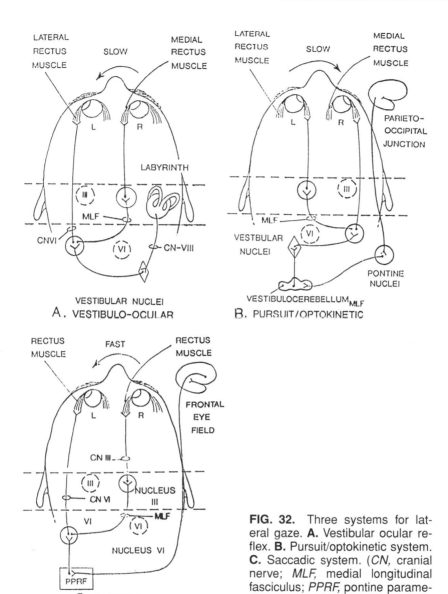

FIG. 32. Three systems for lateral gaze. **A.** Vestibular ocular reflex. **B.** Pursuit/optokinetic system. **C.** Saccadic system. (*CN,* cranial nerve; *MLF,* medial longitudinal fasciculus; *PPRF,* pontine paramedian reticular formation.)

rotation and movement of the visual environment. When the semicircular canals are stimulated by head movement, signals are sent to the appropriate combination of cranial nerves III, IV, and VI for compensatory eye movement in the opposite direction. If one looks at a target and shakes the head from side to side, the eyes can be maintained on the target through this mechanism. It does not require any cortical input and, in fact, can be seen in comatose patients. The pathway from the vestibular nuclei to cranial nerves III, IV, and VI is largely through the medial longitudinal fasciculus (Fig. 32A).

The *smooth pursuit system* keeps the fovea focused on a moving target. In this case, visual input from the retina is integrated, via the thalamus, in both the primary visual cortex and parieto-occipital cortex (Fig. 33) (see Chapter 16). Axons from these cortical re-

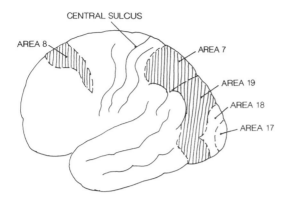

FIG. 33. Cortical eye fields. Area 17 is primary visual cortex. Cortical gaze centers are in areas 8 and 19.

gions descend ipsilaterally to activate neurons in pontine nuclei that project to the contralateral flocculonodular lobe, which in turn projects to the medial vestibular nucleus. The final effect is slow conjugate eye movement *toward* the side of the cortex stimulated (Fig. 32B).

The parieto-occipital eye field is located at the parieto-occipital junction of each hemisphere (Brodmann's area 19) (Fig. 33). This eye field is responsible for involuntary smooth pursuit movements in which the eyes are fixated on an object and maintain visual fixation as the object moves (Fig. 32B). Fibers from area 19 project to nuclei in the pretectal region and to the superior colliculus and from there to the reticular formation. Voluntary fixation on a visual target is broken when the target reaches the limit of the visual field. The eyes then make a quick movement in the opposite direction to fixate on a new target. This movement is called *optokinetic nystagmus* and depends on an intact parieto-occipital eye field.

The *saccadic system* rapidly brings visual images to the fovea. Saccades can be voluntary in response to a command, a remembered target, or a reflex in response to visual, auditory, or somatosensory stimuli. Control of voluntary saccades depends on the *frontal eye fields* (Fig. 33) (see Chapter 16), whereas reflex saccades involve the *superior colliculus.*

The frontal eye fields and superior colliculus project to the brainstem.

When the eyes are still, pause cells located in the raphe nuclei fire tonically and inhibit the burst cells. When the eyes make a rapid movement, or saccade, the pause cells are inhibited. Burst cells then fire briefly, driving the eyes to their new position. Tonic cells also begin to fire, and their discharge frequency is just enough to hold the eye at the new desired position. The pulse created by the burst neuron firing and the step created by the firing of tonic neurons drive the eye to the new position and hold it there. The burst neurons for horizontal saccades are located in the *pontine paramedian reticular formation* near the abducens nucleus, and the burst neurons for vertical eye movements are located in the *rostral interstitial nucleus of the medial longitudinal fasciculus.*

The frontal eye field is in the posterior portion of the middle frontal gyrus, Brodmann's area 8 (Fig. 33), and is responsible for the voluntary control of conjugate saccades (Fig. 32C). Fibers from this region project to the pontine reticular formation and the superior colliculus. Stimulation of the frontal eye field produces conjugate deviation of the eyes to the opposite side and acute destruction results in conjugate deviation of the eyes toward the side of the lesion.

The *superior colliculus* and the pretectal region receive input from the retina, the cortical eye fields, and the inferior colliculus, which is a relay station in the auditory pathway. Fibers from these regions connect with the reticular formation and mediate eye movements in response to targets picked up in the peripheral vision and in response to sound. The superior colliculi map the visual and auditory environment, which helps in the localization of objects and sounds in space.

Eye movements usually have to be conjugate to maintain a visual image on the fovea of both eyes; however, if the object moves closer to the observer, the eyes converge to maintain the image on the fovea. When the object moves away, the eyes diverge. The anatomy and physiology of convergence movements are not well understood. They are slow and seem to be mediated by pontine and medullary structures but *not* by the medial longitudinal fasciculus.

Two other reflexes normally accompany convergence: accommodation and miosis. Both are mediated by the Edinger-Westphal nucleus, the origin of the parasympathetic fibers of the oculomotor nerve. These fibers travel with cranial nerve III to the ciliary ganglion, where they synapse on postganglionic cells that innervate the ciliary muscle. This muscle relaxes the tension on the lens, allowing it to round up and shorten its focal distance. Parasympathetic activity also causes contraction of the circular muscle of the iris, causing constriction of the pupil.

Pathophysiology

Disturbances of ocular movements are important localizing signs in neurologic diagnosis. Lesions of the final common pathway occur at either the posterior fossa level (nucleus or nerve) or the peripheral level (nerve, neuromuscular junction, or muscle) and produce *diplopia.* Supranuclear or prenuclear control over the final common pathway is affected by lesions of the brainstem, vestibular system, cerebellum, or cortical eye fields.

Diplopia, or double vision, occurs when an image no longer falls on exactly corresponding areas of the two retinas. The brain interprets this as seeing two images instead of one (Fig. 34). Diplopia usually occurs secondary to a lesion affecting one or more of the ocular nerves or extraocular muscles. The affected eye shows restricted movement in the field of the weak muscle, and the patient reports maximal separation of the images in the direction of gaze of the weak muscle.

Prenuclear brainstem lesions can produce various gaze disorders. Lesions of the paramedian pontine reticular formation interrupt horizontal conjugate eye movements toward the side of the lesion. This occurs because the pontine paramedian reticular formation sends fibers to the ipsilateral abducens nucleus and from there via the medial longitudinal fasci-

culus to the contralateral oculomotor nucleus, specifically to the neurons innervating the medial rectus muscle. Lesions in the rostral interstitial nucleus of the medial longitudinal fasciculus affect both upward and downward vertical gaze. The fibers from this nucleus that mediate upward gaze pass dorsally through the posterior commissure to the oculomotor nucleus, so that a lesion here may affect only upward gaze.

In addition to lower motor neurons, the abducens nucleus contains *internuclear neurons* that send axons through the contralateral medial longitudinal fasciculus to the oculomotor nucleus. Therefore, a lesion in the medial longitudinal fasciculus prevents adduction of the eye on the side of the lesion when the patient attempts to gaze toward the opposite side. This clinical syndrome is called *internuclear ophthalmoplegia.* A lesion in the abducens nucleus itself, however, will produce an ipsilateral conjugate gaze palsy similar to that caused by a lesion of the pontine paramedian reticular formation. However, the paralysis of the ipsilateral lateral rectus muscle will be disproportionately severe.

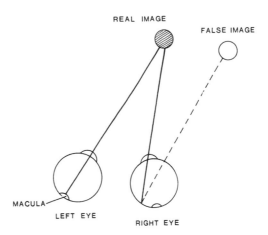

FIG. 34. Diplopia occurs when the images of one object fall on different parts of the two retinas. The brain interprets this as seeing two images. In this example, the right lateral rectus muscle is paretic, and the patient cannot rotate the right eye to the right. The image of the object falls on the nasal aspect of the retina of the right eye, and the brain interprets this as a second image (false image) to the right of the real image.

The interactions between the vestibular and oculomotor systems are most evident clinically in a phenomenon called *nystagmus* (Table 17). Nystagmus is a combination of slow eye movements in one direction followed by quick saccades in the opposite direction. It occurs normally with stimulation of the vestibular system, for example, when a person is rotated rapidly in a circle and then stopped. *Optokinetic nystagmus* is also a normal response to a moving visual environment, for example, when a person watches a passing train. The eyes make a following movement along with the train and then a quick saccade back to the primary position. Nystagmus can also be a sign of disease in the vestibular end-organ or in the vestibulocerebellar pathways in the brainstem.

The most important clinical feature of cortical oculomotor control is the tonic influence of the frontal eye field on the contralateral pontine paramedian reticular formation, causing the eyes to tend to deviate toward the opposite side (see Fig. 32). Normally, the influence from the two sides is balanced. Supratentorial lesions involving the frontal eye fields produce loss of voluntary conjugate gaze to the opposite side. When the lesion is acute, the eyes may be forcefully, conjugately deviated toward the side of the lesion. An irritative lesion, that is, a focal seizure, can cause tonic deviation of the eyes to the opposite side. When lesions affect the parieto-occipital eye field, the optokinetic response toward the side of the lesion is abolished. This is demonstrated by moving a striped tape or rotating a striped drum in front of the patient's eyes. When the stripes move toward the normal side, the eyes follow and then jerk back to pick up the next stripe. When the stripes move toward the abnormal side, the eyes do not move.

The Auditory System

The auditory system is represented at the posterior fossa and supratentorial levels. The auditory structures transform mechanical energy (sound) into action potentials and relay them to the brainstem and cerebral cortex. Auditory information is used for communication.

Sound waves are transformed into electrical signals by the structures in the inner ear. Afferent impulses pass centrally via the acoustic division of cranial nerve VIII and, after synapse in the cochlear nuclei, ascend bilaterally through a multisynaptic brainstem pathway to the primary auditory cortex in the anterior transverse gyrus of Heschl in the temporal lobe. Relay nuclei in the brainstem

TABLE 17. *Examples of nystagmus*

Type of nystagmus	Lesion	Slow eye deviation	Direction of nystagmus (quick phase)
Pendular	Visual system	None	Oscillation to both sides
Optokinetic	None (physiologic)	Toward a moving target	Toward primary position
Vestibular	Vestibular organs or vestibular nerve	Toward the site of the inactive labyrinth, because of predominance of the contralateral vestibular drive to oculomotor neurons	Toward side of more active labyrinth
Cerebellar (gaze-evoked)	Flocculonodular lobe May also occur with muscle fatigue or effects of drugs	Toward the neutral position despite attempt to maintain eccentric gaze, because of inability of ipsilateral cerebellum to provide tonic gaze-holding command ("leaky integrator")	Toward side of cerebellum with lesion Toward direction of gaze
Downbeat	Craniocervical junction	Upward because of lack of tonic stimulation from posterior semicircular canals	Downward
Dysconjugate (internuclear ophthalmoplegia)	Medial longitudinal fasciculus	Inability to adduct ipsilateral eye during attempted lateral gaze	Saccade of abducting eye

include the *superior olivary nuclei,* nucleus of the *lateral lemniscus, inferior colliculus,* and *medial geniculate body.* Although lesions central to the cochlear nuclei result in some alteration of auditory function, unilateral loss of hearing is found only with lesions of cranial nerve VIII or the peripheral receptors.

The Ear

The receptors for the auditory system are in the ear, which is subdivided into three major regions (Fig. 35): (1) the *external ear* consists of the pinna, which collects and directs sounds through the external auditory canal; (2) the *middle ear,* or tympanic cavity, contains the tympanic membrane (eardrum) and the auditory ossicles, which convert sound waves into waves in a fluid-filled chamber; and (3) the *inner ear,* or labyrinth, which is a series of fluid-filled membranous channels in the petrous portion of the temporal bone. The membranous labyrinth duplicates the shape of the bony labyrinth and is divided into two

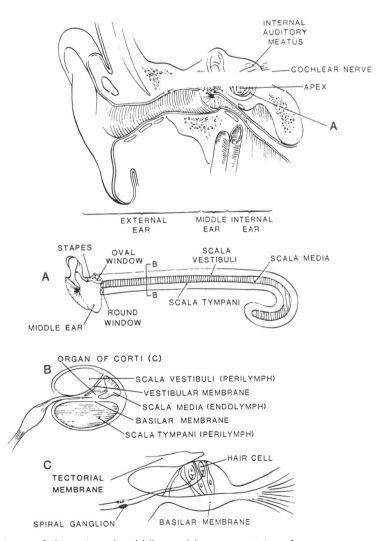

FIG. 35. Structures of the external, middle, and inner ear at top. **A:** Cochlea uncoiled, showing the three chambers. **B:** Cross section of the cochlea (*B-B* in Fig. 35A) showing the three chambers and the basilar membrane. **C:** Close-up view of the organ of Corti.

channels, one containing endolymph and the other containing perilymph. The ionic composition of these two fluids is different. Perilymph is similar to spinal fluid, whereas endolymph has a high potassium and low sodium content. The labyrinth is further divided into the cochlea and the vestibule, which consists of the utricle, the saccule, and the three semicircular canals. The cochlea contains the receptors for sound, and the vestibule contains the receptors of the vestibular apparatus.

Anatomy

The cochlea contains three parallel chambers and is shaped like a snail, coiled 2³/₄ turns from its base to its apex (Fig. 35). The two outer chambers, the *scala vestibuli* and *scala tympani,* contain perilymph and are in continuity at the apex of the coil. The middle chamber, the *scala media* (also called the *cochlear duct*), contains endolymph.

The scala vestibuli and scala media are separated by the vestibular (Reissner's) membrane, and the scala tympani and scala media are separated by the basilar membrane. At the base of the cochlea, the scala vestibuli ends at the oval window, and the scala tympani ends at the round window. The *organ of Corti* lies on the surface of the basilar membrane and contains mechanically sensitive hair cells, the auditory receptors. These cells have processes called *stereocilia* and generate electrotonic potentials in response to movement of the basilar membrane produced by sound waves. The base of the hair cell is enmeshed in a network of nerve endings of the cochlear nerve. The cochlear nerve fibers emerge from the coils of the cochlea in the central axis of the coil and join together to form the acoustic division of nerve VIII. The cell bodies of these first-order neurons for hearing are located in the *spiral ganglion* in the axis of the helix. Fibers pass centrally, enter the brainstem, and synapse in the dorsal and ventral cochlear nuclei (Fig. 36).

From the cochlear nuclei, second-order neurons travel via several pathways to the thalamus. Some fibers enter the reticular for-

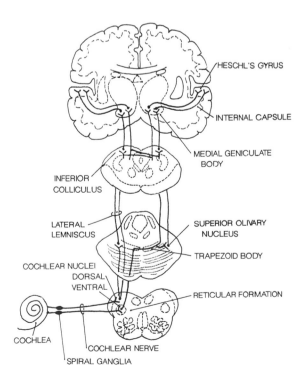

FIG. 36. Auditory pathways. Auditory impulses can ascend directly in the ipsilateral lateral lemniscus or synapse in the trapezoid body or superior olivary nucleus. They also may cross to the opposite side and ascend in the contralateral lateral lemniscus. Fibers thus ascend bilaterally to the inferior colliculus, medial geniculate bodies, and auditory cortex.

mation and participate in the alerting functions of the consciousness system. Some fibers ascend directly in the ipsilateral *lateral lemniscus,* whereas others synapse in the *nuclei of the trapezoid body* or the *superior olivary nuclei* in the ventral tegmentum of the pons (Fig. 36). Many but not all these fibers cross to the opposite side in the trapezoid body before passing rostrally. Thus, in each lateral lemniscus, there are auditory fibers that conduct information from both ears. Some of the fibers synapse in the nucleus of the lateral lemniscus en route to the inferior colliculus. At the inferior colliculus, some fibers again synapse, and a few may pass to the opposite side. Fibers traveling via the brachium of the inferior colliculus end in the medial geniculate body of the thalamus, which gives rise to axons that pass through the sublenticular portion of the internal capsule to go to the auditory cortex of the anterior transverse gyrus (*Heschl's gyrus*) in the temporal lobe (Fig. 36). Because of the partial decussation of auditory fibers, sound entering each ear is transmitted to both cerebral hemispheres.

Physiology

The ear converts sound waves in the external environment into action potentials in the auditory nerves. Sound waves entering the external auditory canal move the tympanic membrane (Fig. 37). This movement is trans-

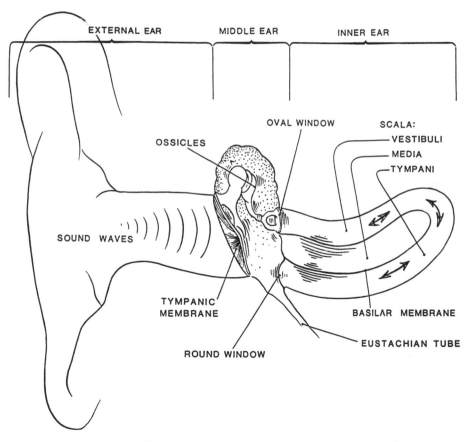

FIG. 37. The sound waves move the tympanic membrane and this mechanical force is transmitted via the ossicles to the footplate of the stapes. The movement of the stapes against the oval window is eventually transmitted to the endolymph, producing movement of the the basilar membrane.

mitted to the ossicles (malleus, incus, and stapes) of the middle ear, which amplify and transform the movements of the eardrum into smaller and more forceful movements of the footplate of the stapes, which rests against the oval window of the inner ear. The movement of the stapes against the oval window produces traveling pressure waves in the perilymph of the scala vestibuli. At the apex of the cochlea, these waves pass into the scala tympani and are dissipated by movement of the round window. As the sound waves enter the perilymph of the scala vestibuli, they are transmitted through the vestibular membrane to the endolymph of the scala media. This causes displacement of the basilar membrane, which in turn stimulates the hair cells in the organ of Corti. The movement of the stereocilia in the hair cells generates electrotonic potentials that are converted into action potentials in the auditory nerve fibers.

From the base to the apex, the basilar membrane gradually decreases in width and increases in tension. Because of this, different portions of the basilar membrane respond to different frequencies. The base responds to high frequencies and the apex to low frequencies. Thus, the cochlea mechanically separates the activation of different hair cells by different frequencies.

Pathophysiology

Patients with disease of the auditory division of cranial nerve VIII or its receptors complain of *tinnitus* (buzzing or ringing sensation in the ear) or loss of hearing. These can be important symptoms and signs in localizing a pathologic process to the posterior fossa level. Lesions within the central nervous system seldom produce a significant alteration in hearing. Therefore, unilateral hearing loss commonly indicates disease in the ipsilateral ear or in cranial nerve VIII. It is important to distinguish between the types of hearing deficit found in ear disease and in neural disease. *Conduction deafness* is due to disease of the external or middle ear that prevents sound waves being transmitted to the cochlea. *Sensorineural deafness* is due to disease of the cochlea or the auditory nerve or its nuclei. The distinction can often be made with a tuning fork, by performing the Weber and Rinne tests, as outlined in Table 18. Audiometric testing identifies the frequencies most impaired. Middle ear disease is associated with low-frequency loss, and nerve damage is associated with high-frequency loss.

Patients with lesions central to the cochlear nuclei do not complain of hearing loss. Although bilateral lesions of the inferior colliculi, medial geniculate bodies, or anterior transverse gyri do produce hearing loss, examples of these are so rare as to be of no practical clinical importance. Unilateral lesions in the region of the auditory receptive areas of the cerebral cortex do not cause hearing loss, but they produce a deficit in sound localization or discrimination. Focal seizures involving the cortical auditory receptive area in the temporal lobe produce hallucinations of sound. Electrical potentials evoked by click stimulation, called *brainstem auditory evoked potentials,* can be recorded on the scalp from

TABLE 18. *The Weber and Rinne tests for unilateral deafness*

Test	Method	Normal response	Conduction deafness	Sensorineural deafness
Weber	Base of vibrating tuning fork placed on vertex of skull	Heard equally in both ears (or center of the head)	Sound louder in abnormal ear	Sound louder in normal ear
Rinne	Each ear is tested separately—base of vibrating tuning fork is placed on the mastoid region until subject no longer hears sound (bone conduction), then held in air next to the ear (air conduction)	Air conduction is better than bone conduction	Bone conduction is better than air conduction in involved ear	Air conduction is better than bone conduction in involved ear

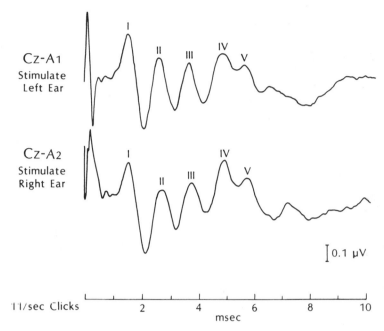

FIG. 38. Normal brainstem auditory evoked potentials *(I–V)* in a 26-year-old man. **Top:** The response of the left ear. **Bottom:** The response of the right ear. (The responses represent an average of 2,048 samples with summation of two superimposed responses.) (*Cz*, central vertex area; *A1*, left ear; *A2*, right ear.)

the structures along the auditory pathway (Fig. 38). Abnormalities in these potentials can identify and localize lesions in the auditory system.

The Vestibular System

The vestibular structures provide the nervous system with information about gravity, rotation, and acceleration that is necessary for maintenance of balance and equilibrium. These structures are located primarily in the posterior fossa.

Receptors that detect gravitational pull, rotational movements, and acceleration are located in the utricle, saccule, and semicircular canals of the inner ear. They transmit information to the central nervous system via the vestibular division of cranial nerve VIII. Numerous connections exist between the vestibular nuclei and the cerebellum, spinal cord, reticular formation, medial longitudinal fasciculus, and cerebral cortex to allow integration of vestibular impulses with other sen-

sory information for normal balance and equilibrium. Lesions affecting the vestibular structures cause a sense of imbalance (dysequilibrium). *Vertigo* is a highly specific symptom of vestibular system dysfunction. Nystagmus also occurs with lesions of the vestibular system or its connections.

Anatomy and Physiology

The receptors for the vestibular system are enclosed in the vestibular portion of the labyrinth in the utricle, the saccule, and the three semicircular canals (Table 19 and Fig. 39). The receptors are *hair cells* that respond to mechanical movement and initiate impulses that are transmitted via the vestibular division of cranial nerve VIII to the vestibular nuclei in the medulla and pons (see Fig. 17). The cell bodies of the first-order neurons are in the vestibular ganglion located in the internal auditory meatus. Movement of the hair cell stereocilia in one direction produces local potentials that increase the frequency of the

TABLE 19. *Vestibular organs, function, and connections*

Organ	Semicircular canals (lateral, superior, posterior)	Otolith organ (utricle and saccule)
Receptor	Hair cells in crista ampullaris	Hair cells in macula
Stimulus	Rotatory (angular) acceleration	Linear acceleration
		Gravity
Afferent	Vestibular nerve	Vestibular nerve
Vestibular nucleus	Superior, medial	Lateral, medial, inferior
Main function	Vestibulo-ocular reflex	Increased tone of antigravity muscles via vestibulospinal tracts
Effects of lesion	Rotational vertigo	Illusion of linear acceleration, loss of postural tone, head and ocular tilt

action potentials in the nerve; movement in the opposite direction inhibits nerve discharge. The hair cells in the utricle and saccule respond to positional and gravitational change, and those in the semicircular canals respond to rotational or angular acceleration.

The utricle and saccule contain endolymph. Specialized areas of epithelium called *maculae* are present in their walls (Fig. 39). Each macula is a tuft of ciliated columnar epithelial cells embedded in a gelatinous matrix containing small calcified particles (*otoliths*).

When the head is tilted from the vertical position, gravitational pull on the otoliths distorts the hair cells and initiates an action potential in the vestibular nerve. The three semicircular canals monitor acceleration in any plane. At one end of each canal is an enlargement called the *ampulla* (Fig. 39). The ampulla contains a specialized region of epithelium, the *crista*, similar to the maculae in the saccule and utricle. The crista is on a transverse ridge that projects into the lumen of the semicircular canal (Fig. 39). During rotational movement,

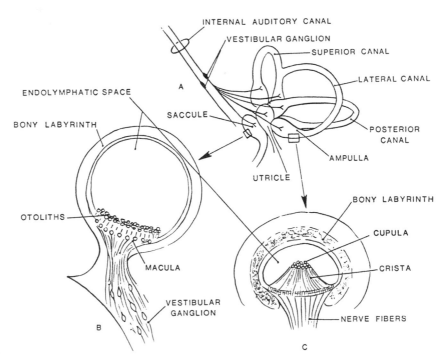

FIG. 39. Vestibular receptors. **A:** Nerve supply to vestibular receptors (utricle, saccule, and semicircular canals). **B:** Macula of utricle and saccule. **C:** Ampulla of semicircular canals.

the endolymph in the semicircular canal moves and distorts the crista, thus stimulating the hair cells and initiating action potentials. Each semicircular canal lies in a different plane so that each one is sensitive to rotation about a different axis.

Fibers of the vestibular division of cranial nerve VIII synapse in the superior, medial, lateral, and inferior *vestibular nuclei* located in the floor of the fourth ventricle. These nuclei have connections with several areas of the central nervous system. Some fibers of the vestibular nerve pass directly to the cerebellum via the inferior cerebellar peduncle. Others synapse in the inferior and medial vestibular nuclei before entering the cerebellum and terminating in the flocculonodular lobe. The flocculonodular lobe, in turn, sends fibers to the lateral vestibular nucleus, the origin of the lateral vestibulospinal tracts and a portion of the medial vestibulospinal tract, to regulate muscle tone in response to changing position. All the vestibular nuclei send fibers to the reticular formation, which can modify activity in the internal regulation and consciousness systems. The medial longitudinal fasciculus receives fibers from the vestibular nuclei for coordination of head and eye movements (Fig. 32). Pathways ascending to the cerebral cortex are not clearly defined. However, vestibular function is represented in the temporal lobes.

Pathophysiology

Input from the vestibular apparatus on each side is continuous and balanced. When receptor activity is altered by motion, the pattern of afferent impulses changes and a subjective sensation of motion is produced. When sensations of motion are in harmony with other sensory input, they are perceived as a correct response to a changing environment. When a lesion renders a portion of the vestibular system either hypoactive or hyperactive, the centrally integrated afferent impulses are not in accord with other sensory stimuli, and dysequilibrium is experienced. Dizziness, light-headedness, giddiness, and wooziness are common but nonspecific examples of dysequilibrium and frequently are not associated with disease of the vestibular system. However, vertigo, the hallucination of rotatory movement, is a highly specific form of dysequilibrium and is suggestive of disease of the vestibular system. Rarely, vertigo is a manifestation of focal seizures involving the temporal lobe; it is more often a manifestation of disease of the peripheral receptors, vestibular nerve, or brainstem. Thus, vertigo is an important neurologic symptom of disease at the posterior fossa level or in the ear. Vertigo caused by disorders of the vestibular system is often accompanied by nausea, vomiting, ataxia, and nystagmus, because of the resulting dysfunction of the reticular, cerebellar, and oculomotor connections of the vestibular system described above.

Vestibular system function is evaluated by caloric stimulation and by testing oculocephalic reflexes. In *caloric testing,* the external canal of each ear is irrigated with either warm or cold water. The temperature gradient of the water causes convection currents and movement of the endolymph in the semicircular canals. If the labyrinth, vestibular nerves, medial longitudinal fasciculus, and oculomotor system in the brainstem are intact, nystagmus occurs. Quantitative electrical measurement of the direction and amplitude of the eye movements produced in caloric testing is used in electronystagmography to help define the location and severity of vestibular lesions. The *oculocephalic (doll's eye) reflexes* are tested by rapidly turning the head from side to side or up and down. This movement stimulates the semicircular canals and causes the eyes to move conjugately in the opposite direction. Clinical caloric testing and doll's eye movements are commonly used to test the integrity of brainstem pathways in patients with altered states of consciousness. Abnormal results are helpful in localizing the responsible lesion to the posterior fossa level.

Clinical Correlations

Lesions that involve the posterior fossa level are associated with abnormalities in cranial nerve, cerebellar, or brainstem function. Because components of each of the major longitudinal systems are found at this level, dysfunction in any of these systems may be present. Lesions in all etiologic categories are found at this level, and the pathologic nature of these lesions can be determined, as at other levels, by applying the general principles of neurologic diagnosis outlined in Chapter 4.

Before the specific manifestations of lesions involving a particular level of the brainstem are described, it is helpful to consider symptom complexes that are common to involvement of multiple levels or of posterior fossa structures as a whole, specifically dysarthria and coma.

Dysarthria

Dysarthria, or motor speech impairment, must be distinguished clearly from *aphasia,* a disorder of symbolic language function discussed in Chapter 16. Clear speech involves closely coordinated and modulated activity of muscles supplied by cranial nerves V, VII, IX, X, and XII as well as the respiratory muscles, especially the diaphragm, innervated by the phrenic nerve (spinal level C-4) (Table 20). The activation, modulation, and coordination of this output are controlled by the direct activation pathway via the corticobulbar tracts, indirect activation via extrapyramidal pathways, and cerebellar control circuits. Thus, dysarthria can take many forms depending on the structures or combination of structures involved.

The most common types are outlined in Table 21. *Flaccid dysarthria* results from

TABLE 20. *Components of speech production*

Component	Nerve	Muscle
Respiration	Phrenic	Diaphragm, intercostal
Phonation	X (inferior laryngeal)	Laryngeal
Resonation	IX, X	Palate
Articulation	V	Masseter, pterygoid
	VII	Orbicularis oris, buccinator
	XII	Tongue

lesions of the final common pathways of cranial nerves V, VII, IX, X, or XII. Although the manifestations vary depending on the specific nerve or combination of nerves involved, typical features include breathy voice, hypernasality, and articulatory imprecision. *Spastic dysarthria* is the result of bilateral corticobulbar tract lesions and is characterized by a strained hoarseness, hypernasality, and a slow articulatory rate. These two speech patterns are typically seen in patients with *bulbar* and *pseudobulbar palsy* (Table 22). *Ataxic dysarthria* occurs with lesions of the cerebellum and produces irregular articulatory breakdowns, and, less frequently, voice tremor and loss of loudness of the voice. *Hypokinetic* and *hyperkinetic dysarthrias* occur with lesions of the basal ganglia circuits. The former is characteristic of Parkinson's disease and related syndromes and features low volume, monotonous, rapid speech with indistinct articulation. The latter is seen in dystonias and choreas in which there are uncontrolled and unpredictable movements of the laryngeal, pharyngeal, lingual, and facial muscles that interrupt and distort phonation, resonation, and articulation.

Coma

The pathophysiology of coma is discussed in Chapter 10. However, because coma is a common result of lesions in the posterior fossa, it is useful to comment on certain specific features of coma of brainstem origin. Coma due to lesions of the brainstem can be identified and localized more precisely by the presence of associated disturbances in brainstem function outside the consciousness system. These include dysfunction of the descending motor pathways resulting in disturbances in posture and tone, dysfunction of the oculomotor system, and disturbances in control of respiratory and cardiovascular functions. The effects on these systems when different levels of the brainstem are involved are outlined in Table 23.

Decorticate and decerebrate posturing involve abnormally increased muscle tone in the extremities mediated by the rubrospinal

TABLE 21. *Types of dysarthrias*

Type	Lesion	Clinical features
Flaccid	X, IX, X, V, VII, XII	Breathy voice, hypernasality, articulatory imprecisions
Spastic	Corticobulbar pathway	Strained voice, hypernasality, slow articulatory rate
Ataxic	Cerebellar control circuit	Irregular articulatory breakdowns (scanning), slow rate
Hypokinetic	Substantia nigra Basal ganglia (parkinsonism)	Reduced voice volume, monopitch, rapid, indistinct articulation
Hyperkinetic	Basal ganglia (dystonia, chorea)	Unpredictable interruptions and distortion of phonation, resonation, and articulation

and vestibulospinal pathways. In *decorticate* posturing due to damage of the rostral brainstem (above the red nucleus), flexor tone is increased more than extensor tone in the upper extremities, resulting in flexion of the arms. *Decerebrate posturing* occurs with lesions below the red nucleus but above the vestibular nuclei. The extensor tone is increased in all four limbs because of the uninhibited influence of the vestibulospinal pathway. Lesions at or below the vestibular nuclei abolish the excitatory influence of all these pathways.

The effects of various lesions on the size and reactivity of the pupil can be deduced from recognizing that the sympathetic influence on pupillary dilatation originates in the hypothalamus and descends the length of the brainstem, whereas the parasympathetic fibers mediating constriction originate in the midbrain and leave the brainstem at that level with cranial nerve III. Any lesion that isolates one or the other results in either abnormally dilated or constricted pupils, whereas a lesion that affects both sets of fibers results in a midposition, unreactive pupil.

The *oculovestibular reflex* refers to effects of caloric stimulation of the labyrinth on eye movements. Caloric stimulation in intact persons produces nystagmus. In coma due to cerebral damage rostral to the midbrain, the refixation, or fast, phase of nystagmus is absent, and the expected response to caloric stimulation, if the brainstem between the vestibular nuclei and the oculomotor nuclei is intact, is conjugate ocular deviation. If the ear is irrigated with cold water, the eyes will deviate slowly toward the stimulated ear. This occurs because cold water inhibits vestibular discharge from the stimulated ear, which results in the relative predominance of the contralateral labyrinth. This drives the eyes toward the side of cold irrigation. With brainstem lesions at or below the level of the oculomotor nuclei, the response will be distorted or absent.

Brainstem centers that participate in the regulation of respiration and cardiovascular reflexes are discussed in Chapter 9. Normal rhythmic respiration appropriately responsive to changes in blood chemistry (especially carbon dioxide level and pH) requires the integrated function of all levels of the nervous system. Loss of cerebral influence because of lesions above the red nucleus results in a periodic breathing pattern characterized by waxing and waning hyperpnea alternating with short periods of apnea. This is called *Cheyne-*

TABLE 22. *Differences between bulbar and pseudobulbar palsies*

	Bulbar	Pseudobulbar
Location of lesion	Lower motor neuron (V, VII, IX, X, XII)	Upper motor neuron (corticobulbar tract, bilateral)
Type of dysarthria	Flaccid	Spastic
Tongue atrophy/ fasciculations	Yes	No
Masseter reflex	Normal or ↓	Exaggerated
Gag reflex	Absent	Exaggerated
Emotional lability	No	Yes

TABLE 23. *Levels of brainstem involvement in patients with coma*

Level	Posture	Pupils	Oculovestibular response	Respiration, blood pressure
Between cortex and midbrain	Decorticate	Miotic, reactive	Slow phase present, fast phase absent	Cheyne-Stokes; normal or elevated
Midbrain (above red nucleus)	Decorticate	Midposition, nonreactive	Slow phase present, fast phase absent	Cheyne-Stokes
Midbrain (below red nucleus) and pons (above vestibular nuclei)	Decerebrate	Pinpoint, reactive	Slow phase present, fast phase absent	Central neurogenic hyperventilation, hypertension, tachycardia, sweating
Caudal pons and rostral medulla (below vestibular nucleus)	Flaccid	Midsize	Absent	Apneustic respiration
Medulla	Flaccid	Midsize, nonreactive	Absent	Irregular, bradycardia, hypotension

Stokes respiration. Midbrain and rostral pontine lesions are suggested by sustained hyperpnea called *central neurogenic hyperventilation.* Lesions in the lower brainstem cause slow, arrhythmic, or periodic breathing patterns, including *apneustic breathing* (long inspiratory pauses), respiration alternans, and ataxic (Biot's) breathing.

Ischemic Lesions of the Brainstem

The blood supply of the brainstem is derived from the vertebrobasilar arterial system. The pattern of supply to each level is relatively constant, with the midline region being supplied by small penetrating paramedian branches of the vertebral and basilar arteries and the lateral area being supplied by larger circumferential branches: the posterior inferior cerebellar artery at the level of the medulla, the anterior inferior cerebellar artery at the level of the pons, and the superior cerebellar artery at the level of the midbrain. Ischemic lesions involving the brainstem usually occur either in the paramedian region or in the lateral region. Infarction of the paramedian region involves the descending motor pathways, medial lemniscus, and the nuclei of cranial nerves III, IV, VI, and XII. Infarction of the lateral region involves the cerebellum, cerebellar pathways, descending sympathetic pathways, the lateral spinothalamic tract, and the nuclei of cranial nerve V, VII, VIII, IX, or X.

Vascular Lesions of the Medulla

The paramedian region of the medulla is supplied by vessels from the anterior spinal and vertebral arteries. Infarction in the paramedian medulla involves the medullary pyramids, medial lemniscus, and cranial nerve XII, resulting in contralateral hemiparesis, impaired conscious proprioceptive sensation, and ipsilateral tongue weakness (Fig. 40).

The lateral regions of the medulla and portions of the cerebellum are supplied by the posterior inferior cerebellar artery. Occlusion or thrombosis of this artery (or its parent vertebral artery) produces infarction of the lateral medulla and results in a constellation of signs and symptoms referred to as *Wallenberg's syndrome* (Fig. 40). This syndrome includes dysarthria and dysphagia due to involvement of the nucleus ambiguus, ipsilateral impairment of pain and temperature on the face due to involvement of the descending nucleus and tract of nerve V, contralateral loss of pain and temperature in the trunk and extremities due to involvement of the spinothalamic tract, ipsilateral Horner's syndrome due to involvement of the descending sympathetic fibers in the lateral part of the brainstem, ipsilateral limb ataxia due to involvement of the inferior cerebellar peduncle, and vertigo due to involvement of the vestibular nuclei or

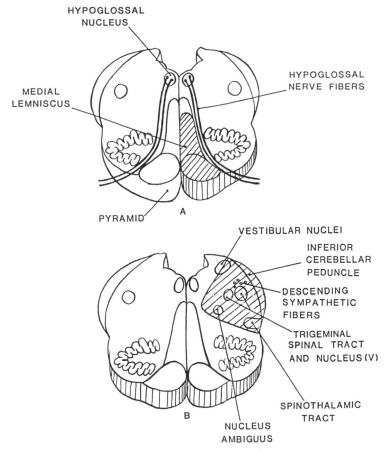

FIG. 40. A: Paramedian infarct of medulla. **B:** Lateral medullary infarct of medulla (Wallenberg's syndrome).

vestibulocerebellar fibers in the tegmentum of the medulla.

Vascular Lesions of the Pons

An infarct of the paramedian area of the pons results in ipsilateral sixth nerve palsy due to involvement of axons arising in the abducens nucleus, ipsilateral facial weakness due to involvement of the facial nerve as it passes around the abducens nucleus, contralateral hemiparesis due to involvement of the corticospinal tracts in the basis pontis, and contralateral impairment of conscious proprioception due to involvement of the medial lemniscus (Fig. 41).

An infarct of the lateral portion of the pons causes ipsilateral facial paralysis due to involvement of the facial nucleus; impairment of touch, pain, and temperature on the same side of the face due to involvement of the main sensory nucleus and descending nucleus and tract of cranial nerve V; loss of pain and temperature on the contralateral side of the body due to involvement of the spinothalamic tract; ipsilateral deafness due to involvement of the nuclei of nerve VIII; ipsilateral Horner's syndrome due to involvement of the descending sympathetic fibers; and ipsilateral cerebellar signs due to involvement of the middle cerebellar peduncle.

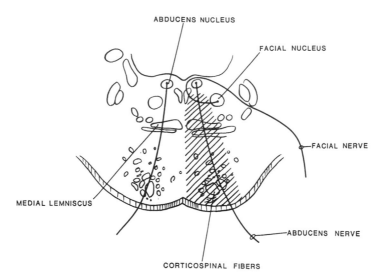

FIG. 41. Paramedian infarct of pons *(shaded area)* with involvement of VI nerve nucleus, facial nerve, medial lemniscus, and corticospinal tract.

Vascular Lesions of the Midbrain

Infarction of the lateral midbrain is uncommon; however, ischemic lesions involving the paramedian region (Fig. 42) are seen occasionally and produce diplopia, ptosis, and mydriasis due to involvement of cranial nerve III and contralateral hemiparesis due to involvement of the cerebral peduncle. This constellation of symptoms is called *Weber's syndrome.*

Neoplasms of the Posterior Fossa

Certain tumors of the posterior fossa are more commonly encountered in children and young adults. Ependymomas and medulloblastomas frequently arise in the region of the fourth ventricle and are associated with ataxia, nausea, and vomiting. As these lesions increase in size, they obstruct the outflow of cerebrospinal fluid from the ventricular sys-

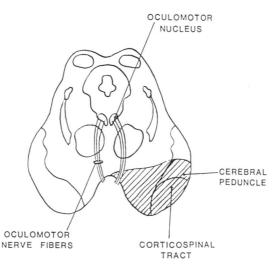

FIG. 42. Paramedian infarct of midbrain—Weber's syndrome *(shaded area)*, with involvement of nerve III and cerebral peduncle.

tem and cause a noncommunicating hydrocephalus and signs of increased intracranial pressure. Astrocytomas of the cerebellum also are common in childhood; they arise in the cerebellar hemisphere (resulting in ipsilateral limb ataxia). These tumors, which are frequently cystic in structure, display a unique biologic behavior; the early diagnosis and surgical removal of cerebellar astrocytomas, in contrast to astrocytomas of other locations, are associated with a good prognosis.

Astrocytomas also arise from glial cells located within the substance of the brainstem and result in a brainstem or pontine glioma (Fig. 43). These tumors involve either the base or the tegmentum and are usually associated with progressive (often bilateral) symptoms of cranial nerve, motor, and sensory dysfunction. If the reticular formation is affected, consciousness is altered.

Certain tumors arise outside the parenchyma of the brainstem (extraaxial tumors), often from the meninges (meningiomas) or from the supporting cells in the cranial nerves. Extraaxial tumors initially produce alteration in cranial nerve function and secondarily affect brainstem function by compression or direct invasion. The most common tumor in this group is the vestibular schwannoma. Although it is commonly referred to as acoustic neuroma, the tumor arises from Schwann cells in the vestibular division of cranial nerve VIII in virtually all cases (Fig. 44). The tumors are frequently bilateral in central, or type II, neurofibromatosis. Early signs of a vestibular schwannoma are unilateral tinnitus, decreased hearing, and disequilibrium. As the tumor enlarges, ipsilateral facial paresis, loss of corneal reflex, and ipsilateral limb ataxia occur. With further increase in size, there may be additional signs of brainstem compression and increased intracranial pressure. These tumors are usually seen with computed tomographic scanning and, even when very small, with magnetic resonance imaging scanning.

Herniations of the Brain

Expanding supratentorial mass lesions may secondarily affect the structures located in the posterior fossa. The cranial cavity is a closed

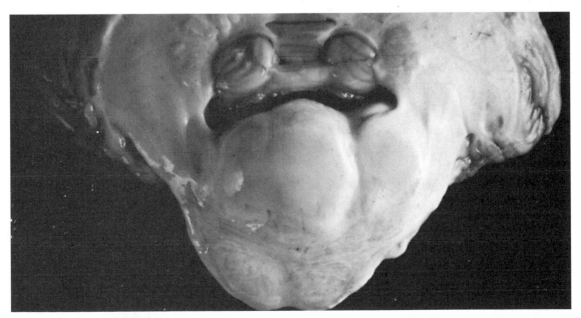

FIG. 43. Gross specimen of brainstem glioma. Transverse section showing diffuse asymmetric enlargement.

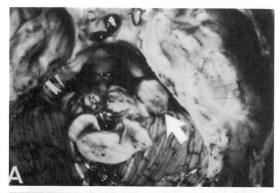

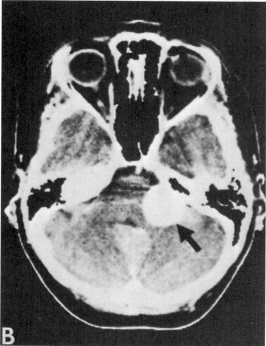

FIG. 44. Vestibular schwannoma. **A:** Gross specimen, with posterior fossa and contents viewed from above with tumor *(arrow)* of cranial nerve VIII. (Note normal cranial nerves VII and VIII on the opposite side.) **B:** Computerized tomographic scan of the posterior fossa at the level of the pons showing a tumor *(arrow)* in the cerebellopontine angle compressing the pons.

space and cannot accommodate to changes in intracranial volume. In the presence of a supratentorial or posterior fossa mass, intracranial pressure increases, and with further expansion the brain adjusts to the increased volume by alteration in shape and slight shifts

in position. With further compression and shift, the function in areas of the nervous system remote from the expanding mass is also compromised, and further deterioration in the clinical condition occurs. The changes in shape and position that occur secondary to intracranial mass lesions are called *herniations of the brain.*

Uncal Herniation

Uncal herniation characteristically occurs when unilateral, expanding supratentorial lesions, especially in the middle fossa, shift the mediobasal edge of the uncus of the hippocampal gyrus toward the midline and over the free edge of the tentorium, compressing the adjacent midbrain (Fig. 45A and Table 24). Cranial nerve III and sometimes the posterior cerebral artery on the side of the herniating temporal lobe are compressed by the overhanging swollen uncus. The clinical sign resulting from compression of cranial nerve III is an ipsilateral third-nerve paresis, usually beginning with dilatation of the pupil. Compression of the contralateral cerebral peduncle against the free edge of the tentorium can cause hemiparesis ipsilateral to the expanding lesion. Midbrain compression also affects the ascending reticular activating system, and there is progressive loss of consciousness. If the posterior cerebral artery is compressed, infarction of the occipital lobe occurs, producing homonymous hemianopia.

Central or Transtentorial Herniation

This type of herniation occurs as a further progression of uncal herniation and in association with parasagittal or bilateral supratentorial masses. It consists of caudal displacement of the diencephalon, midbrain, and pons (Fig. 45B and Table 24). Caudal displacement of the basilar artery (which is attached to the circle of Willis via the posterior cerebral arteries) does not occur to the same degree, resulting in stretching and shearing of paramedian perforating vessels, with secondary infarction and hemorrhage in the brainstem. This type of

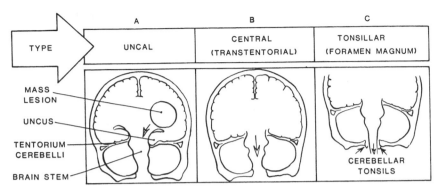

FIG. 45. Herniations of the brain. **A:** Uncal herniation. **B:** Central (transtentorial) herniation. **C:** Tonsillar (foramen magnum) herniation.

herniation blocks the flow of cerebrospinal fluid through the aqueduct of Sylvius, thus further increasing the volume of the supratentorial contents. The clinical signs of central herniation are oculomotor paresis, progressive alteration of consciousness, and decerebrate rigidity. Because mass lesions rarely are directly in the midline, some degree of lateral shift and uncal herniation nearly always accompanies transtentorial herniation.

Tonsillar or Foramen Magnum Herniation

As a result of an expanding mass in the posterior fossa or further progression of uncal or transtentorial herniation, herniation of the cerebellar tonsils through the foramen magnum occurs, with compression of the medulla (Fig. 45C). Signs of tonsillar herniation include neck pain and stiffness, the result of stretching and irritation of the lower cranial

TABLE 24. *Herniations of the brain*

Type	Location	Cause	Anatomical structures involved	Clinical effects
Uncal	Tentorial notch, midbrain	Mass lesion in temporal lobe or middle fossa	Parahippocampal gyrus and uncus	
			Oculomotor nerve	Paresis of nerve III
			Cerebral peduncle	Hemiparesis
			Midbrain ascending reticular activating system	Coma
			Posterior cerebral artery	Homonymous hemianopia
Central (transtentorial)	Tentorial notch, midbrain	Mass lesion in frontal, parietal, or occipital lobe	Midbrain and pons	Decerebrate rigidity
		Progression of uncal herniation	Ascending reticular activating system	Coma
Tonsillar (foramen magnum)	Foramen magnum, medulla	Mass lesion in posterior fossa	Cerebellar tonsils	Neck pain and stiffness
		Progression of uncal	Indirect activation pathways	Flaccidity
		or transtentorial herniation	Ascending reticular activating system	Coma
			Vasomotor centers	Alteration of pulse, respiration, blood pressure

nerves supplying the neck muscles; progressive loss of consciousness secondary to involvement of the ascending reticular activating system; generalized flaccidity; alteration of vital signs, with slowing of the pulse and vasomotor instability; and periodic or irregular respiration, the result of involvement of visceral centers in the medulla.

The three types of herniation of the brain are summarized in Figure 45 and Table 24.

Neurologic Examination of the Posterior Fossa Level

The integrity of the posterior fossa is examined by testing the function of each of the major longitudinal systems found at this level (see Chapters 6 through 11) and the functions associated with the oculomotor, auditory, and vestibular systems and cranial nerves III through XII.

The Oculomotor System and Cranial Nerves III, IV, and VI

Neurologic examination of the eyes begins with observing the size and bilateral symmetry of the palpebral fissures, especially looking for ptosis. The size, shape, and symmetry of the pupils are noted. The pupillary light reflex is tested by shining a light into each eye while observing the direct and consensual pupillary responses. The near reflex is tested by bringing a target toward the patient's nose and by observing pupillary constriction and eye convergence.

The position, alignment, and stability of the eyes when the patient attempts to gaze straight ahead (primary position) are observed. Abnormalities include inability to maintain the primary position because of conjugate deviation, misalignment of the eyes because of monocular deviation, and spontaneous nystagmus. Eye movement is tested in the six cardinal directions, first with both eyes fixing on the target and then testing each eye with the other covered. Subtle muscle weakness can be demonstrated by placing a red glass in front of one eye while the patient follows a white light. This inhibits the reflex tendency of the brain to fuse identical images if possible and allows clearer identification of the field of gaze in which the image separation (diplopia) is greatest, thus identifying the weak muscle. Nystagmus is also looked for in each direction of gaze.

Cranial Nerve V

Sensory function is examined by testing the patient's ability to perceive pinprick and light touch applied to the skin supplied by the three divisions of the trigeminal nerve. The corneal reflex (which also involves cranial nerve VII) is tested by asking the patient to look to one side while the cornea is gently touched with a wisp of cotton, brought toward the cornea from the opposite direction. The normal response is prompt, bilateral blinking.

Motor function is tested by having the patient open the jaw. In the presence of unilateral pterygoid weakness, the jaw deviates to the weak side. The patient is also asked to bite firmly while the examiner palpates the masseter and temporalis muscles on each side. Jaw jerk is tested by placing the examiner's forefinger on the relaxed jaw and by striking the finger with a reflex hammer.

Cranial Nerve VII

Examination of the facial nerve begins with observing the patient's facial expressions. As the patient talks and smiles, facial asymmetry or reduced contraction becomes apparent. Specific muscle groups are then examined. The frontalis muscles are tested by asking the patient to wrinkle the forehead; strength can be assessed by attempting to smooth the wrinkles on each side. The orbicularis oculi can be tested by asking the patient to tightly close the eyes and then to try opening them. The lower facial muscles are tested by asking the patient to smile or show the teeth. Taste is not examined unless a peripheral facial nerve lesion is suspected. It is tested by having the patient protrude the tongue and then asking him or her to identify sugar, salt, or other substances applied to the side of the tongue.

The Auditory and Vestibular Systems and Cranial Nerve VIII

Audiometry provides the best means of examining hearing, but a rough estimate of the functioning of the acoustic system can be made by determining if the patient can hear the sound of a watch or the sound produced by rubbing the forefinger and thumb together in front of the ear. Auditory acuity of one side is compared with that of the other. The Weber and Rinne tests should be performed (see Table 18).

Vestibular function ordinarily is not examined unless disease of cranial nerve VIII, sensory ataxia, or brainstem disease is suspected. Caloric testing (irrigating the outer ear canal with cold water and observing for nystagmus, conjugate deviation of the eyes, or subjective vertigo) is a convenient means of testing vestibular function but usually is reserved for comatose patients.

Cranial Nerves IX and X

The glossopharyngeal and vagus nerves are often tested together by listening to the patient talk and inquiring about difficulty in speaking or swallowing. A soft, breathy voice associated with nasal escape of air is suggestive of weakness in the oropharynx, whereas a hoarse or husky voice suggests a lesion of the nerve supply to the larynx. The patient is also asked to open the mouth and say "ah." Normally, the palate rises in the midline; unilateral palatal weakness causes the uvula to deviate toward the intact side. The gag reflex is examined by touching the back of the throat with a tongue blade and noting the contraction of the pharyngeal muscles.

Cranial Nerve XI

The sternocleidomastoid muscle is tested by asking the patient to turn the head to the side, against resistance applied by the examiner to the patient's jaw. The contracting muscle (on the side opposite the turn of the head) can be observed and palpated. The trapezius muscle is examined by having the patient elevate the shoulders against resistance applied by the examiner.

Cranial Nerve XII

The patient is asked to protrude the tongue in the midline and then to wiggle it from side to side. With upper motor neuron lesions, there is slowing of the alternate motion rate of the tongue. With unilateral lower motor neuron weakness, there are ipsilateral atrophy and fasciculations, and the protruded tongue deviates toward the side of the lesion.

Speech

Verbal communication includes both cognitive and motor skills. The cognitive aspects of verbal communication are considered language and are described in Chapter 16. Some motor speech disorders may result from disease of the brainstem and cranial nerves (flaccid dysarthria) or cerebellum (ataxic dysarthria). Spastic, hypokinetic, and hyperkinetic dysarthrias result from disease at the supratentorial level.

Tests for disorders of speech, the dysarthrias, are commonly administered at the same time as the testing of cranial nerve function. Speech can be evaluated by listening to spontaneous speech or by having the patient repeat the syllables *pa-pa-pa* (facial muscle and nerve function), *ta-ta-ta* (tongue and hypoglossal nerve function), and *ka-ka-ka* (pharyngeal muscle and ninth and tenth nerve function). The syllables *pa-ta-ka-pa-ta-ka* test cranial muscle coordination (cerebellar function).

Clinical Problems ■

1. A 68-year-old woman, previously in good health, suddenly became extremely nau-

seated and dizzy, as if the room were spinning around her. She remained conscious and could describe her symptoms to a companion, who noted that her voice was hoarse. Examination in the emergency room several hours later revealed the following abnormalities: The patient could not sit or stand because of vertigo. She was anxious and perspiring, except on the left side of her face. Her left pupil was small, and her left eyelid drooped slightly. There was horizontal and rotatory nystagmus. The left palate was drooping, and the left gag reflex was absent. There was loss of pain and temperature sensation on the left side of her face. Touch was preserved. Muscle strength and stretch reflexes were normal in the extremities. There was moderate incoordination of her left arm and leg. Sensory examination revealed loss of pain and temperature sensation in her right arm, trunk, and leg.

a. What is the location and type of the abnormality?
b. Specifically, what is the site of the lesion?
c. What artery supplies the involved area?
d. What anatomical structures are responsible for the loss of pain and temperature sensation on the left side of the face and on the right side of the trunk?
e. What is the cause of the ptosis, miosis, and anhidrosis on the left?

2. A 50-year-old man was well until 6 months ago when he noted some difficulty in swallowing. Food seemed to stick in the right side of his throat, and liquids occasionally entered the right side of his nose. In the last 3 months, he has noted progressive hoarseness of his voice and difficulty in reaching overhead with his right arm. Examination revealed that the soft palate sagged on the right side. When the left posterior pharynx was stimulated, the soft palate pulled upward and to the left. When the right side was similarly

stimulated, nothing happened and the patient said he could barely feel the touch. Indirect laryngoscopy revealed that the right vocal cord did not move with phonation. Muscle testing revealed weakness and atrophy of the right trapezius and sternocleidomastoid muscles. Results of the rest of the examination were normal.

a. What is the location and type of lesion?
b. What neural structures are involved?
c. Through what foramen do these structures leave the skull?
d. What other structure also passes through this foramen?
e. Name one lesion that can produce the above syndrome.

3. A 70-year-old woman had sudden onset of weakness of her right arm and leg and difficulty in moving her tongue. When seen in the emergency room a few hours later, she had weakness of her right arm and leg and decreased ability to perceive proprioceptive and tactile stimuli on the right. When her tongue was protruded, it deviated to the left.

a. What is the location and type of lesion?
b. What structures are involved?
c. What is the pathologic nature of the lesion?

4. A 25-year-old man awoke one morning and noted that the left side of his face seemed weak. On looking into a mirror, he noted that he could not retract the left corner of his mouth as well as the right. He also noted that he could no longer close his left eye completely or smile with the left side of his face. Neurologic examination revealed no abnormality except for the following: At rest, the left side of his face drooped, and the left palpebral fissure was wider than the right. The left side of his forehead did not wrinkle when he tried raising his eyebrows. He could not close his left eye completely. When he attempted to show his teeth, his mouth pulled to the right. Results of testing for sensations of pain,

temperature, and touch of the face were normal. Taste was absent on the left side of his tongue. Strips of filter paper were placed in the conjunctival sacs; the one on the right became moist within a few minutes, and the left side remained dry.

a. What is the location and type of lesion?

b. Why was taste involved?

c. Why was there decreased lacrimation?

d. What is the name of this clinical entity?

5. A 60-year-old woman had ringing (tinnitus) in her right ear for the past year as well as intermittent episodes of feeling that the room was spinning around her. In the past 6 months, she began staggering to the right and had difficulty with coordination of her right hand. Three weeks ago, she noted that the right side of her face was weak. Examination revealed a loss of hearing and an absent caloric response on the right. She could not wrinkle her forehead or retract the right side of her face when asked to smile. She had trouble with coordination in her right hand and had an intention tremor on finger-to-nose and heel-to-shin testing of the right upper and lower extremities.

a. What is the location and type of lesion?

b. What specific anatomical structures are involved?

c. What is the general anatomical term used to describe the region of involvement?

d. Name one pathologic lesion that can produce this syndrome.

e. What diagnostic studies might be useful in defining the location of this lesion?

6. A 60-year-old woman had a myocardial infarction. Several days later, however, she complained to the nurse that she had an abrupt onset of seeing double whenever she looked to the left and that she was having some difficulty in using her right arm. Testing of cranial nerves revealed paralysis of the left lateral rectus

muscle. Her speech was slightly slurred, and the left nasolabial fold was flattened. She could not tightly close her left eye, and she could not raise her eyebrow on the left as high as on the right. Facial sensation and taste were normal. Testing of the extremities revealed weakness of the right arm and leg, with hyperactive reflexes and Babinski's sign on the right. There was loss of joint position and vibration sense in the right arm and leg.

a. What is the location and type of lesion?

b. What anatomical structures are involved?

c. What is the pathologic nature of the lesion?

7. A 73-year-old diabetic woman entered the hospital because of abrupt onset of double vision and left-sided weakness. Examination several hours later revealed that her right pupil was 4 mm and her left was 3 mm. The direct and consensual light response of the right pupil was less brisk than the left. There was slight ptosis of the eyelid on the right. On following a light with her eyes, she reported seeing two images when the light was moved directly to her left and to her right and upward. A red glass was placed over her right eye. When the light was moved to the left, the red image was seen to the left of the white image. When the light was moved to her right and upward, the red image was above the white image. In each instance, the separation increased as the light was moved further. The only other abnormalities on neurologic examination were slight drooping of the left corner of her mouth and slight weakness of her left arm and leg, with hyperactive deep tendon reflexes, reduced abdominal reflexes, and Babinski's sign on the left.

a. What is the location and type of lesion?

b. What anatomical structures are involved?

c. Diplopia testing indicated weakness of which muscles?

d. Why was the pupillary light reflex altered?

e. What is the pathologic nature of the lesion?

8. A 10-year-old boy was evaluated because of trouble with coordination of his left side. He had been well until 3 months ago, when he experienced severe headaches. Two months ago, he began to note that his left hand shook when he reached for an object. One month before admission, he noted increasing clumsiness of his left leg. Because of the headaches, nausea and vomiting, and increased clumsiness of the left arm and leg, he was examined. Examination showed that his optic nerve heads were swollen and that he took frequent missteps with his left leg and had an intention tremor on finger-to-nose and heel-to-shin testing. Muscle tone was slightly decreased on the left, but strength and sensation were intact.

a. What is the location and type of lesion?

b. What specific area of the neuraxis seems to be involved?

c. What signs and symptoms suggest the presence of increased intracranial pressure?

d. Name the most common lesion occurring in children that can produce this syndrome.

9. A 55-year-old man had noted progressive difficulty in swallowing and talking during the past year; liquids had tended to go down his windpipe or out his nose, and he had felt that his trouble with speech was due to his tongue "not working right." Examination revealed fasciculations and atrophy of the tongue bilaterally. He had trouble protruding his tongue and moving it from side to side. When he was asked to say "ah," his palate showed only minimal elevation. When asked to say "ka-ka-ka," he had nasal emission of speech. When asked to show his teeth, he was noted to have bilateral facial weakness, left greater than right, and he could not whistle. Slight distal extremity weakness and fasciculations also were seen. Deep ten-

don reflexes were reduced, but Babinski's sign was present bilaterally. Results of the rest of the examination were normal.

a. What is the location and site of the lesion?

b. What system(s) is (are) involved?

c. What component(s) of the system(s) is (are) involved?

d. Name one disorder that can produce this syndrome.

10. A 13-year-old girl awoke one morning complaining of a left earache and a dull generalized headache. Her temperature was 102°F (38.9° C) orally. Her condition did not improve with aspirin and bed rest and that evening she was taken to her family physician, who diagnosed acute otitis media and gave her an injection of penicillin. For the next several days, she continued to have some ear drainage and mild left-sided ear pain and headache. During the next week, she had increasingly severe headaches, with nausea and vomiting. One day before admission, she experienced progressive weakness of the right face, arm, and leg and difficulty in speaking. She also seemed to have difficulty in thinking of what word she wanted to say, and she had difficulty in understanding what people were saying to her.

a. At this point, what is the suspected location and type of lesion?

   When seen at the local hospital, she was stuporous but could be aroused by strong stimuli. Her left pupil was dilated and reacted poorly to light. The right pupillary reflex was intact. The left eye was deviated down and out, and she had ptosis of the left eyelid. During the examination, her right hemiparesis became much worse.

b. What is the reason for her change in level of consciousness?

c. How do you explain the eye findings?

d. Why was there worsening of her hemiparesis?

e. What is the term used to describe the above process?

   It was decided to send the patient to the nearest neurosurgical facility, which was several hours away. On arrival at the second hospital, she was deeply comatose. Respirations were deep and rapid. Her temperature was 105°F (40.6°C). Her pupils were slightly dilated and did not react to light. Her jaw was tightly clenched. Her spine was extended and arched posteriorly. Her arms were stiffly extended and the fists clenched. Her legs were also stiffly extended.

f. The findings present at this point suggest involvement at what level of the neuraxis?

g. What term describes her body position and tone?

h. What term describes the process producing this clinical picture?

Additional Reading ■

Baloh, R. W., and Honrubia, V. *Clinical Neurophysiology of the Vestibular System* (2nd ed.). Philadelphia: F. A. Davis, 1990.

Department of Neurology, Mayo Clinic and Mayo Foundation. *Clinical Examinations in Neurology* (6th ed.). St. Louis: Mosby, 1991.

Hudspeth, A. J. The cellular basis of hearing: The biophysics of hair cells. *Science* 230:745, 1985.

Ito, M. *The Cerebellum and Neural Control.* New York: Raven Press, 1984.

Leigh, R. J., and Zee, D. S. *The Neurology of Eye Movements* (2nd ed.). Philadelphia: F. A. Davis, 1991.

Miller, N. R. *Walsh and Hoyt's Clinical Neuro-Ophthalmology* (4th ed.), vol 2. Baltimore: Williams & Wilkins, 1988.

Schubert, E. D. *Hearing: Its Function and Dysfunction.* New York: Springer-Verlag, 1980.

Wilson-Pauwels, L., Akesson, E. J., and Stewart, P. A. *Cranial Nerves: Anatomy and Clinical Comments.* Toronto: B. C. Decker, 1988.

The Supratentorial Level

Objectives

Diencephalon

1. Name the divisions of the diencephalon, list the components of each division, and localize the structures on a diagram or brain model.
2. List the functional subgroups of the thalamic nuclei and their connections and projections to other parts of the central nervous system.
3. List the regulatory functions of the hypothalamic nuclei.
4. Describe the clinical significance of the pituitary gland, and list the neurohormones secreted by the anterior and posterior lobes and their functions.
5. Describe how a mass lesion in the region of the hypothalamus may affect vision and endocrine function.
6. Describe the clinical significance of the pineal gland.

Telencephalon

1. List the components of the basal ganglia, and identify them on a brain model or diagram.
2. Define projection fibers, commissural fibers, and association fibers.
3. Locate the internal capsule on a gross specimen, and describe what occurs with a lesion involving the internal capsule.
4. Locate on a diagram and describe the functions of the primary motor and premotor areas, frontal eye fields, motor speech area, primary sensory area, primary visual cortex, primary auditory cortex, Broca's area, and Wernicke's area.
5. Define agnosia, and describe its various types.
6. Define apraxia.
7. Define aphasia and its types, and be able to localize the lesion that produces each type. Define motor speech apraxia.
8. List the various types of cortical sensory deficit, and describe how the type of deficit is useful as a localizing sign.
9. Describe the various types of memory, amnesia, dementia, and mental retardation.
10. Differentiate partial from generalized seizures.
11. Describe absence and generalized tonic-clonic seizures.
12. Given the clinical manifestations of a partial seizure, localize the site of origin of the seizure; given the site of origin of a partial seizure, describe the clinical manifestations of the seizure.

Limbic System

1. List the structures of the limbic system.
2. List the functions of the limbic system.
3. List the structures involved with olfaction.

Visual System

1. Describe the anatomy of the optic pathways.

2. Describe what effect a lesion has on the visual fields at the level of the optic nerve, optic chiasm, optic tract, optic radiations, and occipital cortex.
3. Given a visual field defect, localize the lesion.
4. Define and describe the significance of papilledema.
5. Describe the function of the rods and cones.
6. Locate on a diagram: cornea, sclera, iris, ciliary body, lens, vitreous humor, retina, and choroid.
7. Define hemianopia, quadrantanopia, homonymous, macular sparing, scotoma, and visual hallucination.

Introduction

The supratentorial level consists of two main anatomical regions: the diencephalon and the telencephalon. As with other levels, the structures of the supratentorial level include phylogenetically older ("inner tube") and newer ("outer tube") components. The "inner tube" components are classically included in the concept of the limbic system and include the limbic lobe, amygdala, basal forebrain, olfactory structures, hypothalamus, and the thalamic nuclei that interconnect these regions. These structures are involved with the functions of the internal regulation and consciousness systems, emotion, and motivation. The "outer tube" structures include the neocortex of the cerebral hemispheres, the basal ganglia, and the thalamic nuclei that connect these regions. These structures are involved with higher cognitive functions, language, programming of motor function, fine motor control, and processing of sensory information (visual, somatosensory, auditory). Memory is a complex function that involves structures of both the inner and outer tubes.

This chapter discusses the anatomy, physiology, and clinical correlates of the anatomical areas and systems at the supratentorial level.

Overview

The supratentorial level includes all structures located within the skull and above the tentorium cerebelli. These structures develop from the embryonic prosencephalon and, therefore, include derivatives of the diencephalon and telencephalon (Table 1 and Fig. 1). The diencephalon consists of the structures between the midbrain and the cerebral hemispheres that surround the third ventricle.

The diencephalon includes the thalamus, hypothalamus, and surrounding regions. The *thalamus* is the largest structure in the diencephalon and consists of nuclei that act as relay and integrating stations for sensory input to the cerebral cortex and corticosubcortical circuits for motor control and higher cognitive functions.

TABLE 1. *Structures at the supratentorial level*

	"Inner tube" structures (limbic system)	"Outer tube" structures
Diencephalon		
Thalamus	Intralaminar, midline, dorsomedial, and anterior thalamic nuclei	Ventral, geniculate, dorsomedial, and pulvinar thalamic nuclei
Hypothalamus	All hypothalamic nuclei	—
Epithalamus	Pineal gland	—
Telencephalon		
Basal ganglia	Ventral striatum (nucleus accumbens)	Dorsal striatum (caudate, putamen)
Basal forebrain	Amygdala, septal region, nucleus basalis	—
Cerebral cortex	Archicortex/paleocortex (limbic/paralimbic cortex, hippocampus, insula, and cingulate and orbitofrontal gyri)	Neocortex (dorsal prefrontal, lateral frontal, primary motor and sensory, and association cortices)

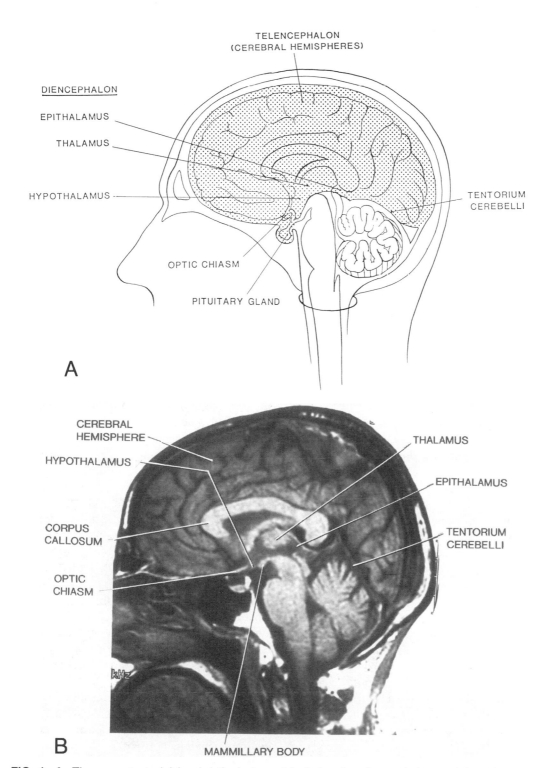

FIG. 1. A: The supratentorial level *(stippled area)* includes the diencephalon and the telencephalon. **B:** Sagittal T1-weighted magnetic resonance image showing some of the components of the supratentorial level. The diencephalon includes the optic chiasm, hypothalamus (including the mamillary bodies), thalamus, and epithalamus (corresponding to the pineal gland). The telencephalon includes the cerebral hemispheres, the corpus callosum, and the basal ganglia. The fornix connects the hippocampal formation (located in the medial portion of the temporal lobe) with the mamillary bodies and thalamus.

The *hypothalamus* is anterior and inferior to the thalamus and contains nuclei involved with the endocrine and autonomic functions important in homeostasis and reproduction. The inferior aspect of the hypothalamus (the ventral surface of the brain) consists of the tuber cinereum and mamillary bodies. The pituitary gland is not part of the hypothalamus but is attached to the tuber cinereum by the pituitary stalk. The hypothalamus regulates visceral and endocrine functions, body temperature, blood osmolality, food intake, and sleep.

The telencephalon consists of the cerebral hemispheres and the basal forebrain. The *cerebral hemispheres* are subdivided into three anatomical regions: basal ganglia, subcortical white matter, and cerebral cortex. The *basal ganglia*—including the striatum and globus pallidus and their connections with the cerebral cortex, thalamus, subthalamic nucleus, and brainstem—form one of the motor control systems.

The *subcortical white matter* is composed of dense fiber tracts connecting cortical and subcortical structures. Projection fibers connect the cerebral cortex with the thalamus, hypothalamus, basal ganglia, cerebellum, and other subcortical structures. Commissural fibers connect homologous areas between the two hemispheres, and association fibers connect areas within one hemisphere.

The *cerebral cortex* is a relatively thin mantle of gray matter covering the outer surface of the cerebral hemispheres; it forms the gyri of the brain. The two main sulci that divide the hemisphere into different lobes are the *central sulcus* and the *sylvian fissure*. Each cerebral hemisphere is divided into five lobes: frontal, parietal, occipital, temporal, and limbic. The frontal lobe, anterior to the central sulcus, has effector (motor) functions. The parietal, occipital, and temporal lobes are posterior to the central sulcus and have receptive and perceptive functions. The sylvian fissure separates the temporal lobe from the frontal and parietal lobes. The right and left hemispheres have specialized functions. The dominant (usually, left) hemisphere is involved with language and calculation, and the right

hemisphere is involved with visuospatial functions.

The *frontal lobe* includes the prefrontal region and the premotor and motor areas. The prefrontal area is involved with motor planning, attention, concentration, and control of affective behavior. The premotor and motor areas are involved with the programming and execution of motor function, oculomotor control, and speech production. The *parietal lobe* is concerned with somatosensory function; the primary somatosensory area is in the postcentral gyrus. Parietal association areas integrate sensory input from several sources. The *occipital lobe* contains the visual areas. The *temporal lobe* consists of a lateral portion, which is the primary sensory area for auditory and vestibular information, and a medial portion, which is involved with memory and is part of the limbic system. The *limbic lobe* is on the medial surface of the hemisphere and includes the orbitofrontal region, cingulate gyrus, and medial portions of the temporal lobe, especially the hippocampus and amygdala. The limbic lobe has an integral role in memory and in visceral and emotional activity.

The *basal forebrain* is an anatomically complex structure that includes the ventral part of the basal ganglia, the amygdala, and the cholinergic neurons of the nucleus basalis.

As is true of other levels, structures at the supratentorial level can be subdivided into inner tube and outer tube components (Table 1). The inner tube structures of this level include what is termed the *limbic system*. The limbic system contains diencephalic and telencephalic structures and consists of the hypothalamus, septal region, basal forebrain limbic cortex (hippocampus and cingulate gyrus), and the thalamic nuclei interconnecting these areas. These structures are involved in high-order autonomic control, neuroendocrine function, homeostasis, emotion, behavioral arousal, motivated behavior, memory, and learning (Table 2). The sensory system associated with the limbic system is the olfactory system.

The outer tube components include the lateral surface of the cerebral hemispheres, the

TABLE 2. *Functions of the supratentorial level*

Inner tube	Outer tube
High-level autonomic control	Motor programming
Homeostasis and reproduction	Fine motor control
Motivated behavior	Sensory discrimination
Behavioral arousal	Visuospatial orientation
Emotion	Vision
Learning	Higher cognitive functions
Memory	Attention
Olfaction	Judgment
	Memory storage and retrieval
	Language

basal ganglia, and the thalamic regions inter-connecting these areas. Functions of these cortical areas include attention, control of behavior, motor programming and execution, sensory processing, perception, language, memory, and visuospatial orientation (Table 2).

Disorders at the supratentorial level may alter motor and sensory functions contralaterally. Disorders involving the diencephalon impair the relay of information to and from the cerebral hemispheres or impair visceral, endocrine, or emotional functions. Disorders involving the cerebral hemispheres may cause general intellectual deterioration (dementia), amnesia, aphasia, agnosia (inability to perceive the meaning of sensory input), apraxia (inability to perform complex motor activities voluntarily), or seizures. In general, lesions of the left hemisphere affect language-related functions, and lesions of the right hemisphere affect visuospatial-related functions.

An important sensory system of the supratentorial level is the visual system. The structures of the visual system—the eye, retina, visual pathway, and occipital cortex—are found at the peripheral, diencephalic, and telencephalic levels.

Diencephalon

The diencephalon is rostral to the brainstem and includes the structures surrounding the third ventricle: thalamus, ventral thalamus, epithalamus, and hypothalamus. The diencephalon is bounded superiorly by the floor of the lateral ventricles, corpus callosum, and fornix and laterally by the internal capsule. Anteriorly, it extends to the region of the foramen of Monro, and caudally, it merges with the tegmentum of the midbrain (Fig. 2).

The thalamus is the largest structure in the diencephalon and consists of several nuclei. The thalamic relay nuclei constitute the dorsal thalamus. The thalamic reticular nucleus is derived from the ventral thalamus. The hypothalamus is inferior and anterior to the thalamus and separated from the thalamus by the hypothalamic sulcus—a groove in the wall of the third ventricle, extending from the foramen of Monro to the aqueduct of Sylvius. The ventral thalamic region lies ventral and posterior to the thalamus and merges with the midbrain. The epithalamus forms part of the roof of the diencephalon and lies superior to the ventral thalamus and posterior to the thalamus.

Thalamus and Related Regions

Anatomy

The thalamus consists of a group of nuclei in the wall of the third ventricle. The thalami sometimes fuse in the midline and form the interthalamic adhesion (or massa intermedia). The anterior end of the thalamus, containing the anterior nucleus, is narrow, and the posterior end, containing the pulvinar and geniculate bodies, is broad. The Y-shaped internal

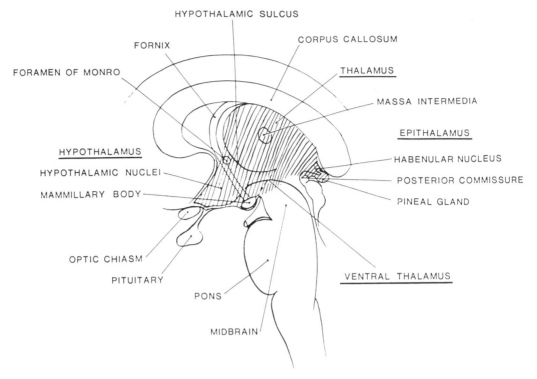

FIG. 2. Diencephalon *(shaded area)* and its four subdivisions: thalamus, ventral thalamus, epithalamus, and hypothalamus.

medullary lamina divides the thalamus into anterior, medial, and lateral areas (Fig. 3).

The anterior nuclear group is in the anterior area, and the dorsomedial and midline nuclei are in the medial area. The lateral nuclei are arranged in two tiers: a dorsal tier and a ventral tier (Table 3). The nuclei in the dorsal tier, from anterior to posterior, are the dorsolateral nucleus, the lateral posterior nucleus, and the pulvinar. The medial geniculate and lateral geniculate bodies extend posteriorly from the ventral surface of the pulvinar. In the ventral tier, from anterior to posterior, are the ventral anterior, ventral lateral, and ventral posterior nuclei (Fig. 3). Between and surrounding these well-defined nuclear groups are layers of cells forming sheetlike nuclei: the intralaminar nuclei in the Y-shaped border between the major groups, the reticular nuclei around the outside, and the midline nuclei.

The *thalamic nuclei* integrate and relay information for the sensory, motor, consciousness, and limbic systems. The ventral posterior (posterolateral and posteromedial) nuclei relay somatic sensory system information to the cerebral cortex. The ventral posterolateral nucleus is the site of termination of the spinothalamic and medial lemniscal pathways from the trunk and limbs. Similarly, axons of the trigeminothalamic pathways from the head terminate in the ventral posteromedial nucleus. Axons from the ventral posterior nuclei project through the posterior limb of the internal capsule to the primary somatosensory cortex in the postcentral gyrus of the parietal lobe.

The ventral lateral nucleus receives input from the cerebellar nuclei and projects to primary motor cortex. The ventral anterior nucleus receives input from the globus pallidus and substantia nigra and projects to the

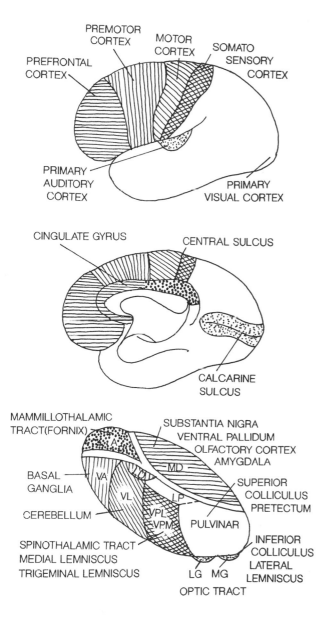

FIG. 3. The major groups of thalamic nuclei and their cortical targets. The medial group includes the midline and dorsomedial or mediodorsal *(MD)* nuclei. The lateral group includes the laterodorsal *(LD)*, lateral posterior *(LP)*, pulvinar *(P)*, medial *(MG)* and lateral *(LG)* geniculate bodies, ventral anterior *(VA)*, ventral lateral *(VL)*, and ventral posterior *(VP)* nuclei.

supplementary motor and premotor cortical areas.

The medial geniculate body receives auditory afferent fibers from the inferior colliculus via the brachium of the inferior colliculus and sends efferent fibers through the auditory radiations in the sublenticular portion of the posterior limb of the internal capsule to the auditory cortex of the temporal lobe. The lateral geniculate body relays visual impulses from the optic tract via the retrolenticular portion of the posterior limb of the internal capsule to the calcarine cortex of the occipital lobe and is part of the visual system.

The pulvinar receives visual information and projects to the posterior parietal cortex and is important in the process of directed visual attention.

The dorsomedial nucleus of the thalamus relays information to the prefrontal cortex. The dorsomedial and midline thalamic nuclei are part of the circuits of the amygdala, hip-

TABLE 3. *Summary of thalamic nuclei*

Nucleus	Input	Cortical target
Ventral anterior	Globus pallidus	Supplementary motor area
Ventral lateral	Cerebellum	Motor cortex
Ventral posterior	Medial lemniscus	Primary sensory cortex
	Spinothalamic tract	
	Trigeminothalamic tract	
Medial geniculate	Inferior colliculus	Primary auditory cortex
Lateral geniculate	Optic tract	Primary visual cortex
Pulvinar	Superior colliculus	Parietotemporo-occipital association cortex
Dorsomedial	Amygdala	Prefrontal cortex
	Prefrontal cortex	Anterior cingulate cortex
	Substantia nigra	
Anterior	Mamillary bodies	Posterior cingulate cortex
	Hippocampus	
Intralaminar	Spinothalamic tract	Striatum
	Reticular formation	Diffuse cortical areas
Midline	Amygdala	Anterior cingulate cortex
	Hypothalamus	Orbitofrontal cortex
	Reticular formation	
Reticular	Other thalamic nuclei	Other thalamic nuclei
	Reticular formation	
	Cerebral cortex	

pocampus, and other parts of the internal regulation system. The intralaminar nuclei are components of the indirect pathway of the sensory system and the consciousness system and have important connections with the basal ganglia. The anterior nuclei, via connections with the hippocampus, mamillary bodies, and cingulate gyrus, are involved with learning and memory.

The reticular nucleus of the thalamus is derived from the ventral thalamus, an embryologically separate component of the thalamus. This nucleus projects to other thalamic nuclei. It is critical in regulating thalamic nuclei that relay information to the cortex, particularly in regard to the wake-sleep cycle. All thalamic nuclei receive projections from the areas of the cerebral cortex to which they project (reciprocal thalamocortical connections).

The subthalamus is a poorly defined area at the mesencephalodiencephalic junction; it includes the *subthalamic nucleus,* which is part of the basal ganglia circuits. A lesion of the subthalamic nucleus causes *hemiballismus,* a movement disorder in which rapid flailing movements occur in one extremity or on one side of the body.

The epithalamus lies in the dorsal wall of the posterior part of the third ventricle beneath the splenium of the corpus callosum. The main structure of the epithalamus is the *pineal gland,* which is formed from an evagination of the roof of the diencephalon. The cavity of the evagination is the pineal recess of the third ventricle. Other structures located in the region include the *habenular nuclei,* which lie in the walls of the epithalamus, and the posterior commissure, which crosses the midline ventral to the pineal gland (Fig. 2).

The pineal gland is part of the circuit for controlling circadian rhythms, which originate in the suprachiasmatic nucleus of the hypothalamus. The circuits are affected by the light cycle. The pineal gland produces melatonin, a hormone that mediates circadian changes, including the wake-sleep cycle.

Physiology

The thalamus acts as both a relay area and a gateway for information transfer to the cerebral cortex. Thalamic relay nuclei contain thalamocortical projection neurons, which send excitatory (glutamatergic) input to the cerebral cortex, and local inhibitory neurons containing γ-aminobutyric acid (GABA). The thalamocortical relay neurons in a thalamic nucleus receive (1) input from the specific sensory system or subcortical structure associated with the nucleus (for example, medial lemniscus or globus pallidus), (2) cortical input from the area of the cortex to which the nucleus projects, and (3) inhibitory input from the reticular nucleus of the thalamus. The reticular nucleus of the thalamus receives input from the cerebral cortex, reticular formation, and thalamic relay nuclei. Unlike other thalamic nuclei, the reticular nucleus does not project to the cerebral cortex but to other thalamic nuclei.

As mentioned in Chapter 10, thalamic neurons exhibit two types of activity: (1) tonic firing that allows precise transmission of information from subcortical sources to the cerebral cortex, typical of active states of the thalamocortical circuits (wakefulness and rapid eye movement [REM] sleep); and (2) rhythmic burst firing that prevents transmission of sensory information to the cerebral cortex and is typical of inactive states, such as non-REM sleep. The transition from one firing pattern to the other depends on the presence or absence of excitatory input from cholinergic and other nuclei of the reticular formation. Thus, the thalamus acts not only as a relay center but also as a gate for sensory information to the cerebral cortex. In addition, the corticothalamocortical loops provide a mechanism by which activity in one area of the cerebral cortex may become synchronized with the activity in another cortical area that is spatially separated but functionally related via the diffuse thalamocortical projection system.

Clinical Correlations

The blood supply to the posterior thalamus is via branches of the vertebrobasilar circulation. Discrete lesions that destroy the ventral posterior nucleus of the thalamus produce a contralateral hemianesthesia, with loss of all sensory modalities in the trunk, limbs, and face. This is often the result of an infarction due to hypertensive vascular disease or thrombosis of one of the branches of the posterior cerebral artery. The initial stage of contralateral hemianesthesia after a thalamic infarct may in turn be followed by a partial return of sensation associated with a very unpleasant burning sensation; this is referred to as the *thalamic syndrome*. Motor function can be altered by lesions of the motor relay nuclei of the thalamus. Discrete neurosurgical lesions in the ventral lateral thalamic nucleus disrupt connections between the cerebellum and the cerebral cortex and thereby decrease tremor in some patients with cerebellar disease, Parkinson's disease, or essential tremor. Lesions of the medial part of the thalamus can produce somnolence and problems with memory.

A prion disease, *fatal familial insomnia,* is associated with selective lesion of the anterior and dorsomedial thalamic nuclei. Its clinical manifestations include progressive intractable insomnia, sympathetic hyperactivity, and disruption of circadian rhythms.

Hypothalamus

Anatomy

The hypothalamus is the main control area of the visceral system. It integrates activity for the limbic, consciousness, internal regulation, and endocrine systems. The hypothalamus includes those structures in the diencephalon anterior and inferior to the thalamus that are separated from it by the hypothalamic sulcus. The hypothalamus consists of the hypothalamic nuclei in the walls of the third ventricle and the tuber cinereum and mamillary bodies in the floor of the third ventricle (Fig. 4).

The hypothalamus extends from the region of the optic chiasm to the caudal border of the mamillary body. The region located in front of the optic chiasm is known as the *preoptic region,* a telencephalic derivative. The preoptic region and hypothalamus form a functional unit.

The hypophysis, or pituitary gland, is functionally related to the hypothalamus and at-

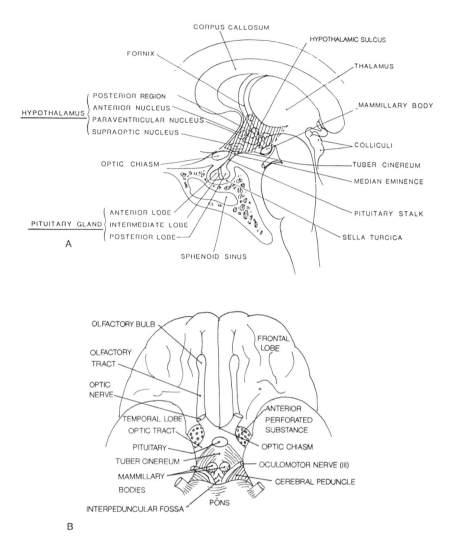

FIG. 4. The hypothalamus. **A:** Midline section of the hypothalamic nuclei *(shaded area)*, the pituitary gland in the sella turcica, and the mamillary bodies. **B:** Base of the brain with the optic chiasm, pituitary stalk, and mamillary bodies.

tached to it at the tuber cinereum by the infundibulum, or pituitary stalk. Other closely related structures not part of the hypothalamus are the optic chiasm, located immediately below the anterior hypothalamus; the internal carotid arteries in the cavernous sinus, located just lateral to the pituitary gland; and cranial nerves III, IV, V, and VI, which lie adjacent to the pituitary gland in the cavernous sinus (Fig. 5). The hypothalamus has fiber connections with all areas of the brainstem and cerebral hemispheres but particularly with the basal

frontal and medial cortical areas and with the reticular formation. The most prominent fiber tracts are the fornix, which ends in the mamillary bodies, and the mamillothalamic tract, which terminates in the anterior nuclei of the thalamus. These tracts and the hypothalamic nuclei are part of the limbic system.

Physiology

The hypothalamic nuclei can be grouped into three functional zones: the periventricu-

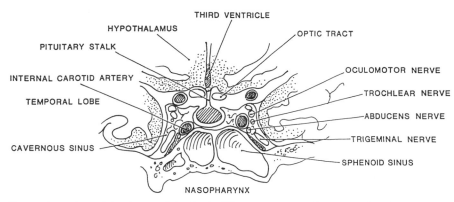

FIG. 5. Coronal section of the base of the brain. The structures adjacent to the pituitary gland are in the cavernous sinus located on either side of the pituitary gland: cranial nerves III, IV, V, and VI and the internal carotid arteries. The optic tracts are adjacent to the pituitary stalk.

lar zone, the medial zone, and the lateral hypothalamic zone (Table 4); also see Chapter 9, Fig. 7).

The nuclei in the periventricular zone are involved in biologic rhythms, neuroendocrine control, and complex autonomic responses. The medial zone contains nuclei involved in homeostasis and reproduction. The lateral zone contains the tuberomamillary nuclei and the medial forebrain bundle, which are involved with arousal mechanisms and motivated behavior. The hypothalamic nuclei and tracts have functional interactions with the limbic system, reticular formation, autonomic centers, and anterior pituitary lobe.

The hypothalamus has the following functions (Table 4):

1. *Neuroendocrine control.* The neuroendocrine functions of the hypothalamus are mediated by two systems: the magnicellular and the parvicellular neurosecretory systems. The magnicellular system consists of the supraoptic and paraventricular nuclei; they secrete vasopressin, or antidiuretic hormone, which controls water metabolism, and oxytocin, which controls uterine contractions and milk ejection. The parvicellular system includes neurons in the paraventricular and arcuate nuclei and the medial preoptic area that secrete releasing or inhibitory hormones controlling anterior pituitary function. The hormones that control anterior pituitary secretion are called *hypo-*

TABLE 4. *Hypothalamic functions and dysfunction*

Nucleus	Function	Dysfunction
Periventricular zone		
Suprachiasmatic	Circadian rhythms	Disruption of circadian rhythms
Supraoptic and paraventricular	Antidiuretic hormone (ADH) and oxytocin	Diabetes insipidus, inappropriate secretion of ADH
Tuberoinfundibular	Releasing factors (regulatory hormones)	Hypopituitarism, Cushing's disease, acromegaly, sexual precocity, amenorrhea, hyperprolactinemia
Medial zone		
Medial preoptic	Thermoregulation	Hyperthermia/hypothermia
Anterior	Osmoregulation, sleep induction	Hypernatremia, thirst disorders, salt wasting syndrome, insomnia
Ventromedial	Food intake	Obesity
Lateral zone	Cortical arousal, motivated behavior	Hypersomnia, aphagia, adipsia

thalamic regulatory hormones, because they regulate the secretions and release of hormones by the anterior pituitary gland. Interruption of hypothalamopituitary connections may cause decreased secretion of all pituitary hormones except *prolactin,* which is *increased.* Failure of secretion of antidiuretic hormone produces *diabetes insipidus,* in which excessive quantities of dilute urine are excreted. Inappropriate secretion of antidiuretic hormone causes retention of water and can produce hyponatremia.

2. *Autonomic control.* The *paraventricular nucleus,* nuclei in the medial zone, and the lateral hypothalamus contain a mixed population of neurons that innervate sympathetic and parasympathetic regions of the brainstem and spinal cord. Autonomic manifestations of hypothalamic disease include the diencephalic syndrome of autonomic hyperactivity, with hyperthermia, hypertension, tachycardia, and sweating.

3. *Thermoregulation.* The *preoptic-anterior hypothalamic region* contains thermosensitive neurons, including warm-sensitive neurons that initiate heat loss responses (skin vasodilatation and sweating) and cold-sensitive neurons that initiate heat gain responses (skin vasoconstriction and shivering). Hypothalamic lesions may cause hypothermia or hyperthermia.

4. *Water metabolism (osmoregulation).* The circuit controlling water metabolism includes the *subfornical organ* and other osmosensitive circumventricular organs in the anterior wall of the third ventricle, the preoptic region, and the magnicellular supraoptic and paraventricular nuclei. These regions exert a major role in water metabolism via two mechanisms: thirst and secretion of antidiuretic hormone. Destruction of the anterior hypothalamic region produces disorders of thirst with hypernatremia, or syndrome of salt wasting.

5. *Food intake.* Several hypothalamic regions contain glucosensitive neurons that also respond to various peptides; these neurons control autonomic output to the endocrine pancreas and adrenal gland, which are important for regulation of energy metabolism. These hypothalamic regions include the paraventricular and the ventromedial nuclei and the lateral hypothalamic area; they are involved in the control of food intake. Lesions of the medial hypothalamus, including the paraventricular nucleus, produce increased appetite and obesity. Lesions of the lateral hypothalamus produce a decrease in the urge to eat or drink.

6. *Reproductive function.* The hypothalamus affects sexual function and reproduction via control of secretion of gonadotropin-releasing hormones and prolactin and control of specific sexual behaviors. Important regions include the medial preoptic area, which contains a *sexually dimorphic nucleus,* and the ventromedial nucleus. These regions contain an abundance of receptors for sex steroids (estrogens and androgens). Hypothalamic disorders may produce precocious puberty, amenorrhea, and other disorders of sexual function.

7. *Wake-sleep cycle.* Two hypothalamic areas control the wake-sleep cycle: the medial preoptic region can initiate non-REM sleep as a part of a thermoregulatory heat loss mechanism, and the lateral hypothalamic area is the rostral part of the reticular activating system and is involved in cortical arousal.

Pituitary Gland

The pituitary gland (hypophysis) lies within a bony-walled cavity, the *sella turcica* ("Turk's saddle"), in the sphenoid bone at the base of the brain (see Fig. 4A). It is connected to the hypothalamus by the *pituitary stalk,* which arises from the median eminence—a midline, ventral projection from the tuber cinereum. The pituitary stalk is located between the optic chiasm and the mamillary bodies. Its relationship with the optic chiasm is clinically important because enlargement of the pituitary gland may compress the visual pathways in the optic chiasm.

The pituitary gland consists of the anterior lobe, or adenohypophysis, and the posterior lobe, or neurohypophysis. Although both lobes are part of a single gland, each has a different embryologic origin. The anterior lobe arises from a neuroectodermal ridge in the oral region, and the posterior lobe arises from a downward evagination of the embryonic diencephalon (see Chapter 2, Fig. 10). The posterior lobe and the pituitary stalk are formed from this evaginated neural process, which serves as the neural connection with the diencephalon in the adult. The anterior lobe, which fuses with the posterior lobe, has no known neural connections with the brain and receives its hypothalamic control through a system of portal vessels. The release of hormones from the pituitary gland is regulated by a vascular mechanism in the case of the anterior lobe (Fig. 6A) and by a neural mechanism in the case of the posterior lobe (Fig. 6B).

The portal circulation connecting the hypothalamus and anterior lobe consists of hypophysial arteries located in the medial eminence that give rise to capillaries that drain into a series of parallel veins coursing down the pituitary stalk (Fig. 6A). On reaching the anterior lobe, the veins form a capillary plexus that supplies blood to the anterior lobe. The release of the anterior pituitary hormones is under the control of neurohumoral substances secreted by the hypothalamus. These substances, the regulatory hormones, are released from nerve endings in the median eminence. They enter the capillaries of the portal circulation, travel down the pituitary stalk through the portal veins, and then empty into the capillary plexus of the anterior pituitary gland, where they stimulate the anterior pituitary cells to release specific hormones.

The posterior pituitary hormones, vasopressin and oxytocin, are synthesized in the cells in the hypothalamus and are transported by axons in the pituitary stalk to the nerve terminals in the posterior lobe for storage or release (Fig. 6B). Vasopressin regulates water metabolism and blood osmolality, whereas oxytocin enhances contractility of uterine musculature during and after delivery and of the myoepithelial cells of the breast ducts in lactating women. This facilitates milk ejection.

As defined by immunostaining and electron microscopy, the anterior lobe of the pituitary gland contains at least five cell types. These cells and their hormones, functions, and hypothalamic regulatory hormones are outlined in Table 5.

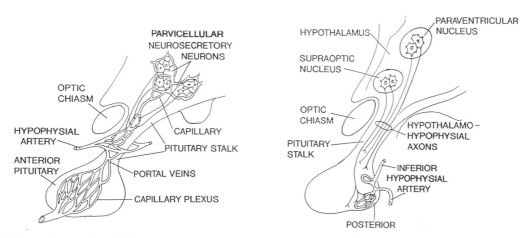

FIG. 6. A: Portal circulation carries releasing factors from the hypothalamus to the anterior pituitary lobe. **B:** Axons carry hormones from the hypothalamic nuclei to the posterior pituitary lobe.

TABLE 5. *Anterior pituitary hormones*

Cell type	Hormone (standard abbreviation)	Hypothalamic regulatory hormone	Function
Somatotroph	Growth hormone (GH)	Growth hormone–releasing hormone	Linear growth
		Somatostatin (inhibits release)	Intermediary metabolism
Lactotroph	Prolactin (PRL)	Vasoactive intestinal peptide (VIP) (stimulates release)	Lactogenesis
		Dopamine (inhibits release)	Breast growth and development
Corticotroph	Corticotropin (ACTH), beta-lipotropin (LPH), beta-endorphin (END)	Corticotropin-releasing hormone (CRH)	Functional integrity and steroidogenic function of adrenal cortex
Gonadotroph	Luteinizing hormone (LH), follicle-stimulating hormone (FSH)	Gonadotropin-releasing hormone (GnRH)	Gonadal function, sexual maturation, reproductive function, gametogenesis, sex steroid production
Thyrotroph	Thyrotropin (TSH)	Thyrotropin-releasing hormone (TRH)	Integrity and function of thyroid gland, secretion of thyroxine and triiodothyronine
		Somatostatin (inhibits release)	

Clinical Correlations

Lesions affecting the hypothalamus and surrounding structures can be seen in any type of medical practice because they cause derangements of visceral, endocrine, visual, or homeostatic functions. Lesions of the hypothalamic nuclei result in a disturbance of visceral and homeostatic functions, such as sleep, appetite, temperature regulation, and water metabolism (see Table 4). Lesions of the pituitary gland cause endocrine disorders due to increased or decreased secretion of pituitary hormones. Examples of endocrine disorders include the following:

1. *Growth hormone.* Increased secretion causes gigantism in children and acromegaly (enlargement of the face, hands, and feet) in adults. Decreased secretion during childhood results in dwarfism.
2. *Thyroid-stimulating hormone.* Decreased secretion results in hypothyroidism, with loss of hair, dry skin, slow pulse, loss of energy, mental apathy, decreased cold tolerance, and slow relaxation of deep tendon reflexes. Increased secretion of thyroid-stimulating hormone can cause goiter and hyperthyroidism.
3. *Adrenocorticotropic hormone* (ACTH) (or *corticotropin*). Increased secretion results

in signs of hyperadrenalism with hirsutism, vascular striae, obesity, and hypertension. Decreased secretion results in hypoadrenalism, with generalized weakness, hypotension, and decreased tolerance to stress.
4. *Gonadotropic hormone.* Decreased secretion results in amenorrhea and decreased libido.
5. *Prolactin.* Prolactin excess causes amenorrhea-galactorrhea syndrome in women and hypogonadism and impotence in men. Lack of prolactin is manifested in postpartum women as inability to lactate.

The visual deficits resulting from involvement of structures adjacent to the hypothalamus serve as additional localizing signs of lesions in this area. A mass lesion in the area of the sella turcica can press on the optic chiasm and cause a characteristic visual field defect, bitemporal hemianopia. A lesion involving the carotid artery or cranial nerves in the cavernous sinus can cause diplopia and loss of sensation over the forehead and cheek. A mass lesion in or near the sella can cause enlargement of the sella or erosion of the bony margins of the sella, which can be seen on radiographs of the skull.

The three most common mass lesions encountered in this region are pituitary adenoma, craniopharyngioma, and aneurysm of the internal carotid artery. A *pituitary adenoma* is a tumor arising from the cells of the anterior pituitary gland. As the tumor expands, it produces enlargement of the sella and compression of the optic chiasm. The demonstration of specific secretory granules by electron microscopy and of hormone content by immunostaining (immunoperoxidase, immunofluorescence) permits classification of these biologically active tumors.

Tumors that are acidophilic on routine stains are most often associated with either somatotropin secretion (which causes acromegaly in adults or gigantism in children) or prolactin secretion (which causes amenorrhea and galactorrhea in women). Tumors that produce corticotropin (ACTH) are usually basophilic and associated with Cushing's syndrome.

Although all the tumors mentioned contain densely granulated cells, similar hormonal activity may occur in much less densely granulated tumors, classed as chromophobe adenomas on routine staining. Many other chromophobe adenomas, although containing identifiable hormone granules, do not result in clinical evidence of trophic hormone excess. These tumors may grow to enormous size and produce clinical effects by compression of the normal pituitary gland and adjacent structures.

Craniopharyngioma is a tumor that arises from an embryonic remnant of Rathke's pouch and is usually located in the region of the pituitary stalk or sella, near the hypothalamus and pituitary gland. It can cause endocrine disturbances, visual symptoms, and erosion of the sella. An *aneurysm* of the internal carotid artery in the region of the sella frequently causes disturbances in extraocular muscle function but rarely disturbs pituitary function.

Telencephalon

The lateral evaginations of the most rostral portion of the embryonic neural tube form the telencephalon, from which the cerebral hemi-spheres arise. The two cerebral hemispheres fill most of the cranial cavity above the tentorium cerebelli and are separated by the falx cerebri. Each cerebral hemisphere contains three layers of tissue surrounding the ventricular cavities deep within the hemispheres (Fig. 7). Immediately adjacent to the ventricles, near the thalamus, are the *basal ganglia.* Surrounding these deep gray nuclei is the *white matter,* a dense intermingling of axons that connect areas within the cerebral hemispheres with each other and with other areas of the nervous system. The outermost layer, the cerebral cortex, contains neurons that have migrated to this location during fetal development. This outer layer of gray matter is referred to as *cortical,* whereas the white matter and deep gray matter are referred to as *subcortical.*

The ventral portion of the telencephalon constitutes the *basal forebrain;* the medial region between the two hemispheres is known as the *septal area.*

The telencephalon can be divided anatomically into the basal ganglia, subcortical white matter, and cerebral cortex.

Basal Ganglia

Anatomy

Basal ganglia is a collective term for several areas of subcortical gray matter, including the caudate nucleus, putamen, and globus pallidus (Fig. 7). The substantia nigra and subthalamic nucleus are also considered part of basal ganglia circuits (see Chapter 8). The caudate, putamen, and nucleus accumbens form the *striatum,* so named because of their striated appearance. The caudate and the putamen are separated by the internal capsule (Fig. 7). The *globus pallidus* ("pale") and putamen together are referred to as the *lenticular nucleus,* because of their shape. The globus pallidus is separated from both the thalamus and the substantia nigra by the internal capsule.

The striatum is the afferent structure of basal ganglia circuits. It receives input from

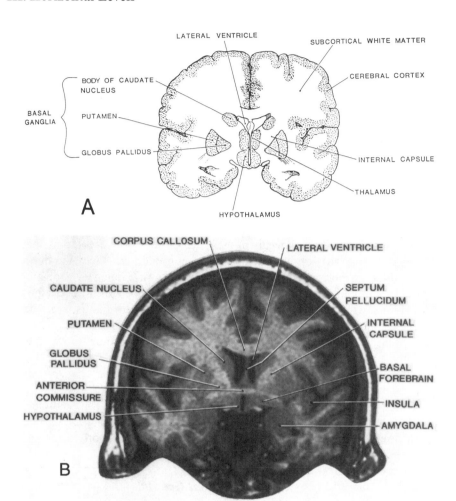

FIG. 7. A: Drawing of a coronal section through the cerebral hemispheres. The three anatomical components of the telencephalon are the cerebral cortex, subcortical white matter, and basal ganglia (caudate nucleus, putamen, and globus pallidus). The internal capsule separates the globus pallidus from the caudate nucleus and the thalamus. **B:** Coronal T1-weighted magnetic resonance image showing several important structures of the cerebral hemispheres. The corpus callosum connects the two cerebral hemispheres. The internal capsule contains all the major interconnections of the cerebral hemispheres with the motor and sensory systems via the thalamus and the corticospinal tract. The caudate and the putamen constitute the striatum. The amygdala is a component of the limbic system. The anterior commissure connects the medial portion of the left and right temporal lobes. The basal forebrain includes the nucleus basalis, which provides cholinergic input to the cerebral cortex. The insula is located in the depth of the sylvian fissure.

most of the cerebral cortex, the intralaminar thalamic nuclei, and the dopaminergic neurons of the substantia nigra pars compacta. The internal portion of the globus pallidus and the nondopaminergic part of the substantia nigra (substantia nigra pars reticulata) are the efferent structures of basal ganglia circuits and project to the thalamus, superior colliculus, and brainstem. The thalamic nuclei to which the globus pallidus and substantia nigra project are connected with different regions of the frontal cortex. The basal ganglia, thalamus, and frontal lobe form parallel *basal ganglia–thalamocortical circuits* that control motor, oculomotor, cognitive, and affective functions. The motor circuit involves the putamen; the oculomotor and cognitive circuits involve the caudate; and the affective, or limbic, circuit involves the nucleus accumbens (Table 6).

Physiology

The physiology of the basal ganglia circuits and their role in motor control are discussed in Chapter 8. Briefly, the striatum receives excitatory input (mediated by L-glutamate) from the cerebral cortex and a modulatory input (mediated by dopamine) from the substantia nigra. On activation by the excitatory corticostriatal pathway, the striatum sends an inhibitory GABAergic projection to both segments of the globus pallidus. The internal segment of the globus pallidus tonically inhibits the thalamus and the thalamocortical circuits from initiating motor programs. The inhibitory activity of the internal segment of the globus pallidus depends on the balance between excitatory input from the subthalamic nucleus and inhibitory input from the striatum. The external segment of the globus pallidus inhibits both the internal segment and the subthalamic nucleus.

The balance between excitation and inhibition of the internal segment of the globus pallidus determines whether a specific motor program triggered by the thalamic input to the supplementary motor cortex will be activated or suppressed. This balance depends on the selective activation of subpopulations of striatal inhibitory neurons, and this is determined by the effects of dopamine. Dopamine activates the striatal neurons that project to the internal segment of the globus pallidus. This allows transient disinhibition of thalamocortical circuits and initiation of a motor program (see Chapter 8).

Clinical Correlations

Disorders of the basal ganglia affect not only motor function but also oculomotor, cognitive, and affective function. Exaggerated inhibition of the thalamus by the basal ganglia results in hypokinetic movement disorders, for example, Parkinson's disease (lack of dopamine, particularly in the putamen) and other forms of parkinsonism. Impaired ability to suppress movements results in hyperkinetic movement disorders, such as chorea, for example, Huntington's disease (severe atrophy of the caudate nucleus). In addition to motor dysfunction, these and other disorders of the basal ganglia are associated with oculomotor abnormalities (for example, inability to initiate saccadic eye movements), cognitive dysfunction (dementia), and psychiatric manifestations (for example, depression, hallucinations).

TABLE 6. *Corticobasal ganglia-thalamocortical circuits*

Circuit	Cortical and subcortical inputs	Striatal component	Output nucleus	Thalamic relay nucleus	Target
Motor	Sensory cortex Motor cortex Intralaminar nuclei	Putamen	Globus pallidus	Ventral anterior	Supplementary motor area
Oculomotor	Frontal eye fields	Caudate	Substantia nigra	Intralaminar Dorsomedial	Frontal eye fields and superior colliculus
Cognitive	Prefrontal cortex	Caudate	Globus pallidus and substantia nigra	Dorsomedial	Prefrontal cortex
Affective	Anterior cingulate cortex Hippocampus Amygdala	Nucleus accumbens	Ventral pallidum	Dorsomedial	Anterior cingulate cortex

Subcortical White Matter

A large proportion of the cerebral hemispheres between the lateral ventricles and the cerebral cortex is composed of myelinated axons that interconnect one area of cerebral cortex with numerous other cortical areas and subcortical areas. These fibers are named on the basis of the areas that they connect. *Projection fibers* travel between the cerebral cortex and the subcortical nuclear structures; *commissural fibers* connect homologous areas in the two hemispheres; and *association fibers* connect cortical areas within one hemisphere.

Projection Fibers

As the axons that connect subcortical and cortical areas pass between the subcortical nuclei, they are collected into a compact structure, the *internal capsule.* The internal capsule is a broad band flanked medially by the thalamus and caudate nucleus and laterally by the globus pallidus and putamen (Fig. 8). In horizontal section, it is a V-shaped structure pointed medially, with an anterior limb, a posterior limb, and a junction called the genu. The caudate is medial to the anterior limb, the thalamus is medial to the posterior limb, and the globus pallidus and putamen are lateral to the genu and both limbs. The axons of the projection fibers carry action potentials either toward the cerebral cortex (afferent) or away from the cerebral cortex (efferent). As the axons of the internal capsule spread out from the internal capsule to reach all areas of cortex, they are known as the *corona radiata.*

The afferent projection fibers arise largely from the thalamus and are called *thalamic radiations.* Fibers traveling to the frontal lobe from the anterior and medial thalamic nuclei, carrying visceral and other information, are located in the anterior limb of the internal capsule. Fibers from the ventral anterior and ventral lateral nuclei of the thalamus, projecting to the motor and premotor areas of the frontal lobe, are in the genu and posterior limb of the internal capsule. Fibers from the ventral posterolateral and posteromedial thalamic nuclei, carrying sensory information to the parietal cortex, travel in the posterior limb of the capsule. Optic radiations, carrying vi-

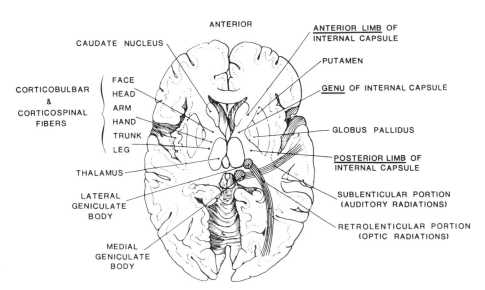

FIG. 8. Internal capsule. The anterior limb carries fibers from the frontal lobe, the genu from the motor areas, and the posterior limb to the sensory areas. The retrolenticular portion of the internal capsule contains the optic radiations; the sublenticular portion contains the auditory radiations.

sual information from the lateral geniculate body and pulvinar to the occipital and parietal cortex, are in the posterior limb behind the globus pallidus and putamen (retrolenticular portion of the internal capsule). Auditory information is carried from the medial geniculate body to the temporal lobe via the fibers in the posterior limb beneath the globus pallidus and the putamen (sublenticular portion of the internal capsule).

The efferent projection fibers have several destinations, including the thalamus, basal ganglia, hypothalamus, red nucleus, and brainstem reticular formation. The largest groups of fibers, however, constitute the direct pathway projecting from the precentral gyrus via the posterior limb of the internal capsule to the motor nuclei in the brainstem (corticobulbar) and the spinal cord (corticospinal). A second large efferent projection contains fibers primarily from the frontal lobe traveling via the internal capsule and cerebral peduncles to the pontine nuclei of the brainstem, which relay information to the cerebellum. All these fibers are involved in the initiation of voluntary movements, integration of motor function, modification of reflex activity, modulation of sensory input, regulation of visceral function, and regulation of states of consciousness and attention.

Commissural Fibers

Commissural fibers connect homologous areas in the two hemispheres to integrate the activity on the two sides (Fig. 9A). Most of the connections pass through the *corpus callosum,* which is a large flat bundle of fibers forming the roof of the lateral ventricles. Two smaller bundles connect areas in the temporal lobes. The *anterior commissure* anterior to the third ventricle interconnects anterior temporal areas, and the *hippocampal commissure* interconnects the hippocampal formation on the two sides.

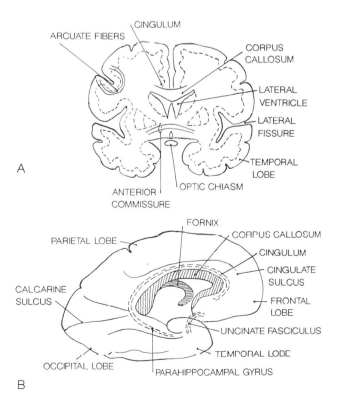

FIG. 9. A: Coronal section of the cerebral hemispheres. Commissural fibers (corpus callosum and anterior commissure) connect the two hemispheres. The arcuate fibers (short association fibers) connect gyri. B: Medial view of the cerebral hemisphere. Examples of long association fibers are the cingulum and uncinate fasciculus.

Association Fibers

Fiber tracts known as association pathways run longitudinally within a single hemisphere to correlate activities in different lobes (Fig. 9B). Two long association tracts are the *uncinate fasciculus,* which joins the temporal and frontal lobes, and the *cingulum,* which interconnects the medial surfaces of the frontal, parietal, and temporal lobes. Short association fibers that connect adjacent gyri are known as *arcuate fibers* (Fig. 9A).

Cerebral Cortex

Anatomy

The cerebral cortex includes the limbic cortex, paralimbic cortex, and neocortex. *Limbic* cortex is the most primitive area of the cerebral hemisphere. The *neocortex* is the most

differentiated area and consists of the primary sensory and motor areas and the association areas. The *paralimbic* cortex is intermediate between limbic cortex and neocortex.

Limbic cortex consists of a group of interconnected structures located on the medial portion of the cerebral hemispheres (Fig. 10). It includes the hippocampal formation, entorhinal cortex, other perihippocampal structures, a portion of the cingulate gyrus, and the primary olfactory cortex. The hippocampal formation includes the dentate gyrus, Ammon's horn, and the subiculum. The entorhinal cortex is the main region that connects the hippocampal formation with the rest of the cerebral cortex. The main output system of the hippocampal formation is the *fornix.*

The paralimbic cortex is located in the basal portion of the cerebral hemispheres between the frontal and temporal lobes and con-

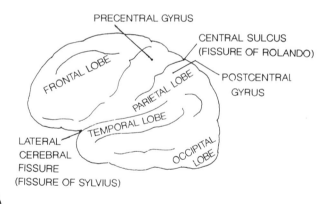

A

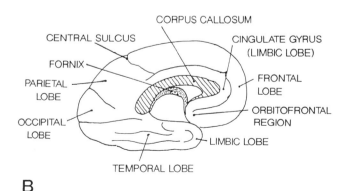

B

FIG. 10. The five lobes of the brain. **A:** Lateral view. **B:** Medial view of limbic lobe structures.

nects limbic and neocortical regions. The paralimbic regions include the parahippocampal gyrus, most of the cingulate gyrus, the orbitofrontal cortex, and the insula. These areas have an intermediate level of differentiation between the limbic cortex and the neocortex and have reciprocal connections with both.

The neocortex occupies the convexity of the cerebral hemispheres. It is a relatively thin mantle of gray matter covering the outer surface of the cerebral hemispheres; it forms the gyri of the brain. Two main sulci, the central sulcus and sylvian fissure, divide each cerebral hemisphere into four lobes: the frontal, parietal, occipital, and temporal lobes (Fig. 10). The frontal lobe is anterior to the central sulcus, and the parietal and occipital lobes are posterior to it. The sylvian fissure separates the temporal lobe from the frontal and parietal lobes. The limbic lobe includes the medial portions of the frontal and temporal lobes: the cingulum, the hippocampus, and the parahippocampal region. The lobes were subdivided into histologically and functionally distinct areas by the German anatomist Brodmann (Fig. 11).

The neocortex includes the primary motor and sensory areas and the association areas (Fig. 12). The primary areas include the primary visual area located in the banks of the calcarine fissure of the occipital lobe (Brodmann's area 17), the primary somatosensory area in the postcentral gyrus of the parietal lobe (areas 3, 1, 2), and the primary auditory area on the transverse gyrus of Heschl (areas 41 and 42). The primary motor area is located in the precentral gyrus of the frontal lobe (area 4). Surrounding these primary areas are association areas. The association areas occupy most of the external surface of the hemispheres and can be divided into (1) *unimodal, or modality-specific, association areas* that surround the primary areas and are intimately related to each sensory modality; and (2) *heteromodal association areas* that receive input from the unimodal association areas. The association areas also serve as a connection between the sensory and motor areas of the brain and the components of the limbic cor-

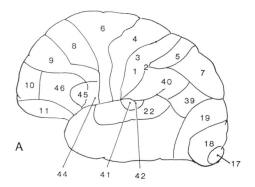

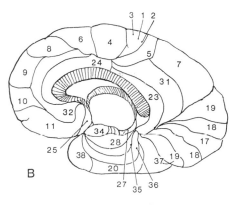

FIG. 11. Brodmann's areas of the cerebral cortex. **A:** Lateral view. **B:** Medial view. (*44,* Broca's motor speech; *11,* orbitofrontal; *6,* premotor; *4,* primary motor; *1, 2,* and *3,* primary somatosensory; *5* and *7,* somatosensory association; *18* and *19,* visual association; *17,* primary visual; *41* and *42,* auditory; *22,* Wernicke's speech; *23* and *24,* cingulate.)

tex. Heteromodal association areas include the parietotemporal regions, the prefrontal cortex, and the paralimbic association areas on the medial surface of the hemisphere.

Development

Cortical neurons are generated by symmetric division of precursor cells in the pseudostratified columnar epithelium lining the ventricular and subventricular zones of the neural tube (see Chapter 2). Phenotypic specificity is restricted at this stage, so that just before the onset of asymmetric division and migration, most progenitor cells can generate pyramidal neurons, nonpyramidal neurons, or glial cells. Neocortical neuron precursors migrate from the site of generation to their final position in the cerebral cortex, undergo further differentiation after migration, and become arranged in cortical layers. In the ontogenesis of the neocortex, the earliest event is the formation of a horizontal layer called the *preplate;* it contains the neurons that are generated first. Subsequent waves of migrating neurons form the *cortical plate* in an inside-to-outside temporal sequence, creating future cortical layers VI to II of the mature cortex (see below). Neurons that migrate into the neocortex move along radial glial cells, and the time of generation of a neuron determines its laminar (vertical) position in the mature cortex. Neocortical development is thought to occur according to the *radial unit hypothesis.* Neurons generated serially in time at the same locus in the germinal epithelium migrate sequentially along the same or an adjacent set of radial glial fibers and settle in an inside-to-outside pattern in a radial column; this radial column constitutes an *ontogenetic unit,* the basic building block of the developing neocortex. The surface area and thus the size of the neocortex is determined by the number of its ontogenetic units, which is set by the number of symmetric divisions of progenitor neurons in the neural epithelium before migration. The tangential (horizontal) spatial origin of the cells in the neural epithelium determines the final tangential position of the cell in the mature neocortex. The cortical parcelation into distinct areas is determined to some degree at the level of the ventricular zone. Humans acquire the full complement of neocortical neurons during the second trimester of pregnancy.

Histology

The cerebral cortex contains large numbers of cells intermingled with axons, dendrites, neuroglia, and blood vessels. The two main types of cortical neurons are projection neurons, represented by *pyramidal cells,* and interneurons, represented by nonpyramidal cells and referred to as *granule* or *stellate cells* (Fig. 13A and B). The cells are organized into horizontal layers and vertical *columns.* The arrangement of these layers and columns varies with the function of each area; thus, differences in function in the lobes of the

FIG. 12. Functional cytoarchitecture of the cerebral cortex. The primary sensory areas include the primary somatosensory area (areas 3, 1, 2) on the postcentral gyrus; the primary auditory area (areas 41, 42) on the transverse gyrus of Heschl, and the primary visual cortex (area 17) on the calcarine cortex. These areas receive input from sensory relay nuclei of the thalamus. The motor areas include the primary motor cortex (area 4) in the precentral gyrus, the lateral premotor area and the frontal eye fields on the convexity of the frontal lobe, the supplementary motor area on the medial aspect of the frontal lobe, and the anterior cingulate motor area. All these motor areas (except the frontal eye fields) are reciprocally connected with specific subdivisions of the basal ganglia (via the thalamus) and contribute to the corticospinal tract. Unimodal sensory association areas include the somatosensory association area in the superior parietal lobe, the visual association areas in the occipital lobe and the inferior parietal and inferior temporal lobes, and the auditory association area in the superior temporal gyrus. All these areas contribute information to the large heteromodal sensory association cortex located in the parietotemporal area. The unimodal and heteromodal sensory association areas receive input from the pulvinar of the thalamus. The sensory association areas project to the prefrontal cortex, which is involved in so-called executive functions (control of behavior and cognitive processing); it is reciprocally connected with the dorsomedial nucleus of the thalamus. The association areas of the cerebral cortex are connected with the limbic system, including the hippocampal formation and the amygdala, via the paralimbic cortical areas. These areas include the cingulate gyrus, parahippocampus, entorhinal cortex, and components of the orbitofrontal, insular, and anterior temporal cortices.

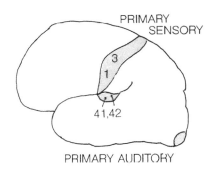

PRIMARY
SENSORY

3

1

41,42

PRIMARY AUDITORY

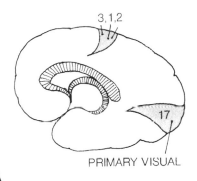

3,1,2

17

PRIMARY VISUAL

A

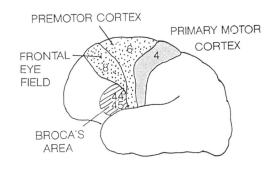

PREMOTOR CORTEX

FRONTAL
EYE
FIELD

PRIMARY MOTOR
CORTEX

6

4

8

44
45

BROCA'S
AREA

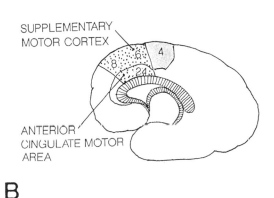

SUPPLEMENTARY
MOTOR CORTEX

8   6   4

24

ANTERIOR
CINGULATE MOTOR
AREA

B

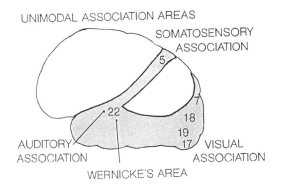

UNIMODAL ASSOCIATION AREAS

SOMATOSENSORY
ASSOCIATION

5

7

22   18

19

17

AUDITORY
ASSOCIATION

VISUAL
ASSOCIATION

WERNICKE'S AREA

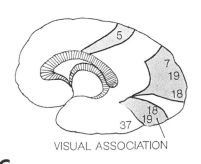

5

7
19

18

18
19

37

VISUAL ASSOCIATION

C

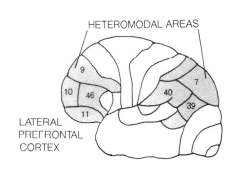

HETEROMODAL AREAS

9

7

10   46

40

11

39

LATERAL
PREFRONTAL
CORTEX

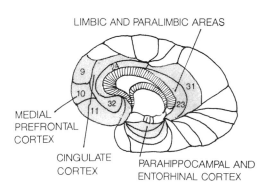

LIMBIC AND PARALIMBIC AREAS

9

24

31

10

32

23

11

MEDIAL
PREFRONTAL
CORTEX

CINGULATE
CORTEX

PARAHIPPOCAMPAL AND
ENTORHINAL CORTEX

D

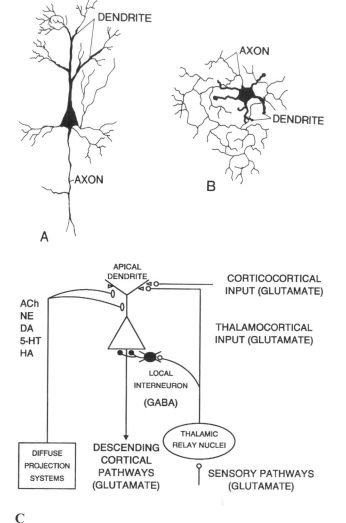

FIG. 13. The two main types of cells of the cerebral cortex and their connections. **A:** Pyramidal cells are the projection neurons and are characterized by a prominent apical and several basal dendrites containing dendritic spines. The neurotransmitter of these neurons is L-glutamate. **B:** Nonpyramidal neurons are aspiny, use γ-aminobutyric acid (GABA), and include several types that participate in local inhibitory circuits. **C:** Pyramidal cells receive excitatory input from the thalamus (thalamocortical axons) and from other cortical areas (corticocortical axons); these axons terminate predominantly on dendritic spines. Nonpyramidal (GABAergic) neurons may synapse on the initial segment of pyramidal cell axons (inhibiting output from the cells) or on the soma, dendritic shafts, or dendritic spines (to inhibit excitatory responses in specific compartments of a pyramidal cell). Input from brainstem and basal forebrain neurons containing acetylcholine *(ACh)*, norepinephrine *(NE)*, dopamine *(DA)*, serotonin *(5-HT)*, or histamine *(HA)* modulate the responses of pyramidal cells to excitatory or inhibitory input.

brain can be correlated with histologic and topographic differences.

A pyramidal cell is triangular, with its upper end giving off an apical dendrite that can extend to the surface of the cortex. The base of the cell gives rise to basal dendrites and a long axon that projects to other cortical areas or to subcortical structures. Pyramidal neurons are excitatory and contain L-glutamate. Dendrites of pyramidal cells contain dendritic spines.

Stellate cells are small multipolar neurons with a dark-staining nucleus, scanty cytoplasm, and a number of dendrites and axons passing in all directions to synapse with other neurons in the cortex. Generally, they are local inhibitory interneurons and use GABA as their neurotransmitter. Nonpyramidal cells (with one exception) lack dendritic spines.

In limbic cortex, the neurons are organized into one or two cell layers, whereas in the neocortex they form six layers (Fig. 14):

I. The molecular (plexiform) layer is the superficial layer. It contains the apical dendrites of pyramidal cells and local interneurons and receives several fiber

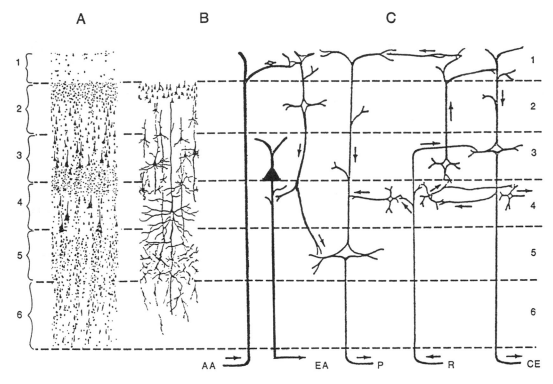

FIG. 14. The six layers of the cerebral cortex: molecular layer *(1)*, external granular layer *(2)*, external pyramidal layer *(3)*, internal granular layer *(4)*, internal pyramidal layer *(5)*, and multiform cell layer *(6)*. **A:** Cells stained by Nissl stain. **B:** Selected cells stained by Golgi stain. **C:** Vertical and horizontal connections of cortical neurons. (*AA,* afferent association fiber; *EA,* efferent association fiber; *P,* efferent projection fiber; *R,* afferent radiation fiber; *CE,* commissural efferent fiber.)

systems, including projections from structures of the consciousness system.

II. The external (outer) granular layer contains many granule (stellate) cells, whose axons synapse in deeper cortical layers, and pyramidal cells, whose axons (commissural fibers) project to contralateral cerebral cortex.

III. The external (outer) pyramidal layer contains mainly pyramidal cells, whose axons are commissural or association fibers.

IV. The internal (inner) granular layer has closely packed granule (stellate) cells and is the main site for termination of thalamocortical fibers.

V. The internal (inner) pyramidal layer contains the large pyramidal cells that project to the basal ganglia, brainstem, and spinal cord. Some of the pyramidal cells give rise to commissural fibers.

VI. The multiform layer contains pyramidal neurons that project back to the same areas of the thalamus that give rise to the thalamocortical projections; others project to layer IV.

The thickness of the cerebral cortex varies (range, 1.3 to 4.5 mm, with the maximal thickness in the calcarine, or primary visual, cortex). The differences in thickness and in cellular composition (for example, the relative number of pyramidal and nonpyramidal neurons) are the basis for the cytoarchitectonic subdivisions of Brodmann described above. The cytoarchitectonic fields can be grouped into several types. *Homotypical* cortical areas have the typical six-layer structure. These areas include most of the cerebral cortex, particularly the association areas in the frontal and parietal lobes. The six layers cannot be clearly discerned in *heterotypical* cortical areas. These areas correspond to the primary (unimodal) sensory and motor cortices. The primary sensory cortices, including the somatosensory (areas 3, 1, 2), visual (area 17, or calcarine cortex), and auditory (areas 41, 42) cortices, are characterized by a prominent layer IV and are referred to as *granular cortex,* or *koniocortex.* Layer IV is the main site of termination of afferents from the thalamus and contains a specific type of nonpyramidal cell, the spiny stellate neuron, that receives input directly from the thalamus. These neurons are glutamatergic. Layer IV reaches maximal thickness in the calcarine cortex, which contains twice as many neurons as other cortical areas. The other heterotypical cortex corresponds to cortical motor areas, including primary motor cortex and premotor cortex, frontal eye fields, and the anterior part of the cingulate gyrus. These areas are referred to as *agranular cortex* and are characterized by a prominent layer V. This layer contains the pyramidal neurons that project to subcortical areas. The most prominent example is primary motor cortex (area 4), which contains the giant pyramidal cells of Betz.

Physiology

Axons in the cortex run vertically and horizontally, mediating both projection and associational activity. An important feature of the neocortex is its organization into functional modules, or columns. A *column* is a vertical cylinder of cortical tissue that includes all six layers and represents the functional unit of cortex. In primary sensory cortices, neurons located in all layers within a column have similar properties: peripheral receptive field, sensory modality, and response characteristic (for example, adaptation). Neurons in the same column receive a cluster of thalamic axons from a particular set of thalamic neurons

and are interconnected by the local excitatory spiny stellate neurons in layer IV (that project vertically across all cortical layers). In primary motor cortex, pyramidal neurons of the same column project to the same pool of spinal motor neurons and receive somatosensory feedback from the same muscle and cutaneous receptors activated by the movement. Columnar organization in the association (homotypical) areas, including posterior parietal and prefrontal cortices, depends on the pattern of intracortical connectivity through corticocortical connections at the level of layer III. For example, neurons in a given column of the posterior parietal cortex respond to a specific combination of stimuli (for example, the position of an object in space and the position of the arm) and project to a column in the prefrontal cortex that drives eye movements according to this information.

Cortical neurons in each column receive input from (1) other columns, (2) local interneurons, (3) the specific thalamic nuclei, and (4) structures of the consciousness system. In general, activation of a column is associated with inhibition of the surrounding columns. This is important for sensory discrimination and for fine motor control. Columns distributed over wide areas of the cortex can be activated simultaneously, a critical feature of cortical function.

The function of the cerebral cortex is characterized by (1) hierarchical, or sequential, processing of information; (2) reciprocal connections between different cortical areas; (3) distributed processing; (4) cortical plasticity; and (5) corticosubcortical interactions. There are close interactions between cognitive processes of the neocortex and the emotional and motivational processes of the limbic cortex.

1. *Hierarchical organization.* An important aspect of cortical function is its activity patterns, that is, what regions of the cortex connect directly with other areas. Cells in a primary sensory area project to their own unimodal, or modality-specific, association areas. For example, primary

visual cortex projects almost exclusively to visual association cortex. Individual cells in this region respond to visual stimuli only. The cells in unimodal association areas react to specific modalities and project to heteromodal association areas, in which inputs from various sensory modalities converge. The heteromodal association areas also project to the paralimbic structures that, in turn, relay the information to the limbic system. The prefrontal association areas send input to the premotor association areas that project to primary motor cortex.

2. *Reciprocal interactions.* Another important feature of cortical function is the reciprocal flow of information between primary and association sensory and motor areas of the neocortex and between neocortical association areas and the limbic system. This allows continuous monitoring of cortical activity in the different areas of the hemisphere.

   Association cortex and paralimbic cortex form a bridge between the primary sensory areas in neocortex and the limbic system. Through the reciprocal connections that form this bridge, the external world communicates with the internal world, and the internal world can affect the processing of external stimuli. For example, an object in the external environment stimulates the retina and produces excitation in primary visual cortex. The information is next transmitted to the visual association cortex, where certain features of the stimulus (such as shape, contour, and color) are abstracted. This information is then transferred to the heteromodal association areas, where the visual information about the object is processed in combination with information from other sensory modalities to produce a more complex perception. This multimodal information is transferred to paralimbic and limbic system structures, where emotional or affective features of the stimulus may be added and where processing of the information for mem-

ory storage takes place. This whole process is dynamic, and the processing that occurs in the limbic system is fed back to the association cortex, thus influencing subsequent processing of incoming stimuli.

3. *Distributed processing.* An important feature of cortical organization is that every cortical function depends on the parallel and simultaneous processing of information by anatomically separate networks that involve different areas of neocortex, limbic cortex, and paralimbic cortex and their respective connections with the basal ganglia and thalamus. For example, processes such as language involve structures in the posterior and anterior regions of neocortex, the caudate nucleus, and the thalamus. Processes such as memory and directed attention involve parallel processing in neocortical, limbic, and paralimbic regions. Therefore, even though a lesion in a specific area of the hemisphere produces a specific deficit, this does not mean that this area is necessarily the seat of the function that is affected. Instead, the area may be part of a more complex network involved in that function.

4. *Cortical plasticity.* Cortical plasticity is the ability of the cerebral cortex to undergo anatomical and functional changes in response to environmental circumstances. This phenomenon occurs even in the cerebral cortex of adults. The cortical representations of sensory and motor maps may change in size and distribution in response to peripheral injury or to effects of training. Cortical plasticity may explain recovery of function after a large hemispheric lesion. Functional plasticity includes long-term increase in efficacy of synaptic transmission in response to repetitive activity in a circuit. This phenomenon, called *long-term potentiation,* occurs in the hippocampus and neocortex and is important for learning and memory.

5. *Corticosubcortical interactions.* The function of the cerebral cortex depends

not only on intracortical connections but also on corticosubcortical circuits that involve the thalamus and basal ganglia.

Important information processing also occurs at the cellular level (Fig. 13C). The pyramidal cells constitute the output of the cerebral cortex. The target of a pyramidal cell varies according to the cortical layer of the pyramidal cell. Activity of the pyramidal cells depends on (1) the intrinsic membrane properties, (2) the pattern of excitatory input, (3) the level of local inhibition, and (4) state-dependent modulation. Pyramidal cells are heterogeneous in regard to ion channel distribution and firing properties, including the ability to originate rhythmic burst activity. Excitatory input to pyramidal cells is mediated by L-glutamate and terminates mainly on dendritic spines. Dendritic spines are functional compartments of dendrites and contain voltage- and glutamate-gated calcium channels. They are the site of use-dependent synaptic plasticity, including long-term potentiation and long-term depression of excitatory neurotransmission. The activity of pyramidal cells is controlled locally by GABAergic inhibitory neurons. There are several types of these neurons, and they synapse on different parts of a pyramidal cell. For example, some neurons control the output of a pyramidal cell via a GABAergic synapse on its initial segment, the site of action potential generation; others control local processing at a single dendritic spine, without affecting excitatory transmission at other sites of the same or other dendrites. Both pyramidal cells and local interneurons receive modulatory input from cholinergic and monoaminergic pathways of the brainstem and basal forebrain. Acetylcholine, norepinephrine, dopamine, serotonin, and histamine, acting through various G-protein–coupled receptors, modify potassium conductance and thus excitability and responsiveness of cortical neurons (see Chapter 12).

Pathophysiology

The anatomical and histologic characteristics and functional organization of the cerebral cortex make it particularly susceptible to the development of excessive paroxysmal synchronized activity that is manifested as seizures.

A *seizure* is a transient disturbance that occurs as a result of an abnormal, excessive discharge of cortical neurons. It represents a specific pathophysiologic expression of abnormality at the supratentorial level.

The two primary factors that produce seizures are (1) increased excitability of cortical neurons and (2) synchronization of neuronal populations. Mechanisms that may cause these processes include (1) alteration of intrinsic membrane properties, (2) impairment of local inhibitory mechanisms, (3) local changes in neuronal environment, and (4) increased recruitment and recurrent excitation of neuronal populations via synaptic input or electrical coupling. Seizures can become generalized as a result of synchronizing mechanisms between the two hemispheres, recruitment of synchronizing thalamocortical circuits, or involvement of subcortical structures. Repeated activation of a neuronal population may produce a persistent increase in neuronal excitability via long-term potentiation, including long-term changes in cytoarchitecture and genetic expression.

Seizures may be manifested in different ways with involvement of different cortical areas. They may be partial (focal) or generalized in distribution. Partial seizures occur with focal lesions such as vascular disorders, neoplasms, abscess, and trauma. Generalized seizures usually occur with metabolic, toxic, degenerative, and traumatic disorders but may also develop from focal seizures.

Functional Organization at the Supratentorial Level ■

Through its connections, the cerebral cortex is the site of the highest order of integration of activities of the sensory, motor, internal regulation, and consciousness systems. In addition to these systems, the limbic, olfactory, and visual systems are located at the supratentorial level. The sensory structures of the cortex are involved with higher order processing of somatosensory, visual, auditory, olfactory, and vestibular sensory functions. The motor system is involved with cortical motor control, motor planning, and oculomotor control. The internal regulation system controls autonomic functions, homeostasis, and emotions. The consciousness system integrates inputs from the brainstem structures involved with cortical arousal and the wake-sleep cycle. The sensory, motor, and visual systems are part of the neocortex. The internal regulation, consciousness, and olfactory systems are components of the limbic system.

Functions that are unique to the telencephalon are attention, control of behavior, language, and memory. Attention, control of behavior, and language are functions of the neocortex, and memory is a function of both the neocortex and the limbic system (Table 7).

Limbic System

The limbic components of the telencephalon include the basal forebrain (amygdala, ventral striatum, and the cholinergic neurons projecting diffusely to the cerebral cortex), the limbic cortex (hippocampus and adjacent structures), and the septal region.

These regions are closely interconnected with limbic components of the diencephalon (dorsomedial and midline thalamic nuclei and hypothalamus) and the structures of the brainstem that correspond to the internal regulation and consciousness systems.

The functions of the limbic system are higher order control of autonomic function, homeostasis, reproduction, emotion, cortical arousal, motivated behavior, and learning.

The limbic system can be subdivided into two main circuits: (1) the anterior limbic circuit includes the amygdala and its connections and is important for the control of homeostasis and affective behavior, and (2) the posterior limbic circuit includes the hippocampal formation and its connections and is important for learning and memory (Table 8 and Fig. 15).

Amygdala

The *amygdala* (from the Greek word for almond) of the temporal lobe is located just anterior to the hippocampus and underlying the uncus. It consists of several nuclei that are divided into a *basolateral nuclear group*, a *centromedial group*, and an *olfactory group*. The amygdala is connected with the neocortex through the external capsule and with the thalamus, hypothalamus, basal forebrain, and

TABLE 7. *Functions of the limbic system and neocortex*

	Function	Dysfunction
Limbic system	Motivated behavior Learning Memory Higher order control of autonomic function Homeostasis Reproduction Emotion Cortical arousal	Inability to learn Amnesia Inappropriate social behavior Emotional disturbances
Neocortex	Control of behavior and motivation Motor programming and execution Processing of sensory information Directed visual attention Oculomotor control Language Memory	Disorder of attention Apraxia Agnosia Visual inattention or neglect Visual field defects Aphasia Memory disorders Seizures Motor and sensory disturbances

TABLE 8. *Comparison of the amygdala and hippocampal circuits*

Feature	Amygdaloid complex	Hippocampal formation
Components	Basolateral nuclear complex Central nucleus	Entorhinal cortex Dentate gyrus Hippocampus proper (areas CA1–CA4) Subiculum

Sensory input	Unimodal, either highly processed
	  from cortical association areas or
	  via direct thalamoamygdala input
		Multimodal

Main receptive component	Lateral nucleus	Entorhinal cortex
Output component	Central nucleus (to subcortical areas) Basal nucleus (to cortex)	Subiculum
Efferent pathway	Stria terminalis Ventral amygdalofugal pathway External capsule	Fornix
Thalamic relay nucleus	Dorsomedial	Anterior
Cortical target	Prefrontal cortex Anterior cingulate cortex Association cortex	Posterior cingulate cortex Entorhinal cortex
Hypothalamic target nuclei	Preoptic Ventromedial Paraventricular Lateral hypothalamic area	Mamillary nuclei
Brainstem connections	Autonomic nuclei Periaqueductal gray Pontine reticular formation	Midbrain tegmentum
Cholinergic input from basal forebrain	Nucleus basalis	Medial septum

Functions	Emotional behavior and
	  emotional memory)
	Fear
		Learning and transient storage of
		  information about facts and events

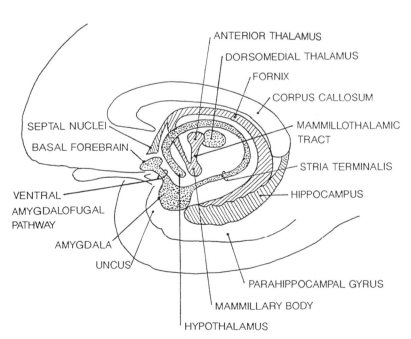

FIG. 15. Medial aspect of the temporal lobe and interconnections with limbic lobe and diencephalic structures in the limbic system. The cerebral cortex of the temporal lobe has been removed to expose the deep fiber pathways. Stippled area indicates the anterior limbic circuit. Hatched area indicates the posterior limbic circuit. These two circuits are intimately connected.

brainstem by the ventral amygdalofugal pathway and the stria terminalis.

The basolateral nuclear group contains both pyramidal and nonpyramidal neurons similar to those in the cerebral cortex. The lateral nucleus is the principal receptive component of the amygdala and receives both highly processed sensory input from unimodal sensory association areas of the cerebral cortex and direct, less elaborated sensory input from the thalamus. The basolateral complex sends axons to the cerebral cortex, including the hippocampal formation and sensory association areas, through the external capsule. It provides input to the prefrontal cortex, both directly and by way of the *dorsomedial nucleus* of the thalamus.

The central nucleus of the amygdala (a component of the centromedial group) is the main source of output to subcortical areas, including the hypothalamus and brainstem autonomic and motor areas. This nucleus is the site of initiation of integrated autonomic, endocrine, and motor responses related to emotion and fear. When an otherwise neutral sensory stimulus (for example, an image, sound, or smell) occurs simultaneously with an emotionally significant experience, either pleasant or unpleasant, it generates not only a cognitive response (recognition of the stimulus) but also emotional autonomic, endocrine, and motor responses. The basolateral amygdala is the site of convergence of the neutral sensory stimulus (via corticoamygdala connections) and the emotionally significant stimulus, such as pain (via direct thalamoamygdala connections). Thus, the amygdala neurons interpret the sensory stimulus in terms of its emotional significance and transfer this information to the central nucleus, which initiates the emotional response. The amygdala is thought to mediate "emotional memory," by which new exposure to the emotionally neutral sensory stimulus alone may generate the emotional response. This is referred to as *classic conditioning.*

Two paralimbic regions, the anterior cingulate and orbitofrontal cortices, are interconnected with the amygdala and are important in the control of motivation and emotional behavior. Lesions of the anterior cingulate cortex can produce decreased psychomotor activity (akinetic mutism) and those of the orbitofrontal cortex can produce inappropriate, impulsive, disinhibited social behavior. Seizure activity that originates in these areas of the frontal cortex or amygdala may be manifested as an emotional experience (fear), excessive autonomic activity (tachycardia), or complex, bizarre motor automatisms, or some combination of these.

Hippocampal Formation

The limbic cortex can be considered as a functional unit involved in the processes of learning and memory. It includes the *hippocampal formation* (that is, the *dentate gyrus, hippocampus,* and *subiculum*) and the *entorhinal cortex,* which are located in the medial aspect of the temporal lobe. The medial temporal lobe structures are part of the reverberatory circuits that allow the formation of persistent associations between stimuli necessary for learning (Fig. 16). Highly processed sensory information from neocortical association areas gains access to the hippocampal circuit via the entorhinal cortex. The entorhinal cortex projects to the hippocampus proper both directly or via the dentate gyrus. The hippocampus proper (also known as the *cornu Ammonis* [CA]) consists of several fields of pyramidal neurons (CA1–CA4); its main projection (axons of CA1 neurons) is to the subiculum. The subiculum, in turn, is the main output structure of the hippocampal formation. Its axons project to subcortical structures, via the *fornix,* and back to the entorhinal cortex. All these connections are excitatory and mediated by L-Glutamate. Parallel entorhinal cortex → dentate gyrus → CA3 → CA1 → subiculum → entorhinal cortex loops act as self-exciting reverberatory circuits and are necessary for phenomena of synaptic plasticity, such as *long-term potentiation* (see Chapter 12), important in memory.

The hippocampal formation has two types of connections, direct cortical connections via

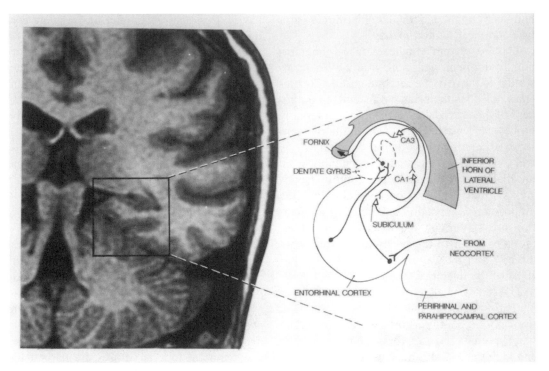

FIG. 16. The intrinsic circuitry of the hippocampal formation. Association areas of the neocortex are connected with the hippocampal formation through the entorhinal cortex. The entorhinal cortex projects via the perforant pathway to the dentate gyrus and hippocampus proper, or cornus Ammonis *(CA),* including pyramidal neurons of the CA3 and CA1 regions. Granule cells of the dentate gyrus project via the mossy fiber system to the CA3 region. Axons from CA3 cells, referred to as Schaffer collaterals, innervate CA1 pyramidal neurons. CA1 neurons project to the subiculum, which contains most of the neurons whose axons form the fornix, the subcortical output of the hippocampal circuits. All these connections are excitatory and mediated by glutamate. Feedback projections from the subiculum and CA1 to the entorhinal cortex provide reentrant excitatory circuits in the hippocampal formation. These circuits are thought to be important for the mechanisms of long-term potentiation involved in memory. Excitability in this circuit is controlled by local GABAergic neurons at each relay station. Abnormal excitability in this circuit may give rise to the paroxysmal discharge and synchronized activity that result in seizures.

the entorhinal cortex to other paralimbic areas, including the cingulate gyrus, and subcortical connections, via the fornix. The fornix, which contains the axons of neurons in the subiculum and, to a lesser extent, those of CA1 and CA3 neurons, projects to the septal area and the mamillary bodies in the hypothalamus. The *mamillary bodies,* in turn, project to the *anterior nucleus* of the thalamus (mamillothalamic tract), and the anterior nucleus projects to the *posterior cingulate cortex.* The posterior cingulate cortex projects back to the hippocampal formation via the *cingulum.* The interconnections of the hippocampal formation, mamillary bodies, anterior thalamic nucleus, and cingulate cortex form the classic *Papez circuit.*

Basal Forebrain and Ventral Striatum

The cholinergic neurons in the nucleus basalis of the basal forebrain project to the neocortex and amygdala, and those in the septal region project to the hippocampus. These projections are involved in arousal and memory mechanisms. The ventral striatum includes the *nucleus accumbens,* which receives input from the amygdala and the limbic cortex. Through projections to the ventral portion of the globus pallidus, the ventral striatum is important in locomotion and motivational aspects of behavior.

Olfactory System

An important sensory system at the supratentorial level is the olfactory system. The receptors for cranial nerve I lie in the superior nasal mucosa and respond to the chemical structures of many agents that are perceived as smells. The *olfactory nerve* is composed of numerous unmyelinated axons from the receptor cells. The axons penetrate the skull through the cribriform plate to end in the olfactory bulb (Fig. 17). The *olfactory bulb* is a small ovoid structure that lies in the anterior end of the olfactory sulcus on the orbital surface of the frontal lobe. Fibers from the olfactory bulb form the olfactory tract, which passes posteriorly and divides into medial and lateral olfactory striae at the end of the olfactory sulcus. The lateral olfactory stria passes into the medial part of the temporal lobe known as the piriform area and ends in the uncus and amygdala (Fig. 17). The medial olfactory stria terminates in the anterior perforated substance and terminal gyri of the medial basal frontal lobe. Most olfactory fibers end in the anterior uncus, the chief cortical olfactory area. (Seizures arising in this area are called *uncinate seizures,* and the aura preceding them may be an abnormal odor.) These connections and those with the amygdala and adjacent hippocampal gyrus link the olfactory structures with the ring of structures forming the rest of the limbic system.

Neocortex

Important functions of the neocortex and associated regions include (1) control of be-

havior and motivation; (2) motor programming and execution; (3) processing of somatosensory, visual, and auditory information; (4) directed visual attention to personal and extrapersonal space; (5) oculomotor control; (6) language; and (7) memory. Higher cortical functions depend on synchronized activity in parallel networks of the cerebral cortex and its connections with the thalamus, basal ganglia, and limbic system. Although damage to a specific area of cortex produces a particular deficit, the networks involved in the affected function are more widespread.

High-Order Control of Behavior

The *prefrontal region* of the frontal lobe is anterior to the motor and premotor areas and is a heteromodal association area critical for attention, motivation, and problem-solving ability. Its functions include short-term, or "working," memory, motor planning, and control of planned behavior. The prefrontal cortex includes two functionally different regions: the dorsolateral convexity and the orbitofrontal and medial frontal regions. Lesions of prefrontal cortex produce two main syndromes. Lesions of the dorsolateral prefrontal cortex produce psychomotor retardation, hypokinesia, and lack of initiative and spontaneity, a condition called *abulia.* Lesions of the orbitofrontal cortex produce behavioral disinhibition, with hyperkinesia, disruption of social behavior, and inappropriate behavior in response to external stimuli.

Cortical Motor Control

Regions of the frontal and parietal lobes are involved in motor control. The motor regions of the frontal lobe include the primary motor area in the precentral gyrus (area 4), the lateral premotor area (area 6), the supplementary motor area on the medial aspect of the hemisphere (also area 6), and regions of the cingulate gyrus. These regions have several characteristics in common: they receive input from the ventral anterior and ventral lateral nuclei of the thalamus (relay

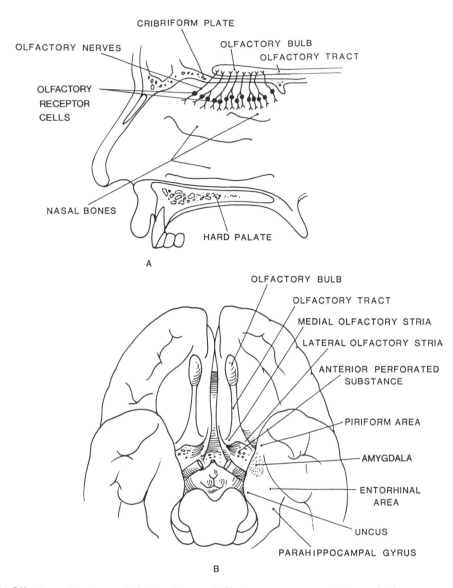

FIG. 17. Olfactory structures. **A:** Lateral view of olfactory nerves penetrating skull through cribriform plate. **B:** Basal view of brain showing termination of lateral olfactory fibers in piriform area of temporal lobe and medial olfactory fibers in the anterior perforated substance.

nuclei for the basal ganglia and cerebellum, respectively), they contain a somatotopic representation of the contralateral body, they project to the spinal cord via the corticospinal tract, and they participate in parallel cortical–basal ganglia–thalamocortical circuits that control different aspects of motor behavior. The primary and secondary somatosensory areas of the parietal lobe are also involved in motor control by providing somatosensory information to premotor and motor regions and contributing fibers to the corticospinal tract for control of sensory processing in the dorsal horn.

The *primary motor area* (area 4) contributes approximately 40% of the fibers of the corticospinal tract. This area integrates cortical and subcortical inputs and then sends signals to spinal motor neurons and interneurons. This area also provides feed-forward information to motor-controlling circuits and mediates long-loop reflexes, which contribute to postural adjustment in response to sensory feedback. The *premotor area* (area 6) is involved in control of proximal limb muscles, regulation of transcortical long-loop reflexes, and mediation of visually guided movements via connections with posterior parietal cortex. The *supplementary motor area* corresponds to the medial aspect of area 6 and is critical in planning voluntary movements and in performing tactilely guided exploratory movements of the limbs. The premotor and supplementary motor areas also contribute axons to the corticospinal tract. The anterior cingulate region is important for motivational aspects of motor behavior.

The corticospinal tract is the direct motor pathway of the outer tube and ends on the opposite side of the spinal cord, mainly on spinal interneurons and motor neurons that innervate distal limb muscles. It is important in producing highly fractionated and independent finger movements and in recruiting motor units for increasing force of contraction. The axon of a single cortical pyramidal neuron innervates motor neurons at different segmental levels, and a spinal motor neuron receives input from different cortical motor fields. Thus, individual pyramidal cells can simultaneously activate several groups of synergistic motor units and, through interneurons, inhibit antagonistic motor units. The corticospinal neurons that affect a specific muscle tend to be clustered together in a cortical column.

A specific disorder of motor control at the supratentorial level is apraxia. *Apraxia* is the inability to perform learned, skilled movements in the absence of an attentional disorder, weakness, sensory abnormality, or incoordination. It is caused by lesions in the supplementary motor area, corpus callosum, or dominant parietal lobe. Testing for apraxia may involve asking the patient to pretend he or she has a hammer in the hand and to pound a nail. A patient with limb apraxia is unable to perform this act yet is able to understand the instruction and has normal strength, sensation, and coordination.

Processing of Somatosensory Information

Neurons in ventral posterolateral and posteromedial nuclei of the thalamus receive tactile and proprioceptive information via the lemniscal, spinothalamic, and trigeminal pathways and project to the primary sensory cortex. The primary somatosensory cortex corresponds to the postcentral gyrus and consists of at least four areas (3a, 3b, 2, and 1). Each of these areas contains a complete somatotopic map of the contralateral body and responds to a specific somatosensory modality (touch or proprioception). For the initial stage of information processing in primary somatosensory cortex, neurons in a cortical column have identical, small receptive fields and respond to a specific submodality. For later stages, the neurons have larger receptive fields and respond to convergent stimulus modalities. Tactile information in combination with proprioceptive information from the fingers during the process of "active touch" (tactile discrimination requiring manipulation of the object) is important for recognition of shapes of objects; this is called *stereognosis.* Information from primary somatosensory cortex is processed further in the secondary somatosensory area (in the region of the insula), the supplementary sensory area (on the dorsomedial surface of the hemisphere), and the somatosensory association areas (in the posterior region of the parietal lobe). The posterior parietal region includes area 5, important in tactile guidance of limb movement, and area 7, important in integration of somatosensory and visual information. Area 7 is also important in directed visual attention and visual control of hand and eye movements.

A disorder of sensory function that is specific to the supratentorial level is agnosia.

Agnosia is the inability to identify the meaning of a stimulus despite being able to perceive it. The patient is alert, attentive, not aphasic, and has intact sensation but is unable to tell what the object is. Agnosias can involve any of the sensory modalities. With tactile agnosia, called *astereognosia,* a patient is unable to tell what the object is by palpating it. With visual agnosia, a patient is unable to recognize an object presented visually yet is able to describe its properties. For example, if shown a toothbrush, such a patient is able to describe its length, texture, and color but is not able to name it or to describe its use. With auditory agnosia, a patient can hear the sound but is unable to describe it. Sensory agnosias occur with lesions in the unimodal sensory association areas.

Other types of cortical sensory disorders include loss of two-point discrimination, right-left disorientation, inability to recognize letters or numbers written on the palm of the hand (agraphesthesia), inability to localize touch (atopognosia), loss of ability to discriminate weights (abarognosia), finger-naming difficulty (finger agnosia), and neglect of a body part or one side of the body. The loss of these cortical sensory functions occurs with lesions of unimodal or heteromodal association areas.

Processing of Visual Information

Most of the visual cortex is devoted to analysis of central vision. Information about form and color, on one hand, and movement, on the other, is transmitted via parallel channels throughout the visual pathway. The cells involved with visual processing in the visual cortex break the image into components, such as form, color, and movement, that are encoded by specific neurons in visual association areas.

The visual association areas that are involved in further processing of visual information include areas 18 and 19 in the occipital lobe and areas of the posterior parietal and inferior temporal lobes. Analysis of form and color occurs in visual association areas in the temporal lobe; analysis of movement is performed in areas in the parietal lobe (see below).

Oculomotor Control

The major function of the extraocular muscles is to move the eyes in such a way that the images of objects in the binocular visual fields always fall on corresponding points in the retinas and to direct the eyes to such images. This requires the coordinated contraction of the muscles of the eyes to produce voluntary and reflex conjugate ocular movements. These movements are under the control of several different regions of the brain, including the brainstem (see Chapter 15), and the frontal and occipital eye fields in the cortex (see The Visual System, below).

Directed Attention

The network for directed attention to extrapersonal space is complex and includes the posterior parietal lobe, frontal eye fields, cingulate gyrus, pulvinar, and caudate nucleus. The posterior region of the parietal lobe directs visual attention, the frontal eye fields are involved in motor exploration, and the cingulate gyrus is involved in motivational components of exploratory behavior. The right hemisphere, particularly the posterior region of the parietal lobe, is dominant for selected attention to extrapersonal or interpersonal space. It controls visual attention to both left and right extrapersonal space or side of the body. The left hemisphere contributes to control of attention to the right side.

Lesions of the right hemisphere produce severe left-side hemineglect, including contralateral visual neglect, anosognosia (lack of awareness of the affected side of the body), dressing apraxia, and constructional apraxia (inability to draw figures). Less severe degrees of right posterior parietal dysfunction can be detected by the phenomenon of extinction, which is elicited by double simultaneous stimulation of visual, auditory, or somatic modalities.

Language

The critical components of language circuits are usually located in the left cerebral hemisphere. The left cerebral hemisphere is dominant for language in almost all right-handed and in more than two-thirds of left-handed persons. Several regions of the left hemisphere are critical for comprehension, production, repetition, or assembly of words into sentences, for naming, writing, reading, and for sign language. The region of cortex around the left sylvian fissure, the *perisylvian region,* includes Broca's area (areas 44 and 45) in the inferior portion of the left frontal gyrus and the underlying white matter and associated basal ganglia, Wernicke's area (area 22) in the posterior aspect of the auditory association area in the superior temporal gyrus, and neocortical regions interconnecting Broca's area and Wernicke's area, particularly the supramarginal gyrus. Coordinated activity of these regions and their subcortical connections is critical for assembling words.

Homologous regions in the right hemisphere are involved in other aspects of language, including production of automatic idioms, prosody (melody and inflection of speech), and musical recognition and expression.

Disturbances of language and speech are divided into three types: disorders of central language processing produce aphasia, disorders of motor programming of language symbols produce apraxia of speech, and disorders of the mechanism of speech produce dysarthrias. Dysarthria occurs with disorders of the direct and indirect motor pathways, the motor control circuits, and the lower motor neuron system.

Aphasia is a disturbance in the dominant hemisphere that produces a defect in the expression or comprehension of any of the forms of language. There are different types of aphasia (Table 9):

Broca's aphasia typically occurs with lesions involving Broca's area, the underlying white matter, and basal ganglia. Specific features include loss of speech fluency, agrammatism (inability to organize words into sentences, "telegraphic speech" (the nonfluent use of content words without connecting words)), and distorted production of speech sounds. Although the patients have normal reception of language, they *cannot convert thoughts into meaningful language.* These patients may also have hemiparesis of the contralateral face and upper extremity.

Wernicke's aphasia occurs with lesions involving Wernicke's area and is characterized by fluent speech that is unintelligible because of errors in phoneme and word choice, causing paraphasia and jargon speech. Patients with this type of aphasia have *impaired comprehension* of verbal and written language but no focal motor deficit.

Conduction aphasia is due to lesions that interrupt the connections between Broca's area and Wernicke's area. It is characterized by impaired repetition. However, patients with this type of aphasia can produce intelligible speech and comprehend sentences.

TABLE 9. *Main types of aphasia*

Type	Clinical correlate	Area involved
Broca's aphasia	Unable to convert thoughts into meaningful language, nonfluent speech, agrammatism, impaired repetition	Broca's area (frontal lobe areas 44 and 45)
Wernicke's aphasia	Impaired comprehension of language, fluent speech, paraphasia, jargon speech, impaired repetition	Wernicke's area (superior temporal gyrus, area 22)
Conduction aphasia	Impaired repetition	Connections between Broca's and Wernicke's areas
Transcortical aphasia	Impaired expression or reception of speech but repetition spared	Arterial border zones
Global aphasia	Impaired comprehension and expression	Perisylvian or central regions
Anomia	Inability to name objects	Left anterior temporal cortex

Global aphasias combine features of Wernicke's aphasia and Broca's aphasia and are commonly associated with a dense contralateral hemiplegia. The perisylvian or central aphasias are commonly due to infarctions in the territory of the left middle cerebral artery, but they may also be an early manifestation of a neoplastic, inflammatory, or degenerative disorder.

Transcortical aphasias result from infarctions in the arterial border zones. These lesions interrupt the connections between the perisylvian language areas and either the anterior (motor) or posterior (sensory) regions of neocortex. With transcortical aphasias, unlike perisylvian aphasias, repetition is spared.

Despite this didactic separation among different types of aphasia, the majority of patients show varied degrees of involvement of expressive or receptive aspects of language, emphasizing the "network" concept of cortical function.

All aphasias are associated with difficulty naming objects, a deficit called *anomia*. Pure anomia occurs with lesions of the left anterior temporal cortex, including the temporal pole. These lesions may impair access to words because of interruption of connections between language and memory areas. Lesions of the left caudate nucleus or the left thalamus may produce subcortical aphasia, characterized by fluent dysarthric speech and hemiparesis.

Aphasia should be distinguished from other disorders of speech production, including speech apraxia, mutism, and dysarthria.

Motor speech apraxia, also called *apraxia of speech,* is a manifestation of lesions restricted to Broca's area (areas 44 and 45). This consists of the partial or complete inability to form the articulatory movements of the lips, tongue, and lower jaw for producing individual sounds that make up words. The patient knows what he or she wants to say but is unable to *execute the motor aspects of speech.*

Mutism is the lack of speech production caused by lesions of the prefrontal areas and the cingulate gyrus.

Dysarthrias, unlike aphasias, are difficulties with speech but not with language. There are several different neuroanatomical subtypes of dysarthria (see Chapter 15).

Memory

Memory is a complex process that involves several structures, including diencephalic and telencephalic components. The term *memory* encompasses several different processes, including the ability to learn, store, and retrieve information about events and facts (*declarative memory*), the ability to hold information to be used for actions planned for a relatively short period in the near future (*working memory*), and the learning of habits and skills (*procedural memory*) (Table 10).

TABLE 10. *Memory systems*

Type of memory	Function	Anatomy
Working memory	Maintains "on-line" information after transient exposure to stimulus	Prefrontal cortex
Explicit, or declarative memory	Conscious awareness and retrieval of past facts and events	Medial temporal lobe (hippocampal formation and surrounding areas)
Episodic	Particular instance of a stimulus or event in personal life	Diencephalon (dorsomedial nucleus of the thalamus)
Semantic	General knowledge, not associated with a particular time and place	Basal forebrain cholinergic system
Priming	Experience of a stimulus influences later processing of the same or related stimulus	Occipital, temporal, parietal, and frontal cortices
Procedural, or explicit memory	Motor skill learning	Striatum, cerebellum
Emotional memory (conditioning)	Learning relationships between perceptual stimuli and emotional significance	Amygdala

Declarative memory involves encoding, learning, storage, and retrieval of information and includes processes of primary and secondary memory. *Primary memory,* also called immediate or short-term memory, refers to the processing done over a brief period during which there is encoding of information for further storage. It depends on distributed and coordinated activity of neocortical association areas. Primary memory has a limited capacity and is generally of short duration; it relies heavily on attentional processes and is disrupted in disorders of attention. For example, primary memory is assessed by asking a patient to remember a short series of digits.

Secondary memory refers to the processing of information for longer retention intervals and involves the processes of learning and storage of information. This is the memory function that most people consider as true memory. There is a temporal gradient of information in secondary memory in that more recently learned events are more labile and subject to disruption. Structures of the medial temporal lobe, including the hippocampus and surrounding regions, diencephalic structures such as the mamillary bodies and the dorsomedial nucleus of the thalamus, and cholinergic neurons of the basal forebrain, are involved in the learning of new information before it is transformed into stable long-term memory.

The hippocampus and related areas of the medial temporal lobe are critical for the process of learning and transient storage before establishment of *long-term memory.* The hippocampus includes an excitatory circuit organized into several parallel loops that allow reverberatory activity. This circuit is characterized by *long-term potentiation,* which increases the efficacy of excitatory transmission in the hippocampal circuits as a consequence of repetitive activation. Cholinergic input from the basal forebrain also facilitates the establishment of long-term memory.

As memory engrams become more firmly consolidated, more of the processing is transferred from the limbic system to the association areas of neocortex. Well-established and old memories (remote memory) are relatively resistant to disruption. This type of information is often of a personal nature and is quite meaningful to the person. Remote memories can be largely preserved even after damage to the hippocampus and limbic system. These memories are also preserved in more general degenerative processes such as Alzheimer's disease.

Memory also includes working memory and procedural memory. *Working memory* involves retaining information for a short time, for example, looking up a telephone number and remembering it briefly before dialing it. It is a function of the prefrontal lobe and depends mainly on attention and ability to prevent interference from other stimuli. Working memory is impaired by lesions of prefrontal cortex. *Procedural memory* (habits and motor skills) involves corticosubcortical circuits that include the caudate nucleus and cerebellum. Working and procedural memory are spared in disorders causing classical memory dysfunction (*amnesia*).

Different clinical conditions selectively affect different aspects of memory. Primary memory is compromised in acute confusional states in which there is impaired attention. Secondary memory, learning, and transient storage of information are selectively affected by lesions of the hippocampus and its diencephalic connections.

Bilateral damage of the hippocampus or the entorhinal cortex and other perihippocampal regions impairs the ability to learn new information. A memory disorder can also occur in patients with midline lesions of the diencephalon, including the dorsomedial nuclei of the thalamus; this is called *diencephalic amnesia.* Korsakoff's syndrome occurs in chronic alcoholics who are often nutritionally deprived and is manifested as a profound inability to learn new information. The pathologic lesions in this condition primarily involve the dorsomedial thalamic nucleus and the mamillary bodies, which are part of the limbic circuits connecting the hippocampus and amygdala with the cortex.

Lesions of lateral temporal association neocortex, including pathways connecting the hippocampus with other neocortical regions, produce not only severe difficulty with learning but also the inability to recall remote events.

In Alzheimer's disease, memory dysfunction reflects inability to learn because of involvement of the hippocampus, inability of the hippocampus to transmit information to the neocortical areas due to involvement of the parahippocampal structures, and impaired cholinergic activation of limbic and neocortical circuits due to loss of neurons in the nucleus basalis.

Acute memory disturbances can also be classified on a temporal dimension if they are caused by an abrupt event. *Anterograde amnesia* is the inability to lay down new memories or to learn new information beginning at the time of the injury. For example, a person who has a head injury may have difficulty remembering events that occur after the injury (this may last for up to several days). Anterograde amnesia usually results from damage to medial temporal lobe structures, medial thalamus, or other limbic system structures. These are the structures involved in the establishment of new memories and of transferring information from primary to secondary memory. They are often affected in head injuries.

In contrast, *retrograde amnesia* is the inability to recall events that occurred before an injury. Typically, there is a temporal gradient to retrograde amnesia, with information learned immediately before the injury being more susceptible to disruption because it is less well established.

Clinical Correlations   ■

Disorders of the cerebral hemispheres may be *diffuse* or *focal* and may be manifested as either *loss of function* (or *deficit*) or *excessive activity* (seizures). Diffuse disorders may consist of an alteration in mentation or consciousness, bilateral motor abnormalities, or generalized seizures. Focal disorders of the cerebral hemispheres produce disturbances that are unique to the supratentorial level. These include apraxia, agnosia, aphasia, dis-

orders of directed attention, visual field defects, motor and sensory disturbances affecting the contralateral body and face, and focal seizures. In addition, lesions of the left hemisphere may affect language-related functions, and lesions of the right hemisphere may affect visuospatial-related functions.

Diffuse Disorders

Diffuse movement disorders include hypokinetic disorders such as parkinsonism and hyperkinetic disorders such as chorea or myoclonus. Generalized seizures may consist of absence or generalized tonic-clonic seizures. Disorders of consciousness or mentation consist of confusional states, dementia, and mental retardation.

Generalized Seizures

Both cerebral hemispheres are involved with abnormal feedback between the cortex and the thalamus to produce widespread discharges in generalized seizures. These seizures are associated with an alteration of consciousness. This may be brief in *absence seizures* or prolonged in *tonic-clonic seizures*. In a *generalized tonic-clonic* (grand mal) *seizure,* the patient abruptly loses consciousness and falls as the body stiffens in a tonic contraction. This is followed by symmetric, clonic jerking of the extremities and head, urinary incontinence, tongue biting, and apnea. After the seizure, the patient is flaccid and unresponsive, with slow return of consciousness through periods of confusion, drowsiness, and headache. The seizure usually lasts 1 to 2 minutes, and the period of altered consciousness after the seizure may last for 10 to 30 minutes. During the seizure, an electroencephalogram shows generalized, repetitive spike discharges in the tonic phase, spike and wave discharges during the clonic phase, and depression of activity followed by slow waves after the seizure (Fig. 18). Repeated seizures are called *status epilepticus.*

Brief generalized seizures lasting 5 to 30 seconds with impaired consciousness but minimal movements are called *absence* (petit

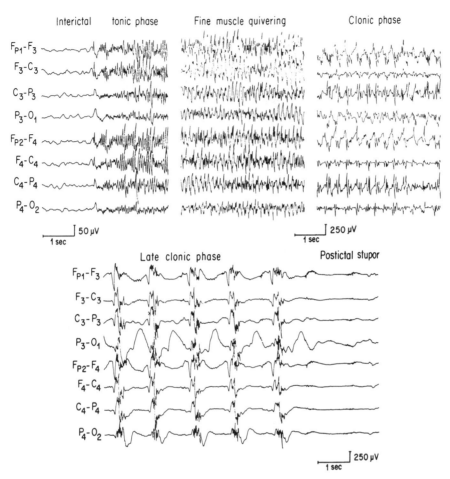

FIG. 18. Electroencephalographic accompaniment to a generalized tonic-clonic seizure. Segments of the recording during different phases of the seizure are shown. Interictal is before the seizure; tonic phase (body stiff) shows repetitive spikes; clonic phase (body jerking) shows spike-and-wave discharges; postictal (after seizure) shows suppression of activity.

mal) *seizures.* Usually, the patient abruptly ceases activity, is unresponsive, and stares, sometimes with mild clonic movements of the face or extremities. These seizures usually occur in children and can be induced by hyperventilation. They are associated with a characteristic bilateral, synchronous, generalized 3-Hz spike-and-wave pattern on the electroencephalogram (Fig. 19).

Confusional State

Confusional state, or *delirium,* is a decrease in awareness of the environment; it typically produces deficits in attention and thus impairs primary memory. In addition to impaired attention, confusional states may be associated with perceptual disturbances (illusions or hallucinations), increased or decreased psychomotor activity, incoherent speech, and disturbances of the wake-sleep cycle. This clinical syndrome commonly develops over a period of hours to days, tends to fluctuate during the day, and may be reversed if caused by a treatable condition. Causes of confusional state include metabolic encephalopathies, drug intoxication or withdrawal states, dementia, infectious processes, head injury, diffuse vascular disease, and nonconvulsive status epilepticus. Generalized motor phenomena

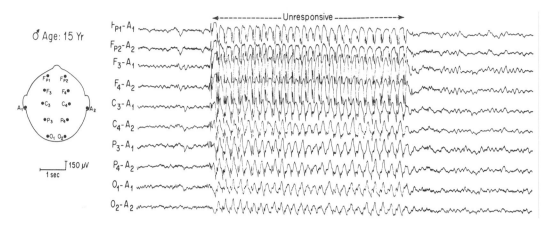

FIG. 19. Electroencephalographic accompaniment during absence seizure consisting of 3-Hz spike-and-wave pattern during which the patient was unresponsive.

such as tremor, myoclonus, or seizures may also be present.

Dementia

Dementia is an acquired condition involving a change in cognitive function from a prior level of performance to the point that social and possibly occupational functions are altered in an alert person. The many causes of dementia include degenerative diseases, vascular insults, toxic or metabolic factors, subdural hematoma, neoplasms, and infections. The most common form of dementia, however, is *Alzheimer's disease.* Typically, the initial finding of patients with Alzheimer's disease is a memory loss that over time progresses to a profound difficulty in learning new information. Often, as the disease progresses, difficulties with language and visuospatial skills develop, and the patient tends to get lost easily, cannot perform household tasks, cannot carry out financial activities, and no longer drives an automobile. In later stages of the illness, the patient no longer recognizes family members and may become mute. The patient usually dies of a complicating illness, such as pneumonia or another type of infection.

The prevalence of Alzheimer's disease increases with age, and 15% to 20% of people older than 80 years are likely to have this dis-order. The pathologic features of Alzheimer's disease include cerebral atrophy with cell loss, particularly in the hippocampus, parahippocampus, and heteromodal association areas (Fig. 20). The motor and sensory areas of cortex are relatively spared. The pathologic hallmarks are neurofibrillary tangles and senile plaques in the cortex, as well as granulovacuolar degeneration, amyloid deposition, and loss of cholinergic neurons in the nucleus basalis (Fig. 21). Several neurotransmitters are depleted in Alzheimer's disease, especially acetylcholine.

Recently, human immunodeficiency virus (HIV-1) has become an important cause of dementia, for example, in *HIV encephalopathy* or the *AIDS dementia complex.*

Mental Retardation

Mental retardation is the failure to develop normal intelligence. It is not a single disease but a group of disorders in which the development of normal intellectual functioning is arrested. Retardation may result from a congenital nonprogressive process, an acquired nonprogressive process, or a progressive disease with onset in infancy or childhood. There are many exogenous causes of mental retardation, such as trauma, anoxia, drugs, toxins, and infections. Three specific examples of endogenous causes are the genetic biochemical

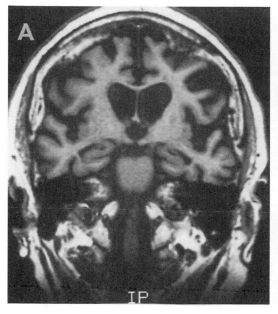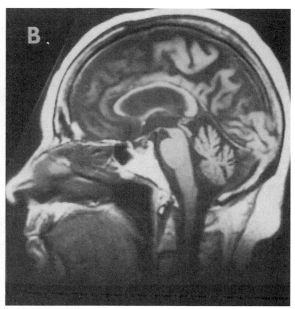

FIG. 20. Magnetic resonance image showing atrophy of the brain of a patient with Alzheimer's disease. **A:** Coronal view. **B:** Sagittal view.

defects of Tay-Sachs disease, phenylketonuria, and the chromosomal abnormality of Down syndrome.

Tay-Sachs disease is an inherited autosomal recessive disorder characterized by an excessive accumulation of the lipid ganglioside in the neurons of the central nervous system (Fig. 22). There is also retinal involvement that produces blindness. Infants with this disorder have normal development during the first few months but then begin to lose previously acquired abilities. The child becomes listless and dull, with weakness, spasticity, and hyperactive reflexes. In the terminal months, there is decerebrate posturing. Death is usually caused by infection.

Phenylketonuria is an inherited autosomal recessive disorder in which an enzymatic defect is associated with inability to convert phenylalanine to tyrosine; the increased levels of phenylalanine produce demyelination in the white matter and ultimately neuronal loss, resulting in retardation and seizures. Fortunately, in contrast to Tay-Sachs disease, the biochemical abnormality of phenylketonuria

can be detected in the blood or urine and treated with a diet low in phenylalanine to prevent mental retardation. If untreated, severe mental retardation occurs.

Down syndrome (mongolism), a chromosomal defect with triplication of chromosome 21, is characterized by mental retardation, heart and bladder defects, and a typical physical appearance of a round face, epicanthal folds, a short neck, and a simian crease on the palms of the hands. Children with this syndrome may survive into adulthood and continue to show moderate to severe retardation.

Focal Disorders

Focal disorders occur as a result of a focal process or lesion involving the cerebral hemispheres; the specific type of deficit or seizure indicates the region or lobe of the brain involved (see Figs. 10 and 12). The following describes the lobes of the brain and the types of dysfunction associated with each.

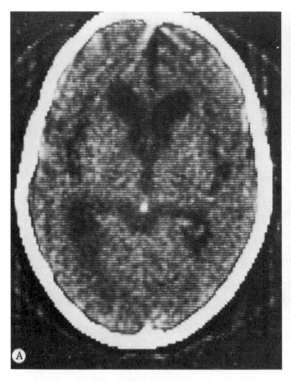

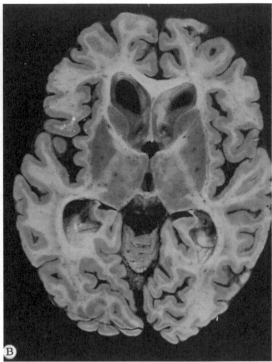

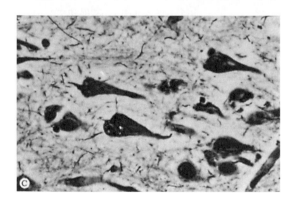

FIG. 21. Alzheimer's disease. **A:** Computed tomogram (CT scan) showing atrophy of the brain with widening of the cerebral sulci and ventricular dilatation. **B:** Corresponding horizontal section of the brain. **C:** Histologic section of cerebral cortex showing dense neurofibrillary tangles in neurons. (Bodian stain; ×400.)

Partial Seizures

Seizures arising from a localized area of the cerebral cortex are called *partial* seizures and are classified as *complex partial seizures* when associated with an alteration of consciousness and as *simple partial seizures* if consciousness is preserved. Partial seizures are often due to a focal pathologic process. The symptoms of partial seizures depend on the site of the discharge (Table 11). Observation of symptoms can localize the pathologic process. Seizures in the precentral gyrus of the frontal lobe are associated with clonic movements of the contralateral side of the face or the contralateral arm or leg. Seizures in the postcentral gyrus of the parietal lobe are accompanied by paresthesias or dysesthesias of the contralateral side of the face or the contralateral extremities. Occipital lobe seizures produce unformed visual im-

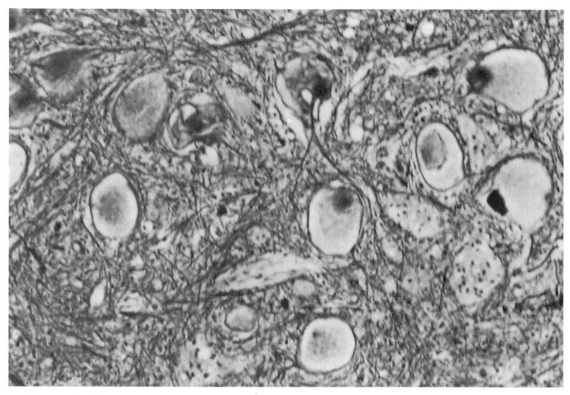

FIG. 22. Tay-Sachs disease. Histologic section of cerebral cortex showing massive ballooning of neurons caused by lipid accumulation. (Bodian stain; ×400.)

ages or impaired vision. Seizures arising from the temporal and limbic lobes are the most common partial seizures. Symptoms are varied and may include strange odors or tastes, formed auditory or visual hallucinations, language and speech disturbances, fear, unusual sensations, mouthing movements, posturing, or automatic behavior. Because there is often an alteration of consciousness, these are complex partial seizures.

TABLE 11. *Features of partial (focal) seizures*

Site of discharge	Clinical correlate
Frontal lobe	
Precentral gyrus (primary motor cortex)	Focal tonic or clonic movements
Supplementary motor cortex	Characteristic posture—elevation of arm and deviation of head and eyes to arm
Frontal eye fields	Deviation of eyes to opposite side
Parietal	
Postcentral gyrus	Paresthesias (tingling) and dysesthesias
(primary sensory cortex)	Numbness
Occipital lobe	Unformed visual hallucinations
Temporal lobe	
Limbic area	Impairment of consciousness, automatisms, language and disturbances, masticatory movements, posturing, affective symptoms, altered sensory perceptions, illusions, hallucinations
Lateral surface	Formed visual and auditory hallucinations, language disturbances
Uncus	Abnormal smell
Dominant lobe	Dysphasia

A partial seizure may remain localized in a single area or may spread to other areas. It may spread sequentially along a gyrus via arcuate fibers and thereby involve the face, arm, or leg sequentially in a so-called *jacksonian march*. It may spread from one lobe to another or from one hemisphere to another via association or commissural fibers. Or it may spread via projection fibers to the thalamus and thereby become generalized. If focal symptoms precede a generalized seizure, the focal symptoms are called an *aura* and provide evidence of the site of seizure origin.

Frontal Lobe Syndromes

The frontal lobe includes the primary motor cortex, premotor area, supplementary motor area, medial motor area, frontal eye fields, Broca's area, dorsolateral prefrontal cortex, and orbitofrontal cortex.

The primary motor cortex contributes most of the fibers in the corticospinal tract. Lesions restricted to this area produce the inability to perform fine finger movements. Acute lesions produce flaccid hyporeflexic paralysis. Seizures in this region consist of focal tonic and/or clonic movements of the contralateral face, arm, or leg.

The premotor area controls proximal limb muscles and transmits activity in other cortical regions to primary motor cortex. Lesions on the left side produce bilateral limb apraxia (inability to perform visuomotor tasks) and forced grasping. Lesions involving this area and area 4 result in a spastic, hyperreflexic paralysis.

The supplementary motor area is involved in motor planning and execution. Lesions of the region produce akinetic mutism, limb apraxia, and forced grasping. Seizures in this area produce a characteristic posturing, with elevation of the arm and deviation of the head and eyes toward the elevated arm.

Involvement of the medial motor area (area 4), which contains the representation of the leg, may produce leg weakness. Bilateral involvement may affect corticoreticulospinal input to motor neurons and cingulate input to pontine micturition centers. Such lesions cause bilateral leg spasticity and an uninhibited bladder, with incontinence.

The frontal eye fields contain neurons controlling voluntary and visually guided saccadic eye movements to the opposite side. Lesions produce transient conjugate deviation of the eyes toward the affected hemisphere and inability to move the eyes past the midline. Partial seizures in this region produce deviation of the eyes to the opposite side.

The motor speech (Broca's area) (areas 44 and 45) is located in the inferior frontal gyrus of the dominant (usually left) cerebral hemisphere; it controls the programming of speech. Lesions in this area produce a motor speech apraxia.

The dorsolateral prefrontal cortex (areas 9, 10, and 46) is involved in attention, working memory, and motor planning. Lesions produce lack of spontaneity and psychomotor retardation, hypokinesia, diminished spontaneity of speech, lack of attention and concentration, and impaired motor planning.

The orbitofrontal and medial prefrontal regions are involved in emotional behavior. Lesions produce behavioral disinhibition and antisocial behavior. Involvement of the olfactory structures in this area produces anosmia (loss of smell). Seizures produce complex automatisms and vocalizations.

Parietal Lobe Syndromes

The parietal lobe is involved in higher order processing of somatosensory and visual information and directed attention to interpersonal and extrapersonal space. It includes primary and association somatosensory cortices.

The primary somatosensory cortex is in the postcentral gyrus. Lesions of this area abolish the basic discriminative somatosensory functions such as touch localization (topognosis), two-point discrimination, weight discrimination (barognosis), joint position sense, the highly discriminative functions of "active touch," and recognition of a number written on the hand (graphesthesia). Seizures in primary somatosensory cortex present with transient symptoms of numbness or tingling sensation of the contralateral face or body.

The unimodal somatosensory association area includes area 5 and part of area 7 in the posterior parietal lobe. Lesions here cause inability to identify objects held in the hand (astereognosia) despite the ability to perceive the objects and disturbance of perception of body image.

The heteromodal association area in the parietal lobe (area 7) processes somatosensory and visual inputs important for directed attention to the interpersonal or extrapersonal space. Lesions on the right side produce severe sensory neglect of the left hemibody or extrapersonal space, resulting in dressing apraxia and constructional apraxia. Lesions in the left inferior parietal lobe may produce a combination of deficits, including *agraphia* (difficulty in writing) with or without alexia; *acalculia* (inability to do arithmetical calculations), *finger agnosia* (finger naming difficulties), and *right/left disorientation;* this combination is called *Gerstmann's syndrome.*

Lesions involving the posterior portion of the superior temporal auditory association area and surrounding parietal lobe produce receptive (Wernicke's) aphasia and conduction aphasia. Bilateral superior parieto-occipital lesions produce severe spatial disorientation, with *ocular apraxia* (inability to voluntarily control the gaze to an object of interest), *simultanagnosia* (inability to integrate the separate components of a complex visual scene), and *optic ataxia* (inability to accurately reach for an object under visual guidance). This constitutes *Balint's syndrome.*

Occipital Lobe Syndromes

The occipital lobe includes the primary visual area in the banks of the calcarine fissure on the medial aspect of the occipital lobe (area 17) and the visual association areas 18 and 19 (peristriate cortex). Peristriate cortex is involved in visuospatial processing, discrimination of movement, and color discrimination. Lesions of the occipital lobe produce visual field defects and scotomas (see The Visual System, below).

Temporal Lobe Syndromes

The temporal lobe includes primary auditory cortex, unimodal auditory and visual association cortices, and limbic cortex. The primary auditory cortex (areas 41 and 42), in the superior temporal gyrus (Heschl's gyrus), receives auditory fibers from the medial geniculate body. Sounds coming into either ear reach the auditory cortex bilaterally. Therefore, unilateral lesions of the auditory cortex cause some difficulty in sound localization, but there is no significant hearing deficit. Bilateral ablation of the auditory cortex does not prevent reaction to sounds but does greatly reduce or abolish the ability to discriminate different patterns of sound.

The superior temporal gyrus (area 22) contains the auditory unimodal association area. Bilateral lesions of this area produce *pure word deafness;* patients react to environmental noise (thus, they are not deaf) and recognize written language but cannot understand or repeat spoken language. Wernicke's area, in the posterior part of the auditory association cortex of the dominant hemisphere, is involved in the processing of written and spoken language. Damage of this area produces Wernicke's aphasia, characterized by comprehension deficit for all modalities. Lesions of the temporal pole or the inferior temporal cortex disconnect the language areas from the limbic structures and produce anomia.

The temporal visual association areas are located in middle and inferior temporal gyri and receive input from the peristriate visual association areas. They project to heteromodal areas involved in language and limbic functions. Lesions of temporal visual association areas may produce achromatopsia, visual agnosia, prosopagnosia, visual anomia, and pure alexia. *Achromatopsia* is the inability to recognize colors. *Visual agnosia* is the inability to recognize an object by sight. *Prosopagnosia* is the inability to recognize familiar faces. *Visual anomia* is the inability to name normally recognized objects. *Pure alexia* is a deficit of visual recognition confined to words and letters and is a visual agnosia for verbal material.

Seizures in the posterolateral part of the temporal lobe are characterized by auditory or visual hallucinations and language disorders and are often associated with automatism and amnesia.

Limbic Lobe Syndromes

The limbic lobe consists of the limbic and paralimbic cortices, portions of the temporal lobe (hippocampal formation), and portions of the frontal lobe (anterior cingulate and medial orbitofrontal regions). Bilateral lesions of the hippocampal formation, particularly those involving the entorhinal and perihippocampal regions, produce severe deficits of learning and memory. Other functions and disorders involving the limbic lobe were described above (see Limbic System). Seizures arising in this region are complex partial seizures and are associated with impairment of consciousness and various symptoms (altered sensory perceptions, hallucinations, illusions, affective or emotional symptoms, cognitive disturbances, automatisms, and speech disturbances).

Focal Lesions

Focal lesions include traumatic, vascular, inflammatory, and neoplastic lesions. As emphasized in Chapter 4, focal disorders are nonprogressive in nonmass lesions and progressive in mass lesions. The most common focal lesions are vascular lesions and mass lesions. One of the most frequent focal lesions is infarction. Infarctions in the distribution of any of the major cerebral arteries produce specific neurologic manifestations (see Chapter 11).

The presence of a mass lesion, however, must always be considered and is suggested by a focal, progressive course, with evidence of increased intracranial pressure or distortion of surrounding tissue (or both). Neoplasm, intracerebral hemorrhage, subdural hematoma, and abscess are examples of supratentorial mass lesions. An important example of a focal, progressive, inflammatory lesion is *herpes simplex encephalitis,* which preferentially affects the temporal lobes. This potentially fatal but treatable condition should be suspected in all patients with fever, changes in mental status, and focal symptoms, including disturbances of language, memory, or behavior. The suspicion is reinforced by the presence of a typical pattern in the electroencephalogram and confirmed by detection of the herpes simplex virus antigen in the cerebrospinal fluid.

A focal, progressive, chronic mass lesion is indicative of a neoplasm, or rarely, a nonneoplastic process such as chronic subdural hematoma or a chronic granulomatous disorder.

Neoplasms in the cerebral hemispheres seldom metastasize to other body tissues and can be categorized into benign or malignant on the basis of their pathologic characteristics and invasiveness. However, whether they are benign or malignant, intracranial neoplasms are a major threat to life because they enlarge within the confined space of the closed cranial cavity and increase intracranial pressure as well as produce local tissue compression. Although any cell type in the nervous system may undergo neoplastic change, three major groups account for most brain tumors.

Gliomas, Meningiomas, and
Metastatic Tumors

Neoplasms arising from glial cells constitute the most common primary neoplasm of the brain. These neoplasms are usually derived from astrocytes and are called *astrocytomas.* Astrocytomas vary in malignancy and may arise anywhere in the nervous system. Low-grade astrocytomas are accumulations of astrocytes with some anaplastic features. Invasion of surrounding tissue by an astrocytoma damages adjacent axons or neurons to produce focal neurologic deficit. As size increases, pressure increases. Compared with low-grade astrocytomas, high-grade astrocytomas evolve more rapidly and show more invasiveness, anaplasia, and areas of hemorrhage (Figs. 23 and 24). Vascularity and surrounding edema in

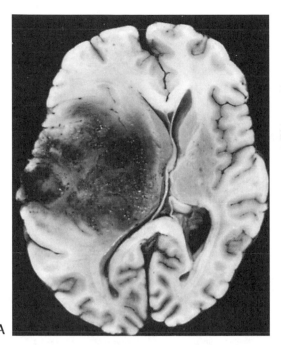

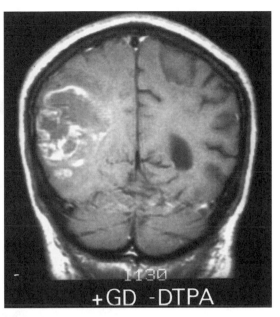

FIG. 23. High-grade astrocytoma. **A:** Horizontal section of the cerebrum showing a massive hemorrhagic-necrotic tumor of the left hemisphere. **B:** Magnetic resonance image in the coronal plane of a typical high-grade astrocytoma.

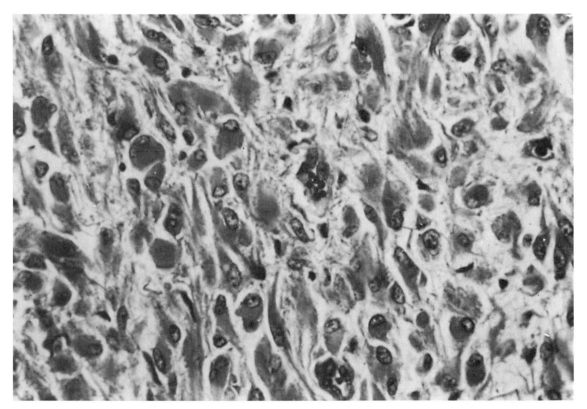

FIG. 24. Astrocytoma. Histologic section of a low-grade astrocytoma. Note the resemblance of cells to reactive astrocytes but with much more irregularity of size, shape, and nuclear morphology. (H&E; ×200.)

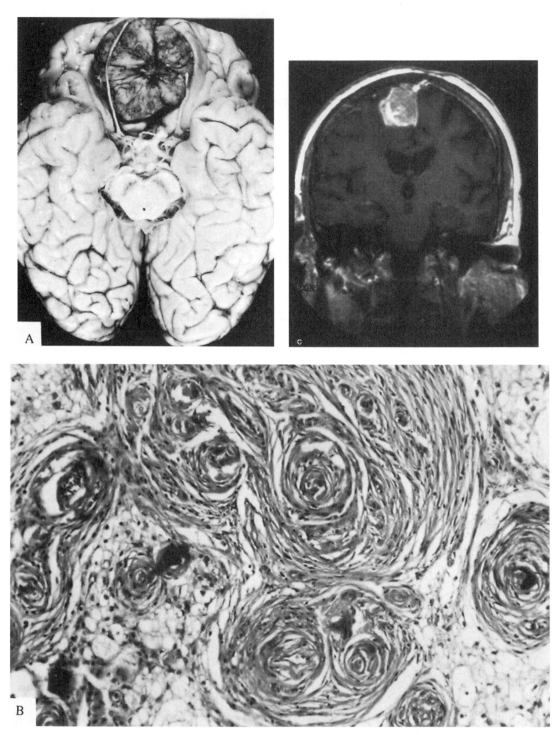

FIG. 25. Meningioma. **A:** Ventral view of the brain showing a large meningioma between the frontal lobes. **B:** Histologic section showing the typical whorl formation of elongated tumor cells. (H&E; ×250.) **C:** Typical appearance and location of a meningioma.

high-grade lesions further increase the size of the tumor.

The neoplastic proliferation of meningothelial cells, the lining cells of the leptomeninges, results in meningiomas. These tumors are almost always histologically benign, slow growing, and produce their clinical effects by compression of the brain and neighboring structures (Fig. 25A). Although they have many different histologic appearances, they typically have whorls of cells, which may degenerate and calcify to form psammoma bodies (Fig. 25B).

Focal accumulations of anaplastic cells within the brain parenchyma may arise from tumors originating elsewhere (Fig. 26). Metastatic tumors invade locally and exert a mass effect on the surrounding tissue. The histologic features resemble those of the primary neoplasm, the most common being lung and breast lesions. Frequently surrounding the tumor cells is a large area of cerebral edema, which increases the mass effect of the lesion (Fig. 27). *Central nervous system lymphoma* is a typical neoplasm in

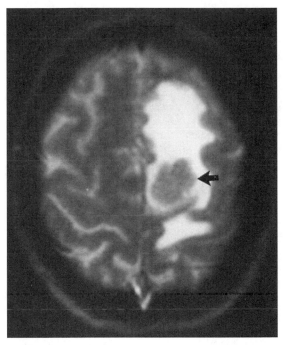

FIG. 27. Magnetic resonance imaging of metastatic adenocarcinoma of the brain with mass effect.

patients with chronic immunosuppression, for example, organ transplant recipients or those with acquired immunodeficiency syndrome.

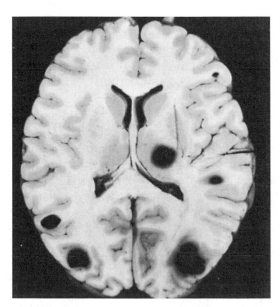

FIG. 26. Metastatic melanoma. Horizontal section of the cerebrum showing multiple pigmented metastatic tumors.

The Visual System

The visual system transforms visual representations of the external world into a pattern of neural activity that the person can use. It has peripheral receptive structures in the eye and central pathways in the diencephalon and telencephalon. The eye is a peripheral receptor organ specialized to respond to visual stimuli. It has nonneural components whose function is the transmission of light stimuli to neural receptors and neural structures that respond to the light. The supratentorial level contains the central neural pathways (in the diencephalon and telencephalon) for vision.

Nonneural Peripheral Structures

Most of the nonneural structures of the eyeball are derivatives of embryonic ectoderm, although the muscles that control the eye are mesodermal in origin. These nonneural structures include the cornea, sclera, anterior chamber, iris, lens, and vitreous humor (Fig. 28).

The *cornea* is a transparent membrane that covers the anterior part of the eye and joins the opaque white sclera at the limbus. The *sclera* is a supporting tissue that covers the rest of the eyeball and to which the extraocular muscles are attached. The *iris* is a circular diaphragm with a central aperture, the *pupil,* through which light projects to the posterior part of the eye. The ciliary body supports the *lens,* a biconvex, transparent, elastic structure that accommodates for vision at varying distances. The *vitreous humor* is a transparent gelatinous material that separates the lens and retina and serves to hold both in place. The *choroid* lies between the sclera and the retina and functions to decrease the scatter of light inside the eye.

These nonneural structures transmit light rays and focus them on the neural structures in the back of the eye. The iris opens or closes in response to varying intensity of light to control the illumination of the retina. The lens inverts the image. The lens also changes its configuration in order to focus the light rays from near or distant objects on the retina.

The Retina

The retina is an extension of the brain and performs the first stages of visual processing. In higher visual centers, coded signals from the retina undergo further processing for perception of contours, colors, textures, and movement of objects.

The embryonic optic vesicle is derived from an evagination of the embryonic diencephalon (see Chapter 2, Fig. 3C and D) and forms a two-layered cup as it grows. The outer layer becomes the retinal pigment epithelium, and the inner layer becomes the neurosensory retina.

Histology

Cells of the neurosensory retina are stratified in well-demarcated layers (Fig. 29). From the outer to inner layers, they are the receptor cell layer, outer nuclear layer, outer plexiform layer, inner nuclear layer, inner plexiform layer, and ganglion cell layer. The ganglion cell layer, the innermost layer, lies adjacent to the vitreous humor. The nerve fiber layer lies just inside the ganglion cell layer and is bounded by the internal limiting membrane. Nuclear layers contain cell bodies, and plexiform layers contain dendrites and synapses. The receptor cell layer is bounded by retinal pigment epithelium and Bruch's membrane. Light has to travel across the inner layers before reaching the receptor cells in the outer layer.

The retina contains five types of nerve cells that interact to convert and encode the image focused on the retina. The *photoreceptor cells,* the rods and cones, are in the outer nuclear layer. They convert light into a trans-

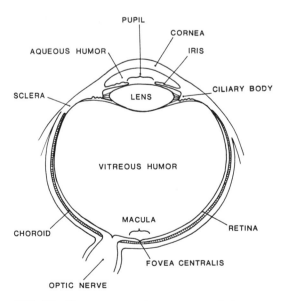

FIG. 28. The nonneural structures of the eye form the anterior portion and the outer coats. The retina and optic nerve are the neural components.

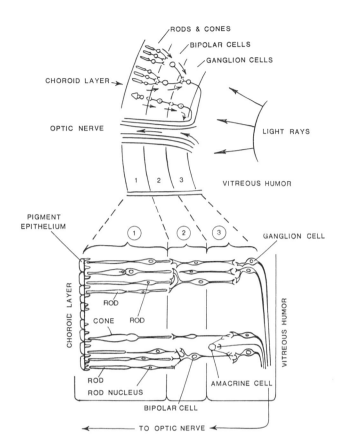

FIG. 29. The retina has three cell layers from outside to inside: rods and cones, the receptor cells *(1)*; the bipolar cells *(2)*; and the ganglion cells *(3)*. Note that the light rays have to pass through the inner layers to reach the receptor cells in the outer layer.

membrane electrical response. Synaptic terminals of receptor cells contact the *bipolar cells,* in the inner nuclear layer. These cells convey information to the *ganglion cells* (ganglion cell layer), the output cells of the retina. Ganglion cell axons collectively form the optic nerve. Two types of interneurons, *horizontal cells* and *amacrine cells,* modify activity of the receptor-bipolar-ganglion cell pathway and provide lateral integration of information.

The thickness of the retina and its cell density vary from the central visual axis to the peripheral regions. The maximal density of cones is in the *macula lutea,* a specialized region of the posterior pole of the eye. The center of the macula, the *fovea centralis,* is responsible for sharpest visual acuity. Unlike peripheral retina, the overlying structures (bipolar cells, ganglion cells, and blood vessels) are swept to the side so light has an un-

interrupted path to the receptor cells. In addition, receptor cells are tightly packed and have nearly a one-to-one ratio to ganglion cells.

Physiology

Rods and *cones* have an outer segment, which consists of membranous disks that contain photopigment, an inner segment, which includes the cell body, and a synaptic terminal. Photopigment consists of a protein, *opsin,* bound to 11-*cis* retinal, a derivative of vitamin A. Rods contain the photopigment *rhodopsin.* These cells are found predominantly in the peripheral retina, are exquisitely sensitive to light, and are used for vision under dim light, *scotopic vision.* Vitamin A deficit causes a deficiency of retinene (a precursor of retinal) and thus rhodopsin, which results in *night blindness,* the inability to see in the dark. Similar symptoms occur with selective degeneration of the rods, as in paraneoplastic retinal degeneration.

Cones are concentrated in the fovea and are involved in vision at high levels of light, *photopic vision,* including color vision. Cones contain one of three different types of visual pigments (opsins) that absorb maximally at the red, green, or blue bands of the spectrum. The red and green opsins are products of two genes located in tandem on chromosome X. Mutations affecting these genes produce X-linked *color blindness.* Visual acuity is greatest in the central fovea, where the density of cones is greatest, and decreases in the peripheral regions.

In darkness, photoreceptor cells are depolarized by a persistent influx of sodium and calcium via a cyclic guanosine monophosphate (GMP)-gated cation channel (see Chapter 7); this is the *dark current.* It is turned off by light. Light produces isomerization of retinal from the 11-*cis* to the all-*trans* form; this results in activation of rhodopsin to *metarhodopsin,* which initiates the receptor transduction cascade. Metarhodopsin has a structure similar to G-protein–coupled receptors (see Chapter 12), and is coupled to the G protein *transducin.* Transducin activates a *phosphodiesterase* that hydrolyzes cyclic GMP and closes its coupled cation channel. This results in hyperpolarization of the photoreceptors and interruption of the tonic release of glutamate from their terminal (that is, at the synapse with bipolar cells). This decrease of L-glutamate initiates the transfer of information within the retinal circuit. The decrease in intracellular calcium initiated by light triggers various mechanisms that block activation of rhodopsin, interrupting the light signal. This is referred to as photoreceptor *adaptation.* Because bright light blocks regeneration of rhodopsin, vision is reduced for 10 to 15 minutes after a person enters a dark room. As rhodopsin regenerates in the rods, the eye becomes adapted to light.

Transmission of the photoreceptor signal within the retinal circuit is a complex process that is summarized only briefly here. The retinal circuit consists of radial channels of information modulated by lateral interactions. In the radial pathway, signals from the photoreceptors are passed through *bipolar cells* to retinal *ganglion cells* whose axons form the optic nerve. The synapses between photoreceptors and bipolar cells occur in the outer plexiform layer, and those between bipolar cells and ganglion cells occur in the inner plexiform layer. All these neurons use L-glutamate. Responses in this radial pathway are regulated by lateral interactions that involve *horizontal cells,* GABAergic neurons that inhibit synaptic transmission at the photoreceptor-bipolar cell synapse, and *amacrine cells,* which modify synaptic transmission at the bipolar cell-ganglion cell synapse. Of all these cells, only the amacrine and ganglion cells are able to generate action potentials. Photoreceptors, bipolar cells, and horizontal cells communicate via local potentials.

The receptive field of a ganglion cell is a circular area on the retina. According to the response to light, ganglion cells are subdivided into *on-center cells,* which respond best to a small spot of light shined on a field surrounded by darkness, and *off-center cells,* which encode for the brightness of a small region in comparison with its surround. Thus, the visual system is designed to respond to contrast rather than to absolute light intensity. The retinal circuits activating the on and off ganglion pathways differ in important respects, including the type of bipolar cell involved, the type of glutamate receptor, and the effects of amacrine cells.

The ganglion cells are the output cells of the retina. Their axons go to the *lateral geniculate nucleus.* From its initial stages in the retina, the visual pathway is segregated into various subsystems involved in analysis of different aspects of an image, such as form and color and position and movement. The retinal ganglion cells that respond primarily to object motion project to specific regions of the lateral geniculate nucleus and form the *magnicellular* component of the visual pathway (*M pathway*). Ganglion cells that respond primarily to shapes and color project to other regions of the lateral geniculate nucleus and constitute the *parvicellular* component (*P pathway*). These two components remain segregated in the visual pathway until very late stages of processing in the cerebral cortex, when the visual image is again bound together.

Central Neural Structures

The visual structures within the cranial cavity at the supratentorial level include the optic nerve and optic chiasm, the optic tracts, and the lateral geniculate bodies in the diencephalon and the optic radiations and occipital cortex in the telencephalon.

Diencephalic Structures

The optic nerve consists of axons arising from ganglion cells in the retina. These axons converge at the optic disk, become myelinated, and then leave the back of the eye through the lamina cribrosa. The optic nerve leaves the orbit and enters the cranial cavity through the optic foramen. Although the optic nerve is considered one of the cranial nerves (cranial nerve II), it is actually a nerve tract similar to tracts in the central nervous system and consists of axons with myelin sheaths formed by oligodendroglia cells rather than by Schwann cells. Thus, disease processes such as multiple sclerosis that affect myelin of the central nervous system produce similar lesions in the optic nerve.

After the optic nerves pass through the optic foramen, they unite to form the *optic chiasm,* beyond which the axons continue as the *optic tracts.* Within the chiasm, a partial decussation occurs: the fibers from the nasal half of each retina cross to the opposite side and those from the temporal halves of the retina remain uncrossed. As the fibers from the inferior nasal retina cross, they loop forward for a short distance into the opposite optic nerve.

In binocular vision, each visual field, right and left, is projected upon one-half of both right and left retinas. Thus, the images of objects in the right field of vision are projected on the right nasal and the left temporal halves of the two retinas. In the chiasm, the fibers from these two retinal segments are combined to form the left optic tract, which then represents the complete right field of vision. By this arrangement, the whole right visual field is projected upon the left hemisphere, and the left visual field is projected upon the right hemisphere (Fig. 30).

After the partial decussation in the optic chiasm, the visual pathways, now corresponding to the optic tracts, course laterally and posteriorly to terminate in the lateral geniculate bodies in the thalamus. A few fibers leave the optic tract before it reaches the lateral geniculate bodies. Some of these fibers go to the pretectal area and form the afferent limb of the light reflex; others end in the suprachiasmatic nucleus of the hypothalamus to control circadian rhythms. Finally, other ganglion cell axons end in the superior colliculus to control reflex saccadic eye movements and to provide, through connections with the pulvinar nucleus of the thalamus, input to visual association cortex.

The *lateral geniculate body* receives the fibers from the optic tract and gives rise to the *geniculocalcarine tract,* which forms the last relay of the visual pathway.

Telencephalic Structures

The geniculocalcarine tract arises from the lateral geniculate body, passes through the retrolenticular portion of the internal capsule, and forms the *optic radiations.* The upper or dorsal fibers of the optic radiations run posteriorly in the parietal lobe and terminate in the superior part of the calcarine cortex of the occipital lobe. The lower or ventral fibers loop anteriorly and laterally around the temporal horn in the temporal lobe (Meyer's loop) before turning posteriorly to end in the inferior calcarine cortex (Fig. 31).

The primary visual (calcarine) cortex is organized into columns of cells running from the surface to the white matter. These columns function as units that respond to specific pat-

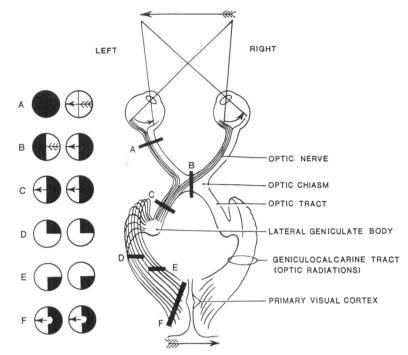

FIG. 30. Visual pathways as seen from the base of the brain. The visual impulses from the right half of the visual field project to the left half of each retina and to the left occipital lobe. On the **left** are the visual field defects *(black areas)* produced by lesions affecting the optic nerve **(A)**, optic chiasm **(B)**, optic tract **(C)**, optic radiation in temporal lobe **(D)**, optic radiation in parietal lobe **(E)**, or occipital cortex **(F)**.

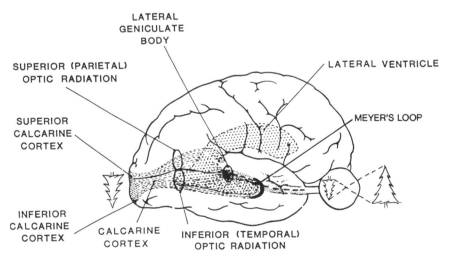

FIG. 31. The course of the superior and inferior optic radiations. Fibers from the upper part of the retina (which receive impulses from the inferior visual field) form the superior optic radiations (located in the parietal lobe) and terminate in the superior calcarine cortex. Fibers from the inferior half of the retina (which receive impulses from the superior visual field) form the inferior optic radiations (located in the temporal lobe) and terminate in the inferior calcarine cortex.

terns of visual stimuli, such as moving lines or bars. Each column is activated by a particular pattern or array of cells in the lateral geniculate body, which in turn is activated by retinal ganglion cells.

The visual images impinging on the retina are inverted so that the superior part of the visual field projects to the inferior part of the retina and the inferior visual field projects to the superior part of the retina. Fibers from the upper part of the retina form the superior part of the optic radiations, which run in the parietal lobe and terminate in the superior calcarine cortex. Fibers from the lower part of the retina form the inferior optic radiations, which run in the temporal lobe to terminate in the inferior calcarine cortex (Fig. 31).

The calcarine cortex thus has a topographic organization such that the superior part of the visual field terminates in the inferior calcarine cortex and the inferior visual field terminates in the superior calcarine cortex (Figs. 31 and 32). In addition, the posterior portion of the occipital pole is primarily concerned with macular (central) vision, and the more anterior parts of the visual cortex are concerned with peripheral vision. The final processing of the visual image occurs in the primary and visual association areas of the cerebral cortex (Fig. 32).

The primary visual cortex (area 17) is located in the walls of the calcarine fissure. The visual association areas (areas 18 and 19) are lateral to the primary visual area and are called the peristriate cortex. The peristriate cortex has two outflow pathways: a dorsal outflow pathway directed to the posterior parietal lobe is predominantly involved in visual spatial processing, and a ventral outflow pathway directed to the inferior temporal visual association areas is involved in the discrimination and identification of colors and visual-limbic interactions (Table 12).

The visual association areas synthesize visual impressions, integrate visual impressions with other sensory modalities, and help form visual memory traces. The visual association areas are also responsible for eye movements induced by visual stimuli.

The different modalities within the visual system remain separated in the primary visual cortex. Axons from the parvicellular and magnicellular regions of the lateral geniculate nucleus terminate in different sublayers of layer IV of primary visual area. (Layer IV is especially prominent in primary visual cortex.) Each sublayer projects to separate sectors in the immediate visual association cortex. From there, the flow of visual information follows two different streams in the cerebral cortex. The M pathway follows a dorsal stream through the medial temporal and medial superior temporal cortex to reach the posterior parietal cortex. This motion pathway is used to

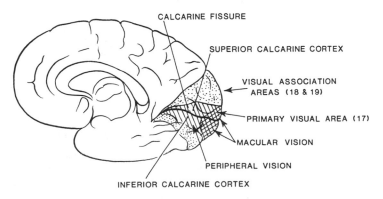

CALCARINE FISSURE
SUPERIOR CALCARINE CORTEX
VISUAL ASSOCIATION AREAS (18 & 19)
PRIMARY VISUAL AREA (17)
MACULAR VISION
PERIPHERAL VISION
INFERIOR CALCARINE CORTEX

FIG. 32. Medial aspect of the occipital lobe showing the superior and inferior calcarine cortices separated by the calcarine fissure, the location of the primary visual area *(17)*, and the visual association areas *(18* and *19)*.

TABLE 12. *Processing of visual information*

System	Magnicellular (M) "dorsal stream"	Parvicellular (P) "ventral stream"
Function	Perception of motion and localization in space	Perception of shape and color
Retinal ganglion cells	Extramacular M cells	Macular P cells
Lateral geniculate cells	Magnicellular	Parvicellular
Other input	Superior colliculus	
	Pulvinar	
Primary visual cortex	Calcarine cortex (area 17)	Calcarine cortex (area 17)
Association areas	Medial temporal	Inferior temporal
	Medial superior temporal	
	Posterior parietal cortex (area 7)	Anterior inferior temporal cortex
Connection	Dorsolateral prefrontal cortex	Ventrolateral prefrontal cortex
	Frontal eye fields	Medial temporal lobe
Effect	Visual guidance of eye and hand movement	Object recognition
Effect of lesion	Simultanagnosia	Visual agnosia
	Ocular apraxia	Achromatopsia
	Optic ataxia (Balint's syndrome)	Alexia

localize objects in space, direct visual attention, and guide reaching movements. Lesions involving the dorsal stream or posterior parietal cortex affect motion detection (*akinetopsia*) and perception of different components of the image as a whole (*simultanagnosia*) and result in the inability to direct gaze in response to visual stimuli (*ocular apraxia*) and impairment of visually guided reaching and grasping movements (*optic ataxia*).

The P pathway goes ventrally along the inferior temporal gyrus. Along this pathway, analysis of form and color becomes increasingly more complex and involves neurons that increasingly respond more selectively to a particular combination of features (for example, faces). Lesions involving this ventral stream may be manifested as the inability to recognize colors (*achromatopsia*), objects as a whole (*visual agnosia*), words presented visually (*alexia*), or faces or objects of a particular category (*prosopagnosia*).

The *frontal eye fields* are responsible for voluntary control of conjugate gaze. One such center is located in the posterior portion of the middle frontal gyrus (area 8 [see Fig. 11]) of each frontal lobe, immediately rostral to the precentral gyrus. Stimulation of this center causes the eyes to move conjugately to the opposite side; that is, if the right frontal field is stimulated, the eyes turn to the left. If one center is acutely destroyed, the unbalanced activity of the other center causes the eyes to deviate to the side of the lesion; that is, if the right side is destroyed, the eyes deviate to the right.

The *parieto-occipital centers* are responsible for involuntary visual pursuit. These centers are located in each hemisphere in the visual association area (area 19 [see Fig. 11]) at the parieto-occipital junction. Stimulation of this area causes contralateral deviation of the eyes in a similar fashion to that outlined for the frontal fields. The involuntary visual pursuit center is responsible for fixing the eyes on an object in the visual field and maintaining that visual fixation as the object moves through the visual field. Because of the action of this center, the eyes of a person casually looking out the window of a moving car will automatically fix on some point in the environment and follow the object involuntarily until it approaches the limits of the person's visual fields. Then visual fixation is broken, and the eyes make a quick conjugate movement in the opposite direction to fix on a new point of interest. Such involuntary visual pursuit of a moving target is the basis for the optokinetic nystagmus produced by a rotating drum containing dark bands alternating with white bands (optokinetic nystagmus is the nystagmus produced by looking at a moving object).

Voluntary movement of the eyes to a point of interest in the visual fields occurs via the frontal eye centers. The parieto-occipital centers help keep the eyes fixed on an object after it has been located.

Clinical Correlations

Disorders of the visual system produce specific, readily identifiable visual defects that depend on the part of the visual system damaged. Knowledge of these defects permits precise localization of many lesions involving the visual system. Damage may occur at any site along the visual pathways and will be considered in terms of the observed differences between lesions at each site.

Eye Disease

Most visual system disorders are due to abnormalities in the nonneural structures of the eye and are seen as abnormalities in visual acuity due to inability to focus visual images properly. Common examples are nearsightedness or farsightedness; distortion of light rays by diseases of the cornea or lens, such as a cataract; and glaucoma, in which there is increased pressure within the eye. Each of these causes monocular visual loss (unless both eyes are involved) and can be identified by tests of visual acuity and direct inspection of the eye.

Retinal Disease

Disorders of the retina also cause monocular visual loss, often with reduced visual acuity. Retinal detachment and retinal degeneration are associated with progressive loss of vision. A focal lesion of the retina causes a *scotoma,* or blind spot. Vascular diseases involving the retina are also reflected in visible changes in the retinal arteries with arteriosclerosis, small emboli, or hemorrhages. *Amaurosis fugax* is a transient loss of vision in one eye due to reduced blood supply (see Chapter 11). In elderly persons, it is most often the result of atherosclerotic disease in the ipsilateral internal carotid artery.

Optic Nerve

Focal lesions may involve a single optic nerve to produce a *negative scotoma,* in which part of the visual world is missing. Some dis-

orders of the optic nerve head may be seen with the ophthalmoscope. *Optic atrophy* is seen as a pale disk and occurs with degenerative diseases of the retina or nerve. *Optic neuritis* is an inflammation of the optic nerve and may be associated with blurring of the disk margin and decreased visual acuity. *Papilledema,* a sign of increased intracranial pressure, is seen as swelling and elevation of the disk, with blurring of the disk margin (see Chapter 6).

Optic Chiasm

Lesions of the optic chiasm cause several kinds of defects. Most commonly, the crossing fibers from the nasal portions of the retina are involved, with consequent loss of the two temporal fields of vision (bitemporal hemianopia) (see Fig. 30). Rarely, both lateral angles of the chiasm are compressed; in such cases, the nondecussating fibers from the temporal retinas are affected, and the result is loss of the nasal visual fields (binasal hemianopia).

Optic Tract and Optic Radiations

Lesions affecting the optic tract, the lateral geniculate body, or optic radiations on one side produce homonymous defects in the opposite visual field (see Fig. 30). For example, a lesion affecting the optic tract or radiations on the right side results in a homonymous field defect in the left visual field of both eyes. Complete destruction of the optic tract or radiation on one side produces a complete *homonymous hemianopia,* that is, complete loss of vision in the opposite half of the visual field of each eye. A lesion in the temporal lobe on one side destroys the fibers running in the lower portion of the optic radiation and results in a *superior quadrantic field defect,* that is, loss of vision in the superior portion of the visual fields of the opposite side. A lesion in the parietal lobe destroys the superior optic radiations and results in an *inferior quadrantic field defect,* that is, loss of vision in the inferior visual fields of the opposite side.

Axons mediating the pupillary light reflexes and other visual reflexes leave the optic tract at or before the lateral geniculate to terminate in the pretectal area. Therefore, optic radiation lesions differ from optic tract lesions in that the pupillary light reflex is preserved in the former.

Occipital Lobe

Lesions affecting the visual cortex in the occipital lobe on one side also cause homonymous loss of vision in the contralateral visual field (see Fig. 30). Because the visual fibers are topographically ordered in the occipital lobe, lesions here cause congruent visual field defects, that is, exactly the same loss in the fields of the two eyes. Bilateral destruction of the occipital lobes produces a form of blindness in which the visual loss is often denied. Disorders of occipital cortex can be associated with subjective transient anomalies of vision such as scintillating scotomata, visual hallucinations, and illusions. *Scintillating scotomata* are sensations of flashing lights in a field of vision. This condition commonly accompanies migraine headache. *Visual hallucinations* are perceptions of visual images for which there is no external stimulus. These may be unformed in nature and consist of flashing or twinkling lights or they may be formed visual hallucinations in which an actual scene or picture is visualized. Such hallucinations may occur as part of a seizure involving the posterior temporal lobes or as an imagined phenomenon in psychotic states. *Visual illusions* are distorted perceptions of external visual stimuli; they include macropsia (objects appear larger than normal), micropsia (objects appear smaller), achromatopsia (objects lack color), and erythropsia (objects appear to have a red tinge).

Neurologic Examination   ■

Assessment of functions specific to the supratentorial level includes tests of cranial nerves I and II; evaluation of intellectual function, particularly memory and language; and tests of cortical motor and sensory functions. In addition, the distribution of findings with involvement of longitudinal systems can aid in the localization of supratentorial damage. For example, the presence of weakness in the face, arm, and leg on one side is evidence of a unilateral cerebral lesion.

Cranial Nerve I (Olfactory)

Olfaction is tested by having the patient sniff a substance that has an odor (camphor, coffee, wintergreen) with each nostril separately while the other nostril is held closed. Because it is not possible to quantitate this sensation, the appreciation of the odor is sufficient to exclude anosmia. Intranasal disease is a common cause of impaired olfactory sensation and must be excluded before a diagnosis of neurogenic anosmia is made.

Cranial Nerve II (Optic)

Visual system testing requires attention to four aspects of visual function: the appearance of the nonneural components of the eye, visual acuity, visual field, and ophthalmoscopic examination of the optic fundus. The nonneural structures are examined by direct inspection of the external appearance and by visualization of internal features, such as the lens, with the ophthalmoscope. Tests of the extraocular muscles are described in Chapter 15.

Visual Acuity

The resolving power of vision depends on the ability of the retina to distinguish a separation between two images, and it is measured as acuity. Visual acuity is tested separately in each eye for near and distant vision. A patient who wears glasses should be tested with and without the glasses. Eye charts (Snellen's chart) are available that are read at fixed distances. The smallest size of print the patient can read is compared with what a person with normal vision can read at the same distance, and acuity is reported as a comparison of these numbers. For example, visual acuity of 20/200 means that the patient can read at 20 feet what a person with normal vision can read at 200 feet. With major visual loss, acuity can be tested with large objects such as fingers or hands.

Visual Field

Localized loss of vision in one area of the field of vision is tested by confrontation in which the examiner faces the patient and compares his or her visual field with the patient's. Each eye is tested separately by having the patient look straight ahead at the examiner's nose while a target (usually a finger) is moved in the field of vision. Two methods of testing can be used. In one, a finger is wiggled and gradually brought in from the periphery in all four quadrants of the visual field to determine where it is first seen. In the second, one to four fingers are briefly extended in each of the four quadrants, and the patient is asked to identify the number of fingers shown. With uncooperative patients or those who cannot respond directly, the field can be tested grossly by swiftly moving the hand toward the eye from one direction and looking for defensive blinking. Very precise plots of the visual field can be obtained with a perimeter or tangent screen.

Funduscopic Examination

Both optic fundi should routinely be examined with an ophthalmoscope as part of a neurologic examination. The optic disk, blood vessels, and retina should be examined. The disk should be examined for variation from its usual yellow color and for flat appearance with distinct margins. In papilledema, the margins are blurred and elevated; in optic atrophy, the disk is pale. The arteriolar caliber and appearance and the venous pulsation should be examined. Areas of exudates, hemorrhage, and abnormal pigmentation may be seen in the retina.

Visual Evoked Potentials

A low-amplitude, surface-positive electrical potential can be recorded over the occipital areas in response to a visual stimulus. The best stimulus for eliciting a consistent visual evoked response is a black and white checkerboard pattern with rapid reversal of the black and white checks. With amplification and computer averaging of a hundred or more successive responses, the evoked response is clearly distinguished from random background electroencephalographic activity (Fig. 33). The major surface-positive potential occurs approximately 100 milliseconds after the stimulus. A latency of the response prolonged beyond the upper limit of normal is suggestive of delayed conduction in the visual pathway of that eye.

Cortical Functions

The specific functions mediated by the cerebral cortex are tested as a group in the *mental status examination*. The mental status examination is an essential component of the neurologic examination and includes assessment of the level of consciousness, cognitive functions, cortical motor and sensory functions, and language.

Level of Consciousness

Evaluation of the level of consciousness is performed by testing the patient's awareness of (or response to) the external environment, by stimulating him or her with verbal, visual, tactile, and painful stimuli. The responses allow the patient to be characterized as alert, confused, somnolent, stuporous, or comatose (see Chapter 10). As part of the assessment of the level of consciousness, the patient's orientation and affect also should be noted. Does the patient know who he or she is, where he or she is, and what the date is? Is his or her emotional state one of anger, hostility, fear, suspicion, or depression?

Cognitive Functions

The patient's intellectual functions are tested with a series of specific tests, most of

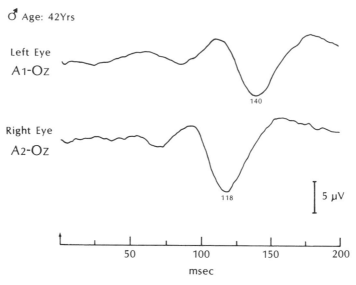

FIG. 33. Visual evoked responses to television pattern reversal stimuli in a 42-year-old man with multiple sclerosis. Stimulation of the left eye **(top segment)** shows an abnormal peak-positive response of 140 milliseconds due to demyelination of the left optic nerve. Stimulation of the right eye **(bottom segment)** shows a normal response of 118 milliseconds. Responses represent an average of 128 responses. (Recording electrodes: *A1*, left ear; *A2*, right ear; *Oz*, midline occipital.)

which depend on diffuse cortical processes. The tests can be helpful in determining the extent of dementia or retardation or in distinguishing organic intellectual impairment from psychiatric diseases. The evaluation should include memory, fund of knowledge, calculation, ability to think abstractly, and judgment. *Memory function* should be tested in the three memory modes of short-term, recent, and long-term memory. Short-term memory is tested by having the patient repeat a sequence of digits of increasing length and recall the names of items after 5 minutes. Normal subjects can readily repeat up to six digits immediately and can recall the names of three cities or objects after 5 minutes. Recent memory is tested by having the patient recall events of the past few days, such as where he or she has been, whom he or she has seen, or what he or she has eaten. Long-term memory is tested by asking about events, such as date of birth and marriage, or overlearned material, such as the alphabet or names of the months.

The *general fund of information* should be tested in the light of the patient's intellectual level, cultural background, and geographic origin. Inquiry can be made into knowledge of the presidents, other public figures, dates of major events such as world wars, or knowledge of geographic features such as rivers, lakes, and distances. Ability to *calculate* is usually tested by serial 7's, in which the patient is asked to subtract 7 from 100 and then from each subsequent answer. For some patients, simpler tasks such as simple addition or serial 3's may be more appropriate for their level of education. The *ability to abstract* is tested by determining the patient's ability to detect similarities such as those between gold and silver or a book and a newspaper. It also may be tested by asking for an interpretation of a well-known proverb such as "People who live in glass houses shouldn't throw stones." A patient's *judgment* is tested by asking such questions as "Why are laws needed?" or "What would you do if there were a fire in a theater?"

Cortical Sensory Function

The general tests for agnosias include assessment of stereognosis, graphesthesia, two-point discrimination, tactile localization, and visual or auditory agnosia. These tests might include tests of ability to recognize visual objects, to identify sounds, to recognize parts of the body, or to know right from left. The last may be tested with commands such as "Show me your thumb" or "Touch your left ear with your right thumb."

Cortical Motor Function

The general tests of motor function have been described in Chapter 8, but additional special tests may be needed if disease in the frontal association areas and a resultant apraxia are suspected, particularly if the results of standard tests of strength and coordination are normal. The patient's motor activities during the entire examination should be observed, and comparisons should be made between facility in performing automatic acts and facility in performing voluntary acts. In addition, asking the patient to demonstrate how to drink a cup of water or light a match may reveal apraxia that is not apparent on routine testing.

Language

The four modalities of central language processing are listening, speaking, reading, and writing. Each should be tested in a patient if a language disorder is suspected. Listening is evaluated by judging a patient's ability to recognize and respond appropriately to verbal input. The patient may be asked to perform acts, point to objects, move part of the body, and so forth. If there is a defect of speaking, the patient should be asked to respond in ways other than with language. Speaking is evaluated through conducting an ordinary conversation, but it also may be specifically tested by having the patient repeat certain phrases or name objects.

Reading should be evaluated by having the patient either read a paragraph silently and explain what was in the paragraph or, if speech is significantly impaired, to ask the patient to point to words and sentences on the printed page spoken by the examiner. Writing can be tested by having the patient write something from dictation or copy a written message.

Additional Tests of Cortical Function

Additional tests of cortical function include neuropsychologic testing, electroencephalography, and functional imaging studies. *Neuropsychologic* assessment involves psychometric testing of cortical function with procedures that have a standardized administration and normative references. In general, neuropsychologic testing is used to detect impairment of cognitive abilities, including learning, memory, attention, language, visuospatial skills, and executive or reasoning functions. Neurocognitive testing is commonly used in evaluating such central nervous system disorders as diffuse encephalopathies, dementia, vascular disorders, stroke, epilepsy, and head injury.

The *electroencephalogram* (EEG) records the electrical activity of the cerebral cortex and can be used to detect abnormalities of cerebral function and indicate whether the disturbance is focal or generalized. The EEG is particularly helpful in evaluating patients with seizures, altered states of consciousness, and focal cortical lesions. It is described in more detail in Chapter 10.

Activity in specific brain regions in humans performing specific sensory, motor, or verbal tasks can be studied with *noninvasive imaging techniques*. These techniques include positron emission tomography (PET), single-photon emission computed tomography (SPECT), and functional magnetic resonance imaging (MRI). The principle underlying these techniques is that increased neuronal activity in a particular brain region is coupled with a local increase in cerebral blood flow, oxygen consumption, and glucose metabolism. Thus, changes in blood flow or metabolism detected with PET, SPECT, or MRI reflect activation of cortical regions during specific tasks or in pathologic conditions (Fig. 34). PET depends on the use of short-lived isotopes that contain an extra proton and label biologically relevant molecules such as carbon dioxide, oxygen, 2-deoxyglucose, or drugs that bind to specific membrane receptors. The isotopes are administered to the subject within a few minutes before performance of the task and allow measurement of blood flow (carbon dioxide), oxygen consumption (oxygen), or glucose metabolism (2-deoxyglucose). For example, motor tasks in response to visual commands increase activity in the posterior parietal cortex, cortical motor areas, basal ganglia, and contralateral cerebellum. Tasks involving language increase cerebral blood flow predominantly in the left hemisphere; hearing words produces increased activity in Wernicke's area.

Functional MRI detects changes in signal intensity in specific brain regions during performance of a task. The changes reflect either local changes in blood volume or in oxygen concentration in cerebral veins, both of which are proportional to the degree of neuronal activation and oxygen consumption.

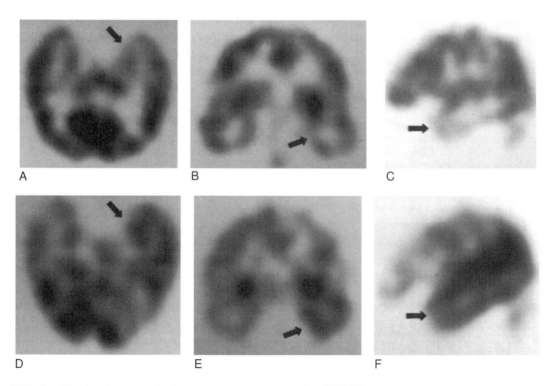

FIG. 34. Single-photon emission computed tomography (SPECT) scan in a patient with a left temporal lobe seizure. Images show the distribution of intravenously administered radioactive tracer, which reflects the regional cerebral blood flow. Because regional cerebral blood flow is directly related to the energy metabolism of cells, in turn dependent on adenosine triphosphate (ATP) consumption for maintenance of the sodium pump, SPECT as well as other functional studies is used to assess the degree of electrophysiologic activity in specific brain regions. **Top:** Interictal SPECT in horizontal **(A)**, coronal **(B)**, and sagittal **(C)** planes. Note the reduced perfusion on the **left,** as compared with the right anterior temporal lobe. **Bottom:** Ictal SPECT in horizontal **(D)**, coronal **(E)**, and sagittal **(F)** views. Note that during the seizure there is a significant increase in cerebral perfusion in the left anterior temporal lobe, indicating a focal exaggerated increase in neuronal activity in this region.

Clinical Problems ■

1. A 30-year-old woman noted the onset of amenorrhea 1 year ago. In the last 6 months, she noted that she tired easily, could not tolerate stress or cold weather, and had lost weight. Physical examination revealed a dull, apathetic, thin woman with low blood pressure, slow pulse, bitemporal hemianopia, and deep tendon reflexes with a slow relaxation phase.
   a. Where is the primary lesion?
   b. What structures are affected by the lesion?
   c. What are the two lobes of the pituitary gland?
   d. Which lobe of the pituitary gland is involved?
   e. What hormones are secreted by this lobe? What regulates the release of these hormones?
   f. Which hormones are affected in this patient?
   g. How do you explain the visual symptoms?
   h. What might you expect a radiograph to show?
   i. What structures are near the pituitary gland?
   j. What is the lesion?
2. A 10-year-old boy had become fat and listless during the last year. He also drank water and urinated excessively. For the last several months, he complained of headaches and experienced nausea and vomiting on arising in the morning. Neurologic examination revealed an obese boy with papilledema and bitemporal hemianopia.
   a. Where is the primary lesion?
   b. What regulates the release of the hormones?
   c. Which hormone is affected in this patient?
   d. What are the functions of the hypothalamic nuclei?
   e. What is the lesion?

3. A 65-year-old man had sudden onset of numbness of the right side of his face and body, and he noted difficulty in seeing in his right visual field. Neurologic examination performed 2 hours later revealed that he could not identify objects or written numbers in his right hand, or localize sensory stimuli on the right side, or distinguish right from left. Further testing revealed that he had difficulty with arithmetic calculations and writing his name.
   a. Where is the lesion?
   b. What is the lesion?
   c. What kinds of agnosia are manifested by this patient?
   d. What are the other types of agnosia, and where would the lesion be located to produce these?
   e. What type of visual field defect might be expected in this patient?
4. A 50-year-old woman had gradual onset of memory loss 3 years ago. This loss has become progressively worse, so that now she cannot remember from one minute to the next what she has been doing. She also has had difficulty in carrying out various household activities such as sewing, cooking, and washing dishes, even though she denies being weak or having trouble with coordination. Neurologic examination revealed that she could not recall numbers just presented to her, what she had had for breakfast, or even where she was born. She was unable to perform activities such as pretending to light a cigarette or showing how a key would work.
   a. Where is the lesion?
   b. What is the disease process?
   c. What types of memory functioning were affected in this patient?
   d. What is the difference between dementia and mental retardation?
   e. What is the name given to the inability to perform learned complex motor activities in the absence of weakness?
   f. Name three other types of neurologic dysfunction that signify a lesion or disease process affecting cortical structures.

5. Three years ago, a 28-year-old man had onset of transient spells lasting 1 to 2 minutes in which he experienced an unpleasant odor. Immediately after the odor, he felt as if he were in a dream state in which he saw and heard things that he had experienced before. He also was aware that he was unable to understand what other people were saying to him during these episodes. In the last year, the spells have changed somewhat, in that he now hears the sound of a bell and at the same time experiences a mental picture of a country scene from his childhood. In the last 3 months, he has been bothered by increasingly severe headaches, nausea, and vomiting. He has difficulty understanding what people are saying to him even when he is not having his spells. Neurologic examination showed bilateral blurring of the disk margins, a visual field defect, aphasia, and Babinski's reflex on the right.

   a. Where is the lesion?
   b. What is the lesion?
   c. What visual field defect would you expect this patient to show?
   d. What do the transient spells represent?
   e. What was the initial site of origin for the spells?
   f. What clues are present that show progression of the underlying process?
   g. What tests would be most helpful for this patient?
   h. What might these tests show?
   i. What type of language problem did the patient have?
   j. The olfactory structures are part of what system? Name the other structures that are associated with this system. What are the functions of this system?

6. What type of visual field defect might be expected in each of the following clinical situations?

   a. A 47-year-old woman with a large tumor protruding from the pituitary fossa and pushing the optic chiasm forward.
   b. An 81-year-old man who had an occlusive vascular event involving the right posterior cerebral artery.
   c. A 44-year-old woman with a right parietal lobe tumor.
   d. A 14-year-old boy with an abscess of the left temporal lobe after a chronic infection of the left middle ear.

Additional Reading

Alexander, G. E., and DeLong, M. R. Central mechanisms of initiation and control of movement. In Asbury, A. K., McKhann, G., and McDonald, W. I. (eds.), *Diseases of the Nervous System: Clinical Neurobiology,* vol 1 (2nd ed.). Philadelphia: W. B. Saunders, 1992, pp. 285–308.

Aronson, A. E. *Clinical Voice Disorders: An Interdisciplinary Approach* (3rd ed.). New York: Thieme, 1990.

Becker, K. L. Principles and practice of endocrinology and metabolism. In Robertson, G. L. (ed.), *The Endocrine Brain and Pituitary Gland.* Philadelphia: J. B. Lippincott, 1990, pp. 92–261.

Department of Neurology, Mayo Clinic and Mayo Foundation. *Clinical Examinations in Neurology* (7th ed.). St. Louis: Mosby, 1998.

Devinsky, O., Morrell, M. J., and Vogt, B. A. Contributions of anterior cingulate cortex to behaviour. *Brain* 118:279, 1995.

Engel, J., Jr. *Seizures and Epilepsy.* Philadelphia: F. A. Davis, 1989.

Mesulam, M.-M. *Principles of Behavioral Neurology.* Philadelphia: F. A. Davis, 1985.

Mountcastle, V. B. The columnar organization of the neocortex. *Brain* 120:701, 1997.

Warwick, R. *Eugene Wolff's Anatomy of the Eye and Orbit* (7th ed.). Philadelphia: W. B. Saunders, 1976.

Answers to Clinical Problems

Chapter 1
Integrated Neuroscience for the Clinician

Questions 1 and 2 are both "thought questions," and the "correct" answers will differ for each individual. As you review your answers ask yourself: What type of reasoning did I use to generate hypotheses? Was there any difference between the way I approached question 1 and question 2? What past experiences helped me to understand the problems? What background knowledge did I use? What additional knowledge do I need to understand this problem? Where can I obtain that knowledge?

Chapter 2
Developmental Organization of the Nervous System: Neuroembryology

1. a. Fusion of neural tube, posterior neuropore.
   b. Neural tube at 4 weeks of development.
   c. Motor, sensory, and visceral.
   d. Neural tube and somites (myotome, sclerotome, dermatome).
   e. Ependymal, mantle, and marginal.
   f. Myelomeningocele.
2. a. Tumor formation in ectodermal derivatives: skin, eye, brain.
   b. Ectoderm and diencephalon.
   c. Neuroblast and spongioblast.
   d. Special somatic afferent.
   e. Tuberous sclerosis.

Chapter 3
Diagnosis of Neurologic Disorders: Anatomical Localization

1. Supratentorial, focal-left.
2. Supratentorial, focal-left.
3. Posterior fossa, focal-left.
4. Posterior fossa, focal-right.
5. Spinal, focal-midline.
6. Peripheral, focal-right.
7. Spinal, focal-left.

Chapter 4
Diagnosis of Neurologic Disorders: Neurocytology and the Pathologic Reactions of the Nervous System

1. Supratentorial, focal-right, nonmass, vascular.
2. Supratentorial, focal-right, mass, inflammatory.
3. Supratentorial, focal-left, mass, neoplastic.
4. Multiple levels, nonfocal-diffuse, nonmass, vascular.
5. Multiple levels, nonfocal-diffuse, nonmass, inflammatory.
6. Supratentorial, nonfocal-diffuse, nonmass, degenerative.
7. Posterior fossa, focal-left, nonmass, vascular.
8. Multiple levels, nonfocal-diffuse, nonmass, degenerative.
9. Spinal, focal-right, nonmass, vascular.
10. Peripheral, focal-right, mass, neoplastic.

Chapter 5
Diagnosis of Neurologic Disorders: Transient Disorders and Neurophysiology

1. a. Ischemia or anoxia impairs production of ATP and blocks the sodium pump; extracellular potassium accumulates. A decrease in the potassium concentration gradient reduces the resting membrane potential, and this depolarization inactivates the voltage-gated sodium channels responsible for generating action potentials, making the cell inexcitable.
    b. Recovery occurs with restoration of blood flow and recovery of aerobic metabolism in neurons.
2. a. Both would be reduced, with possible block of action potential conduction.
    b. It would reduce the resting potential.
3. By slowing or blocking conduction in optic nerve axons and thus causing decreased visual acuity.
4. a. The resting potential moves closer to threshold.
    b. Increased extracellular potassium concentration.
5. a. Decreased
    b. None
    c. Decreased
    d. None
6. a. Partial depolarization due to failure of the sodium pump, increased excitatory postsynaptic potentials, or reduced inhibitory postsynaptic potentials.
    b. Prolonged neuronal depolarization leads to energy failure and depolarization block.
    c. Blockade of sodium channels, blockade of calcium channels, opening of potassium channels, opening of chloride channels, decreased excitatory transmission by L-glutamate or increased inhibitory transmission by GABA.
7. a. Equilibrium
    b. Steady state
    c. Active transport

Chapter 6
The Cerebrospinal Fluid System

1. a. By comparison with standardized tables of normal head circumference, 50 cm at 10 months is more than 2 standard deviations above the norm.
    b. An increase in the volume of any of the constituents of the skull. At this age, subdural hematomas and hydrocephalus due to several causes are common.
    c. Computed tomography and magnetic resonance imaging are safe, noninvasive procedures. This patient had aqueductal stenosis.
    d. Noncommunicating hydrocephalus.
    e. i. Enlargement of the lateral and third ventricles with obstruction at the aqueduct. The fourth ventricle would not be visualized.
       ii. Uniform dilatation of the ventricular system proximal to the blockage (of the lateral and third ventricles, aqueduct, and fourth ventricle).
      iii. Uniform dilatation of the entire ventricular system.
       iv. Usually no changes (but the cerebrospinal fluid would probably be bloody).
2. In the infant, intracranial volume can be increased by modest expansion of the sutures, which increases the head size and results in a less significant increase in intracranial pressure. In the adult, such compensation is impossible, and intracranial pressure increases.
3. a. Spinal, focal-midline, mass, neoplastic.
    b. Assuming that the lesion is at the midthoracic level, producing near complete blockage of CSF pathways, then the opening pressure in the lumbar sac would be low normal; some respiratory pulsations transmitted via the abdomen would be seen but cardiac pulsations would not; compression of abdominal contents would result in an increase in pressure transmitted to the lumbar sac below the blockage.

c. Skin, subcutaneous tissues, intraspinous ligaments, epidural space, dura mater, subdural space, and arachnoid and subarachnoid spaces.

d. Myelography. MRI of the spine.

4. a. Multiple levels, diffuse, nonmass, an unidentified inflammation.

b. An inflammatory process and a traumatic tap.

c. Possibly bacteria; growth of the offending organism.

d. In the presence of bacterial meningitis, the cerebrospinal fluid glucose level is often significantly lowered due to impaired transport.

Chapter 7
The Sensory System

1. a. Peripheral, focal-right, nonmass, traumatic or vascular.

b. The lateral femoral cutaneous nerve (refer to Fig. 14).

c. Refer to Fig. 14.

2. a. Spinal, focal-midline and bilateral, mass, neoplastic.

b. Dorsal roots or spinal nerves of the C-2 segment.

c. Structures listed in 2b and dorsal columns (fasciculus cuneatus and fasciculus gracilis) bilaterally.

d. The segmental loss at C-2 suggests that this is the level of the lesion.

e. Meningioma, neurofibroma.

f. The segmental sensory loss would be at the level of the nipples, and the dorsal column deficit would spare the upper extremities and be present in the lower extremities.

3. a. Spinal, focal-midline, mass, neoplastic.

b. The second-order axons transmitting pain and temperature impulses (bound for the spinothalamic tracts bilaterally), as they decussate in the ventral white commissure at the involved levels.

c. Syringomyelia; but the same clinical pattern could be produced by an intramedullary neoplasm at that level.

4. a. Spinal, focal-left, nonmass, traumatic.

b. T-10 (refer to Fig. 15).

c. Brown-Séquard syndrome.

d. The lesion involves only the left side of the spinal cord, affecting the spinothalamic and dorsal column tracts on that side. The sensation of touch ascends via both tracts and, thus, is maintained by the intact tracts on the right side of the cord.

e. Wallerian degeneration occurs in the distal axon when it is severed from its cell body of origin. Above the level of the lesion, the left spinothalamic tract would show degeneration up to the level of the thalamus. The left fasciculus gracilis would show degeneration only to the level of its second-order neuron—the nucleus gracilis. The left corticospinal tract would show degeneration below the lesion.

5. a. Supratentorial, focal-right, nonmass, vascular.

b. Thalamus (ventral posterolateral nucleus).

c. In the right thalamocortical radiations.

6. a. Supratentorial, focal-right, mass, neoplastic.

b. Focal sensory seizures.

c. The lesion is in the primary sensory cortex (postcentral gyrus), producing a cortical sensory loss. Crude perceptions of touch, pain, temperature, and vibration are also intergrated in other cortical areas, while discriminative sensations require processing in the parietal sensory cortex.

Chapter 8
The Motor System

1. a. Supratentorial, focal-right, mass, neoplastic.

b. Corticospinal.

c. It is higher than normal.

d. Focal clonic seizures secondary to local ionic changes in the area of the tumor.

e. No. It would be dangerous and perhaps fatal to the patient.

2. a. Multiple levels, diffuse, nonmass, degenerative.

b. Basal ganglia control, cerebellar control.

c. It is degenerative according to temporal profile, so toxic and metabolic causes must be considered. This is a case of hepatolenticular degeneration, or Wilson's disease, a genetic error in copper metabolism.

d. Basal ganglia—caudate nucleus, putamen, globus pallidus, thalamus, and cortex; cerebellum—dentate nucleus, red nucleus, thalamus, cortex, and pons.

e. Hypokinesia, hyperkinesia, athetosis, dystonia, tremor, and rigidity.

3. a. Multiple levels, diffuse, nonmass, vascular.

b. Traumatic and toxic. This is an example of carbon monoxide poisoning.

c. Corticospinal and brainstem motor pathways.

d. By damage at midbrain level with release of vestibulospinal and excitatory reticulospinal activation of lower motor neurons.

e. Type II (secondary) muscle spindle endings and muscle nociceptors.

4. a. Multiple levels, diffuse, nonmass, inflammatory.

b. Yes, typical of viral infection—in this case, poliomyelitis.

c. Final common pathway.

d. Weakness, atrophy, hypotonia, hyporeflexia, and fasciculations.

e. Sensory from peripheral afferents, corticospinal, vestibulospinal, reticulospinal, rubrospinal, tectospinal, and input from other cord levels.

5. a. Supratentorial, left, nonmass, vascular.

b. Corticospinal and corticobulbar, precentral gyrus inferiorly on the left, including Broca's area.

c. Babinski's sign present, abdominal reflexes absent.

d. Speech apraxia and aphasia.

e. Lower motor neurons to upper facial muscles receive bilateral cortical innervation.

6. a. Posterior fossa, right, mass, inflammatory.

b. Cerebrospinal fluid pressure might be increased, and cerebellar tonsil herniation might occur.

c. Cerebellar control circuit.

d. Superior cerebellar peduncle in the midbrain, pontocerebellar fibers entering the middle cerebellar peduncle, olivocerebellar fibers entering the inferior cerebellar peduncle.

e. Flocculonodular lobe (vestibulocerebellum) is involved in equilibrium and oculomotor control; the anterior lobe and vermis (spinocerebellum) control posture and gait; the posterior lobe (hemisphere, pontocerebellum) controls skilled movements of the limbs.

Chapter 9
The Internal Regulation System

1. a. Multiple levels, diffuse.

b. Nonmass, degenerative.

c. Orthostatic hypotension, lack of sweating.

d. It would produce sweating.

e. All four.

2. a. Spinal, focal-midline.

b. Mass, neoplastic.

c. Nonreflex, autonomic neurogenic bladder dysfunction (flaccid bladder).

d. Impotence.

3. a. Peripheral, focal-left.

b. Mass, neoplastic.

c. Superior cervical ganglion or sympathetic trunk.

d. Sympathetic.

e. Hypothalamus, midbrain, pons, medulla, cervical cord, T-1 spinal nerve, sympathetic trunk, carotid plexus.

f. Postganglionic or ganglionic lesion.

g. Preganglionic lesion.

4. a. Peripheral, diffuse.

b. Nonmass, other (toxic).

c. Parasympathetic.

d. Mushroom poisoning (muscarine).

e. It would enlarge the pupils.

f. i., ii., iii., iv., altered by fear; iv., by blushing; v., by crying.

5. a. Supratentorial, focal-midline.

b. Mass, neoplastic.

c. Hypothalamus and optic chiasm.

d. Neurosecretory systems, nutrient homeostasis systems, and possibly osmoreceptors and temperature receptors.

e. Blocking of regulatory hormones that control the pituitary gland, and optic chiasm compression, producing visual loss.

Chapter 10
The Consciousness System

1. a. Multiple levels (supratentorial and posterior fossa), nonfocal and diffuse, nonmass, metabolic.

   b. Widespread areas of cerebral cortex and portions of the ascending reticular activating system in the cerebral hemispheres, thalamus, and brainstem.

   c. Hypoglycemia.

   d. Diffuse slow-wave abnormality.

2. a. Supratentorial, focal-right, mass, vascular.

   b. Intracerebral hemorrhage.

   c. Although unilateral cerebral lesions do not ordinarily cause a loss of consciousness, a mass lesion (as present in this case) may compress diencephalic structures bilaterally or produce herniation of the supratentorial structures (or do both) with secondary involvement of diencephalic and brainstem structures bilaterally.

   d. In addition to the focal slow-wave abnormality present over the right cerebral hemisphere, a more diffuse slow-wave disturbance may be seen.

3. a. Supratentorial, nonfocal-diffuse, indeterminate. The only abnormalities present were transient symptoms. As noted in Chapter 5, transient symptoms alone may be associated with various disorders and do not allow a pathologic diagnosis to be established.

   b. Generalized epileptiform abnormalities occurring in repetitive and rhythmic fashion.

   c. Inflammatory (encephalitis), vascular, neoplastic, degenerative, toxic-metabolic, traumatic.

d. The presence of focal seizures would increase the likelihood of an underlying structural lesion involving one cerebral hemisphere. In a patient of this age, a neoplasm should be suspected.

Chapter 11
The Vascular System

1. a. Supratentorial, focal-right, nonmass, vascular.

   b. Vertebrobasilar system. The complete loss of vision suggests involvement of both posterior cerebral arteries; with resolution, only the distribution of the right posterior cerebral artery was involved.

   c. Infarction (right occipital lobe).

   d. Embolization from the heart.

   e. Decrease in PaO_2, increase in $PaCO_2$, increase in lactic acid, decrease in pH.

2. a. Supratentorial, focal-right, nonmass, vascular.

   b. Right carotid system–middle cerebral artery distribution.

   c. Infarction.

   d. May be related to extracranial carotid artery disease: thrombosis or embolization.

   e. True.

3. a. Supratentorial, focal-left, mass, vascular initially. (The loss of consciousness and bilateral Babinski's signs suggest secondary bilateral involvement at supratentorial or posterior fossa levels.)

   b. Intracerebral hemorrhage (with secondary early herniation).

   c. Hypertension, rupture of a vascular anomaly (arteriovenous malformation), trauma.

   d. Focal signs, headache, alteration in consciousness.

   e. Magnetic resonance imaging.

4. a. Posterior fossa, focal-left, nonmass, vascular.

   b. Vertebrobasilar system, left posterior inferior cerebellar artery distribution.

   c. Infarction (in the left lateral medulla).

d. Mechanism indeterminate; many patients have thrombotic occlusion of the vertebral artery.

e. Vertigo—vestibular nucleus involvement; dysarthria, dysphagia, and left palatal weakness—left cranial nerves IX and X; loss of pain sensibility over left face—left descending tract and nucleus of cranial nerve V; loss of pain sensibility of the right limbs and trunk—left spinothalamic tract; left Horner's syndrome—left descending sympathetic fibers.

5. a. Multiple levels, diffuse, nonmass, vascular. There are no focal abnormalities. The loss of consciousness suggests diffuse involvement of supratentorial and posterior fossa levels. Full recovery suggests no pathologic change in the central nervous system.

b. Diffuse ischemia (syncope)—secondary to decreased cardiac output.

c. The ability of an organ to maintain a constant blood supply in spite of variations in blood pressure. This regulation applies for all but the widest extremes in pressure.

d. Only inhalation of carbon dioxide.

e. Transient ischemic attacks are episodes of focal neurologic dysfunction; syncope is diffuse ischemia.

6. a. Multiple levels (supratentorial, posterior fossa, and spinal), diffuse, nonmass, vascular. The diffuse involvement, meningeal signs, and bloody cerebrospinal fluid suggest subarachnoid hemorrhage.

b. At this age, rupture of an intracranial aneurysm is suspected.

c. Immediate centrifugation of the specimen. The presence of a xanthochromic supernatant would suggest that it was not a traumatic puncture.

Chapter 12
The Neurochemical Systems

1. a. Diffuse.

b. Nonmass, metabolic (hypoxia, global ischemia).

c. Excitatory amino acid (glutamate).

d. Excitotoxicity, mediated by calcium-triggered cascades: phospholipases, proteases, nitric oxide.

e. Layers III to V of cerebral cortex, hippocampus, cerebellum, striatum. These areas have selective vulnerability to hypoxic injury.

f. Blockade of excitatory amino acid receptors and calcium ion channels.

2. a. Supratentorial.

b. Nonmass, toxic-metabolic.

c. GABA.

d. Withdrawal of GABA inhibition in setting of downregulation of receptors due to chronic exposure.

3. a. Supratentorial

b. Nonmass, degenerative, toxic-metabolic.

c. Acetylcholine.

d. Decreased memory and learning due to blockade of cortical muscarinic cholinergic receptors.

4. a. Supratentorial.

b. Nonmass, toxic-metabolic.

c. Dopamine.

d. Parkinson-like features due to blockade of dopaminergic receptors in the striatum.

e. Chorea-like features, called tardive dyskinesia, due to supersensitivity of striatal dopaminergic receptors caused by chronic pharmacologic blockade by the antipsychotic drug.

f. Neuroleptic malignant syndrome, with hyperthermia, rigidity, and autonomic hyperactivity, due to dopaminergic blockade in the hypothalamus and basal ganglia.

5. a. Multiple levels, diffuse.

b. Toxic-metabolic.

c. Opioids.

d. An opioid antagonist (naloxone).

Chapter 13
The Peripheral Level

1. a. Peripheral (motor, sensory, and visceral), diffuse, nonmass, degenerative (metabolic).

b. Peripheral neuropathy.

c. They indicate loss of nerve or muscle fibers.

d. It indicates loss of innervation of muscle fibers.

e. Fibrillation is repetitive, rhythmic discharge of single muscle fiber. Fasciculation is single, spontaneous discharge of a motor unit.

f. Loss of pinprick and temperature sensation, orthostatic hypotension, dry skin.

g. Normal

2. a. Peripheral (motor and sensory), diffuse, nonmass, inflammatory.

b. Large myelinated, sensory and motor.

c. Demyelination.

d. Segmental demyelination.

e. Remyelination.

3. a. Size of quanta and number of quanta.

b. Number of quanta released.

c. 11.

d. End-plate potential below action potential threshold; no muscle fiber contraction.

e. Lambert-Eaton myasthenic syndrome associated with carcinoma of the lung.

4. a. Myositis.

b. Peripheral, diffuse, nonmass, inflammatory.

c. Muscle and nerve.

d. Increased rate of firing, recruitment of more motor units.

e. By making them of lower amplitude and shorter duration.

f. Inflammatory cells, fiber degeneration, central nuclei.

g. No.

h. Neurogenic atrophy.

i. As a result of collateral sprouting of intact axons.

j. They all mediate excitation-contraction coupling.

k. Because of leakage of enzyme from damaged muscle fibers.

Chapter 14
The Spinal Level

1. a. Spinal, midline, nonmass, vascular.

b. L-1 to L-3, all of spinal cord except dorsal columns.

c. No.

d. Reflex (spastic) bladder and nonreflex (flaccid) bladder, respectively.

e. Anterior spinal artery occlusion.

2. a. Spinal, midline, mass, neoplastic.

b. Motor: final common pathway, direct and indirect activation pathways. Sensory: spinothalamic.

c. C-4 to T-1: central gray matter affecting commissural fibers, ventral horn cells, and corticospinal tracts.

d. Spinal cord mass—tumor or syrinx (possible syringomyelia).

3. a. Multiple levels, diffuse, nonmass, degenerative.

b. Dorsal columns.

c. Peripheral and spinal cord involvement.

d. Biochemical (vitamin B_{12} deficiency in this patient).

4. a. Spinal, right, mass, traumatic.

b. Right L-5 spinal nerve.

c. Peroneal nerve, sciatic nerve, sacral plexus, L-5 spinal nerve, L-5 ventral roots, lumbar spinal cord, and paracentral lobule.

d. Traction on sacral spinal nerves.

Chapter 15
The Posterior Fossa Level

1. a. Posterior fossa, left, nonmass, vascular.

b. Left lateral medulla.

c. Left posterior inferior cerebellar artery—a branch of the left vertebral artery (which is often the site of occlusion in this syndrome).

d. The left descending tract of cranial nerve V, the left spinothalamic tract.

e. Involvement of the descending sympathetic pathways en route to the spinal cord (producing Horner's syndrome).

2. a. Posterior fossa, right, mass, neoplastic.

b. Cranial nerves IX, X, and XI on the right.

c. Jugular foramen.

d. Jugular vein.

e. Chemodectoma.

3. a. Posterior fossa, left, nonmass, vascular.

   b. Left medullary pyramid (weakness), left medial lemniscus (decreased proprioception), left hypoglossal nerve (tongue weakness).

   c. Infarction of left medial medulla in the paramedian zone.

4. a. Posterior fossa, left, nonmass, vascular.

   b. Special visceral afferent fibers of the facial nerve supply taste to the anterior two-thirds of the tongue.

   c. General visceral efferent fibers of the facial nerve supply the lacrimal gland.

   d. Bell's palsy.

5. a. Posterior fossa, right, mass, neoplastic.

   b. Auditory division of cranial nerve VIII (decreased hearing, tinnitus), vestibular division of cranial nerve VIII (absent caloric response, dysequilibrium), facial nerve (weakness of muscles of facial expression), cerebellar control circuit (decreased coordination).

   c. Cerebellopontine angle.

   d. Acoustic neuroma.

   e. Skull radiograph and petrous tomograms (enlargement of the internal auditory meatus), computed tomography, magnetic resonance imaging.

6. a. Posterior fossa, left, nonmass, vascular.

   b. Cranial nerve VI (lateral rectus weakness), cranial nerve VII (facial weakness), medial lemniscus (loss of joint position and vibratory sense), descending (direct and indirect activation) motor pathways (hemiparesis).

   c. Infarction, left paramedian region of the pons.

7. a. Posterior fossa, right, nonmass, vascular.

   b. Cranial nerve III on right (diplopia, ptosis, mydriasis), right cerebral peduncle (left hemiparesis).

c. Right medial and superior rectus muscles.

d. The efferent limb of the pupillary light reflex travels via general visceral efferent fibers contained in cranial nerve III.

e. Infarction, right paramedian region of the mesencephalon.

8. a. Posterior fossa, left, mass, neoplasm.

   b. The left cerebellar hemisphere (ataxia).

   c. Headache, nausea, vomiting, papilledema.

   d. Cerebellar astrocytoma. (These tumors are often cystic and have a good prognosis.)

9. a. Multiple levels, diffuse, nonmass, degenerative.

   b. Motor system only, at the posterior fossa and spinal levels.

   c. Final common pathway (weakness, fasciculations), direct activation pathways (bilateral Babinski's signs).

   d. Motor neuron disease (amyotrophic lateral sclerosis).

10. a. Supratentorial, left, mass, inflammatory (abscess).

    b. Secondary involvement of the consciousness system by the expanding mass lesion causing herniation.

    c. Compression of cranial nerve III on the left by an expanding temporal lobe mass.

    d. With increasing herniation, there is also secondary compression of the cerebral peduncle.

    e. Uncal herniation.

    f. Mesencephalon, below the red nucleus.

    g. Decerebrate posturing.

    h. Transtentorial or central herniation.

Chapter 16
The Supratentorial Level

1. a. Supratentorial, midline (region of pituitary gland).

   b. Pituitary gland and optic chiasm.

   c. Anterior lobe and posterior lobe.

d. Anterior lobe.

e. TSH, GH, ACTH, gonadotropins (FSH, LH), and prolactin; regulatory hormones from the hypothalamus, which descend to the anterior lobe via a portal circulation.

f. TSH, ACTH, and gonadotropin.

g. Compression of the optic chiasm by the lesion.

h. Enlarged sella.

i. Optic chiasm; internal carotid artery; cavernous sinus with cranial nerves III, IV, V, and VI.

j. Mass, neoplastic (chromophobe adenoma).

2. a. Supratentorial, midline (in the region of the hypothalamus).

b. Hypothalamus via nerve fibers.

c. Vasopressin.

d. Regulation of visceral functions, regulation of releasing factors for the anterior pituitary lobe, regulation of water metabolism, regulation of food intake, regulation of body temperature, regulation of sleep, reproduction, and emotion.

e. Mass, neoplastic (craniopharyngioma).

3. a. Supratentorial, left (left parietal cortex).

b. Nonmass, vascular (infarct).

c. Astereognosia, graphesthesia, atopognosia, right-left disorientation.

d. Visual agnosia, occipital lobe. Auditory agnosia, temporal lobe.

e. A right inferior homonymous quadrantanopia.

4. a. Supratentorial, diffuse (cerebral cortex).

b. Nonmass, degenerative (Alzheimer's disease).

c. Short-term, recent, and long-term memory.

d. Mental retardation is the failure to develop normal intelligence; dementia is the loss of cognitive processes after these have developed.

e. Apraxia.

f. Seizures, aphasia, agnosia.

5. a. Supratentorial, left (left temporal lobe).

b. Mass, neoplastic (glioma).

c. Right superior homonymous quadrantanopia.

d. Complex partial seizures arising from the temporal lobe.

e. Uncus.

f. Change in the seizures with involvement of more posterior portions of the temporal lobe, the development of aphasia, increasingly severe headaches, and nausea and vomiting.

g. EEG, magnetic resonance imaging, computed tomographic scan, and arteriogram.

h. EEG: focal showing and spike discharges over the left temporal region. Magnetic resonance imaging and computed tomographic scan: mass lesion, left temporal lobe. Arteriogram: mass lesion, left temporal lobe.

i. Receptive aphasia.

j. Limbic system. Anatomical structures: telencephalic structures—hippocampus, amygdala, part of the cingulate gyrus, basal forebrain, septal region, fornix; diencephalic structures—hypothalamus and anterior, dorsomedial, midline thalamic nuclei. Functions: learning, memory, emotion, affective behavior, control of autonomic function and homeostasis, cortical arousal, motivated behavior, olfaction.

6. a. Bitemporal hemianopia.

b. Left homonymous hemianopia with macular sparing.

c. Left inferior homonymous quadrantanopia.

d. Right superior homonymous quadrantanopia.

Subject Index

Page numbers in *italics* indicate figures. Page numbers followed by "t" indicate tables.

A

Abarognosia, 566
Abdomen, spinal nerve distribution to, 430*t*
Abdominal reflex, 243
Abducens nerve, 45, 487
Abnormal movements, examination of, 244
Abscess formation, 82
Acalculia, 577
Accessory nerve, spinal, 475–476
  anatomical relationship, function of, 45
Acetyl coenzyme A, 400
Acetylcholine, 111, 194–195, 199, 354–355, 360–363, 375, 399–400
  anatomical distribution, 361, *362*
  biochemistry, 360–361, 361*t*
  functions, 363
  inactivation of, 271
  internal regulation, 266
  receptor mechanisms, 361–363
  sudomotor axon reflex test, 285
Achromatopsia, 577, 590
Acoustic division, auditory nerve, 483–484
Acoustic meatus, internal, associated structures, 35*t*
Acquired immunodeficiency syndrome
  bacterial meningitis with, 141
  pathologic reactions in, 82
Action potential, 89, 103–115, *110,* 111–112, *113*
  components of, 104

conductance changes during, *104*
consciousness, 299, *299*
current flow, in axon, *108*
defined, 104
excitability changes during, *106*
firing pattern, 108–109
G-protein-coupled receptors, 112
ionic basis, 103–106, *104–105,* 105*t*
ligand-gated receptors, 112
local potential, compared, 105*t*
membrane, excitability of, 106–107, *106–107*
neurochemical transmitters, *110,* 111–112, *113*
  postsynaptic effects, 112–114, 113*t*
neuromodulation, 113*t*
neurotransmission
  classic, 112–114, 113*t*, *115*
  electrical synapses, 114–115
  neuromodulation, 114
patterns of activity, 108–111
  synaptic transmission, 110–111, *110–111*
postsynaptic potentials, 114*t*
propagation of, 107–108, *108–109*
recording of, 387–388
threshold, *101,* 103
triggering of, *90*
voltage changes, in axon, *108*
Active transport, cell membrane, 92
Adenoma sebaceum, neuroectodermal dysplasia, 27*t*

Adenosine triphosphate, 94, 280, 406
  in active transport, 92
  bindings, 88–89
  internal regulation, 266
  membrane potential, 116
  sodium-potassium pump, 116
  vascular system, 330
Adrenocorticotropic hormone, 544
Adventitia, arterial wall, *334*
Afferents
  fibers
    peripheral level, 383
    primary, 179
  in formation of nervous system, 14–15
  glossopharyngeal, 263
  nociceptive, pain, 169*t*, 175
  pathways, 152. *See also* Sensory system
  sensory system, 161*t*, 164, 169*t*, 169–170
  somatic, 264
    special impulse, 152
  spinal, reflex connections of, *449*
  tissue innervated, tissue origin, 25
  vagal, 263
  visceral, 260–263
    brainstem, 262*t*, 263
    connections in spinal cord, *262*
    special impulse, 152
    spinal, 261–263, *262 263*
Afterhyperpolarization, action potential and, 109
Afterpotential, 106
Agnosia, 565–566
Agraphesthesia, 566
Agraphia, 577